THE 5 MINUTE CLINICAL CONSULT FOR DENTAL PROFESSIONALS

JAMES R. HUPP, DMD, MD, JD, FACS

Professor & Chair, Department of Oral-Maxillofacial Surgery
University of Maryland Dental School
Chair, Department of Dentistry
University of Maryland Medical System
Baltimore, MD

THOMAS P. WILLIAMS, DDS

Private Practice, Oral-Maxillofacial Surgery
Dubuque, Iowa
Adjunct Associate Professor
University of Iowa
Iowa City, Iowa

WARREN P. VALLERAND, DDS

Clinical Associate Professor of Oral-Maxillofacial Surgery
University of Medicine and Dentistry of New Jersey
New Jersey Dental School
Newark, NJ

THE 5 MINUTE CLINICAL CONSULT FOR DENTAL PROFESSIONALS

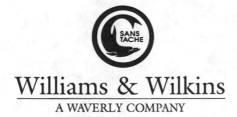

Williams & Wilkins
A WAVERLY COMPANY

BALTIMORE • PHILADELPHIA • LONDON • PARIS • BANGKOK
BUENOS AIRES • HONG KONG • MUNICH • SYDNEY • TOKYO • WROCLAW

1996

Editor: Darlene Cooke
Senior Managing Editor: Sharon R. Zinner
Production Manager: Laurie Forsyth
Book Project Editor: Robert D. Magee
Designer: Susan Blaker
Typesetter: Port City Press
Printer: Port City Press

Accurate indications, adverse reactions, and dosage schedules for drugs are provided in this book, but it is possible that they may change. The reader is urged to review the package information data of the manufacturers of the medications mentioned.

Printed in the United States of America

Library of Congress Cataloging-in-Publication Data

5 minute clinical consult For dental professionals / [edited] by James R. Hupp.
    p.   cm.
  Includes index.
  ISBN 0-683-04279-3
    1. Oral manifestations of general diseases—Handbooks, manuals, etc.   2. Sick—
Dental care—Handbooks, manuals, etc. I. Hupp, James R.
  [DNLM: 1. Clinical Medicine—handbooks. WB 39 Z9991 1996]
RK305.A14 1996
616'.00246176—dc20
DNLM/DLC
for Library of Congress   95-41086
                                      CIP

The Publishers have made every effort to trace the copyright holders for borrowed material. If they have inadvertently overlooked any, they will be pleased to make the necessary arrangements at the first opportunity.

96 97 98 99
1 2 3 4 5 6 7 8 9 10

Reprints of chapters may be purchased from Williams & Wilkins in quantities of 100 or more. Call Isabella Wise in the Special Sales Department, (800) 358-3583.

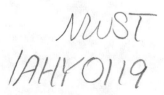

DEDICATION

To the love of my life, Carmen, our wonderful children, Jamie, Justin, Joelle, and Jordan, and the parents we love, Lucie, Rose, Richard and Günther

James R. Hupp

To my loving wife, April Hazard, PhD, RN, and to the memory of my brother, Ronald Vallerand, RN. Both have been invaluable role models from whom I have learned the importance of compassion and humor in patient care. And to my wonderful children Ben and Kate who, along with their mom, give me unconditional love and support through all my endeavors

Warren P. Vallerand

To my mother and father

Thomas P. Williams

Preface

Dental practice and the educational process required to become a dental professional have always been time-intensive activities. Dental practice has increasing business management demands; and as financial pressures increase, less time will be available to confer with consultants or to find needed information in comprehensive reference texts. Similarly, changes in dental education are placing strains on student and resident time. This is occurring because of the need to learn new concepts and clinical techniques as an addition to an already packed curriculum. These realities of time constraints in modern dental practice and education threaten to encroach upon the most central goal of dentistry: quality patient care.

The 5 Minute Clinical Consult for Dental Professionals is specifically designed to address this problem by providing ready access to the specific information the dentist requires quickly about topics she or he would otherwise need to consult other health care providers or search for in a regular textbook. Topics chosen for inclusion in this book relate to areas of a clinical practice or patient conditions most dentists are unlikely to manage frequently enough to carry important details at their fingertips or unlikely to be able to remain abreast of new developments.

Thus, when the busy practitioner or student is confronted with a patient with a medical condition, a suspected pathologic entity, or an unusual symptom, he or she can quickly find the information they need to safely proceed with patient care or direct the patient to the appropriate health care colleague. And because the book was authored entirely by dental professionals, the coverage of each entity contains the amount of detail and attention to dental relevance not seen in texts prepared for, and by, physicians.

The editors selected and provided coverage for over 250 topics believed to be of greatest interest to dental professionals and students of dentistry. If readers find coverage gaps that should be included in future editions, we request readers to forward their ideas to us, along with any other suggestions for which the utility of this book can be enhanced.

HOW TO USE THIS BOOK

The book is organized with the busy practitioner and student in mind. The entities are arranged alphabetically to permit rapid location. Major headings and subheadings are clearly visible, permitting users of the book to quickly scan the contribution for the information they seek. The information is presented in outline or brief sentence form, speeding the process of assimilation by the reader.

Guides to basic background information, etiology, diagnosis and therapy are provided, including early steps to take if emergency care is required, as well as recommendations for consultations and referral when appropriate. When indicated, therapy that will be delivered by other health care providers is outlined to permit the dentist to better understand the patient's total care needs and then be able to adjust dental care in response, thereby lessening the chance of causing problems in patients treated by multiple doctors or getting uncoordinated health care.

A special feature of the book is the provision of diagnostic and treatment codes using the ICD diagnostic and CPT treatment coding systems. These codes, which accompany each contribution are used by most North American health care providers, managed care groups, government agencies and insurance companies. Although essentially all dental practitioners are familiar with the ADA coding process, few agencies outside of dentistry recognize ADA codes, and for the types of entities with which the book deals, practitioners will be better served by having access to and using ICD and CPT codes when communicating with managed care groups, government agencies and health insurance companies. Some dentists fail to realize that many procedures that relate to oral-facial pathology or medical conditions in the dental patient are and deserve to be compensated for by patients and their health care insurers or other third party payors.

Many CPT (treatment) codes relate to procedures applicable to a portion of the entities covered in the book. Those are placed in the "coding" section of those entities. For example, the code for diagnostic TMJ arthroscopy is provided only in the text for those few entities that relate to conditions for which this procedure would be relevant. However, codes for procedures such as an office visit or a hospital consultation could apply to almost all entities in the book. Those codes are provided in a separate section that is located on the following pages to make retrieval simple. It is important for dentists not accustomed to using medical codes that in comparison to dental coding, medical coding provides much more ability to code and therefore justify reimbursement for procedures that are not specific operations. Examples are codes for certain levels of consultations such as for consultative visits to the hospital emergency room, codes for transporting patient specimens to a facility outside of the office, or for interpretation of radiographs. In many cases, patients with medical problems or tissue pathology that impact upon dental care or that require dental expertise may be reimbursable through medical insurance. And, with the spread of degree of provider antidiscrimination laws, dentists are permitted and should use all legal and ethical means available to maximize a patient's access to their health care reimbursement benefits. ICD-9 and CPT coding will assist in this endeavor. Practitioners also need to use the most current codes available. CPT treatment codes are updated on an annual basis, although most of the codes do not change regularly. ICD-9 diagnosis codes change more slowly, but in the next couple of years it is likely that the ICD-10 codes will appear.

Each entity ends with a list of synonyms and suggestions for other entities in the book that the reader may also want to see for related information. For practitioners seeking in-depth coverage of a topic, recommended contemporary references are given. Finally, the author or authors who did the background research and prepared the contribution for the book are given.

James R. Hupp

USEFUL CPT CODES THAT DO NOT RELATE TO ANY SPECIFIC ENTITY

Code	Description
99201	New patient, office visit, about 10 minutes
99202	about 20 minutes
99203	about 30 minutes
99204	about 45 minutes
99205	about 60 minutes
99211	Established patient, office visit, about 5 minutes
99212	about 10 minutes
99213	about 15 minutes
99214	about 25 minutes
99215	about 40 minutes
99221	Initial hospital care, about 30 minutes
99222	about 50 minutes
99223	about 70 minutes
99231	Subsequent hospital care, about 15 minutes
99232	about 25 minutes
99233	about 35 minutes
99238	Discharge patient from hospital
99241	Office consultation, about 15 minutes
99242	about 30 minutes
99243	about 40 minutes
99244	about 60 minutes
99245	about 80 minutes
99251	In-patient initial consultation, about 20 minutes
99252	about 40 minutes
99253	about 55 minutes
99254	about 80 minutes
99261	In-patient follow-up consultation, about 10 minutes
99262	about 20 minutes
99263	about 30 minutes
99271	Second opinion, focused history/exam, straightforward decision
99272	expanded but focused history/exam, straightforward decision

Code	Description
99273	detailed history/exam, decision of low complexity
99274	comprehensive history/exam, decision of moderate complexity
99275	comprehensive history/exam, decision of high complexity
99281	Emergency dept. visit, focused history/exam, straightforward decision
99282	expanded but focused history/exam, decision of low complexity
99283	expanded but focused history/exam, decision of moderate complexity
99284	detailed history/exam, decision of moderate complexity
99285	comprehensive history/exam, decision of high complexity
99354	Prolonged doctor service in out-patient setting, 1st hour
99355	each additional 30 minutes
99356	Prolonged doctor service in in-patient setting, 1st hour
99357	each additional hour
99361	Conference with interdisciplinary team of health professionals lasting about 30 minutes
99362	lasting 60 minutes
99371	Telephone call to patient or for consultation or for coordinating health care management, simple or brief
99372	intermediate
99373	complex
99382	Initial preventive health care, ages 1–4
99383	ages 5–11
99384	ages 12–17
99385	ages 18–39
99386	ages 40–64
99387	age 65 and over

Code	Description
99392	Periodic preventive health care, ages 1–4
99393	ages 5–11
99394	ages 12–17
99395	ages 18–39
99396	ages 40–64
99397	age 65 and over
00100	Anesthesia for procedures on integumentary and salivary glands of head including biopsy
00160	Anesthesia for procedures on nose and accessory sinuses
00170	Anesthesia for intraoral procedures
00190	Anesthesia for procedures on facial bones
00192	radical facial bone surgery, such as orthognathics
40490	Lip biopsy
40800	Drainage of abscess, vestibule of mouth, simple
40801	complicated
40806	Incision of labial frenum
40808	Biopsy, vestibule of mouth
40810	Excision of lesion of mucosa, without repair
40812	with simple repair
40814	with complex repair
40818	Excision of oral mucosa as donor graft
40819	Excision of labial or buccal frenum
40820	Destruction of lesion of oral mucosa with laser, cryo or cautery
40899	Unlisted procedure, vestibule of mouth
41000	Intraoral incision and drainage of abscess of tongue/floor of mouth
41005	sublingual, superficial
41006	sublingual, deep
41007	submental
41008	submandibular
41009	masticator space
41010	Incision of lingual frenum
41100	Biopsy of tongue, anterior two-thirds
41105	posterior one-third
41110	Excision lesion of tongue without closure
41112	with closure, anterior two-thirds
41250	Repair of tongue/floor of mouth laceration ≤ 2.5cm
41252	≥ 2.6
41800	Drainage of abscess from dentoalveolar structure

Code	Description
41820	Gingivectomy, each quadrant
41821	Operculectomy, excision of pericoronal tissues
41822	Excision of fibrous tuberosity
41823	Excision of osseous tuberosity
41828	Excision of hyperplastic alveolar mucosa
41830	Alveolectomy
41870	Periodontal mucosal grafting
41872	Gingivoplasty, each quadrant
41874	Alveoloplasty, each quadrant
41899	Unlisted procedure, dentoalveolar structures
64400	Injection, anesthetic agent, trigeminal nerve, any division/branch
70100	Radiologic examination, mandible, partial, less than 4 views
70300	Single periapical radiograph
70310	periapicals, less than full mouth
70320	periapicals, full mouth
70328	Radiologic examination, TMJ, open/closed, unilateral
70330	bilateral
70350	Cephalogram
70355	Panorex
70390	Sialography
90780	IV infusion for therapy under direct doctor supervision
90782	Therapeutic injection/sub Q or IM
90784	IV
90788	IM injection of antibiotic
99000	Handling or conveyance of specimen from doctor's office to lab
99050	Services requested after hours
99052	Services requested between 10pm and 8am
99054	Services requested on Sundays and holidays
99056	Services requested in location other than doctor's office
99058	Services provided on an emergency basis
99070	Supplies and materials provided by doctor over and above those usually included in office visit
99071	Educational supplies provided by doctor to patient, at cost to doctor
99075	Medical testimony
99100	Anesthesia for patient of extreme age, ≤ 1 yr or ≥ 71 yrs
99140	Anesthesia complicated by emergency condition

ACKNOWLEDGMENTS

I wish to thank several individuals for their special efforts in preparing this book: my wife, Carmen, for her untiring assistance in word processing every entry in this book; Darlen Barela Cooke and Sharon Zinner for shepherding me through the preparation process; Shane Decker, for the unique graphics he created; Laurie Forsyth and Bob Magee for their production talents; and Doctors Michael Siegel, Bernard Levy, James Karesh, and Bruce Harswell for sharing photographs used in the CD-ROM version of this work.

James R. Hupp

I would like to thank Dr. M. Franklin Dolwick and Dr. Matthew B. Hall who have been mentors, friends, and professional colleagues and who have always served as sources of inspiration and direction. I would also like to acknowledge my students and residents whose inquisitiveness and enthusiasm make the challenge of teaching worthwhile and enjoyable.

Warren P. Vallerand

I would like to thank the Department of Oral Pathology at the University of Iowa for their assistance and support. In addition, I would like to thank my mentors at Bellevue Hospital in New York City for their guidance and instruction during my training in Oral & Maxillofacial surgery. Last, I would like to thank my family for their love and support.

Thomas P. Williams

CONTRIBUTORS

ROGER BADWAL, MD, DMD
Senior Resident
Department of Oral-Maxillofacial Surgery
University of Medicine and Dentistry of New Jersey
University Hospital
Newark, NJ

HILLARY BRODER, PhD, MEd
Associate Professor in the Department of General and Hospital
    Dentistry
Division of Behavioral Science at New Jersey Dental School
University of Medicine and Dentistry of New Jersey
Newark, NJ
Consultant at Montefiore Medical Center
Center for Craniofacial Disorders
New York City, NY

MICHAEL J. BUCKLEY, MS, DMD
Associate Professor
Director of Research for the Department of Oral-Maxillofacial Surgery
University of Pittsburgh Medical Center
Pittsburgh, PA

FRANK CATALANOTTO, DMD
Dean and Professor of Pediatric Dentistry
New Jersey Dental School, College of Dentisry
University of Florida
Gainesville, Fl

ROBERT CHUONG, MD, DMD
Private Practice, Maxillofacial Surgery
Institute of Florida
St. Petersburg, FL

MICHAEL J. DALTON, DDS
Private Practice, Oral-Maxillofacial Surgery
Dubuque, IA

PAUL DANIELSON, DMD, FACD
Director, American Board of Oral-Maxillofacial Surgery
Fellow, American Association of Oral-Maxillofacial Surgeons
Diplomate, American Board of Oral-Maxillofacial Surgery
Fellow, American College of Dentists
Associate Clinical Professor
University of Vermont College of Medicine
Department of Surgery
Attending Physician
Department of Surgery
Fletcher Allen Health Care
South Burlington, VT

JEFFREY B. DEMBO, DDS, MS
Associate Professor, Oral-Maxillofacial Surgery
University of Kentucky College of Dentistry
Lexington, KY

ERIC J. DIERKS, MD, DMD, FACS
Clinical Associate Professor of Oral-Maxillofacial Surgery
Oregon Health Sciences University
Staff Head and Neck Surgeon
Legacy Portland Hospitals
Portland, OR

ALAN L. FELSENFELD, MA, DDS
Adjunct Assistant Professor
Section of Oral-Maxillofacial Surgery
UCLA School of Dentistry
Los Angeles, CA

MICHAEL FINKELSTEIN, DDS, MS
Professor, Department of Oral Pathology, Radiology and Medicine
University of Iowa
College of Dentistry
Iowa City, IA

PETER G. FOTOS, DDS, MS, PhD
Professor of Oral Medicine
University of Iowa
College of Dentistry
Iowa City, IA

JOHN W. HELLSTEIN, DDS, MS
Lieutenant Colonel U.S. Army Dental Corps
Sugar Creek, MO

LAWRENCE T. HERMAN, DMD
Assistant Clinical Professor of Oral-Maxillofacial Surgery
Boston University and Tufts University
Chief of Department of Dental Medicine
Norwood Hospital
Norwood, MA

BRUCE B. HORSWELL, MD, DDS, MS
Assistant Professor, Oral-Maxillofacial Surgery
University of Maryland Medical Center
Baltimore, MD

Contributors

JAMES R. HUPP, DMD, MD, JD, FACS
Professor & Chair, Department of Oral-Maxillofacial Surgery
University of Maryland Dental School
Chair, Department of Dentistry
University of Maryland Medical System
Baltimore, MD

JOHN JANDINSKI, DMD
Specialty License in Oral Pathology (NJ)
Clinical Professor, Division of Oral Medicine
New Jersey Dental School
Attending Physician
University Hospital
Clinical Associate Professor, Department of Pediatrics
New Jersey Medical School
Director of Dental Services
Children's Hospital AIDS Program
United Hospital Medical Center
Newark, NJ

DENNIS JOHNSON, DDS, MS
Private Practice, Oral-Maxillofacial Surgery
Crystal Lake, IL

JERRY L. JONES, DDS, MD
Private Practice, Oral-Maxillofacial Surgery
Albuquerque, NM

MYUNG-RAE KIM, DDS, MSD PhD
Associate Professor, Chairman
Department of Dentistry, College of Medicine
Director, Department of Dentistry & Oral Surgery
EWHA Womans University
Mok-dong Hospital
Seoul, KOREA

PETER E. LARSEN, DDS
Associate Professor & Director of Residency Program
Department of Oral-Maxillofacial Surgery
The Ohio State University
Columbus, OH

JANET E. LEIGH, BDS, DMD
Associate Professor of General Dentistry & Oral Medicine
Clinical Director at Infectious Disease
Dental Clinic at Charity Hospital
New Orleans, LA

SAMUEl J. McKENNA, DDS, MD
Associate Professor, Oral-Maxillofacial Surgery
Director, Residency Training
Vanderbilt University School of Medicine
Nashville, TN

MICHAEL MILORO, DMD, MD
Assistant Professor, Department of Oral-Maxillofacial Surgery
Director, Dentofacial Deformities Program
The Ohio State University, College of Dentistry
Columbus, OH

DALE J. MISIEK, DMD
Professor, Coordinator of Advanced Education Program in
  Oral-Maxillofacial Surgery
Louisiana State University Medical Center
School of Dentistry
Director, Oral-Maxillofacial Surgery
Medical Center of Louisiana
Charity Hospital
New Orleans, LA

ANDRE MONTAZEM, DMD, MD
Oral-Maxillofacial Surgery Resident
The Mount Sinai Medical Center
New York, NY

KANI NICOLLS, DDS
Certified in Hospital Dentistry and Geriatrics
Medical Staff at Memorial Mission Hospital
Asheville, NC

ROBERT ORD, MD, DDS, FRCS, FACS
Associate Professor and Residency Program Directory,
  Oral-Maxillofacial Surgery
University of Maryland
Associate Professor, Oncology Program
University of Maryland Cancer Center
Baltimore, MD

C. DANIEL OVERHOLSER, Jr, DDS, MSD
Professor & Chairman, Department of Oral Medicine & Diagnostic
  Sciences
Professor, Program of Oncology
University of Maryland School of Medicine
Baltimore, MD

ROBERT A. RUDMAN, DDS, MS
Assistant Professor
Department of Oral-Maxillofacial Surgery
University of Florida
Gainesville, FL

JOSEPH J. SANSEVERE, DMD
Clinical Assistant Professor
Oral-Maxillofacial Surgery
University of Medicine and Dentistry of New Jersey
Newark, NJ
Private Practice
Flemington, NJ

DANIEL SARASIN, DDS
Assistant Professor of Oral-Maxillofacial Surgery
University of Iowa Hospitals & Clinics
Iowa City, IA

JONATHAN SASPORTAS, DMD, MD
Resident Oral-Maxillofacial Surgery
University of Medicine and Dentistry of New Jersey
Newark, NJ

VIVEK SHETTY, DDS, Dr Med Dent
Assistant Professor
Section of Oral-Maxillofacial Surgery
UCLA School of Dentistry
Los Angeles, CA

MICHAEL A. SIEGEL, DDS, MS
Associate Professor of Oral Medicine
School of Dentistry
Associate Professor of Dermatology
School of Medicine
University of Maryland
Baltimore, MD

SHARON CRANE SIEGEL, DDS, MS
Assistant Professor
Department of Restorative Dentistry
Baltimore College of Dental Surgery
University of Maryland
Baltimore, MD

DAVID SIROIS, DMD, PhD
Director, Division of Oral Medicine
University of Medicine and Dentistry of New Jersey Dental School
Chief, Hospital Dentistry, University of Medicine and Dentistry of
    New Jersey
University Hospital
Newark, NJ

IRENE H. S. So, DMD
Private Practice, Limited to Orthodontics
Berkeley Heights, New Jersey
Clinical Assistant Professor, Department of Orthodontics
University of Medicine and Dentistry of New Jersey
Newark, NJ

THOMAS P. SOLLECITO, DMD
Assistant Professor, Oral Medicine
School of Dental Medicine
University of Pennsylvania
Director of Academic Programs
Hospital of The University of Pennsylvania
Philadelphia, PA

WARREN P. VALLERAND, DDS
Clinical Associate Professor of Oral-Maxillofacial Surgery
University of Medicine and Dentistry of New Jersey
New Jersey Dental School
Newark, NJ

STEVEN D. VINCENT, DDS, MS
Professor, Department of Oral Pathology Radiology and Medicine
The University of Iowa
College of Dentistry
Diplomate, American Board of Oral Pathology
Iowa City, IA

JAMES VOPAL, DDS, MD
Private Practice, Oral-Maxillofacial Surgery & General Surgery
Stuart, FL

MARK WAGNER, AB, DMD, FACD, FICD
Professor of Dentistry
Department of Pediatric Dentistry
Consulting Staff:
University of Maryland Medical System
Kennedy-Kreiger Institute
Anne Arundel County Health Department
Baltimore, MD

MARIA ROSA WATSON, DDS, MS, MPH
Clinical Assistant Professor
Department of Pediatric Dentistry
University of Maryland Dental School
Baltimore, MD

THOMAS P. WILLIAMS, DDS
Private Practice, Oral-Maxillofacial Surgery
Dubuque, Iowa
Adjunct Associate Professor
University of Iowa
Iowa City, IA

CHRISTINE WISNOM, CDA, BSN, RN
Department of Oral and Diagnostic Sciences
University of Maryland School of Dentistry
Member, "The Expert Review Panel for Infected Dental
    Health Care Workers"
Maryland State Board of Dental Examiners
Mid-Atlantic Regional AIDs Education Trainer
Baltimore, MD

DEBORAH ZEITLER, DDS, MS
Professor and Vice Chair
Department of Hospital Dentistry
Division of Oral-Maxillofacial Surgery
University of Iowa Hospitals and Clinics
Iowa City, IA

Contents

Contents

THE 5 MINUTE CLINICAL CONSULT FOR DENTAL PROFESSIONALS

Acromegaly

BASICS

DESCRIPTION
A chronic and debilitating disease caused by growth hormone (GH) hypersecretion, usually from a pituitary adenoma.

ETIOLOGY

• Most common etiology is a benign pituitary adenoma.
• Less frequently is ectopic production of growth hormone-releasing hormone (GHRH) from a carcinoid or other neuroendocrine tumor resulting in pituitary hyperplasia and GH hypersecretion.
• Even rarer, hypothalamic and/or pituitary gangliocytoma production of GHRH; a GH-producing adenoma in an ectopic pituitary gland or ectopic tumor of nonpituitary origin.

SYSTEMS AFFECTED
• Classically, hands and feet spade-like, fleshy, moist with thickened heel pad.
• Progressive facial disfigurement: frontal bossing, coarsening of facial features, and macrognathism. Dental underbite.
• Dental disease, including increased space between the teeth.
• Multiple organ systems, including cardiac, pulmonary, and musculoskeletal systems.

DIAGNOSIS

SYMPTOMS AND SIGNS
• Arthralgias and severe osteoarthritis common.
• Dermatologic changes, including skin tags, excessive skin oiliness with cystic acne, frequent.
• Carpal tunnel syndrome (35 to 50%).
• Complaints of muscle weakness and decreased exercise capacity common.
• Daytime somnolence due to obstructive sleep apnea (60%), due to airway obstruction, including deformity, and enlargement of the tongue, jaw, and epiglottis.
• Malignancy including colon cancers, as well as benign colonic polyps.
• Headaches severe (60%) and visual field defects.
• Amenorrhea, impotence, decreased libido resulting from hypogonadotrophic hypogonadism.
• Euthyroid goiter (10 to 40%)
• Abnormal glucose tolerance test (up to 50%)
• Hypertension (33%)
• Hyperphosphatemia and hypercalciuria
• Associated cardiovascular disease such as congestive and cardiac hypertrophy, including concentric left ventricular hypertrophy and asymmetric septal hypertrophy.

LABORATORY
• Elevated plasma somatomedin C (IGF-I/SM-C insulin-like growth factor I), the single best diagnostic test. If IGF-I mildly elevated, a 2-hour oral glucose tolerance test with concurrent measurements of plasma GH.
• Second line tests based on paradoxical GH responses to administration of thyrotrophin-releasing hormone (TRH), gonadotrophin-releasing hormone (GnRH) or levodopa.
• Also may see hypercalciuria, hyperphosphatemia, and hyperprolactinemia.

IMAGING/SPECIAL TESTS
• Magnetic resonance imaging (MRI) or computerized tomography (CT) of pituitary and hypothalamus gland.

TREATMENT

MEDICATIONS
Drug therapy: bromocriptine or octreotide.

SURGERY
Surgical resection of GH-producing tumor, radiation therapy sometimes in conjunction with surgery.

IRRADIATION
Heavy particle irradiation occasionally used.

CONSULTATION SUGGESTIONS
Endocrinologist

REFERRAL SUGGESTIONS
Primary Care Physician, Oral-Maxillofacial Surgeon and Orthodontist (for jaw deformity)

COURSE/PROGNOSIS
If left untreated, significant morbidity. Treatment halves the mortality rate; prevention or reversibility of many of the systemic complications after therapy repeatedly documented.

CODING

ICD-9-CM
253.0 Acromegaly
524.1 Mandibular prognathism
524.4 Malocclusion
524.8 Dentofacial abnormality

CPT
21085 Oral surgical splint
21139 Recontouring forehead
21144 Le Fort I, single piece
21193 Reconstruction of mandibular ramus, vertical
21195 Reconstruction of mandibular ramus, sagittal split without rigid fixation
21196 Reconstruction of mandibular ramus, sagittal split with rigid fixation
41120 Glossectomy, less than one-half tongue
70240 Radiologic exam, sella turcica
70350 Cephalogram, orthodontic
70355 Panorex

MISCELLANEOUS

SYNONYMS
Acromegalia
Eosinophilic adenoma syndrome

REFERENCES
Jaffe CA, Barkan AL: Acromegaly. Drugs 47:425-455, 1994.

Melmed S: Medical management of acromegaly – what and when? Acta Endocrinologica 129:13-17, 1993.

Daniels GH, Martin JB: Neuroendocrine regulation and diseases of the anterior pituitary and hypothalamus. In: Harrison's Principles of Internal Medicine, 13th ed. Isselbacher KJ, et al (eds), NY, McGraw-Hill, 1994, pp. 1897-1902.

AUTHOR
Irene H.S. So, DMD

Actinomycosis

BASICS

DESCRIPTION
A chronic, suppurative, and granulomatous infection of soft tissue and bone of endogenous origin. Its nonspecific presentation and relatively difficult diagnosis make actinomycosis an important consideration in the differential diagnosis of head and neck swelling.

ETIOLOGY

• Actinomyces and arachnia species are constituents of normal oral flora. The organisms are gram-positive, microaerophilic, nonspore-forming, nonacid-fast bacteria. The organisms can assume both filamentous and coccal forms, and collect into filamentous masses, appearing clinically as sulfur granules.
• Found in periodontal pockets, carious teeth, plaque, calculus, and tonsillar crypts. Usually due to A. israelii, but may be due to such other Actinomyces species as naeslundii that are found as normal saprophytes in the human oral cavity.
• Infections result opportunistically with organisms taking advantage of concomitant tissue injury such as can accompany restorative dental procedures, oral surgery, infection by other organisms, or trauma.

SYSTEMS AFFECTED
• Three clinical presentations of actinomycoses have been observed:
   cervicofacial (55%)
   pulmonary-thoracic (25%)
   abdominal-pelvic (20%)
• Cervicofacial spreads unimpeded by traditional anatomic barriers and may involve regional bone and soft tissues, skullbone, and CNS. When facial bones involved, mandible much more frequent than other bones.

DIAGNOSIS

• Presentation is variable and often eludes the doctor.
• Fewer than 10% of the patients presenting with actinomycosis infection are diagnosed correctly on initial presentation.

SYMPTOMS AND SIGNS
• History of recent facial infection, surgery, or trauma with a slow growing mass (chronic) or faster growing swelling (acute).
• Both chronic and acute presentation of cervicofacial actinomycosis may be, but is frequently not, associated with pain.
• Patient may have low-grade fever, and when the mandible is involved, paresthesias.
• "Woody" fibrosis with swelling of the face (lumpy jaw) may appear, frequently in the submandibular or parotid region.
• Pain to palpation, while lymphadenopathy not common.
• Cutaneous or intraoral sinus tracts may occur-resolve and recur that are preceded and surrounded by dark red or purple discoloration of the skin.
• Yellow, thick-to-serous exudate from sinus tract(s) that may contain "sulfur granules" of 1 to 4 mm in size may be present.
• Associated dental disease and poor oral hygiene.

LABORATORY
• Growth of actinomyces in anaerobic media such as thioglycolate or brain-heart infusion agar with 5% CO_2 for 4 to 6 days.
• Frequently no growth if patient on antibiotics.
• Only 30% of cultures will be positive.
• Identification of sulfur granules in specimens stained with hematoxylin-eosin or a Gram stain.
• Sulfur granules are colonies of filamentous bacteria found within purulent drainage. White cells adherent to filaments may give them a club-like appearance.
• Culture and sensitivity may need to be performed on tissue specimens rather than from aspirate to obtain adequate numbers of organisms.

IMAGING/SPECIAL TESTS
• Plain radiographs of mandible may reveal periosteal elevation, destruction, and sclerosis. If neurologic signs or symptoms, consider MR imaging.
• Immunofluorescence may be useful for early identification of organisms in exudate or tissue specimens.

DIFFERENTIAL
Other infections:
    Nocardiosis, tuberculosis, deep fungal infections, osteomyelitis due to other causes, and dental abscess of bacterial origin.
Tumors:
    Metastatic carcinoma involving cervical lymph nodes, benign or malignant salivary gland tumors, and lymphoma.
Other processes:
    Wegener's granulomatosis, branchial cleft cyst, chronic sialoadenitis.

TREATMENT

MEDICATIONS
• Long-term antibiotic therapy with penicillin.
• Penicillin G, 10 to 20 million units per day IV for 2 to 6 weeks followed by penicillin V, 2 to 4 grams per day orally, along with probenecid, 0.5 grams q.i.d.
• Oral penicillin should be continued for 3 to 12 months.
• Alternate antibiotics include minocycline, erythromycin, or clindamycin.

SURGERY
Drain abscess(es).
Debride necrotic bone and soft tissue, and other identified sources of infection.

IRRADIATION
Not indicated.

CONSULTATION SUGGESTIONS
Infectious Disease Specialist

REFERRAL SUGGESTIONS
Oral-Maxillofacial Surgeon

PATIENT INSTRUCTIONS
Adhere strictly to antibiotic regimen.

COURSE/PROGNOSIS
Compliance with chronic antibiotic therapy difficult, but if there is compliance, prognosis is good.
Left untreated, the process can spread locally and to distant sites.

CODING

ICD-9-CM
039.0 Actinomycosis, cervicofacial
730.1 Osteomyelitis (chronic)
730.2 Osteomyelitis (acute, subacute)
906.0 Late effect of open wound of head

CPT
21026 Excision of bone (non-neoplastic), facial bones
41800 Drainage of abscess from dentoalveolar structures
87070 Culture bacterial, definitive, any source
87075 Culture bacterial, any source, anaerobic
87205 Smear with interpretation
99000 Transport of specimen to outside laboratory

MISCELLANEOUS

SYNONYMS
Lumpy jaw

SEE ALSO
Nocardiosis

REFERENCES
Lerner PI: The lumpy jaw. Cervicofacial actinomycosis. Infect Dis Clin N Am 2:203-220, 1988.

Deloach-Banta LJ, Barber FA: Non-healing mass of the right cheek and submandibular area. Arch Dermatol 127:1831-1834, 1991.

Actinomycosis. In: Oral Pathology:Clinical-Pathologic Correlations. 2nd ed. Regezi JA, Sciubba J. (eds), Philadelphia, WB Saunders Co., 1993, pp. 45-47.

AUTHOR
Peter E. Larsen, DDS

Addison's Disease (Adrenocortical Insufficiency)

BASICS

DESCRIPTION
Chronic adrenal insufficiency from hypofunction of the adrenal cortex. A related condition can occur in hypopituitarism in which adrenocorticotropic hormone (ACTH) levels are abnormally low, or in polyendocrine deficiency syndromes in which a number of different endocrine glands are affected (eg, adrenal, thyroid, pancreas). Affects females more than males. Occurs at all ages.

ETIOLOGY

• Autoimmune disease with the production of anti-adrenal antibodies.
• Granulomatous infection of the adrenal gland such as tuberculosis or histoplasmosis.
• A component of a hereditary disease of progressive myelin degeneration in the brain (adrenoleukodystrophy) or spinal cord (adrenomyelodystrophy).
• A complication of acquired immunodeficiency syndrome (AIDS) with involvement of the adrenal glands by opportunistic infection and/or Kaposi's sarcoma.
• Metastatic infiltration of the adrenal glands.
<u>Drugs</u>
◊ Etomidate (anesthetic), ketoconazole (antifungal).
• Adrenal crisis may be precipitated by physiologic stress from surgery or infection.

SYSTEMS AFFECTED
All systems influenced by adrenal cortical hormones (cortisol, androgens, aldosterone) with effects on:
• Blood glucose
• Hemostasis
• Appetite
• Heart rate and contractility
• Synthesis of sex steroids by liver
• Blood volume
• Electrolyte levels
• Blood cell function
• Protein synthesis
• Cerebral function
• Immune reactivity

DIAGNOSIS

SYMPTOMS AND SIGNS
• Weakness, anorexia, fatigue, nausea, vomiting, fever, dizziness, diarrhea, abdominal pain, weight loss, cold intolerance, hypotension.
• Skin pigmentation over palmar and other body creases, over pressure points, and around areolas of nipples (tanning, freckles, vitiligo).
• Mucosal blue-black pigmentations (oral, conjunctiva).

LABORATORY
<u>Serum chemistry</u>
◊ Decreased Na^+, increased K^+, increased BUN, decreased glucose, moderate neutropenia.
• Decreased plasma cortisol level, high renin level.
• Elevated ACTH levels.

IMAGING/SPECIAL TESTS
• Chest radiograph may reveal adrenal calcification and decreased heart size.
• Abdominal CT scan for adrenal masses.
• Decreased plasma cortisol and urinary metabolic by-products of cortisol and androgens after challenge with ACTH (Cosyntropin 0.25 mg).

DIFFERENTIAL
• Secondary adrenocortical insufficiency (due to exogenous steroid use)
• Autoimmune disease
• Granulomatous disease
• Metastatic disease
• Other hypoglycemic conditions
• AIDS
• SIADH

Addison's Disease (Adrenocortical Insufficiency)

 TREATMENT

 CODING

 MISCELLANEOUS

MEDICATIONS
• Maintenance replacement therapy-daily cortisone (hydrocortisone 10 mg in AM and 5 mg in PM q.d.), fludrocortisone (mineralocorticoid) (0.1-0.2 mg q.d.).
• Increased steroid dose during exposure to major stress.
• Adrenal crisis-medical emergency intravenous fluid resuscitation (5% dextrose). Intravenous hydrocortisone hemisuccinate (100 mg IV bolus), treat trigger of crisis.

SURGERY
If surgery on patient with adrenal insufficiency required, consider exogenous steroid supplementation.

CONSULTATION SUGGESTIONS
Primary Care Physician, Endocrinologist

REFERRAL SUGGESTIONS
Primary Care Physician

FIRST STEPS TO TAKE IN AN EMERGENCY
• Activate EMS
• Administer hydrocortisone (100 mg IV bolus)
• Monitor vital signs
• Fluids intravenously (normal saline, Ringers lactate)

PATIENT INSTRUCTIONS
Wear identification jewelry to identify them as needing steroids in an emergency.

COURSE/PROGNOSIS
Satisfactory course if adequate daily replacement of cortisone and mineral-corticoid. Doses must be adjusted during periods of physiological stress or adrenal crisis may result.

ICD-9-CM
255.4 Adrenocortical insufficiency

CPT
90780 IV infusion

SYNONYMS
Adrenocortical insufficiency (primary)
Corticoadrenal insufficiency

REFERENCES
Federman DD: The adrenal. In: Scientific American Medicine, Section 3, Subsection 4. Rubenstein E, Federman DD (eds). New York, Scientific American Inc., 1994, pp. 11-13.

McKenna SJ, Roser SM, Werther JR: Management of the Medically Compromised Patient. In: Impacted Teeth. Alling CC, Helfrick JE, Alling RD (eds), Philadelphia, WB Saunders Co, 1993, pp. 86-87.

Gann DS: Adrenal Insufficiency. In: Scientific American Surgery, Section VII, Subsection 9, Wilmore DW, Brennam MF, et. al. (eds). New York, Scientific American Inc., 1989, pp. 1-8.

AUTHOR
Samuel J. McKenna, DDS, MD

Adenovirus Infections

BASICS

DESCRIPTION
Complex DNA viruses that are 70 to 80 nm in diameter. Cause a variety of clinical syndromes. Most common is an acute, self-limited upper respiratory tract infection with prominent rhinitis.

ETIOLOGY

• Belongs to genus Mastadenovirus of which there are 47 stereotypes recognized.
• The replicative cycle of adenovirus may result in lytic infection of cells.
• Can establish latent infection involving lymphoid cells.
• Infections occur most frequently in infants and children from fall to spring. Occur in epidemic patterns. Types 1, 2, 3, and 5 are the most frequent isolates in children.
• Less frequent infection in adults (less than 2% of respiratory illnesses).
• Types 3, 4, 7, and 21 are associated with outbreaks of acute respiratory disease (ARD) in military recruits.
• Transmission can occur by inhalation of aerosolized virus, inoculation of virus in conjunctival sacs, and probably by the fecal-oral route.
• Type-specific antibody develops after infection and is associated with protection against infection with the same stereotype.

SYSTEMS AFFECTED
Upper respiratory tract
  ◊ Occasionally, lower respiratory tract.
• Whooping cough with or without Bordetella pertussis.
• Can be suspect for pneumonia in immunocompromised patients.
Eyes
  ◊ conjunctivitis
  ◊ sometimes associated with types 3 and 7, which cause pharyngo-conjunctival fever among children in summer camps. Other sources are from contaminated ophthalmic solutions and roller towels.
GI
Urinary

DIAGNOSIS

SYMPTOMS AND SIGNS
• Rhinitis
• Coryza (sneezing and rhinorrhea)
• Pharyngitis, tonsilar enlargement with little or no exudate.
• Diarrhea
• Headache
• Nausea/vomiting
• Malaise
• Cough
• Conjunctivitis
• Fever
• Lymphadenitis
• Mucosa may show patches of white exudate
• Hemorrhagic cystitis

LABORATORY
See Special Tests

IMAGING/SPECIAL TESTS
Viral culture
  ◊ Detection of virus from sites such as the conjunctiva, oropharynx, sputum, and urine. Viral culture techniques involve inoculation of the virus into cell cultures. Immunofluorescence or other immunologic techniques are most commonly used. A special viral transport medium such as veal infusion broth or Hank's or Earle's balanced salt solution is used to preserve the specimen. Antibiotics are added to inhibit bacterial overgrowth. The media is kept refrigerated and should be transported on ice to the laboratory. Usually 3 to 14 days are required to isolate or identify the virus.
• Adenovirus types 40 and 41, which are associated with diarrhea illnesses, require special tissue culture cells for isolation, most commonly detected by ELISA of stool.
• Serum antibody rises can be demonstrated by complement fixation or neutralization, ELISA, or AI.
• Biopsy may be needed when presentation atypical.

DIFFERENTIAL
Other viral respiratory agents.
Mycoplasma pneumoniae
  ◊ especially in acute respiratory disease.

Adenovirus Infections

 TREATMENT

General
◇ Only symptomatic and supportive therapy is available for adenovirus infection. Live vaccines have been developed against adenovirus types 4 and 7, which are used in military recruits. These vaccines consist of live, unattenuated virus that are administered in enteric coated capsules. Vaccines prepared from purified subunits of adenovirus are currently under investigation.

MEDICATIONS
• No clinically useful antiviral agents have been successful.
• Acetaminophen (10 to 15 mg/kg/dose) for fever control. Avoid aspirin in children.
• Topical corticosteroids may be used for conjunctivitis.
• Use over-the-counter cough suppressants as necessary.

CONSULTATION SUGGESTIONS
Primary Care Physician, Infectious Disease Specialist, Ophthalmologist

REFERRAL SUGGESTIONS
Primary Care Physician

PATIENT INSTRUCTIONS
Rest, plenty of oral fluids, wash hands frequently.

COURSE/PROGNOSIS
In children the most common form of disease is an acute upper respiratory tract infection that resolves in a few days. Pharyngo-conjunctival fever persists for 1 to 2 weeks with its associated rhinitis, sore throat, and cervical adenopathy. In adults, the most frequently reported illness is acute respiratory disease that is marked by a prominent sore throat and the gradual onset of fever, often reaching 39 degrees celcius on the second or third day of illness. The disease is self-limiting.

 CODING

ICD-9-CM
079.0 Adenovirus infection
462.0 Pharyngitis
480.0 Adenoviral pneumonia

 MISCELLANEOUS

SYNONYMS
Conjunctivitis sometimes referred to as "pink eye"

SEE ALSO
Conjunctivitis
Pneumonia

REFERENCES
Dolin R: Common viral respiratory infections. In: Harrison's Principles of Internal Medicine, 13th ed. Isselbacher KJ, et. al. (eds.) New York, McGraw-Hill, Inc., 1994, pp. 803-808.

McDowell PR, et al: Adenovirus infection of the adenoids. Arch Otolaryngol Head Neck Surg 120: 668-671, 1994.

Hodge WG, et al: Adenoviral keratoconjunctivitis precipitating Steven-Johnson syndrome. Can J Ophthalmal 29: 198-200, 1994.

AUTHOR
Jonathan S. Sasportas, DMD, MD

Airway Obstruction

BASICS

DESCRIPTION
An acute or chronic process by which air exchange between the environment and the alveolar membrane is impeded.

ETIOLOGY

Can result from physical obstruction of the naso-, oro-, or hypopharynx, change in effective diameter of the tracheobronchial tree, or loss of alveolar volume. In the anesthetized patient the most common causes of airway obstruction are hypopharyngeal obstruction by the tongue and laryngospasm. Foreign body obstruction and bronchospasm can occur both in the conscious and unconscious state. Spread of fascial space infections is another cause of airway obstruction (ie, Ludwig's angina).

SYSTEMS AFFECTED
Upper airway and/or tracheobronchial tree.

DIAGNOSIS

SYMPTOMS AND SIGNS
• Dyspnea or apnea with or without ventilatory effort.
• Obvious use of accessory muscles, especially retraction of the sternocleidomastoid, absence or diminished breath sounds on auscultation, tracheal descent ("tugging") upon respiration, tachypnea (respiratory rate > 30), expiratory abdominal tensing, cyanosis, dyspnea, stridor, agitation, diaphoresis, wheezing, "rocking" motions of chest and abdomen upon inspiration and expiration. Note: all noisy breathing indicates obstruction; however, the totally obstructed airway makes no noise at all.

LABORATORY
Arterial blood gases and measures of oxygen saturation may be helpful after the acute episode has passed.

IMAGING/SPECIAL TESTS
For chronic obstruction, spirometry can help in the diagnostic process. If the forced vital capacity (FVC), or forced expiratory volume in 1 second (FEV1) is less than 50% of predicted, there is significant disease and risk to the patient. Improved pulmonary function tests in response to bronchodilators indicate the need to maximize bronchodilator therapy prior to dental treatment.

DIFFERENTIAL
Loss of muscle tone in the anesthetized patient with loss of the ability to maintain airway patency, foreign body aspiration, silent emesis with aspiration, laryngospasm, bronchospasm, anaphylaxis, allergic laryngeal (angioneurotic) edema, opioid-induced chest wall rigidity, pneumothorax. If during a general anesthetic with intubation, consider equipment failure (kinked tube or hoses, displacement of the endotracheal tube, ventilator malfunction, mucous plugging of the tube) or insufficient anesthetic plane.

TREATMENT

MEDICATIONS
• Laryngospasm
◊ If positive pressure ventilation is unsuccessful, succinylcholine 10 to 20 mg IV may break the spasm if given early and if only partial laryngospasm is present. If there is a delayed diagnosis or presence of complete laryngospasm, 60 to 80 mg succinylcholine IV (100 mg IM) should be given. In either case, controlled ventilation will be needed until the neuromuscular block has subsided (3 to 5 min).
• Bronchospasm
◊ With mild to moderate bronchospasm in the awake patient, use of a beta-2 agonist inhaler (albuterol, salmeterol) should be administered. With moderate to severe bronchospasm or with bronchospasm in the unconscious patient, epinephrine (1:10,000 dilution) should be titrated IV up to 0.5 mg as the initial dose, repeated as necessary. If intravenous access is not established, 0.3 mg IM or 0.5 mg subcutaneously is given using a 1:1000 dilution. If bronchospasm was associated with anaphylaxis, medications also to be given include hydrocortisone 100 mg IV immediately and diphenhydramine (Benadryl) 50 mg IV immediately and at 6 hour intervals over the next 24 hr. (See anaphylaxis contribution in book.)

SURGERY
Acute total airway obstruction that cannot be corrected by conservative measures may require emergency cricothyrotomy or tracheotomy.

CONSULTATION SUGGESTIONS
Oral-Maxillofacial Surgeon, Anesthesiologist, Otolaryngologist

REFERRAL SUGGESTIONS
Oral-Maxillofacial Surgeon, Anesthesiologist, Otolaryngologist

FIRST STEPS TO TAKE IN AN EMERGENCY
1. Terminate treatment and remove materials from the mouth.
2. Position patient supine if unconscious, or reclining/upright if conscious and indicating this would be more comfortable.
3. Administer 100% oxygen.
4. Call for assistance: other nearby personnel and emergency response team if needed.
5. Initially assess airway and determine cause of obstruction.
6. Begin initial treatment; calm and reassure patient.
Conscious:
◊ Heimlich maneuver/abdominal thrusts to clear foreign body if unsuccessful coughing attempts.
• Calm and reassure if due to anxiety.
• Administer bronchodilator if bronchospasm, consider presence or absence of anaphylaxis.
• Suction if vomitus is present.
• If opioids were recently administered parenterally and there is suspicion for chest wall rigidity, naloxone (Narcan) should be slowly titrated (0.1 to 0.4 mg IV)
Unconscious:
◊ Administer positive pressure ventilation.
• If laryngospasm, administer succinylcholine and provide positive pressure ventilation.
• If bronchospasm or anaphylaxis, administer epinephrine.
• If emesis, place in Trendelenburg with head down at least 15°, roll on right side, suction, be prepared to treat laryngospasm or bronchospasm.
• If foreign body can be visualized, attempt to retrieve the object; if not seen, perform abdominal thrusts/ Heimlich maneuver.
7. Monitor vital signs, reassess airway. Maintain suspicion for recurrence of symptoms, especially with bronchospasm or laryngospasm.
8. Begin cardiopulmonary resuscitation if needed.
9. Consider emergency cricothyrotomy or endotracheal intubation if continued efforts at ventilation are unsuccessful.

PATIENT INSTRUCTIONS
Patients with history of laryngospasm or bronchospasm (ie, asthmatics) should bring inhaler to appointments.

COURSE/PROGNOSIS
If the clinical course is of low severity, self-limiting, and resolves without incident, the procedure should be terminated and the patient observed in the waiting area. If no further sequelae exist, the patient can be discharged with follow-up by phone over the next 12 to 24 hours. If greater severity exists, the patient should be transferred to the local Emergency Department for observation and treatment.

CODING

ICD-9-CM
478.75 Laryngospasm
493.9 Asthma
933.1 Foreign body aspiration
995.0 Anaphylaxis

CPT
31231 Nasal endoscopy, diagnostic
31500 Emergency endotracheal intubation
31505 Laryngoscopy, indirect
31515 Laryngoscopy, direct
31530 Laryngoscopy, direct, foreign body removal
31603 Emergency tracheostomy
31605 Emergency cricothyrotomy
70360 Radiologic exam neck, soft tissue

MISCELLANEOUS

SEE ALSO
Asthma
Aspiration
Anaphylaxis

REFERENCES
Office Anesthesia Evaluation Manual (4th ed), Chicago, American Association of Oral and Maxillofacial Surgeons, 1991. Malamed SF: Medical emergencies in the dental office (4th ed). St. Louis, CV Mosby, 1993.

AUTHOR
Jeffrey B. Dembo, DDS, MS

Alcoholism

BASICS

DESCRIPTION
• Condition that results from chronic, compulsive over-consumption of ethanol-containing substances that leads to deleterious effects on the body and personal life.
• Estimates as high as 7% of the U.S. population fit the diagnosis of alcoholism.

ETIOLOGY

The cause of alcoholism is unknown but is likely the result of genetic, psychologic, and environmental factors that combine to cause the disease. Compulsive nature of the drinking separates the alcoholic from the heavy drinker.

SYSTEMS AFFECTED
Central Nervous System
◇ Primary system affected. Limited withdrawal of ethanol usually results in minor tremors, while more severe condition of delirium tremens occurs with acute alcohol withdrawal. DT's include severe tremors, severe hallucinations and, often, seizure activity.
Peripheral nervous system
◇ Peripheral neuropathies are often seen. (Wernicke-Korsakoff syndrome).
Gastrointestinal
◇ Anorexia, nausea and vomiting, abdominal pain, peptic ulcer disease, GI bleeding.
Oral Cavity
◇ Xerostomia and decreased ability to taste.
Liver
◇ Fatty and fibrous tissue invasion (called cirrhosis) causing significant decrease in function.
Heart
◇ Fat infiltration resulting in cardiomyopathy, palpitations.
Other systems affected to a varying degree include renal, skin, musculoskeletal, endocrine, and immune systems.

DIAGNOSIS

SYMPTOMS AND SIGNS
Symptoms of alcoholism related to the damage done to various organ systems:
General
◇ Family and social problems common.
CNS
◇ tremors, memory loss, confusion, blackouts, difficulty with speech (dysarthria), unstable gait (ataxia).
Liver
◇ hepatomegaly.
Skin
◇ jaundice, rhinophyma (enlarged, engorged nose with prominent vascular markings), spider angiomata.
Oral
◇ frequently have poor oral hygiene and advanced periodontal disease, xerostomia. Vitamin and nutritional deficiencies lead to significant oral changes, including tongue enlargement, hyperesthesia of the mucosa, burning tongue, diminution of taste, glossitis, and angular cheilosis.

LABORATORY
Liver functions abnormal (all increased)
Elevated:
    Gamma-glutamyl transferase (GGT)
    Alanine aminotransferase (ALT) (SGPT)
    Aspartate aminotransferase (AST) (SGOT)
    Prothrombin time (PT)
    Bilirubin (total)
Elevated amylase
High blood ethanol levels
Decreased hematocrit and platelets
Serum proteins decreased

IMAGING/SPECIAL TESTS
Liver biopsy
◇ fibrosis and fatty replacement

DIFFERENTIAL
Depression
Senile dementia
Seizure disorders
Psychiatric diseases
Alzheimer's
Other chemical dependencies

TREATMENT

General
◇ Abstinence from drinking an absolute requirement.
◇ Vitamins, particularly thiomine
◇ Nutritional support
Social
◇ Alcoholics Anonymous or other psycho/social therapy.

MEDICATIONS
• Use tranquilizers and sedatives during the withdrawal period. Benzodiazepines, such as Librium, commonly used to manage tremors.
• Disulfiram (Antabuse) causes nausea and vomiting when ethanol consumed, used to discourage ethanol intake.
• Use care if prescribing acetaminophen and other drugs requiring hepatic metabolism.

SURGERY
In presence of signs of severe liver disease, obtain coagulation studies, including platelet count, pre-operatively.

CONSULTATION SUGGESTIONS
Primary Care Physician, Mental Health Professional, Social Services

REFERRAL SUGGESTIONS
Primary Care Physician, Social Services

FIRST STEPS TO TAKE IN AN EMERGENCY
• If patient has bleeding problem after surgery, consider giving dose of aquamephyton (Vitamin K) and factor replacement. Treat thrombocytopenia with platelet transfusion.
• If patient shows signs of delirium tremors, administer large dose of benzodiazepine, such as Librium.
• If patient has signs of hepatic insufficiency, swallowing large amounts of blood or other high nitrogen substances can lead to hepatic coma. Warn patient/caregivers to seek medical attention if mental status decreases.

PATIENT INSTRUCTIONS
Consider obtaining help from Alcoholics Anonymous.

COURSE/PROGNOSIS
If the alcohol abuse stops early, most of the symptoms are reversible.
Untreated, the disease is progressive and fatal.

CODING

ICD-9-CM
291.0	Alcohol withdrawal delirium
291.1	Amnestic disorder
291.3	Hallucinosis
291.9	Psychosis
303.90	Alcohol dependence
305.0	Acute intoxication
527.7	Xerostomia
571.2	Chronic liver disease

MISCELLANEOUS

SYNONYMS
Ethanolism
Alcohol abuse

SEE ALSO
Hepatic failure

REFERENCES
Scheff S: Nutritional Disorders of the Nervous System. In: Internal Medicine for Dentistry, Rose L., Kaye D. (eds) St. Louis, CV Mosby, 1990, pp. 743-746.

Alcoholic liver disease. In: Dental Management of the Medically Compromised Patient. 4th ed. Little JW, Falace DA (eds). St. Louis, CV Mosby Co. 1993, pp. 269-275.

McMilken DB, et al: Alcohol-related seizures. Emerg Med Clin North Am 12: 1057-1079, 1994.

AUTHOR
Michael J. Buckley, DMD, MS

Alzheimer's Disease

 BASICS

 ETIOLOGY

 DIAGNOSIS

DESCRIPTION
• A generally progressive, deteriorating dementia for which all other specific causes have been excluded by history, physical examination, and laboratory tests. In the majority of cases the brain atrophies, with widened cortical sulci and enlarged cerebral ventricles.
• Accounts for about 70% of dementias.
Prevalence
◇ between 2 to 4% of the population over 65 years of age, increasing after 75; 45% over 85.
• Onset usually in the elderly, although certain specific etiologic factors may cause dementia at any age.

Unknown; familial patterns reported with linkage to chromosomes 14, 19, and 21; possible slow virus, metal (aluminum) intoxication; possibly head trauma.

SYSTEMS AFFECTED
Nervous:
◇ Neurologic increased muscle tone in approx. 33%.
   Myoclonus in approx. 10 to 15%.
   Seizures approx. 20%.
Mental:
◇ May have depression, insomnia, incontinence, delusions, hallucinations, illusions, catastrophic verbal, emotional, or physical outbursts, sexual disorders, inability to tolerate change.
Musculoskeletal:
◇ May have weight loss.

Usually found with absence of other physical disease.

SYMPTOMS AND SIGNS
Multifaceted cognitive impairment: Early stages
◇ memory loss and subtle personality changes such as apathy, lack of spontaneity, and a quiet withdrawal from social interaction, occasional irritability.
With progression
◇ behavior and personality changes are more obviously affected; depression, insomnia, poor problem solving and judgment, increased disorientation.
Later stages
◇ myoclonus and gait disorder may appear, approximately 20% develop seizures, may become completely mute and inattentive, incapable of self-care.

LABORATORY
No consistent peripheral marker available; diagnosis made by exclusion. Thyroid function test, CBC, Sequential Multiple Analyzer tests, folate and B_{12} levels, urinalysis, blood count, screening metabolic profile, syphilis serology.
Pathological Findings: Gross
◇ diffuse cerebral atrophy in hippocampus, amygdala, in some subcortical nuclei; Micro-pyramidal cell loss, decreased cholinergic innervation, senile plaques, degeneration of locus ceruleus, degeneration of basal forebrain nuclei of Meynert, neurofibrillary tangles, astrocytic gliosis, and amyloid angiopathy. Definitive diagnosis is made postmortem. Indicators include senile plaques with amyloid protein, neurofibrillar tangles in neocortex, and loss of neurotransmitter markers.

IMAGING/SPECIAL TESTS
MRI and CT used to rule out other diseases.
Assessment: mental status testing, neuropsychological testing, EEG, ECG, and or cerebrospinal fluid; intellectual testing
◇ short and long-term memory testing
◇ naming objects, tests of common facts, similarities subtests, block designs
◇ copying three dimensional figures.

DIFFERENTIAL
Hypothyroid, stroke, tumor, meningitis, nonAlzheimer's-type dementia, brain tumor, end-stage sclerosis, subdural hematoma, mental hormonal dementia (hypothyroidism), drug reactions, alcoholism, and other drug abuse, other dementias, depression, toxicity from liver or kidney failure, vitamin and other nutritional deficiencies, delirium, schizophrenia.

Alzheimer's Disease

TREATMENT

General
◇ Neglect of personal appearance, poor oral hygiene, and dehydration are common. Oral injuries common from falls. When dementia is mild, the individual has knowledge of their memory loss. Marked anxiety and depression are often associated features. Failed appointments can be problematic. Individuals may need assistance to get to appointments on time as well as find the location.
◇ Transportation arrangements are needed and patients should be accompanied to their appointments by significant others.
◇ Treatment is generally experimental.

MEDICATIONS
• May include antipsychotics such as neuroleptics. For restlessness, give benzodiazepine. For persistent agitation haloperidol or phenothiazine. Avoid anticholinergic drugs, such as antidepressants and antihistamines.
• Neuroleptic medications may induce agranulocytosis, leukopenia, and thrombocytopenia (rule out with CBC) with secondary ulceration, infection, bleeding, candida, or stomatitis.
• Dental treatment should not be undertaken if there is significant bone marrow suppression (WBC < 3000 per mm or granulocyte count < 1500 per mm). Neuroleptics induce extrapyramidal side effects including, xerostomia and movement disorders (tardive dyskinesia, mandibular tics, spasm of perioral and jaw muscles, and dysphagia with secondary drooling). High dose or long-term use of neuroleptics may cause tachycardia, orthostatic hypotension or blood pressure fluctuations. Anticholinergics, antihistamines, and beta blockers may be used to control these side effects. Anticholinergic properties may contribute to sedation, hypotension, and body temperature elevations.

CONSULTATION SUGGESTIONS
Geriatric Specialist, Mental Health Professional

REFERRAL SUGGESTIONS
Primary Care Physician, Geriatric Specialist, Mental Health Professional

FIRST STEPS TO TAKE IN AN EMERGENCY
• Extrapyramidal reaction may respond to administration of anti-Parkinsonian drug benztropine (Cogentin).

PATIENT INSTRUCTIONS
Ask patient to do only one thing at a time; always reintroduce yourself and staff; use concrete expressions and short phrases to communicate; use the same operatory; be as consistent, as possible; approach patient slowly, use visual cues, and explain all procedures. Be aware of potential signs of elder abuse and neglect.

COURSE/PROGNOSIS
May progress slowly or have rapid decline. With senile onset, the average duration of symptoms, from onset to death, is about 8 to 10 years. Potential long life expectancy (>10 years) necessitates comprehensive dental care with aggressive preventive regimen early in disease while patient is still able to cooperate and adapt to new regimen. Once oral health function is restored, caregivers (spouses) should be told to initiate aggressive preventive modalities. Caregiver may need to assist or provide oral hygiene.

CODING

ICD-9-CM
331.0 Alzheimer's disease

MISCELLANEOUS

SYNONYMS
Presenile dementia
Primary degenerative dementia

SEE ALSO
Dementia
Alcoholism
Hypothyroidism

REFERENCES
Papas A, Niessen L, Chauncey H: Geriatric dentistry: aging and oral health. St. Louis, CV Mosby, 1991, pp. 34-36.

Hazzard W, et al.: Principles of Geriatric Medicine and Gerontology. 2nd ed. New York, McGraw Hill, 1990, pp. 934-1096.

Scully C, Cawson PA: Medical problems in dentistry. Oxford. Butterworth-Heinemann, 1993.

American Psychiatric Association. Diagnostic and statistical manual of mental disorders, DSM-IV, Washington, DC, 1994.

Sigal MJ, et al: Down's syndrome and Alzheimer's disease. J Can Dent Assoc 59: 823-825, 1993.

Roth ME: Advances in Alzheimer's disease. J Fam Pract 37:593-607, 1993.

Authors
Hillary Broder, PhD, MEd
Kani Nicolls, DDS

Amalgam Tattoo

BASICS

DESCRIPTION
• An asymptomatic gray to blue-black macule ranging from a few millimeters to 2 cm.
• The most common pigmented lesion of the oral mucosa.
• Most frequently found on the buccal mucosa, gingiva, and alveolar mucosa; often located adjacent to a tooth with an amalgam restoration.
• Inflammation or changes of the lesion are rarely seen.

ETIOLOGY

• Implantation of silver amalgam into the tissues from oral surgical or operative dental procedures.
• Fracture of amalgam restorations during trauma with incorporation of amalgam into lacerations.
• Introduction of particles into adjacent tissues during apicoectomy and retrograde amalgam procedures.
• Corrosion of endodontic silver points or retrograde amalgam restorations.

SYSTEMS AFFECTED
Pigmentation of oral mucosa only; no systemic affects.

DIAGNOSIS

SYMPTOMS AND SIGNS
• The only clinical finding is a pigmented macule; the lesions are asymptomatic.
• Findings of amalgam particles around blood vessels and along collagen fibers with few inflammatory cells, except when particles are large.

IMAGING/SPECIAL TESTS
Demonstration of radiopacities on radiograph if particles are of sufficient size.

DIFFERENTIAL
Addison's disease
Peutz-Jeghers syndrome
Melanotic macule
Oral pigmented nevus
Radial pigmentation
Heavy metal pigmentation
Drug induced pigmentation
Hemangioma
Varix
Kaposi's sarcoma
Melanoma

Amalgam Tattoo

 TREATMENT

General
◇ Observation if amalgam implantation into tissues documented by history or if amalgam particles(s) demonstrated radiographically.

SURGERY
Any questionable lesions require surgical incision/excision with microscopic examination and tissue diagnosis.

CONSULTATION SUGGESTIONS
Oral Medicine

REFERRAL SUGGESTIONS
Oral-Maxillofacial Surgeon

PATIENT INSTRUCTIONS
Reassurance lesion benign with no tendency toward malignant change.

COURSE/PROGNOSIS
Benign course with no untoward sequelae.

 CODING

ICD-9-CM
709.0 Tattoo
935.0 Foreign body in mouth

CPT
40804 Removal of embedded foreign body, vestibule of mouth; simple
40808 Biopsy, vestibule of mouth
40810 Excision of lesion of mucosa and submucosa, vestibule of mouth; without repair
40812 With simple repair
41100 Biopsy of tongue; anterior two-thirds posterior one-third
41105 Posterior one-third
41108 Biopsy of floor of mouth
41112 Excision of lesion of tongue with closure; anterior two-thirds
41113 Posterior one-third
41116 Excision, lesion of floor of mouth
42100 Biopsy of palate
42104 Excision, lesion of palate; without closure
42106 With simple primary closure

 MISCELLANEOUS

SYNONYMS
Focal argyrosis

SEE ALSO
Kaposi's sarcoma
Melanoma

REFERENCES
Owens BM, Johnson WW, Schuman NJ: Oral amalgam pigmentations (tattoos): a retrospective study. Quintessence Int. 23:805-810, 1992.

Shiloah J, Covington JS, Schumann NJ: Reconstructive mucogingival surgery: the management of amalgam tattoo. Quintessence Int. 19:489-492, 1988.

Regezi JA, Sciubba J: Oral Pathology, Clinical

Pathologic Correlations, 2nd ed. Philadelphia. WB Saunders, 1993, pp. 171-175.

AUTHOR
Dennis L. Johnson, DDS, MS

Anaphylaxis

 BASICS

DESCRIPTION
A serious, life-threatening hypersensitivity reaction brought about by exposure of a sensitized person to an antigen such as a drug, foreign protein or toxin. Shock occurs due to failure of cardiovascular system to maintain blood pressure.

 ETIOLOGY

Occurs within minutes after exposure to foreign antigen. Antibodies (IgE) attach to mast cells which release histamine and other mediators that act on the heart, lungs, and vessels to cause the symptoms. Referred to as type I hypersensitivity reaction.

SYSTEMS AFFECTED
Lungs
 ◇ bronchospasm produced by smooth muscle contraction.
Heart
 ◇ decreased cardiac output progressing to heart failure secondary to venous pooling.
Skin
 ◇ flushing and edema secondary to capillary dilatation and increased permeability.
Mouth
 ◇ copious secretions due to a generalized salivary stimulation.

 DIAGNOSIS

SYMPTOMS AND SIGNS
General
 ◇ apprehension, malaise
Skin
 ◇ urticaria (hives), pruritus (itching)
Lungs
 ◇ cough, wheeze, dyspnea (difficulty breathing)
Neurologic
 ◇ incontinence, dilation of pupils, loss of consciousness, convulsions, shivering
Skin
 ◇ wheezing, respiratory failure, rhonchi
Heart
 ◇ tachycardia, hypotension
Gastrointestinal
 ◇ nausea and vomiting, difficulty swallowing

LABORATORY
Arterial blood gases
 ◇ hypoxemia, hypercarbia

IMAGING/SPECIAL TESTS
Skin testing with antigen to predict hypersensitivity by allergist.

DIFFERENTIAL
Asthma
Vasovagal reactions
Hereditary angioedema

TREATMENT

General
◇ Prevention is the best treatment. A thorough questioning of allergies is important.
◇ Activate EMS. BLS as needed.

MEDICATIONS
• Diphenhydramine (Benadryl) 25 to 50 mg IM or IV
• Epinephrine 0.3 ml of 1:1000 (0.3 mg) IM
• Dexamethasone (Decadron) 2 to 8 mg IM or IV.
• Start IV fluids
• Oxygen, at least 6 liters per minute nasally, may need intubation.
• Aminophylline 6 mg/kg IV over 10 to 20 minutes.

CONSULTATION SUGGESTIONS
Allergist

REFERRAL SUGGESTIONS
Primary Care Physician, Allergist

FIRST STEPS TO TAKE IN AN EMERGENCY
• Stop all drugs
• Activate EMS
• If hypotensive
◇ place in head down position and begin IV fluids
• Administer oxygen, epinephine, corticosteroids and antihistamine
• Monitor vital signs
• Transport to emergency facility

PATIENT INSTRUCTIONS
Medic-alert bracelets if drugs known to cause reactions.

COURSE/PROGNOSIS
Usually reversible if treated appropriately, but can often progress to shock and death.

CODING

ICD-9-CM
977.9 Anaphylaxis due to wrong drug
995.0 Anaphylactic shock
995.2 Anaphylaxis due to correct drug
995.6 Anaphylaxis due to food

CPT
31500 Emergency intubation
31603 Emergency tracheostomy
31605 Emergency cricothyrotomy
90780 IV infusion
90799 Unlisted therapeutic injection

MISCELLANEOUS

SYNONYMS
Type I hypersensitivity
Anaphylactic shock

SEE ALSO
Cardiac arrest

REFERENCES
Murasko DM, Kay D. Immunologic and Allergic Disease. In Internal Medicine for Dentistry, 2nd ed. Rose LF, Kaye D (eds) St. Louis, C.V. Mosby, 1990, pp. 13-17.

Atkinson TP, Kaliner MA. Anaphylaxis. Med Clin N Am 76:841, 1992.

AUTHOR
Michael J. Buckley, DMD, MS

Anemia, Iron Deficiency

 BASICS

DESCRIPTION
Decreased numbers, size, and hemoglobin content of red blood cells due to inadequate availability of stored iron. Also seen with poor utilization of iron, such as occurs in anemia of chronic disease, which presents in similar fashion without depleted iron stores. It is much more frequent in women during ages of menstruation.

 ETIOLOGY

Usually due to chronic, insidious blood loss such as seen with slow GI bleeds or excessive menstrual blood loss. Also frequently seen in normally menstruating women who consume inadequate amounts of dietary iron. Similar mechanism for iron deficiency occurs in infants and pregnant patients who have increased demand for iron that may not be met by iron consumption. May also occur when rapid blood loss occurs and insufficient iron is consumed during recovery from the blood loss. Poor absorption of iron may occur postgastrectomy leading to anemia. Rarely may occur with chronic dietary inadequacy of iron.

SYSTEMS AFFECTED
Hematopoiesis:
  ◇ decreased
General
  ◇ weakness, fatigue
Skin, mucous membranes
  ◇ pallor
Neurologic
  ◇ headache, poor concentration

 DIAGNOSIS

SYMPTOMS AND SIGNS
• May be asymptomatic, especially if anemia develops slowly.
• Dyspnea on exertion
• Fatigability
• Headaches
• Pallor
• Peripheral neuropathy
• Pica (craving for eating ice, dirt, clay, paint, etc.).
Oral changes
  ◇ glossitis, angular cheilitis.
Koilonychia (spoon-shaped nails)
Menorrhagia

LABORATORY
• Decreased serum ferritin.
• Elevated total iron binding capacity (TIBC).
• Microcytic, hypochromic red blood cells.
• Poikilocytosis (bizarre shaped red cells).
• Decreased total red cell count.
• Absence of reticulocytosis in response to anemia.
• Normal hemoglobin electrophoresis.
• Decreased hemoglobin A_2.

IMAGING/SPECIAL TESTS
• Low or absent stainable iron on bone marrow aspirate. Ringed sideroblasts absent.
• Elevated number of transferrin receptors.

DIFFERENTIAL
• Anemia due to causes other than iron problems such as renal disease, bone marrow depression, hemolytic anemias, etc.
• Anemia due to defective iron utilization such as thalassemia, sideroblastosis, etc.
• Anemia of chronic disease.
• Dietary deficiency of iron.
• Defective iron utilization such as cancer, infection, etc.
• Iron deficiency due to chronic blood loss.

TREATMENT

General
◇ Reversal of iron deficiency characterized by marked reticulocytosis 3 to 4 days after iron therapy begins.

MEDICATIONS
• Ferrous sulfate 325 mg PO t.i.d. taken between meals. If gastric irritation occurs, can use ferrous gluconate or lactate. Iron dextran can be used in patients unable to take oral preparations.
• Avoid concurrent administration of antacids or tetracyclines.

CONSULTATION SUGGESTIONS
Hematologist, Primary Care Physician

REFERRAL SUGGESTIONS
Primary Care Physician

FIRST STEPS TO TAKE IN AN EMERGENCY
• Serious anemia can be mitigated by blood transfusion.

PATIENT INSTRUCTIONS
Maintain dietary iron intake, particularly menstruating females and infants.

COURSE/PROGNOSIS
Cure depends on correcting cause of iron deficiency or the body's inability to utilize iron.

CODING

ICD-9-CM
280.0 Anemia due to chronic blood loss
280.9 Iron deficiency anemia
648.2 Iron deficiency anemia complicating pregnancy

CPT
36430 Blood transfusion
99000 Transport specimen to laboratory

MISCELLANEOUS

SEE ALSO
Sickle cell anemia
Vitamin deficiency

REFERENCES
Lee RG, Bithell TC, et al: Wintrobe's Clinical Hematology, 9th ed. Philadelphia, Lea & Febiger, 1993.
Bridges KR, Bunn HF: Anemias with disturbed iron metabolism. In: Harrison's Textbook of Internal Medicine, 13th ed. Isselbacher KJ, et al (eds), New York, McGraw-Hill, 1994, pp. 1721-1725.

AUTHOR
James R. Hupp, DMD, MD, JD

Anemia, Sickle Cell

BASICS

DESCRIPTION
• A genetically determined hemoglobinopathy most commonly seen in Blacks, that causes red blood cells to assume a sickle shape and become lodged in vascular beds when cells are in a hypoxic environment. Homozygous condition produces sickle cell disease, while the heterozygous condition produces sickle cell trait. Most of the severe morbidity and mortality associated with sickle cells is seen with the disease, rather than trait condition.
• May also occur in combination with thalassemia.
• Affects 1 in 500 Blacks in U.S.

ETIOLOGY

• Sickle form of hemoglobin (HbS) has a valine substituted for a glutamate in the beta hemoglobin chain. This type of hemoglobin polymerizes when in hypoxic environment, forcing red cells to assume a sickle shape.
• Sickle shaped cells are rigid and obstruct small vessels leading to ischemia of downstream tissue. Sickled cells are also fragile and hemolyze more easily.
• Ischemia due to sickled cell obstruction causes painful crises, splenic infarcts with destruction of splenic function impairing immune defenses, aplastic crisis due to bone marrow infection, and hemolytic crisis due to massive red cell hemolysis.
• Sickling triggered by hypoxia, dehydration, infection, fever, acidosis, hypothermia, exercise.

SYSTEMS AFFECTED
Hematologic
  ◊ anemia
Spleen
  ◊ infarcts
Pulmonary
  ◊ infections
Joints
  ◊ pain during crisis
Bone marrow
  ◊ infection, suppression
Abdominal pain
Renal
  ◊ microinfarcts
Neurologic
  ◊ headache, seizures, coma

DIAGNOSIS

SYMPTOMS AND SIGNS
Constitutional
  ◊ growth disturbance, frequent infections.
Anemia
  ◊ fatigue, weakness, pallor.
Cardiovascular
  ◊ hyperdynamic circulation, systolic ejection murmur.
Pulmonary
  ◊ pneumonia (fever, pleuritic pain).
Abdominal
  ◊ pain, jaundice
Skeletal
  ◊ bone pain, joint pain
Skin
  ◊ chronic leg ulcers

LABORATORY
Peripheral blood smear
  ◊ normochromic, normocytic anemia. May see sickled cells. If splenic infarction has occurred will see:
    Howell-Jolly bodies and siderocytes
Reticulocytosis
Serum bilirubin elevation, high urinary urobilinogen

IMAGING/SPECIAL TESTS
Metabisulfite prep or solubility test indicates presence of hemoglobin S.
Hemoglobin electrophoresis
  ◊ examined for hemoglobin A & S or other types. Sickle cell disease is SS, sickle cell trait is AS.

DIFFERENTIAL
Anemia due to other etiologies, other hemoglobinopathies, iron deficiency, hemolytic anemias, etc.

TREATMENT

General
◊ Hydration
◊ Improve oxygenation
◊ Promptly and aggressively treat infections

Transfusion
◊ to increase amount of normal hemoglobin
Bedrest during crisis

MEDICATIONS
• Analgesics
◊ narcotics for severe pain but avoid creating excessive respiratory depression.
• Some recommend use of prophylactic antibiotics for those with splenic dysfunction.
• Hydroxyurea therapy shows promise in preventing painful crises by increasing fetal hemoglobin production.

CONSULTATION SUGGESTIONS
Hematologist, Primary Care Physician

REFERRAL SUGGESTIONS
Primary Care Physician

FIRST STEPS TO TAKE IN AN EMERGENCY
• Rapid IV hydration, analgesics, oxygen therapy.

PATIENT INSTRUCTIONS
Avoid dehydration or hypoxia-producing situation. Sickle cell disease patients may also need to avoid strenuous exercise.
Genetic counseling important.

COURSE/PROGNOSIS
Those with sickle cell disease begin to show severe complications in second decade and beyond. Most live to early- to mid-adulthood. Few live over age 50. Sickle cell trait patients have few problems except in situations causing hypoxia or dehydration.

 ## CODING

ICD-9-CM
282.4 Thalassemia
282.60 Sickle cell disease
282.62 Sickle cell crisis

 ## MISCELLANEOUS

SYNONYMS
S/S disease
Hb S disease
Sickle cell disease
Sickle cell crisis

SEE ALSO
Iron deficiency anemia

REFERENCES
Bunn HF: Disorders of hemoglobin. In: Harrison's Textbook of Internal Medicine 13th ed. Isselbacher KJ, et al (eds), New York, McGraw-Hill, 1994, pp.1734-1743.

Charache S. et al: Effect of hydroxyurea on the frequency of painful crises in sickle cell anemia. N Engl J Med 332:1317-1322, 1995.

AUTHOR
James R. Hupp, DMD, MD, JD

Angina Pectoris

BASICS

DESCRIPTION
The symptom of chest pain and/or pressure/tightness caused by myocardial ischemia.

ETIOLOGY

- Narrowing of coronary artery from atherosclerosis.
- Platelet thrombi superimposed on atheromatous coronary artery narrowing.
- Inflammation of coronary artery (systemic lupus erythematosus, polyarteritis nodosa, rheumatoid arthritis, etc.).
- Coronary artery spasm (usually superimposed on atherosclerotic coronary artery disease).
- Prinzmetal's variant angina caused by coronary artery spasm, rather than fixed intraluminal obstruction.

SYSTEMS AFFECTED
Myocardium

DIAGNOSIS

SYMPTOMS AND SIGNS
- Substernal chest pain, pressure, or tightness usually precipitated by physical activity. Other precipitating factors include emotional stress, cold exposure, or a large meal. Anginal equivalents include pain in other locations such as the mandible, neck, left shoulder and/or arm, and rarely epigastric and/or back. Pain is relieved by rest and/or sublingual nitroglycerin.
- Patient denial, distress.
- Possible transient S3, S4 gallop or heart murmur from left ventricular dysfunction.

LABORATORY
No laboratory abnormalities unless myocardial ischemia progresses to myocardial infarction. Cardiac enzyme studies may be helpful in determining status of myocardium.

IMAGING/SPECIAL TESTS
- Electrocardiogram (ECG) may reveal evidence of old myocardial infarction and/or myocardial ischemia during the anginal attack.
- Exercise electrocardiogram (stress test).
- Radioisotope imaging (Thallium scan/ stress test).
- Coronary artery angiography (catheterization).

DIFFERENTIAL
Myocardial ischemia
Musculoskeletal pain (TM joint, neck, shoulder, arm, chest)
Pulmonary disease
Pericarditis

TREATMENT

General
◇ Terminate dental procedure
◇ Reassure/comfort patient (nitrous oxide safe to use for anxiety control).
Supplemental oxygen
◇ nasal cannula or hood at 3-6 L/minute.
Summon paramedics if angina persists. Confer with family physician before subsequent treatment.
Prevention
◇ Avoid exogenous vasoconstrictors.
• Patient should not skip usual anti-anginal medication prior to dental treatments.
• Use conscious sedation in anxious, at-risk patient.
• Defer treatment, refer to family physician if progressive angina or angina at rest.

MEDICATIONS
• Nitroglycerin 0.4 mg sublingual or spray, repeat in 5 to 10 minutes.
• Nitrates, beta blockers, calcium channel blockers can also be used to decrease likelihood of recurrent angina. Calcium antagonists particularly useful for Prinzmetal's variant angina.

SURGERY
Coronary artery angioplasty
Coronary artery bypass

CONSULTATION SUGGESTIONS
Cardiologist

REFERRAL SUGGESTIONS
Primary Care Physician

FIRST STEPS TO TAKE IN AN EMERGENCY
• Stop procedure, check vital signs, if not hypotensive administer 0.4 mg nitroglycerin, sublingual tablet or oral spray.

PATIENT INSTRUCTIONS
If any change in frequency, severity of angina, response to medication, or unstable angina present, patient should see primary care physician immediately.

COURSE/PROGNOSIS
Atherosclerotic coronary artery disease is a progressive disease. Risk of death is based on location and magnitude of coronary artery narrowing. Prognosis is greatly affected by left ventricular function with increased mortality when ventricular function is compromised. In properly selected groups, coronary angioplasty and coronary artery bypass decrease anginal symptoms and improve survival.

CODING

ICD-9-CM
410.9 Acute myocardial infarction
412.0 Previous myocardial infarction
413.9 Angina
411.1 Unstable angina
413.1 Prinzmetal's angina

MISCELLANEOUS

SYNONYMS
Myocardial ischemia
Angina

SEE ALSO
Myocardial Infarction
Pericarditis

REFERENCES
Hutter AM. Ischemic Heart Disease: Angina Pectoris. In: Scientific American Medicine, Section 1, Subsection IX.

Rubenstein E, Federman DD (eds), New York, Scientific American, Inc., 1991, pp. 1-15.

McKenna SJ, Roser SM, Werther JR: Management of the Medically Compromised Patient. In: Impacted Teeth. Alling C, Helfrick JF, Alling RD (eds), Philadelphia, WB Saunders Co, 1993, pp. 69-70.

AUTHOR
Samuel J. McKenna, DDS, MD

Angioneurotic Edema, Hereditary

BASICS

DESCRIPTION
Uncommon disorder characterized by rapid onset of nonpitting edema with diffuse borders involving the lips, face, tongue, or periorbital region with a high incidence of potentially lethal airway/laryngeal edema. Involvement of the extremities and gastrointestinal tract is common. The mortality rate among patients with untreated hereditary angioneurotic edema (HAE) is about 30%. The symptoms are typically triggered by stress or trauma and last for 1 to 3 days. The disorder usually appears during childhood or adolescence, although adult-onset does occur.

ETIOLOGY

Unlike angioedema, which is a hypersensitivity reaction, HAE is an inherited (autosomal dominant) disorder characterized by a quantitative or qualitative defect in the level of the complement inhibitor C1-esterase. This deficiency allows the C1-esterase to react with subsequent components of the complement cascade, resulting in kinin production and edema due to increased capillary permeability. The most common triggers to complement activation and HAE are trauma and stress (physiologic or psychologic). An acquired (adult) form of C1-esterase inhibitor deficiency has been associated with benign or malignant lymphoproliferative disease or autoimmune disease, resulting from immune complex formation and activation of the complement pathway.

SYSTEMS AFFECTED
Face
  ◇ lips, perioral skin, oral mucosa
Airway
  ◇ bronchitis, asthma, rhinitis
Extremities
  ◇ nonpitting edema
Abdomen
  ◇ inflammation, colitis, pain, nausea, vomiting, diarrhea

DIAGNOSIS

SYMPTOMS AND SIGNS
• Sudden onset edema involving the lips, tongue, extremities, or airway, with or without gastrointestinal symptoms, lasting for 1 to 3 days. Typically provoked by stress or trauma, including dental manipulation or contact with antigens (AE). Usually evident before adolescence. Recurrence is common.
• There may be a family history.
• May also have stinging or burning sensation, but minimal, if any, itching.

LABORATORY
Immunohistochemical assay of C1-esterase inhibitor and C4 levels. Low C1-esterase inhibitor level indicates a quantitative defect; a normal C1-esterase inhibitor with a low C4 level suggests a qualitative defect and a functional C1-esterase inhibitor test should be performed.

IMAGING/SPECIAL TESTS
Biopsy of little help. Reveals edema, vasculitis and perivasculitis of submucosal/subcutaneous tissues.

DIFFERENTIAL
Angioedema
  ◇ hereditary vs. hypersensitivity
Anaphylaxis
Cellulitis
Erysipelas
Contact dermatitis
Lymphedema

TREATMENT

General
◇ HAE may be life threatening. Any patient with HAE who requires dental surgery should have treatment provided in a hospital setting with the appropriate life support services.
◇ Hospitalization for airway management, including possible intubation or tracheostomy, is essential.

MEDICATIONS
• Acute attack: Epinephrine, antihistamines, and steroids used in an acute attack of HAE. They are of limited value. Acute abdominal pain is managed with nonsalicylate narcotics (NSAIDs and aspirin are CONTRAINDICATED in patients with HAE because they increase histamine release and lead to breakdown of arachidonic acid, resulting in chemical mediators that exacerbate mast cell degranulation. Similarly, histamine-releasing narcotics such as meperidine (Demerol) should be avoided. Although purified C1-esterase inhibitor is useful in an acute attack, it is not readily available).
• Long-term preventive therapy: Indicated for patients who experience more than one attack per month. The synthetic androgen Danazol (200 mg t.i.d.) increases C1-esterase inhibitor levels and activity several fold and C4 levels 15 fold after about 1 week of therapy. Epsilon amino caproic acid (Amicar) is an antifibrinolytic that also blocks plasmin activation, leading to a reciprocal increase in C1-esterase inhibitor levels. However, the patient must be closely watched for thromboembolisms or phlebitis.
• Short-term preventive therapy: In anticipation of traumatic surgical or dental procedures, Danazol and Amicar can be prescribed about 1 week before the procedure. Alternatively, two units of fresh frozen plasma (FFP) 12 hours before the procedure will increase C1-esterase levels for about 10 days. However, FFP should never be given during a acute attack because it will supply the necessary complement components to fuel an attack.

CONSULTATION SUGGESTIONS
Allergist

REFERRAL SUGGESTIONS
Primary Care Physician

FIRST STEPS TO TAKE IN AN EMERGENCY
• If any sign of airway compromise, administer epinephrine (1:1000) 0.2 to 0.3 mL IV or SQ. Transport to emergency facility.

PATIENT INSTRUCTIONS
If angioedema due to known factor advise patient to wear medical alert bracelet.

COURSE/PROGNOSIS
An acute attack can be life threatening. Time intervals between attacks can vary widely. Any patient with a history must be considered at lifetime risk for another attack and the appropriate preventive and management measures taken.

CODING

ICD-9-CM
277.6 Hereditary angioneurotic edema
995.1 Angioneurotic edema

CPT
99000 Specimen handling

MISCELLANEOUS

SYNONYMS
Angioneurotic edema

SEE ALSO
Angioneurotic edema, nonhereditary
Contact allergy
Cellulitis
Erysipelas

REFERENCES
Nusinow SR, Zuraw BL, Curd JG: The hereditary and acquired deficiencies of complement. Med Clin N Am 69:487-503, 1985.
Sim TC, Grant JA: Hereditary angioedema: its diagnosis and management perspectives. Am J Med 88:656-662, 1990.

AUTHOR
David A. Sirois, DMD, PhD

Angioneurotic Edema, Nonhereditary

BASICS

DESCRIPTION
• Angioneurotic edema consists of nonpitting edema of skin, respiratory and GI tract. Most incidents are acute and self-limited.
• Angioneurotic edema has hereditary and nonhereditary forms.
• The inherited form is an autosomal dominant and is less common.
• Affects both sexes equally, and all ages are affected.

ETIOLOGY

• May result from many different stimuli. It may be immunologic or nonimmunologic in nature. Immunologic mechanism is deficiency of C1 inhibition of complement.
• The nonhereditary form is more common and may be due to food allergies, although the trigger in most cases is unknown. Rarely can be seen in patients with lymphoproliferatic malignancies.
• Local traumatic injury, such as tooth removal, may precipitate an acute attack in the hereditary form.

SYSTEMS AFFECTED
• Manifests as a smooth, diffuse edematous swelling particularly involving the face around the lips, chin, and eyes, the tongue, and sometimes the hands and feet, as well as larynx, pharynx, esophagus, or intestines.
• Eyes may be puffy and swollen shut.
• The symptoms appear rapidly.
• Frequently accompanied by urticaria.
• Usually lasts 48 to 72 hours.

DIAGNOSIS

SYMPTOMS AND SIGNS
• Smooth, diffuse, edematous swelling of the face around the lips, chin, eyes, tongue, and sometimes the hands and feet. Skin of normal color or pink.
• Vomiting and abdominal pain may be present. If edema of the epiglottis is present, severe airway embarrassment may occur.
• Laryngeal compromise manifests with stridor (crowing sound).

LABORATORY
C4 assay (low in hereditary form). If low, do C1 inhibitor assay.

IMAGING/SPECIAL TESTS
Serum levels of C2 and C1s substrates depressed.

DIFFERENTIAL
Contact dermatitis
Urticaria
Erysipelas
Cellulitis

TREATMENT

If the etiologic agent can be identified, such as a food allergy or reaction to chemicals, then elimination will prevent recurrence.

MEDICATIONS
Androgens such as stanozolol used to prevent recurrences.

SURGERY
Tracheotomy if indicated for laryngeal or pharyngeal involvement.

CONSULTATION SUGGESTIONS
Allergist

REFERRAL SUGGESTIONS
Oral Medicine, Primary Care Physician

FIRST STEPS TO TAKE IN AN EMERGENCY
Monitor airway and activate EMS if airway involved.

PATIENT INSTRUCTIONS
Avoid triggering substances or inciting trauma.

COURSE/PROGNOSIS
Self-limited, will usually respond over 36 to 72 hours.
Life-threatening if air embarrassment occurs.
Recurs on repeat of triggering substance or trauma.

CODING

ICD-9-CM
995.1 Angioneurotic edema

CPT
99000 Transport of specimen to outside laboratory

MISCELLANEOUS

SYNONYMS
Hereditary angioedema
Angioedema
Quincke's Edema (when uvula involved)

SEE ALSO
Angioneurotic edema (hereditary)
Cellulitis
Erysipelas

REFERENCES
Rocklin RE: Inherited complement and immunoglobulin deficiencies. In: Textbook of Internal Medicine. Kelley WN (ed), Philadelphia, JB Lippincott, 1989, p. 1012.

Tierney, McPhee, and Papadakis. Current Medical Diagnosis & Treatment. Norwalk, CT, Appleton and Lange. 1994, pp. 121-123.

Cooper KD: Urticaria and angioedema: diagnosis and evaluation. J Am Acad Dermatol 25:166, 1991.

AUTHOR
Michael J. Dalton, DDS

Angular Cheilitis

 BASICS

DESCRIPTION
Inflammation of the lips or labile commissures with cracking, ulceration, excoriation, and secondary infection (most commonly by Staphylococcus aureus or Candida albicans). There is often a thick, white membrane covering the area involved.

 ETIOLOGY

• Angular cheilitis may result from a number of local or systemic factors. The majority of cases occur in patients with denture stomatitis and reduced vertical dimension resulting in chronic wetting of the commissures and secondary infection by Candida albicans. Habitual lip licking or sucking may also lead to angular cheilitis.
• Impaired immune surveillance resulting from diabetes mellitus, neutropenia, AIDS, or therapeutic immunosuppression can also result in angular cheilitis due to secondary infection with Candida albicans or Staphylococcus aureus.
• Finally, and least common, anemia resulting from iron, vitamin B_{12}, or folate deficiency can lead to angular cheilitis, sometimes also referred to as perleche.

SYSTEMS AFFECTED
• The lips and labial commissures are the primary site of angular cheilitis. However, because the condition is often associated with other local and systemic factors, signs and symptoms related to those factors may be found elsewhere (ie, denture stomatitis, oral candidiasis, mucosal atrophy associated with gastrointestinal disorders, and other intraoral abnormalities associated with diabetes, AIDS, etc.).
• Less commonly, when the condition is due to systemic factors, there are extraoral signs or symptoms such as chronic paronychial (nail bed) infection and koilonychia (striated, brittle, spoon-shaped nails), intertriginous candidiasis (especially the ano-genital regions), fatigue, or gastrointestinal symptoms.

 DIAGNOSIS

SYMPTOMS AND SIGNS
A presumptive diagnosis is usually straightforward based on the location and appearance of the lesion and identification of other local factors such as reduced vertical dimension, denture stomatitis, or poor denture hygiene. The lesion appears as painful, cracked, ulcerated labial commissures and/or lips.

LABORATORY
• Confirmatory exfoliative cytology from a simple lesional smear will identify yeast and hyphae when there is secondary infection by Candida albicans.
• When an underlying systemic disorder is suspected, a screening examination consisting of a CBC with differential and red cell indices, SMA12, and serum B12, folate, and iron will identify abnormalities associated with anemia, immunosuppression, or diabetes. Referral to a internist is essential for further evaluation.

IMAGING/SPECIAL TESTS
Elimination of the condition after a simple treatment trial with topical antifungal-antibacterial ointment confirms a presumptive diagnosis. Biopsy is rarely helpful except when the lesions do not respond to conventional therapy.

DIFFERENTIAL
The lesion itself is usually straightforward. Identification of the etiology can be more difficult:
• Reduced vertical dimension and denture stomatitis.
• Immunosuppression due to diabetes, AIDS, medications.
• Long-term antibiotic use.
• Anemia
• Xerostomia due to medications or systemic illness.
• In nonresponsive, chronic forms:
• Cheilitis granulomatosis ("oral" Crohn's).
• Chronic mucocutaneous candidiasis (many other symptoms present).

TREATMENT

General
◇ Any associated local or systemic factors must be addressed for successful long-term management. Correction of vertical dimension and adequate denture hygiene is essential. Management of the systemic disorders mentioned above should be performed with the assistance of the appropriate medical specialist.

MEDICATIONS
• Angular candidiasis secondary to local factors is treated with a topical antifungal-antibacterial ointment or cream applied 3 times daily. Several creams are available: nystatin, clotrimazole, and miconazole.
• When there is concomitant oral candidiasis or denture stomatitis, an antifungal solution such as nystatin oral suspension or pastille, miconazole troche, or clotrimazole troche should be used with the dentures removed. Caries-prone patients should avoid sucrose-containing solutions or troches; the vaginal clotrimazole troche is best to use for these patients. Dentures should be cleansed and soaked in chlorhexidine. Dentures should be removed from the mouth for several hours every day, typically while sleeping.
• Systemic antifungals should be used when there is inadequate response to topical treatment. Fluconazole is the drug of choice, 100 mg per day for 10 to 14 days.

CONSULTATION SUGGESTIONS
Oral Medicine Specialist, Prosthodontist, Oral-Maxillofacial Surgeon

REFERRAL SUGGESTIONS
Oral Medicine Specialist

PATIENT INSTRUCTIONS
Correction of underlying disorder critical to success.

COURSE/PROGNOSIS
Angular cheilitis due to local factors responds well to local treatment. When systemic factors are involved, the prognosis will depend on the degree to which the underlying disorder is corrected.

CODING

ICD-9-CM
112.0 Candidiasis
265.2 Cheilosis with pellagra
266.0 Angular cheilosis due to vitamin deficiency
527.2 Xerostomia
528.5 Angular cheilosis

CPT
40490 Biopsy, lip
87205 Exfoliative cytology
99000 Specimen handling

MISCELLANEOUS

SYNONYMS
Perleche
Cheilo-candidiasis

SEE ALSO
Anemia
Candidiasis
Xerostomia

REFERENCES
Mooney M, Sirois D: Oral Candidiasis. Int J Derm. In Press.

Davenport J: The oral distribution of Candida in denture stomatitis. Br Dent J 129:151-155, 1970.

Reade PC, Rich AM, Hay KD, Radden BG: Cheilo-candidiasis – a possible clinical entity. Br Dent J 152:305-309, 1982.

AUTHOR
David A. Sirois, DMD, PhD

Ankylosing Spondylitis

 BASICS

DESCRIPTION
• One of the spondyloarthropathies (inflammation of the spine) that primarily affects the axial skeleton, and, to a variable extent, peripheral joints and extra-articular structures. Back pain and limited spinal mobility caused by sacroiliitis, in addition to ascending spinal inflammation, dominate the clinical disease.
• Male to female ratio is 3:1.

 ETIOLOGY

• Associated with HLA-B27 gene product in 90 to 95% of white patients. Association is less marked in nonwhite populations.
• Up to 20% of patients with HLA-B27 markers eventually develop symptomatic disease.
• Autosomal transmission suspected, but the concordance rate in identical twins is estimated to be 60% or less; therefore, both genetic and environmental factors may play a role in the pathogenesis of the disease.
• Immune-mediated mechanisms are theorized to be important.

SYSTEMS AFFECTED
Axial skeleton involvement
◇ symmetrical inflammation of the sacroiliac joints. Calcification of the spinal ligaments and the intervertebral zygoapophyseal joints causes limited spinal mobility.
Peripheral joint involvement
◇ erosive hip and shoulder lesions.
• Distal joint synovitis less common.
Extra-articular
◇ acute anterior uveitis, aortic insufficiency, heart block, inflammation in the colon or ileum, upper lobe pulmonary fibrosis, and chronic prostatitis.

 DIAGNOSIS

SYMPTOMS AND SIGNS
• Gradual onset of low back pain, persisting for months, is usually noticed in late adolescence or early adulthood. Unlike mechanical low back pain, the sacroiliitis is prolonged with rest and relieved with exercise. Spinal mobility is lost with limitation of anterior flexion, lateral flexion, and extension of the lumbar spine. Eventually, pain tends to become intermittent, with alternating exacerbations and quiescent periods.
• Severe progression leads to syndesmophyte formation and the patient's posture undergoes characteristic changes. The lumbar lordosis is obliterated with accompanying atrophy of the buttocks. Thoracic kyphosis is accentuated.
• Bony tenderness may accompany the back pain stiffness. Common sites of tenderness include the costosternal junctions, spinous processes, iliac crests, greater trochanters, ischial tuberosities, tibial tubercles, and heels. Occasionally, chest pain is the presenting complaint. May see osteoporosis.
• Peripheral pain and stiffness usually involves the cervical spine; a serious complication is cervical fracture.
• Limitation or pain with motion of the hips and shoulders may be present.
• Acute anterior uveitis typically attacks unilateral and tends to recur causing pain, photophobia, and increased lacrimation.
• Aortic insufficiency can cause symptoms and signs of congestive heart failure.

LABORATORY
• Antigenic testing most often demonstrates the HLA-B27 antigen (present in 90% of patients compared to 5 to 8% in nonaffected population) and elevated serum IgA levels.
• Absence of rheumatoid factor in the serum.
• Elevated erythrocyte sedimentation rate and an elevated C-reactive protein.
• Mild normochromic, normocytic anemia may be present.
• Possible increase of alkaline phosphatase level.

IMAGING/SPECIAL TESTS
AP radiograph of the pelvis demonstrates changes in the sacroiliac joints and blurring of the cortical margins of the subchondral bone. Eventually, erosions and sclerosis are visualized. Progression of the erosions leads to "pseudowidening" of the joint space and then bony ankylosis occurs.
Spinal x ray
◇ flowing calcifications that bridge the intervertebral disk which appear as a "bamboo" spine on the film.

Pulmonary function tests may demonstrate decreased vital capacity and increased functional residual capacity.

Schober test
◊ measure forward flexion of the lumbar spine. Less than 4 cm of spinal lengthening measured in the region of the lumbosacral junction denotes a positive finding of decreased flexion.

Synovial fluid
◊ mild leukocytosis and decreased viscosity

DIFFERENTIAL
Mechanical low back pain
Diffuse idiopathic skeletal hyperostosis (DISH)
Sacroiliitis due to Reiter's syndrome
Psoriatic arthritis
Rheumatoid arthritis

TREATMENT

General -
◊ In general there is no cure for ankylosing spondylitis. Patients are encouraged to exercise to improve posture and range of motion to save spinal function. Education as to protection of a brittle spine is imperative. Adjunctive use of soft collars and a firm mattress are helpful.

MEDICATIONS
• NSAIDs are used to reduce inflammation and provide pain relief for therapy. Indomethacin is most often effective as a 75-mg slow-release preparation b.i.d. Recent trials are examining sulfasalazine in doses of 2 to 3 g/d.
• Attacks of acute anterior uveitis are managed with topical glucocorticoids in conjunction with mydriatic agents.

SURGERY
Surgery is indicated for patients with severe hip joint arthritis.
Cardiac disease may necessitate implantation of a pacemaker or aortic valve replacement.

CONSULTATION SUGGESTIONS
Primary Care Physician, Rheumatologist, Cardiologist

REFERRAL SUGGESTIONS
Primary Care Physician, Rheumatology

PATIENT INSTRUCTIONS
Use firm mattress and sleep without pillow.
Exercise regularly.
Stop smoking.

COURSE/PROGNOSIS
Prognosis is dependent upon the rate at which the disease is progressing. Most patients remain employable and continue to function well. The progression to severe, deforming disease cannot be predicted on the basis of HLA-B27 status or other criteria. Those with more severe disease seem to be more prone to the extra-articular sequellae which may serve to decrease life span.

CODING

ICD-9-CM
720.0 Ankylosing spondylitis

MISCELLANEOUS

SYNONYMS
Marie-Strumpell disease
Rheumatoid spondylitis

SEE ALSO
Rheumatoid arthritis

REFERENCES
Taurog JD, Lipsky PE. Ankylosing spondylitis, reactive arthritis and undifferentiated spondyloarthropathy. In: Harrison's Principles of Internal Medicine, 13th ed., Isselbacher KJ, et. al. (eds.) N.Y., McGraw-Hill, Inc., 1994, pp. 1664-1669.

Bakker C, et al: Measures to assess ankylosing spondylitis. J Rhematol 20: 1724-1730, 1993.

Turner JF: Bronchiolitis obliterons organizing pneumonia associated with ankylosing spondylitis. Arthritis Rheum 37: 1557-1559, 1994.

AUTHOR
Jonathan S. Sasportas, DMD, MD

Anorexia Nervosa

BASICS

DESCRIPTION
Eating disorder characterized by refusal to maintain body weight over a minimal normal weight for age and height (eg, 15% below that expected); intense fear of gaining weight or becoming fat; disordered body image; and amenorrhea (in females absence of at least three consecutive menstrual cycles when otherwise expected to occur). Weight loss is usually accomplished by a reduction in total food intake, often with extensive exercising and self-induced vomiting, use of laxatives, enemas, or diuretics. Mean age of onset is 17 years. Predominantly seen in females (95%).

ETIOLOGY

Unknown; typically emotional
◇ self-reported psychosocial stressors

SYSTEMS AFFECTED
Nervous/psychiatric
Cardiovascular
◇ due to malnutrition
◇ hypokalemia
Immune secondary to malnutrition
GI
◇ especially oral cavity (see dental considerations below)

DIAGNOSIS

SYMPTOMS AND SIGNS
• Severe weight loss
• Parotid enlargement
• Anemia, leukopenia
• Hypokalemia
• Cardiac dysrhythmias
• Hypotension
• Body image disturbance
• Peripheral edema
• Hypothermia
• Depression
• Cracked, dry skin, sparse scalp hair
• Dental Manifestations: dry mouth, dehydration, acid stains from vomiting. Oral lesions may result from malnutrition.

LABORATORY
• Diminished plasma luteinizing and follicle stimulating hormones, T3 and T4
• Elevated growth hormone and cortisol levels
• Positive dexamethasone suppression test
• Decreased fasting blood glucose

IMAGING/SPECIAL TESTS
• Psychological screening; Eating Attitudes Test
• Pathological Findings: Related to starvation and dehydration

DIFFERENTIAL
Bulimia nervosa, depressive disorders, body dysmorphic disorder, bipolar disorder, substance abuse disorder, borderline personality disorder, brain tumor, food phobia, schizophrenia.

TREATMENT

Majority are treated as outpatients. Hospitalize if weight loss is greater than 50% in 6 months, if patient has suicide ideation, or lab findings indicating electrolyte imbalance.

MEDICATIONS
• Often heterocyclic antidepressants (HCA) used, or short-term anxiolytic therapy (oxazepam 15 mg or alprazolam 0.25 mg) before meals to lessen anxiety about weight gain. Low dose phenothiazines (thorazine 10 to 25 mg/day) for inpatients. Precautions of dangerous or lethal side effects due to compromised liver and kidney function. Oxazepam for anxiety; tricyclics (Tofranil) for resistance, therapeutic vitamin-mineral supplement. Metoclopramide (Reglan) 10 to 40 mg before meals for abdominal distension; antidepressants (Prozac) when obsessive compulsive symptoms dominate.
• HCA's side effects include xerostomia, stomatitis, bad taste, parotid swelling, black tongue. Drug interactions with HCA's: epinephrine
◊ increase hypertensive response and dysrhythmia.
• Sedative/hypnotics
◊ increased CNS depression

CONSULTATION SUGGESTIONS
Mental Health Professional

REFERRAL SUGGESTIONS
Most patients deny anorectic behavior when confronted, but referral to a Mental Health Professional is recommended.

PATIENT INSTRUCTIONS
Seek care of Primary Care Physician or Mental Health Professional.

COURSE/PROGNOSIS
Highly variable; mortality 6%.

CODING

ICD-9-CM
307.1 Anorexia nervosa

CPT
21080 Custom preparation, fluoride applicator

MISCELLANEOUS

SEE ALSO
Depression
Xerostomia
Obsessive-compulsive disorder

REFERENCES
Scully C, Cawson RA: Medical problems in dentistry. Oxford. Butterworth-Heineman, 1993.

Little J, Falace D: Dental Management of the Medically Compromised Patient. 4th ed. St. Louis, CV Mosby, 1993, pp. 483-511.

American Psychiatric Association. Diagnostic and statistical manual of mental disorders, DSM-IV, Washington, DC, 1994.

Fletcher MM: Bulimia Nervosa. NY: John Wiley and Sons. 1990.

Tougz SW, et al: Oral and dental complications in dieting disorders. Int J Eat Disord 14: 341-347, 1993.

Kinzl J, et al: Significance of vomiting for hyperamylasemia and sialadenosis in patients with eating disorders. Int J Eat Disord 13: 117-124, 1993.

AUTHORS
Hillary Broder, PhD, MEd
Kani Nicolls, DDS

Anxiety Disorders

 BASICS

DESCRIPTION
• Psychiatric disorder consisting of group of mental problems that produce anxiety without delusional ideations. Anxiety appears disproportionate to the stimulus, arises without apparent threat, and persists when the stimulus is withdrawn.
• The following disorders are in this group:
  Acute Stress Disorder
  ◇ symptoms similar to post-traumatic stress disorder that occur immediately after the traumatic event.
  Generalized Anxiety Disorder
  ◇ at least 6 months of persistent and excessive anxiety and worry.
  Anxiety Disorder associated with or due to a general medical condition
  ◇ anxiety as a direct physiologic consequence of a medical condition.
  Panic Attack
  ◇ sudden onset of intense apprehension, fearfulness, or terror, often associated with feeling of impending doom, shortness of breath, chest pain, fear of "going crazy" or losing control, chills or hot flashes, feeling of choking, trembling, paresthesia, dizziness, nausea (peaks within 10 minutes). Thirty to forty percent of population report one or more panic attacks.
  Agoraphobia
  ◇ anxiety about or avoidance of places or situations from which escape might be difficult or embarrassing.
  Obsessive Compulsive Disorder
  ◇ fifteen to thirty percent of those with panic disorder.
  Post-traumatic Stress Disorder (PTSD)
  ◇ re-experiencing an extremely traumatic event accompanied by symptoms of increased arousal and avoidance of stimuli associated with the trauma.

 ETIOLOGY

Unknown but some evidence may be due to neurochemical abnormalities in brain.

SYSTEMS AFFECTED
• Nervous/Mental
• GI
• Cardiac
• Respiratory

 DIAGNOSIS

SYMPTOMS AND SIGNS
General
  ◇ insomnia, sweating, dizziness, trembling, fatigue, irritability, restlessness, cold clammy hands, difficulty concentrating.
GI
  ◇ xerostomia, dysphagia, abdominal pain, nausea, vomiting.
Cardiac
  ◇ chest tightness (pain), tachycardia
Respiratory
  ◇ hyperventilation, dyspnea

LABORATORY
CBC and urinalysis
Toxicology screen
Thyroid function tests

IMAGING/SPECIAL TESTS
Personality testing, psychiatric interview
EEG, ECG
PET scan looking for sites of abnormal metabolism

DIFFERENTIAL
• Cardiovascular disease (ie, dysrhythmias)
• Respiratory disease (ie, asthma)
• CNS (ie, transient cerebral insufficiency)
• Metabolic and hormonal disorders (ie, hypothyroidism, myasthenia gravis)
• Nutritional (ie, iron deficiency anemia)
• Substance abuse disorder (ie, alcohol addiction)
• Substance withdrawal
• Depression

TREATMENT

General
◇ Psychotherapy, biofeedback, relaxation, hypnosis

Before Medications
◇ Careful questioning and listening to establish nature of the anxiety and establish avenues of communication. Consider use of relaxation techniques (hypnosis, biofeedback, or progressive relaxation), combined with desensitization.
Emergency treatment may require use of pharmacosedation.
Use anxiety reduction protocols prior to and during dental care.

MEDICATIONS
• Typically used in treatment are benzodiazepines, heterocyclic antidepressants (HCA), monoamine oxidase (MAO) inhibitors, buspirone, beta-adrenergic blockers, and antihistamines.
• HCAs may cause xerostomia, hypotension, tachycardia, dysrhythmias. If patient using HCAs, avoid use of atropine (increased ocular pressure), epinephrine (potential for hypertensive crisis), and narcotics, sedatives, hypnotics, or barbiturates (increases respiratory depression).
• MAO inhibitors may cause xerostomia, hypotension, manic reactions, nausea, constipation, or anorexia. If patient taking MAO inhibitors, avoid use of atropine, sedatives, narcotics, hypnotics, and barbiturates.
• Xerostomia may occur secondary to many psychiatric medications.

CONSULTATION SUGGESTIONS
Mental Health Professional

REFERRAL SUGGESTIONS
Primary Care Physician, Mental Health Professional

FIRST STEPS TO TAKE IN AN EMERGENCY
• Gentle reassurance
• Refer to Primary Care Physician

PATIENT INSTRUCTIONS
For literature contact: National Institute of Mental Health, Anxiety Awareness Program, 9000 Rockville Pike, Bethesda, MD 20892

COURSE/PROGNOSIS
Variable, good prognosis for short-term anxiety disorders but more chronic problems such as post-traumatic stress disorder more difficult to resolve.

CODING

ICD-9-CM
300.3 Anxiety states

MISCELLANEOUS

SYNONYMS
Panic disorder

SEE ALSO
Obsessive Compulsive Disorder
Phobias
Hypothyroidism

REFERENCES
Scully C, Cawson RA: Medical problems in dentistry. Oxford. Butterworth-Heinemann, 1993.

American Psychiatric Association. Diagnostic and statistical manual of mental disorders, DSM-IV, Washington, DC, 1994.

AUTHORS
Hillary Broder, PhD, MEd
Kani Nicolls, DDS

Aortic Valvular Disease

BASICS

DESCRIPTION
Aortic valvular lesions are manifested by valvular narrowing or incompetence. Severity of valve disease determines whether cardiac function will be adversely affected. Diseased, deformed or prosthetic valves are at risk of infective endocarditis.

ETIOLOGY

• Rheumatic fever remains an important cause of aortic valve disease in adults.
• Isolated aortic stenosis usually results from progressive narrowing of a congenitally bicuspid aortic valve or from degenerative thickening and progressive calcification of normal valve leaflets.
• Isolated aortic valve incompetence is usually secondary to disease affecting the aorta (syphilis, ankylosing spondylitis, inherited connective tissue diseases or aneurysm formation).
• Infective endocarditis can produce aortic valve perforation or incompetence.

SYSTEMS AFFECTED
Heart
   ◇ both stenosis and incompetence increase the demands placed on the heart to pump an adequate volume of blood, leading eventually to heart failure.
Lungs
   ◇ as a late event, pulmonary edema will result from heart failure.
Other
   ◇ any organ system may be adversely affected by inadequate cardiac output in the failing heart.

DIAGNOSIS

SYMPTOMS AND SIGNS
General
   ◇ if cardiac output is compromised; poor exercise tolerance. If appearing pale, possibly diaphoretic from cardiac failure.
Heart
   ◇ angina from superimposed myocardial ischemia. Irregular heart beat from conduction abnormalities. Syncope due to dysrhythmias or other causes of impaired cardiac output.
Heart murmur
   ◇ used to differentiate stenosis from incompetence. Other abnormal heart sounds may be heard such as S3 or S4, clicks (ejection sounds).
Pulse
   ◇ characteristic alteration in arterial pulse wave-form. Irregularly, irregular beat from conduction disturbance.
Lungs
   ◇ congestion, cough, asthma from heart failure.

LABORATORY
No specific abnormalities

IMAGING/SPECIAL TESTS
Electrocardiogram
   ◇ changes may reflect ventricular hypertrophy (aortic stenosis) or ventricular enlargement (aortic incompetence).
Chest radiograph
   ◇ heart enlargement in regurgitation and with heart failure in aortic stenosis.
Echocardiogram
   ◇ will demonstrate abnormal valve function.
Cardiac catheterization
   ◇ definitive test to determine the severity of valve stenosis or incompetence. Transvalvular pressure gradients, ejection fractions, and coronary patency can be evaluated.

DIFFERENTIAL
Rheumatic valvular disease
Congenital bicuspid aortic valve
Progressive thickening/calcification of normal valve
Hypertrophic obstructive cardiomyopathy

TREATMENT

General
◇ Supportive medical management of heart failure, when present.
Prevention of infective endocarditis.

MEDICATIONS
• Coumadin
◇ lifelong anticoagulation required for prosthetic/mechanical valves. Anticoagulants should not be stopped. Confer with patient's physician before any extractions or other surgery.
• Prophylactic antibiotics required for dental extractions to minimize risk of infective endocarditis.

SURGERY
Commissurotomy for aortic stenosis with balloon or finger in pediatric patients or in elderly that are not likely to tolerate valve replacement.
Valve replacement (porcine or mechanical/prosthetic).

CONSULTATION SUGGESTIONS
Primary Care Physician

REFERRAL SUGGESTIONS
Primary Care Physician, Cardiologist, Cardiothoracic Surgeon

FIRST STEPS TO TAKE IN AN EMERGENCY
• If signs of heart failure, transport to emergency facility on oxygen and sitting semi-erect.

PATIENT INSTRUCTIONS
Always remind patients of the need for antibiotics prior to invasive dental procedures.

COURSE/PROGNOSIS
Variable depending on degree of stenosis/incompetence.
Valve replacement before significant heart failure improves prognosis.
Heart failure may persist or recur after valve replacement. Prognosis also influenced by co-existing coronary artery disease.

CODING

ICD-9-CM
746.4 Aortic insufficiency
746.9 Aortic stenosis

CPT
90780 IV infusion for therapy

MISCELLANEOUS

SYNONYMS
Aortic regurgitation
Aortic Stenosis
Aortic Insufficiency

SEE ALSO
Mitral valvular disease
Congestive heart failure
Endocarditis

REFERENCES
McKenna SJ, Roser SM, Werther JR: Management of the Medically Compromised Patient. In: Alling CC, Helfrick JF, Alling RD (eds). Impacted Teeth. Philadelphia, WB Saunders Co, 1993. pp. 70-71.

Hupp JR. Medical management of the surgical patient. In: Principles of Oral and Maxillofacial Surgery. Peterson LJ, et. al. (eds). Philadelphia, JB Lippincott Co. 1992, pp. 21-27.

AUTHOR
Samuel J. McKenna, DDS, MD

Aphthous Stomatitis

BASICS

DESCRIPTION
• An idiopathic, noninfectious, recurrent, ulcerative disease affecting nonkeratinized oral mucous membranes, including buccal, labial, ventral surface of tongue, floor of mouth, soft palatal, and oropharyngeal mucosa.
• Minor aphthae can occur as single or multiple ulcers, measuring less than 1.0 cm in diameter, and healing without treatment in 10 to 14 days.
• Herpetiform aphthae measure about 1 to 2 mm in diameter, and can occur in groups which may coalesce. The ulcers usually heal in 7 to 10 days.
• Major aphthae (Sutton's disease, periadenitis mucosa necrotica recurrens) are greater than 1.0 cm in diameter and may take more than 2 to 4 weeks to heal, often with scarring.

ETIOLOGY

• The cause of aphthous is unknown but numerous "triggers" have been reported to include specific foods and beverages, mechanical trauma, hormonal changes, illness, and undefined stress.
• Some cases show a familial pattern.
• There is an inverse relationship between aphthous ulcers and smoking.

SYSTEMS AFFECTED
• Nonkeratinized oral and oropharyngeal mucosa show single or multiple ulcerations with rims of erythema. The ulcers are typically nonindurated, without purulence. Major aphthae, if present for several weeks, may become clinically firm due to a buildup of scar and granulation tissue. Mucosa is predisposed to secondary infection.
• Oral hygiene is compromised because use of brush, floss, and mouth rinses cause increased discomfort.
• In severe cases, multiple systems may be affected due to dehydration and lack of nutritional intake.

DIAGNOSIS

SYMPTOMS AND SIGNS
• Patients will present with a chief complaint of recurrent severe oral discomfort, in many cases for months or years, with each episode or lesion lasting a few days to a few weeks followed by complete remission.
• Circumscribed, nonindurated (unless chronic) ulcers with surrounding erythematous borders, currently or by history, involving nonkeratinized mucosa which includes buccal, labial, tongue, floor of mouth, soft palatal, and oropharyngeal mucosa. Ulcers may begin on nonkeratinized oral mucosa, and as they enlarge, may involve a keratinized mucosal border, (eg, lateral tongue).

LABORATORY
• No clinical laboratory findings of diagnostic significance.
• Biopsies are seldom necessary and are only used to rule out other diseases.
• Histopathologic features of an aphthous biopsy specimen show only nonspecific ulceration.

IMAGING/SPECIAL TESTS
None are of diagnostic significance.

DIFFERENTIAL
Recurrent herpes
    Ruled out by occurrence on keratinized mucosa, usually vermilion, gingiva, and hard palate.
Lichen planus
    Shows mucosal erythema remote from ulceration and hyperkeratotic striations.
Pemphigus/Pemphigoid
    Involves keratinized and nonkeratinized mucosa. Nikolsky's sign helps differentiate.
Traumatic/Factitial/Iatrogenic ulcer
    Usually can be ruled out by pattern of occurrence and history.
Behcet's syndrome
    Eye and genital lesions

Aphthous Stomatitis

TREATMENT

General
◇ Avoid triggers if identified

MEDICATIONS
• Topical steroid suspensions: triamcinolone acetonide 0.1% aqueous suspension, Disp 200 ml, Sig 5 ml oral rinse and expectorate q.d. PC and hs NPO 1 hr.
• (Directions to the Pharmacist: Injectable triamcinolone QS into water for irrigation, add 5 ml of ethanol to increase solubility) May alter suspension to include viscous lidocaine as a topical anesthetic.
• Prednisone burst therapy, 40 mg q.d. in the morning 30 minutes after arising for 5 days, then 20 mg q.o.d. also 30 minutes after arising for an additional 1 to 2 weeks.
• Dapsone
• Colchicine
• Imuran

SURGERY
Excision not indicated.

CONSULTATION SUGGESTIONS
Oral Medicine, Oral-Maxillofacial Surgeon

REFERRAL SUGGESTIONS
Oral Medicine

PATIENT INSTRUCTIONS
• If unable to tolerate until resolution, consider use of topical steroid/anesthetic combination.
• Patient education is important because therapy may promote healing of current ulcers and if used at subtherapeutic doses, can prevent recurrences but cannot "cure" the patient of the disease. Long-term management is aimed at finding the minimum amount of therapy that will keep the ulcers from recurring. This can be accomplished usually by using the topical triamcinolone t.i.d., b.i.d., o.d., q.o.d., or even p.r.n.
• The most common complication/side effect of long-term topical triamcinolone use is oral candidosis. In these cases, an antifungal such as nystatin can be used in the topical triamcinolone suspension (replacing the water).

COURSE/PROGNOSIS
Lesions tend to recur throughout life. Typically leave no scars.

CODING

ICD-9-CM
528.2 Aphthous

CPT
11900 Intralesional injection
40808 Biopsy, vestibule of mouth
40812 Incisional biopsy with simple repair
41108 Biopsy of floor of mouth
42110 Biopsy of palate
87252 Culture isolation
88160 Cytologic preparation

MISCELLANEOUS

SYNONYMS
Canker sores

SEE ALSO
Lichen planus
Pemphagoid
Herpes simplex
Behcet's syndrome

REFERENCES
Vincent SD, Lilly GE: Clinical, historic and therapeutic features of aphthous stomatitis. Oral Surg Oral Med Oral Path, 74:79-86, 1992.

Regezi JA, Sciubba JJ: Ulcerative conditions. In: Oral Pathology: Clinical-Pathologic Correlations. Philadelphia, WB Saunders, 1989, pp. 29-68.

Eversol LR, Shopper TP, Chambers DW: Effects of suspected foodstuff challenging agents in the etiology of recurrent aphthous stomatitis. Oral Surg Oral Med Oral Path, 54:33-38, 1982.

Vincent SD, Finkelstein MW: Differential diagnosis of oral ulcers. In: Principles of Oral Diagnosis. Coleman GC, Nelson JF (eds), St. Louis, Mosby-Year Book Co., 1993, pp. 328-351.

AUTHOR
Steven Vincent, DDS, MS

Asthma

BASICS

DESCRIPTION
• A heterogeneous group of illnesses causing reversible airway obstruction present in five percent of the United States population. Asthma is most common in young children, least common in late adolescence, and the incidence again increases in early adult life.
• Intrinsic form due to poorly identified triggering factors that do not arise from environment.
• Extrinsic form due to environmental irritants, usually antigens, that trigger hyperresponsive airways to spasm.

ETIOLOGY

• Ninety percent of asthmatics under the age of 30 have a coexisting allergic condition.
• Only fifty percent with onset of asthma after age 40 have an allergic condition, but many have a history of previous bronchial irritation.
• In susceptible individuals, asthma may be precipitated by upper respiratory infection, cold exposure, exercise, chemical irritants, and medications such as aspirin and other nonsteroidal anti-inflammatory agents. Antigens such as pollen, molds, mites, animal fur, and feathers may also trigger asthmatic attacks.
Emotional stress may trigger an asthmatic event.

SYSTEMS AFFECTED
Lungs
◇ primary obstruction occurs in those reactive airways containing smooth muscle.
Paranasal sinuses
◇ sinusitis and asthma will often co-exist.
Hypothalamic-Pituitary-Adrenal Axis
◇ may be suppressed in those asthmatics who are receiving or have received corticosteroids.

DIAGNOSIS

SYMPTOMS AND SIGNS
Lungs
◇ recurrent intermittent wheezing, shortness of breath, cough, and sputum production. Wheezing, increased respiratory expiratory phase, respiratory distress, decreased breath sounds, hyperresonance, use of accessory respiratory muscles.
Sinus
◇ nasal/sinus congestion in those with sinusitis. In allergic individuals, rhinitis, nasal congestion, sinus congestion, drainage.
Cardiovascular
◇ cyanosis from hypoxemia with acute episode, tachycardia, pulsus paradoxus.

LABORATORY
Skin testing
◇ may show allergies to any number of environmental allergens.
Theophylline level
◇ used to monitor therapy with methylxanthene bronchodilators.
Serum IgE
◇ usually elevated in allergic individuals.
Arterial blood gas
◇ will show hypoxia and hypocarbia in asthmatic attack. Hypercarbia is a late event with respiratory fatigue.

IMAGING/SPECIAL TESTS
Spirometry will show decreased airflow.
Chest radiograph
◇ may show areas of pulmonary consolidation from mucous plug formation but usually normal. Flattening of diaphrams.
Sinus radiographs
◇ may show opacification of paranasal sinuses in some asthmatics.

DIFFERENTIAL
Allergic condition including drug allergy .
Chemical airway irritant
Upper respiratory infection
Sinusitis, chronic bronchitis
Emphysema (irreversible obstructive lung disease)
Cardiac disease

Asthma

TREATMENT

General
◊ Avoid known triggers, including allergens, chemical irritants, stress.
◊ Patient should take all usual asthma medications up to time of dental treatment.
◊ Avoid elective treatments during upper respiratory infection when symptoms poorly controlled.

MEDICATIONS
Maintenance:
• Bronchodilators (beta-adrenergic agonist, anticholinergics, methylxanthines).
• Anti-inflammatory (cromolyn, medocromil, corticosteroids)
• Antigen desensitization therapy in allergic individuals. (controversial efficacy)
• Respiratory therapy to mobilize secretions.
Acute Bronchospasm:
• Aerosolized bronchodilator
◊ Metaproterenol or albuterol inhaler 2 puffs q 6 hours.
• -Supplemental oxygen

CONSULTATION SUGGESTIONS
Pulmonologist, Allergist

REFERRAL SUGGESTIONS
Primary Care Physician

FIRST STEPS TO TAKE IN AN EMERGENCY
• Use of inhaled bronchodilator such as beta-agonist.
• Summon paramedics if poor response to inhaled bronchodilator.

PATIENT INSTRUCTIONS
Carry inhaler, avoid respiratory irritants. Contact American Lung Association (212)315-8700 or Asthma Foundation (800)727-8462 for printed information.

COURSE/PROGNOSIS
Usually adequately controlled especially with simultaneous management of allergic conditions, sinusitis, and strict avoidance of known precipitants. Acute bronchospasm is a life-threatening condition and requires prompt aggressive therapy with bronchodilator drugs.

CODING

ICD-9-CM
493.0 Extrinsic asthma
493.1 Intrinsic asthma
493.9 Unspecified asthma

CPT
90780 IV infusion for therapy

MISCELLANEOUS

SYNONYMS
Reactive airway disease

SEE ALSO
Bronchitis
Anaphylaxis
Airway obstruction
COPD

REFERENCES
McKenna SJ, Roser SM, Werther JR: Management of the Medically Compromised Patient. In: Impacted Teeth. Alling CC, Helfrick JR, Alling RD (eds). Philadelphia, WB Saunders Co., 1993, pp. 76-78.

Barnes PJ: A new approach to the treatment of asthma. N Engl J Med 321:1517, 1989.

Goldstein RA, et al: NIH conference. Asthma. Ann Intern Med 121: 698-708, 1994.

Leatherman J: Life-threatening asthma. Clin Chest Med 15:453-479, 1994.

AUTHOR
Samuel J. McKenna, DDS, MD

Atrial Bradycardia

BASICS

DESCRIPTION
• Cardiac dysrhythmia in which rate of atrial contractions is less than 60 beats per minute. The normal atrial rhythm is set by the sinoatrial (SA) node, which lies at the junction of the right atrium and superior vena cava. The SA node has a regular spontaneous discharge, the impulse of which traverses the atrium until it reaches the atrioventricular (AV) node, which lies at the base of the interatrial septum. The impulse is somewhat delayed in the AV node and then exits into the bundle of His which transmits the electrical pulse to the ventricular conduction system.
• The SA and AV nodes are significantly influenced by autonomic tone. Vagal activity depresses SA node automaticity (slows rate), and prolongs the refractory period of atrial and AV nodal tissue. Sympathetic activity has the opposite effect.
• Normal sinus node discharge rate is 60 to 100 beats per minute.
• Types of bradycardia include:
  1) Sinus bradycardia
  2) First degree heart block
  ◇ prolonged PR interval (greater than or equal to 0.2 seconds).
  3) Second degree heart block
  ◇ intermittent failure of sinus node discharge, causing intermittent absence of P waves.
  4) Third degree heart block
  ◇ lack of atrial activity or presence of ectopic atrial pacemaker(s).
  5) Sick sinus syndrome
  ◇ SA node dysfunction with marked sinus bradycardia, SA block or sinus arrest.

ETIOLOGY

Advanced age, amyloidosis, hypothyroidism, advanced hepatic disease, hypothermia, vasovagal syncope or other forms of hypervagotonia, severe hypoxia, hypercapnia, acidemia, acute hypertension, antidysrhythmic, or beta or calcium antagonist medications, or ischemic heart disease affecting coronary artery supply to node.

SYSTEMS AFFECTED
Cardiovascular
  ◇ impaired cardiac output, heart failure.
Neurologic
  ◇ syncope, confusion, fatigue

DIAGNOSIS

SYMPTOMS AND SIGNS
Dizziness, fatigue, syncope, confusion, hypotension, cardiac failure, cardiac arrest, palpitations, irregular pulse, signs of congestive heart failure, signs of hypothyroidism.

LABORATORY
Thyroid function studies
Arterial blood gas determination
Liver function studies

IMAGING/SPECIAL TESTS
ECG
Holter monitoring
Chest radiograph
Electrophysiologic testing

DIFFERENTIAL
See etiology section

TREATMENT

General
◇ The first steps in management of sinus node dysfunction are to precisely diagnose the underlying problem and correct it if possible.

◇ If problem cannot be corrected, no treatment is necessary unless the patient is symptomatic.

MEDICATIONS
• Vasovagal syncope treated with placing patient in head position that places their head below the level of the heart and/or legs. It can also be managed or prevented with vagolytic drugs such as atropine 0.5 to 2 mg or glycopyrrolate (Robinul) 0.1 mg IV. In life-threatening situations, isoproterenol (Isuprel) 1 to 4 µg/min IV can be used.

SURGERY
Symptomatic sinus node dysfunction usually requires temporary or permanent pacemaker insertion.

CONSULTATION SUGGESTIONS
Cardiologist, Primary Care Physician

REFERRAL SUGGESTIONS
Primary Care Physician

FIRST STEPS TO TAKE IN AN EMERGENCY
• Place patient in head-down, Trendelenberg position.
• Administer 0.5 mg atropine. May be repeated every 5 minutes up to maximum of 2 mg.

PATIENT INSTRUCTIONS
If symptoms occur, the patient's primary care physician should be notified. Pacemakers do not mandate use of prophylactic antibiotics prior to invasive dentistry.

COURSE/PROGNOSIS
If underlying problem is correctable or pacemaker inserted, prognosis excellent. Uncorrected sick sinus can lead to congestive heart failure. Pacemaker problems can appear as fatigue, dizziness, syncope or abnormal pulsations in the neck veins.

 ## CODING

ICD-9-CM
426.0   3rd degree heart block
426.11 1st degree heart block
426.12 2nd degree heart block Mobitz II
426.13 2nd degree heart block Mobitz I
427.81 Chronic bradycardia
427.89 Sinus or vasovagal bradycardia (acute)

 ## MISCELLANEOUS

SYNONYMS
Vasovagal syncope
Vagal reaction
Sick sinus syndrome

SEE ALSO
Atrial tachycardia
Hypothyroidism

REFERENCES
Josephson ME, Marchlinski FE, Buxton AE: The bradyarrhythmias. In: Harrison's Principles of Internal Medicine. Isselbacher KJ, et al (eds), New York, McGraw-Hill, 1994, pp. 1011-1019.

AUTHOR
James R. Hupp, DMD, MD, JD

Atrial Flutter, Atrial Fibrillation

 BASICS

DESCRIPTION
Abnormal heart rhythms originating in the atria and characterized by disorganized electrical activity without discrete P waves on ECG. Atrial flutter is characterized by an increased rate of atrial activity, typically 250 to 350 bpm, with a characteristic "saw tooth" pattern on ECG. Either condition may be paroxysmal or persistent.

 ETIOLOGY

• Paroxysmal form is typically related to inciting events such as stress, exertion, anxiety, hypoxia, hypocapnea, acute metabolic or hemodynamic derangements or acute alcohol intoxication (in so-called "holiday heart syndrome").
• Persistent forms are generally due to structural or organic heart disease, most commonly rheumatic heart disease, mitral valve disease, hypertensive heart disease, myocardial infarction, thyrotoxicosis, and in chronic lung diseases.
• Both atrial fibrillation and atrial flutter are common after open heart surgery.
• Paroxysmal forms may convert to persistent forms, and often do if the rhythm is sustained. In addition, chronic atrial flutter often degenerates into atrial fibrillation.

SYSTEMS AFFECTED
Cardiovascular
  ◇ rapid ventricular rates may lead to ischemic heart disease due to increased myocardial oxygen demand.
Hypotension from inadequate ventricular filling, ventricular fatigue may also occur.
CNS
  ◇ systemic embolization particularly to the brain may result in stroke. TIAs, syncopal episodes, amaurosis fugax or frank ischemic stroke may result from emboli depending upon the size of the embolus and the vessel in which it lodges.
Patients with other concomitant heart disease, especially rheumatic heart disease, are particularly prone to stroke.

 DIAGNOSIS

SYMPTOMS AND SIGNS
• Palpitations, syncope, dizziness, transient ischemia attack, amaurosis fugax, angina, fatigue, dyspnea.
• Irregularly, irregular heart beat (pulse).
• Heart rate greater than 250 seen on ECG, although the ventricular rate is usually much less due to atrioventricular block 2:1, 3:1, 4:1, etc.

LABORATORY
Thyroid function tests to rule out thyrotoxicosis.

IMAGING/SPECIAL TESTS
• Chest radiograph (for cardiomegaly)
• ECG
• Transthoracic or transesophageal echocardiogram may be used to detect thrombi or diseased valves.

DIFFERENTIAL
• Anxiety
• Sinus tachycardia
• Paroxysmal supraventricular tachycardia
• Thyrotoxicosis
• Acute alcohol intoxication ("holiday heart syndrome")
• Congestive heart failure

TREATMENT

Nonpharmacologic Approaches
  ◇ Direct current cardioversion is a highly effective method of restoring sinus rhythm with a success rate of approximately 85%, particularly if done soon after atrial rhythm abnormality appears. Failed initial attempts at cardioversion may succeed after initiation of anti-dysrhythmic therapy. Disadvantages of direct current cardioversion include the usual requirement of general anesthesia and necessity of anti-coagulation prior to cardioversion due to risk of thromboembolism.

MEDICATIONS
  • Antidysrhythmic drugs:
  ◇ Intravenous procainamide used in acute management to restore and maintain sinus rhythm.
  • Oral antidysrhythmics: quinidine can be given to restore and maintain sinus rhythm when the restoration is not urgent. Quinidine is also used to maintain sinus rhythm after restoration with direct current cardioversion. Disopyramide has also been shown to be effective in maintaining sinus rhythm.
  • Control of ventricular rate: Digoxin is most useful to control ventricular rate in acute situation.
  • Beta-blockers and calcium channel blockers are being used more frequently to control ventricular rate because they have a quicker response than does digoxin.
  • Class IC anti-dysrhythmics; flecainamide, moricizine, and propafenone have proven to be effective both in restoration of sinus rhythm and in maintenance.
  • The newer class III agents, sotalol and amiodarone, have also proven effective particularly in refractory atrial fibrillation.
  • It should be noted that all antidysrhythmic therapy carries a potential risk as a prodysrhythmic.
  • Aspirin and coumadin: have been used to reduce the risk of stroke in patients with atrial fibrillation. Coumadin has been proven to be the more effective agent; however, the side effect profile is certainly less safe.

SURGERY
Surgical techniques aimed at ablation of the AV conduction pathway have been described but usually require pacing, transient or permanent.

CONSULTATION SUGGESTIONS
Cardiologist

REFERRAL SUGGESTIONS
Primary Care Physician, Cardiologist

FIRST STEPS TO TAKE IN AN EMERGENCY
  • Stop dental care
  • Administer oxygen
  • Monitor vital signs
  • Transport to emergency facility as indicated

PATIENT INSTRUCTIONS
Seek evaluation by primary care physician.

COURSE/PROGNOSIS
Prognosis related to etiology. Stroke risk low if anticoagulated.

CODING

ICD-9-CM
427.3   Atrial fibrillation and flutter
427.31 Atrial fibrillation
427.32 Atrial flutter

MISCELLANEOUS

SYNONYMS
A. fib.

SEE ALSO
Congestive heart failure
Cerebrovascular accident

REFERENCES
Josephson ME, Buxton AE, Marchlinski FE: The Tachyarrhythmias. In: Harrison's Principles of Internal Medicine. 13th ed.

Isselbacher KJ, et al, (eds), New York, McGraw Hill, 1994, pp. 1022-1024.

Pritchett EL: Management of atrial fibrillation. N Engl J Med, 326:1264-1271, 1992.

Murgatroyd FD, Camm AJ: Atrial arrhythmias. Lancet 341 (8856):1317-1322, 1993.

AUTHOR
André Montazem, DMD, MD

Atrial Tachycardias

BASICS

DESCRIPTION
Cardiac dysrhythmias with three or more atrial complexes at rate exceeding 100 beats per minute.
Types of atrial tachycardias -

Sinus tachycardia (ST)
◊ rate 100 to 200 beats per minute. Usually represents a physiologic response to stresses such as fever, exercise, anxiety, anemia. ECG shows P wave with sinus contour prior to each QRS complex.

Atrial flutter (AF)
◊ range 250 to 350 beats per minute. Seen in patient with pericarditis or respiratory failure. Will eventually deteriorate to fibrillation if allowed to persist.

Atrial fibrillation (A. fib.)
◊ rate 350 to 600 beats per minute. Seen most commonly associated with congestive heart failure, chronic lung disease, thyrotoxicosis or acute ethanol intoxication. Produces irregularly, irregular heart rhythm.

Paroxysmal supraventricular tachycardia (PSVT).
◊ Re-entry type abnormality, occurring in situations that produce prolongation of PR interval. Presents with rapid rhythm without P waves.

ETIOLOGY

ST
◊ fever, exercise, anxiety, anemia, hypoxia, intravascular volume depletion, thyrotoxicosis, hypotension, heart failure.
AF
◊ pericarditis, acute respiratory failure.
A. fib.
◊ emotional stress, acute ethanol intoxication, acute hypoxia, hypercapnia, congestive heart failure, valvular heart disease, chronic lung disease, thyrotoxicosis.

SYSTEMS AFFECTED
Cardiovascular
Pulmonary

DIAGNOSIS

SYMPTOMS AND SIGNS
Palpitation, light-headedness, hypotension, syncope, symptoms and signs of underlying disease or condition. A. fib. produces irregularly, irregular pulse.

LABORATORY
Digoxin level
Thyroid function studies
Toxin screening including ethanol
WBC
Arterial blood gas

IMAGING/SPECIAL TESTS
ECG
Chest radiograph
Thyroid scan
Echocardiogram

DIFFERENTIAL
Etiologies possible
◊ fever, exercise, congestive heart failure, sick sinus syndrome, caffeine, anxiety, anemia, thyrotoxicosis, chronic lung pathology, acute ethanol intoxication.

TREATMENT

General
◇ Management depends on identifying underlying cause of dysrhythmia.
◇ PSVT can sometimes be stopped with carotid sinus massage. If drugs do not work, pacemaker use may be necessary.
◇ AF is treated with direct current cardioversion at 10 to 50 Watt-sec under mild sedation. Use of a pacemaker may be necessary.
◇ A. fib. resistant to medical therapy may respond to cardioversion using 100 to 200 Watt-sec of energy. Anticoagulation should be begin 2 weeks prior and continue for 2 weeks after electrically cardioverting A. fib.

MEDICATIONS
• Tachycardia due to catecholamines can be treated with cardioselective beta antagonist.
• PSVT can usually be successfully stopped with administration of adenosine (6 to 12 mg IV) or verapamil (2.5 to 10 mg IV).
• AF may respond to digoxin, a beta sympathetic antagonist, or a calcium antagonist.
• A. fib. may respond to digoxin, a beta sympathetic antagonist, or a calcium antagonist. Quinidine-like drugs or flecainide may be successful in converting A. fib. Patients with chronic A. fib. need anticoagulation with Coumadin to limit formation of a thrombus in the left atrium.

CONSULTATION SUGGESTIONS
Cardiology

REFERRAL SUGGESTIONS
Primary Care Physician

FIRST STEPS TO TAKE IN AN EMERGENCY
• If tachycardia symptomatic and causing physiologic compromise, consider immediate cardioversion or pacemaker insertion. PSVT may convert with carotid sinus massage.

PATIENT INSTRUCTIONS
If chronically anticoagulated, warn doctors before any surgery.

COURSE/PROGNOSIS
If underlying cause corrected, cure possible. If patient with A. fib. not converted, a thrombus may form in left atrium that sends emboli to central nervous system.

CODING

ICD-9-CM
427.2 Paroxysmal supraventricular tachycardia
785.0 Tachycardia

M   MISCELLANEOUS

SEE ALSO
Congestive heart failure
Hyperthyroidism
Atrial fibrillation

REFERENCES
Pieper JS, Stanton MS: Narrow QRS Complex Tachycardias. Mayo Clin Proc 70:371-375, 1995.

Josephson ME, Buxton AE, Marchlinski FE: The Tachyarrhythmias. In: Harrison's Principles of Internal Medicine. Isselbacher KJ, et al (eds), N.Y. McGraw-Hill, 1994, pp. 1019-1029.

AUTHOR
James R. Hupp, DMD, MD, JD

Basal Cell Carcinoma

 BASICS

DESCRIPTION

• A slow-growing, locally invasive malignant tumor of skin that arises from basal cells of the epidermis and appendages and almost never metastasizes. It is the most prevalent cancer in humans and adequate excision is usually curative. Large and/or recurrent lesions can require aggressive therapy.

• Nodular (most common) variant demonstrates a flesh-colored nodule within the skin.

• Morpheaform variant presents as an indurated superficial lesion that is ill-defined.

• Basosquamous skin cancer has histologic features of both basal cell and squamous cell carcinoma.

 ETIOLOGY

Ultraviolet sunlight exposure is the primary etiologic factor

SYSTEMS AFFECTED

Integumentary
Other systems depending upon specific site of physical invasion.

 DIAGNOSIS

SYMPTOMS AND SIGNS

Skin

◇ nonhealing, skin ulceration that can intermittently bleed and crust over. Persistent scaly or crusted nonulcerated skin lesion.

◇ Slow-growing mass lesion within skin.

◇ Ulceration with rolled border is classical, but is not always seen.

◇ Superficial telangiectasia overlying skin nodule.

◇ Slow destruction of eyelid, ear, nose or other sun-exposed skin area suggests a neglected basal cell carcinoma.

IMAGING/SPECIAL TESTS

Biopsy demonstrates basaloid epithelial malignancy with local invasion.
CT scan for evaluation of large lesions

DIFFERENTIAL

Cutaneous squamous cell carcinoma
Benign nevus
Traumatic ulcer
Malignant melanoma
Skin adnexal tumor

TREATMENT

MEDICATIONS
• Topical 5-fluorouracil can be used for chemoexfoliation of high-risk, sun-damaged skin.

SURGERY
• Thorough excision is the cornerstone of treatment. Larger and/or recurrent lesions require wider margins as well as resection of adjacent underlying bone.
• Mohs micrographic surgery is used for lesions in areas of embryologic fusion and for recurrent lesions.
• Large defects of the face and other sites often require flap reconstruction.

IRRADIATION
Not indicated

CONSULTATION SUGGESTIONS
Oral-Maxillofacial Surgeon, Plastic Reconstructive Surgeon, Dermatologist (Mohs Surgeon)

REFERRAL SUGGESTIONS
Oral-Maxillofacial Surgeon, Plastic Reconstructive Surgeon, Dermatologist (Mohs)

PATIENT INSTRUCTIONS
Avoid continued exposure to sun without sunscreen.

COURSE/PROGNOSIS
Prognosis is excellent for lesions that undergo timely and thorough removal. Large, neglected lesions or those that have recurred on multiple occasions can require extensive surgery and reconstruction.

CODING

ICD-9-CM
173 Unspecified basal cell carcinoma
239.2 Neoplasm of uncertain nature of bone, soft tissue or skin

CPT
11052 Biopsy skin
11640 Excision malignant lesion face, lips 0.5 cm or less
11641 Excision malignant lesion face, lips 0.6-1 cm
11642 Excision malignant lesion face, lips 1.1-2 cm
17304 Mohs chemosurgery
40490 Biopsy lip
40510 Wedge excision of lip, primary closure
99000 Transport of specimen to outside laboratory.

MISCELLANEOUS

SYNONYMS
"Rodent ulcer"
Basal cell nevus syndrome

SEE ALSO
Basal cell nevus syndrome
Squamous cell carcinoma

REFERENCES
Friedman RF, et al: Skin cancer: basal cell and squamous cell carcinoma. In: American Cancer Society Textbook of Clinical Oncology, Atlanta, American Cancer Society, 1991.

Swanson NA, Johnson TM. Management of basal and squamous cell carcinoma. In: Otolaryngology-Head & Neck Surgery. 2nd ed, Cummings CW, et al (eds), St. Louis, Mosby Year Book Publ. 1993, pp. 403-418.

Derrick EK, et al: The use of cytology in the diagnosis of basal cell carcinoma. Br J Dermatol 130: 561-563, 1994.

Lang PG, et al: The management of non-melanoma skin cancer of the head and neck. J S C Med Assoc 90: 455-473, 1994.

AUTHOR
Eric J. Dierks, DMD, MD

Basal Cell Nevus Syndrome

 BASICS

DESCRIPTION
A complex syndrome with multiple manifestations of the skeletal, integumentary, and endocrine systems. The most notable presentations for the dental practitioner are jaw cysts, basal cell carcinomas, and a characteristic facial appearance.

 ETIOLOGY

The syndrome is a hereditary condition that is transmitted as an autosomal dominant trait with high penetrance and variable expressivity.

SYSTEMS AFFECTED
Skin
◇ multiple basal cell carcinomas develop from existing nevi that most commonly occur on the face, neck, upper extremities, and upper trunk. Palmar and plantar pits occur on the hands and feet. Epidermal cysts, lipomas, and milia are common findings.
Facies
◇ there is frontal and temporoparietal bossing with prominent supraorbital ridges. Hypertelorism and a broad nasal root is the result of an enlarged sphenoid bone. Mandibular prognathism is a common finding.
Endocrine disorders
◇ abnormal calcium excretion is due to hyporesponsiveness to parathyroid hormone and results in calcifications and osteomas of the dura mater, the falx cerebri, and the retroclinoid ligaments. Endocrine disorders in females include ovarian fibromas, and ovarian and uterine cysts with calcifications. Male disorders include missing testicles, hypogonadism, female pubic hair distribution, and sparse facial hair.
Skeletal disorders
◇ odontogenic keratocysts of the maxilla and mandible are present in approximately 70% of affected individuals. Other skeletal anomalies include bifid ribs, rudimentary cervical ribs, cervical and upper thoracic vertebral fusion, and shortened metacarpals.
Neurologic anomalies
◇ includes mental retardation, dural calcification, agenesis of corpus callosum, congenital hydrocephalus, and a high frequency of medulloblastomas.
Ophthalmic abnormalities
◇ manifested by hypertelorism, dystopia canthorum, congenital blindness, and internal strabismus.

 DIAGNOSIS

SYMPTOMS AND SIGNS
Most often the patient is asymptomatic, but may notice the enlargement of nevi on the face, arms, or trunk.
Oral Cavity
◇ expansion of the alveolar ridges by enlarging keratocysts of the maxilla and/or mandible.
Dermatologic
◇ presence of flesh-colored to brownish dome-shaped papules, soft nodules or flat plaques measuring up to 1 cm in diameter. Ulcerations may occur in long-standing lesions.

IMAGING/SPECIAL TESTS
A panorex is a useful screening radiograph for the diagnosis of cysts of the jaws. Large cysts with cortical perforation and soft tissue extension may best be evaluated with a CT scan. A chest radiograph will illustrate the presence of bifid ribs.
Rubbing carbon paper on the palms of the hands and soles of the feet can aid in the demonstration of pitting.

DIFFERENTIAL
Odontogenic keratocysts or basal cell nevi not associated with syndrome.

TREATMENT

SURGERY
Jaw Cysts
◊ odontogenic keratocysts are treated with enucleation and curettage. These lesions have a recurrence rate of up to 60%, and chemical cautery (Carnoy's solution) or a peripheral ostectomy are advocated to lessen the chance of recurrence.
Basal Cell Carcinoma
◊ these lesions are malignant, but with little to no chance of metastasis. Treatment is local excision. Large lesions may best be excised with the Moh's technique in which margins are checked with thin sections. Local flaps may be necessary to close the surgical defects.

CONSULTATION SUGGESTIONS
Oral-Maxillofacial Surgeon

REFERRAL SUGGESTIONS
Oral-Maxillofacial Surgeon

PATIENT INSTRUCTIONS
Keratocysts have relatively high likelihood of recurrence, particularly if resection with margins not performed.

COURSE/PROGNOSIS
Jaw Cysts
◊ patients should be followed for 10 years following the removal of keratocysts. A yearly panorex is essential for the first 5 years and every other year for the next 5 years.
Basal Cell Carcinoma
◊ a complete dermatologic evaluation is recommended on a yearly basis. These patients require very close follow-up because both odontogenic keratocysts and basal cell carcinomas may result in extensive destruction if not discovered early.

CODING

ICD-9-CM
214.9   Lipoma
257.2   Hypogonadism
318.0   Mental retardation
369.0   Congenital blindness
378.9   Strabismus
524.0   Mandibular sagittal hyperplasia
526.0   Odontogenic keratocyst
620.8   Uterine cyst
705.1   Milia
706.2   Epidermal cysts
742.3   Hydrocephalus
756.0   Frontal bossing/prominent supraorbital ridge
756.0   Hypertelorism
756.15 Vertebral fusion; congenital
756.2   Cervical rib
756.3   Bifid rib
759.89 Basal cell nevus syndrome
M809013 Basal cell carcinoma
170.0   face
195.0   neck
195.4   upper extremity
195.8   trunk

CPT
11640 Excision, malignant lesion of face (0.5 cm or less)
11641 0.6 to 1 cm
11642 1.1 to 2.0 cm
1730H Moh's micrographic surgery
20220 Biopsy, bone, needle (aspiration)
20240 Biopsy, excisional, bone
21030 Excision of cyst of facial bone other than mandible
21040 Excision of cyst of mandible; simple
21041 Excision of cyst of mandible; complex
41899 Extraction of tooth
70100 Radiologic exam, mandible; partial, less than four view
70110 Radiologic exam, mandible; complete minimum of four views
70355 Panorex
70486 Computerized axial tomography, maxillofacial area

MISCELLANEOUS

SYNONYMS
Gorlin's syndrome
Jaw cyst-basal cell nevus-bifid rib syndrome
Hereditary cutaneomandibular polyoncosis
Nevoid basal cell carcinoma syndrome

SEE ALSO
Odontogenic keratocyst
Basal cell carcinoma

REFERENCES
Carl W, Helm F, Wood R: Disorders involving medicine and dentistry: The basal cell nevus syndrome. Quint Int 10:1041-1047, 1982.

Gorlin RJ, Goltz RW: Multiple nevoid basal-cell epithelioma, jaw cysts and bifid rib. New Engl J Med 262:908-912, 1960.

Regezi JA, Sciubba JJ: Cysts of the Oral Region. In: Oral Pathology Clinical Pathologic Correlations, 2nd ed. Philadelphia, WB Saunders, Co., 1993, pp. 337-343.

AUTHOR
Robert Rudman, DDS

Behcet's Syndrome

BASICS

DESCRIPTION
A rare, multisystem disease characterized by oral, ocular, and genital ulcers. Males twice more common than females, and occurs in 3rd to 4th decades.

ETIOLOGY

Although the cause of Behcet's syndrome is unknown, much information points to an autoimmune vasculitis. Some evidence suggests a viral trigger. A genetic predisposition due to the frequent finding of HLA-B51 in those affected has been proposed.

SYSTEMS AFFECTED
• Oral manifestations include ulcers, usually less than 1 cm in diameter involving, at the time of clinical examination or historically, the nonkeratinized mucosa including labial, buccal, ventral surface of the tongue, floor of mouth, and soft palate.
• Ocular changes can include uveitis, conjunctivitis, and retinitis.
• Genital lesions consist of single or multiple ulcers involving skin or mucosa.
• Perianal ulcers have been reported, as well as inflammatory bowl disease.
• Other, less often involved features include vasculitis related CNS alterations to include headaches and infarcts, recurrent arthritis multiple joints including wrists, knees, and ankles, and cardiovascular insufficiency as a result of vasculitis and thrombosis, polychondritis, and pustules of the skin.

DIAGNOSIS

SYMPTOMS AND SIGNS
• Recurrent pain in the above described locations, sometimes to include headaches and symptoms of cardiovascular insufficiency.
• Recurrent ulcerations that may involve several areas including oral, genital, and ocular mucosa.
• Other signs include epidermal erythema and pustules, uveitis, retinitis, bloody diarrhea secondary to inflammatory bowel disease, arthritis, cardiovascular insufficiency, and polychondritis, often involving auricular and nasal cartilage.

LABORATORY
• No laboratory tests produce specific, diagnostic results.
• ESR elevated, hypergammaglobulinemia
• Histopathologic features include nonspecific ulcers infiltrated with T lymphocytes. Some lesions will show neutrophils and immunoglobulin within vessel walls.

IMAGING/SPECIAL TESTS
• None are of diagnostic value other than to rule out other diseases.
• Depression of antithrombin III levels. Antibodies to endothelium and cardiolipin.

DIFFERENTIAL
• Aphthous stomatitis
• Erythema multiforme
• Idiosyncratic drug reaction
• Primary herpes
• Recurrent herpes with immunosuppression
• Reiter's syndrome

Behcet's Syndrome

TREATMENT

General
◊ Prevent dehydration by increasing fluids.

MEDICATIONS
• Systemic burst therapy of prednisone followed by alternate day maintenance dosing.
• Other immunosuppressants, including chlorambucil and azathioprine, as well as dapsone, cyclosporine and interferon, may be of value.
• Topical anesthetic ointments and creams.

CONSULTATION SUGGESTIONS
Oral Medicine, Ophthalmology

REFERRAL SUGGESTIONS
Primary Care Physician, Oral Medicine

FIRST STEPS TO TAKE IN AN EMERGENCY
• If severe involvement of eyes, refer to ophthalmology immediately.

PATIENT INSTRUCTIONS
Contact American Behcet's Association (507) 281-3059 for helpful information.

COURSE/PROGNOSIS
Unpredictable, usually characterized by exacerbations and relative or absolute periods of remission. Possible permanent vision impairment.

CODING

ICD-9-CM
136.1 Behcet's syndrome

CPT
11900 Intralesional injection
40808 Biopsy, vestibule of mouth
40812 Incisional biopsy with simple repair
41108 Biopsy, floor of mouth
42100 Biopsy of palate
87252 Culture isolation
88160 Cytologic preparation
99000 Transport specimen to outside laboratory

MISCELLANEOUS

SYNONYMS
MAGIC syndrome (Mouth And Genital ulcers with Inflamed Cartilage)
Mucocutaneous ocular syndrome

SEE ALSO
Aphthous stomatitis
Primary and recurrent herpes simplex
Erythema multiforme

REFERENCES
Jorizzo J: Behcet's Disease. Arch Dermatol, 122:556-558, 1986.

O'Duffy J: Behcet's Syndrome. N Engl J Med 323:326-327, 1990.

Vincent SD, Finkelstein MW: Differential Diagnosis of Oral Ulcers. In: Principles of Oral Diagnosis. Coleman GC, Nelson JF (eds), St. Louis, Mosby-Year Book Co., 1993, pp. 328-351.

AUTHOR
Steven Vincent, DMD, MS

Bell's Palsy

 BASICS

DESCRIPTION

Partial or complete unilateral paralysis of the muscles of facial expression. The incidence of Bell's palsy is equal in males and females, and can occur at any age.

 ETIOLOGY

The majority of cases are idiopathic. However, there are several known causes that must be considered and investigated, including:
- intracranial processes such as neoplasm, multiple sclerosis, cerebellopontine lesions, and brainstem infarction.
- intratemporal processes such as otitis media, neurofibroma, carcinoma, Ramsey-Hunt syndrome, and herpes zoster.
- extracranial processes such as parotid carcinoma, infectious mononucleosis, sarcoidosis, and trauma.

In all cases, injury to the facial nerve leads to muscle paralysis. The location of the nerve involvement will determine the signs and symptoms.

SYSTEMS AFFECTED

Unilateral paresis or paralysis of the muscles of facial expression is the hallmark finding. However, depending on the location of the nerve involvement, there can be taste deficits (chorda tympani involved), hearing deficits (if cranial nerve VIII is involved), eye involvement (lacrimal gland, intra- and extra-ocular muscles with brainstem involvement), or multiple cranial nerve deficits (with posterior fossa tumors). When herpes zoster or otitis media is involved, there are peri- or intra-auricular lesions. Bell's palsy due to multiple sclerosis will be associated typically with other symptoms such as impaired vision, muscular incoordination, and bladder dysfunction, as well as fine rippling activity of the facial muscles.

 DIAGNOSIS

SYMPTOMS AND SIGNS

- Sudden onset unilateral facial paralysis characterized by a sensation of facial stiffness, facial asymmetry, drooping of the eyelid and corner of the mouth on the affected side, displacement of the mouth to the opposite side, and altered taste. Patient cannot close the eyelids or wrinkle the forehead on the affected side, and facial asymmetry is pronounced when asked to smile. Facial skin wrinkles may be smoothed and the palpebral fissure widened.
- The majority of patients have lower motor neuron (ie, peripheral) disease with symptoms involving the upper and lower face on the same side. When there is upper motor neuron (ie, central) disease, the lower 2/3 of the face is more commonly involved due to the bilateral projections from motor cortex to the facial motor nucleus.

LABORATORY

Increased protein and lymphocytosis may be present on examination of cerebral spinal fluid.

IMAGING/SPECIAL TESTS

- CT or MR scan of the cranium to detect intracranial mass(es).
- Electromyography (EMG) revealing absence of function of facial motor units.
- Nerve conduction studies may show altered evoked potentials in facial nerve.

DIFFERENTIAL

Majority of cases are idiopathic. Other causes include:
- otitis media or herpes zoster oticus
- intracranial mass
- brainstem infarction
- multiple sclerosis
- Melkersson-Rosenthal syndrome (with recurrent oral or peri-oral swelling and fissured tongue).

Rule out:
- meningitis
- parotid tumors
- base of skull tumors or osteomyelitis
- sarcoidosis
- temporal bone fracture
- Guillain-Barre syndrome
- facial hemiatrophy of Romberg

TREATMENT

General
◇ Prompt referral for a complete neurological examination is essential. Most idiopathic cases improve without treatment within 2 to 6 weeks.

MEDICATIONS
• Most patients receive moderate to high-dose oral systemic corticosteroid (prednisone) for the first 5 to 10 days to reduce neuritis and minimize nerve injury.

SURGERY
In some cases with incomplete recovery, cosmetic surgery has improved appearance; males can often hide the asymmetry by growing a beard. Anastomosis between the hypoglossal and facial nerves can restore partial function to the muscles of facial expression. When an intracranial or infratemporal disorder is the source of the Bell's palsy, appropriate neurosurgical intervention may be indicated.

CONSULTATION SUGGESTIONS
Neurologist, Neurosurgeon

REFERRAL SUGGESTIONS
Neurologist, Primary Care Physician

PATIENT INSTRUCTIONS
Reassurance that complete return of nerve function expected.

COURSE/PROGNOSIS
Most idiopathic cases resolve with weeks. Treatment must be started promptly (within 5 days of onset) to be maximally effective. Prompt referral and investigation are essential. Poorest prognosis is seen in patients who present with early pain and complete paralysis. Advanced age is also associated with a poorer prognosis.

 ## CODING

ICD-9-CM
053.19 Herpes Zoster
351 Bell's Palsy
907.1 Late CN Injury
951.4 CN VII Injury

CPT
64402 Block, CN VII
64505 Sphenopalatine block
70355 Panoramic x-ray
95831 Muscle testing
95851 Range of motion testing

 ## MISCELLANEOUS

SYNONYMS
Facial palsy
Idiopathic facial paralysis

SEE ALSO
Guillain-Barre
Multiple Sclerosis

REFERENCES
Facer GW: Facial nerve paralysis. Is it always Bell's palsy? Postgrad Med 69:206-216, 1981.

Ludman H: Facial palsy. Br Med J 282:545-547, 1981.

Wiet RJ, Lotan NA, Monsell EM, Shambaugh GE: Tumor involvement of the facial nerve. Laryngoscope 93:1301-1309, 1983.

Victor M, Martin JB: Disorders of the cranial nerves. In: Harrison's Principles of Internal Medicine,13th ed. Isselbacher KJ, et. al. (eds), New York. McGraw-Hill, Inc., 1994, pp. 2349-2350.

AUTHOR
David A. Sirois, DMD, PhD

Benign Jaw Tumors

 BASICS

DESCRIPTION
Variety of lesions that range from tumors developed from the odontogenic tissues to regular neoplasms derived from other tissue types located in or near the jaws.

 ETIOLOGY

For most of these lesions the etiology is unknown. Though there is no clear cut instigating event or agent involved in the formation of any of these lesions, the quality of the tumor itself is a reflection of the tissue line of origin. The following two categories outline the types of lesions included here:
Odontogenic Tumors
◇ Epithelial Tumors
  • Ameloblastoma
  • Squamous odontogenic tumor
  • Calcifying epithelial odontogenic tumor
  • Clear cell odontogenic tumor
  • Adenomatoid odontogenic tumor
◇ Mesenchymal Tumors
  • Odontogenic myxoma
  • Central odontogenic fibroma
  • Cementifying fibroma
  • Cementoblastoma
  • Periapical cemental dysplasia
◇ Mixed (epithelial and mesenchymal) tumors
  • Odontoma
  • Ameloblastic fibroma and ameloblastic fibro-odontoma
◇ Nonodontogenic Tumors
  • Ossifying fibroma
  • Fibrous dysplasia
  • Osteoblastoma
  • Chondroma
  • Osteoma
  • Central giant cell granuloma
  • Hemangioma of bone
  • Idiopathic histiocytosis (Langerhans' cell disease)
  • Tori and exostoses
  • Coronoid hyperplasia
  • Brown tumor (hyperparathyroidism)

SYSTEMS AFFECTED
Bone
  ◇ the maxilla and mandible have both seen involvement from these lesions. The amount of tissue destruction present is dependent upon the aggressiveness of the lesion and the length of its duration.
Oral mucosa
  ◇ often involved when these lesions have perforated bone and periosteum.
Teeth
  ◇ may be involved in the lesion when the origin is odontogenic. Displacement of teeth with malocclusion can be seen in some cases of fibrous dysplasia.

 DIAGNOSIS

SYMPTOMS AND SIGNS
Depending upon the lesion, patient may experience pain, gingival bleeding, loosening of teeth, paresthesia, visual disturbances, or oral and craniofacial swelling with or without concomitant malocclusion.
Facial
  ◇ distorted anatomy often associated with lesion such as fibrous dysplasia.
Vision
  ◇ can be altered when pressure applied to optic nerve.
Oral hard tissues
  ◇ distortion or swelling often seen.
Oral Mucosa
  ◇ usually intact and of normal quality but expanding with underlying bony changes. Can be involved in lesional changes when perforation of bone and periosteum has occurred.
Gingiva
  ◇ bleeding inflammation and ulceration often seen in cases of idiopathic histiocytosis. Involvement seen when perforation of bone and periosteum has occurred.
Teeth
  ◇ loosening or displacement with malocclusion can occur depending upon the tumor involved.

LABORATORY
• Most common laboratory tests are nondiagnostic for this group of lesions.
• Hypercalcemia may indicate hyperparathyroidism causing a giant cell tumor (Brown's tumor) of the jaws. Elevated parathyroid hormone levels confirm this diagnosis.

IMAGING/SPECIAL TESTS
Radiographically, these lesions can have various patterns from uni- to multilocular, and from radiolucent to radiopaque.
Panoramic and periapical radiographs
  ◇ often give the first indication of these pathologic changes.
Head and jaws radiographs
  ◇ used to better delineate the extent of the lesion.
CT
  ◇ study of choice to determine the full extent of lesion and evaluate potential perforation of bone.
CT with contrast or MRI
  ◇ can be helpful to evaluate soft tissue involvement.
Tissue biopsy
  ◇ most important method of establishing definitive diagnosis.
Aspiration
  ◇ helpful in ruling out a vascular lesion.

DIFFERENTIAL
Odontogenic tumors
  ◇ epithelial, mesenchymal, mixed type

Nonodontogenic tumors
Cysts
Malignant neoplasms
Lymphoma
Abscess

TREATMENT

MEDICATIONS
• Chemotherapeutic agents
◊ often useful in the management of idiopathic histiocytosis.

SURGERY
Odontogenic tumors
◊ complete surgical excision is the treatment of choice. This may involve enucleation or resection depending upon the type and size of the lesion. Ameloblastoma and myxoma require resection with 1 cm margins to decrease recurrence rate.
Nonodontogenic tumors
◊ treatment here can vary widely depending upon the lesion involved. The range may not involve treatment for things such as tori and exostoses, to complete excision, recontouring, resection, sclerosing, cryotherapy, presurgical embolization, radiation therapy, and chemotherapy. These lesions, therefore, vary greatly in the treatment of choice. Each entity should be viewed individually when planning comprehensive treatment.

CONSULTATION SUGGESTIONS
Oral Pathologist

REFERRAL SUGGESTIONS
Oral-Maxillofacial Surgeon

PATIENT INSTRUCTIONS
Alert patient that certain benign tumors, even though not usually life-threatening, can create significant destruction leaving aesthetic and functional defects in facial region.

COURSE/PROGNOSIS
Extremely variable depending upon the lesion involved. Though most of these lesions do not recur after excision, some can be more aggressive and require future resection with reconstruction. Some, such as idiopathic histiocytoses, can be life-threatening.

CODING

ICD-9-CM
213.0 Bones of skull and face benign neoplasms
213.1 Lower jaw bone benign neoplasms

CPT
20130 Excision of benign tumor cyst of facial bones other than mandible
20140 Excision of benign cyst or tumor of mandible, simple
20141 Excision of benign cyst or tumor of mandible, complex
20170 Coronoidectomy
20220 Biopsy, bone; trocar or needle
20240 Biopsy, excisional; superficial
20245 Biopsy, excisional, deep
21031 Excision of torus mandibularis
21032 Excision of torus palantinus
70100 Radiologic exam of mandible
70140 Radiologic exam of facial bones
70310 Radiologic exam teeth, less than full mouth
70320 Radiologic exam teeth, full mouth
70355 Panorex

MISCELLANEOUS

SYNONYMS
Odontogenic tumors
Nonodontogenic tumors

SEE ALSO
Odontogenic tumors
Nonodontogenic tumors
Ameloblastoma

REFERENCES
Regezi JA, Sciubba J: Oral Pathology 2nd ed. Philadelphia, WB Saunders, 1993, pp. 362-420.

Hjorting-Hansen E: Benign tumors of the jaws. Curr Opin Dent 1:296-304, 1991.

Batsakis JG, Hicks MJ, Flaity CM: Peripheral epithelial odontogenic tumors. Ann Otol Rhinol Laryngol 102:322-324, 1991.

Ulmansky M, et al: Benign cementoblastoma, A review and five new cases. Oral Surg Oral Med Oral Path 77:48-55, 1994.

AUTHOR
Lawrence T. Herman, DMD

Bleeding, Post-extraction

 BASICS

DESCRIPTION
Hemorrhage from the extraction socket, flap, or surrounding tissue after surgical extraction of teeth; primary hemorrhage defined as direct bleeding from the injured vessels, and secondary hemorrhage is due to clot lysis or biochemical deficit of the clotting factors.

 ETIOLOGY

• Direct injuries to the underlying vascular bundle, intra-bony nutrient artery.
• Unexpected injury to telangiectatic lesions such as hemangiomas.
• Intermediate, recurrent hemorrhage within 24 hours due to loose ligatures, returned high blood pressure.
• Secondary hemorrhage after 24 hours; fibrinolysis as result of infection.
• Biochemical bleeding; prolonged bleeding due to abnormal blood elements or vascular system.
• Abnormal clotting and coagulation of blood such as hemophilia, hepatic disorders, blood dyscrasias (leukemia, anemia, thrombocytopenia, etc.)

SYSTEMS AFFECTED
Maxillary and mandibular skeletal and soft tissue structures

 DIAGNOSIS

SYMPTOMS AND SIGNS
• Bleeding, pulsating arterial flow, or continuous venous oozing.
• Blood-tinged saliva, filling of mouth with blood clots.
• Prolonged bleeding, arterial bleeding with bright red pumping flow, venous bleeding with dark red steady flow, and capillary hemorrhage with steady oozing of bright red blood.
• Sudden swelling and tenderness of surrounding soft tissues, mouth floor, retromandibular, and cheek spaces.
• Diffuse subcutaneous swelling, edema, hematoma with ecchymosis.
• Pallor, cold, sweating skin, rapid weak pulse, lowered blood pressure (< 80 mm Hg, systolic) with rapid weak pulse as the clinical signs of hypovolemic shock.

LABORATORY
• Complete blood count (differential and hemoglobin), platelet count.
• Lee-White coagulation time, bleeding time.
• Prothrombin time, partial thromboplastin time.
• Liver function test; if history or physical suggestive of severe liver dysfunction with decreased clotting factor production.

IMAGING/SPECIAL TESTS
• CT for localization of the hemorrhage fields and hematoma in the profuse bleeding.
• Arteriogram if arterial bleeding present and cannot be controlled with local measures.

DIFFERENTIAL
Differentiate biochemical bleeding from mechanical bleeding.

TREATMENT

General
◇ Basic procedures to control the post-extraction bleeding:
• Preparations: proper illumination, adequate suction, gauze sponges, adequate retraction, hemostatic instruments, sutures, local anesthetics and syringes, other basic surgical instruments.
• Suction the mouth free of all blood clots, ensure a patent airway.
• Local anesthesia containing a vasoconstrictor.
• Ascertain the exact bleeding point and place a pressure pack on it.
• Re-inspection in 5 minutes to determine the type of bleeding.
• Isolation of the bleeding area and temporary arrest of hemorrhage.
• Proper control of bleeding; packing, clamping, tying or suturing.
• Immediate control of post-extraction bleeding:
• Direct pressure over the socket with gauze firmly for 45 minutes.
• Pressure packs with a hemostatic agent such as oxidized cellulose (Surgical, Hemopak) or gelatin sponge saturated in epinephrine or thrombin.
• Clamping and ligation of visible, isolated bleeding vessel.
• Electro-coagulation of the bleeding vessels.
• Crushing the nutrient foramen that houses the intrabony vessels.
• Sterile bone wax to control capillary oozing from the alveolar bone.
• Suture the flap, or place a deep stay suture.
• "Stick tie" (circumferential suture) through the palatal flap.
• Placement of modeling compound, or soft relining materials beneath immediate temporary dentures.
• Removal of the infected hematoma.
• Bimanual pressure and ligation of sublingual artery.
• More central exposure and ligation of arteries may be necessary. Consider arteriogram with selective catheterization and embolization prior to surgery.
• Screening for possible bleeding disorder including checking for a history of prolonged bleeding or use of medications known to interfere with hemostasis such as NSAIDs.
Prevention -
• Clean, meticulous dissection to avoid tissue tears and bony fragmentation.
• Careful subperiosteal dissection when possible to preserve the lamina propria and the periosteum, thereby gaining access through a relative avascular plane.

• Preoperative preparation for the patients who have been on anticoagulant therapy; vitamin K against coumarin series of drugs, protamine as antagonist for heparin.
• Preoperative screening for the patient who has a history of bleeding.
• Avoid use of NSAIDs for 10 days prior to extensive dental surgery.

MEDICATIONS
• Local agents; thrombin, fibrinogen, epinephrine injection, collagen, oxidized cellulose.
• Place patient on antibiotic for oral organisms if hematoma occurs.

SURGERY
See general treatment section.

CONSULTATION SUGGESTIONS
Oral-Maxillofacial Surgeon, Hematologist

REFERRAL SUGGESTIONS
Oral-Maxillofacial Surgeon

FIRST STEPS TO TAKE IN AN EMERGENCY
• See general treatment section.

PATIENT INSTRUCTIONS
If bleeding occurs at home, can first attempt to control with 45 minutes of biting pressure on moist gauze.
Can also try to bite on tea bag (supplies vasoconstricting tannic acid) to gain hemostasis.
If bleeding fails to stop, see dentist as soon as possible while continuing to bite on gauze. Do not rinse or spit.

COURSE/PROGNOSIS
Hematoma formation, ecchymosis. Infection and clot lysis may occur. Hypovolemic shock if bleeding is profuse or prolonged.

CODING

ICD-9-CM
523.8 Bleeding from gingiva
528.9 Bleeding from mouth
998.1 Postoperative bleeding

CPT
35800 Exploration postoperative hemorrhage, neck
37204 Transcatheter embolization
37600 Ligation, external carotid artery
37799 Unlisted procedure, vascular surgery
40800 Drainage of hematoma, vestibule of mouth
41000 Intraoral drainage of hematoma, floor of mouth
41015 extraoral
41800 Drainage of dentoalveolar hematoma
41899 Unlisted procedure, dentoalveolar structures
85002 Bleeding time

MISCELLANEOUS

SEE ALSO
Coagulopathies
Hemophilia

REFERENCES
Pogrel MA: Complications of third molar surgery. Oral Maxillofac Surg Clin N Am 2:441-448, 1990.

AUTHOR
Myung-Rae Kim, DDS, PhD

Brain Abscess

 BASICS

DESCRIPTION
A localized, suppurative infection of the brain that may be caused by a variety of organisms through a number of mechanisms.

 ETIOLOGY

• Most commonly a result of extension from sinus infection, otitis media, or mastoiditis. The organisms responsible are those normally causing the above mentioned infections: Strep. pneumoniae, Strep. viridans, Staph. aureus, and H. influenzae, as well as anaerobic species including anaerobic streptococci, bacteroides, and fusobacterium.
• Hematogenous spread is less common and is related to lung abscess, congenital right to left cardiac shunts, vegetations of endocarditis, or bacteremia. In addition to the above mentioned organisms, Gram negative rods including Pseudomonas and E. coli may cause hematogenous brain abscess, as well as unusual organisms such as Nocardia, primarily from lung abscess.
• The least common cause of brain abscess is traumatic injury due to penetrating intracranial injury. S. aureus and Gram negative rods are the most likely pathogens in this circumstance.

SYSTEMS AFFECTED
<u>CNS</u>
◊ may result in altered mental status, seizures, focal and/or nonfocal neurologic deficits.

 DIAGNOSIS

SYMPTOMS AND SIGNS
Altered mental status, headache, nausea, vomiting, fever, leukocytosis, seizures, papilledema, focal or nonfocal neurologic deficits. Occasionally, no systemic signs are present if the abscess is well walled off.

LABORATORY
• Gram stain, culture and sensitivity of facial infection, sinuses, or middle ear fluid.
• Lumbar puncture for CSF cytology, cell counts, culture and sensitivity.
• Direct antigen studies.

IMAGING/SPECIAL TESTS
CT scan of the head is mandatory in patients with altered mental status. The lesion may present as an expanding mass with cerebral edema and mass effect. A contrast exam will reveal enhancing lesions with central hypodensity. CT scan will be used to monitor response to therapy in addition to diagnosis. EEG may demonstrate a seizure focus.

DIFFERENTIAL
• Viral encephalitis with cyst formation.
• Brain tumor, cyst, hematoma
• Protozoan infection eg, toxoplasmosis
• Fungal infection eg, Cryptococcal meningitis
• HIV infection
• Stroke

TREATMENT

MEDICATIONS
• High-dose antibiotic therapy directed at the offending organism. Treatment is started empirically until definitive culture and sensitivity is received. Therapy may be directed by lumbar puncture with CSF culture and sensitivity or by aspiration of the abscess cavity. The efficacy of antibiotic therapy alone decreases with increasing size of the abscess.
• Corticosteroids may be used if significant cerebral edema is evident to lessen intracranial swelling and pressure to reduce the risk of herniation. Osmotic diuresis with mannitol may also be used to reduce intracranial pressure. Success of antimicrobial therapy can be appraised by periodic repeat CT scans. Because a large percentage of patients will develop seizure activity, prophylactic anticonvulsants are recommended.

SURGERY
CT-guided needle aspiration (especially in cases of multiple abscesses).
• Stereotactic localization guided by CT or real time ultrasound.
• Craniotomy with drainage and possible excision of the abscess cavity and necrotic tissues.

CONSULTATION SUGGESTIONS
Neurosurgeon, Otolaryngologist

REFERRAL SUGGESTIONS
Neurosurgeon, Neurologist

PATIENT INSTRUCTIONS
Contact Brain Research Foundation (312) 782-4311 for patient literature.

COURSE/PROGNOSIS
• With prompt recognition and treatment, therapy has a high level of success. However, if there is intraventricular rupture of an abscess, the course is rapidly fatal.
• Depending upon location, surgical therapy may result in significant neurologic morbidity.

CODING

ICD-9-CM
324.0 Brain abscess

MISCELLANEOUS

SYNONYMS
Cerebral abscess

SEE ALSO
Seizure disorders
Meningitis

REFERENCES
Haines SJ, Mampalam T, Rosenblum ML, Nagib MG: In: Neurologic Surgery, 3rd ed. vol. 6, London, Harcourt Brace Jovanovich Inc. 1990.

Luby JP: Infections of the central nervous system. Am J Med Sci 304:379-391, 1992.

Vallee L, et al: Brain abscess complicating dental caries in children. Arch Pediatr 1:166-169, 1994.

Wispelwey B, et al: Brain abscess. Semin Neurol 12: 273-278, 1992.

AUTHOR
André Montazem, DMD, MD

Branchial Cleft Cysts

BASICS

DESCRIPTION
Cysts, sinuses, and fistulae of the neck that develop from embryologic branchial arch proliferation and subsequent epithelial entrapment.

ETIOLOGY

• Many head and neck structures derive from five branchial arches during 2nd to 7th week embryologically.
• Branchial arches contain endodermal, mesodermal, and ectodermal elements, which are the structural precursors for some cartilaginous, muscular, neurovascular, and epithelial tissues of the head and neck.
• During development, the arches form clefts that may result in preauricular or cervical sinus tracts, blind pouches or cysts.

Classification
Branchial cleft cysts are classified according to which arch is affected:

First Branchial Cleft
◇ preauricular region with attachment to or close association with the external auditory canal.

Second Branchial Cleft
◇ most common, typically found along the anterior border of the sternomastoid muscle with tracts coursing between the internal and external carotids.

Third Branchial Cleft
◇ rare; cysts also appear on the anterior border of sternomastoid; however, the tract courses deep and posterior to the internal carotid artery.

Fourth Branchial Cleft
◇ very rare; found deep in lower neck with loop around aortic arch; usually on left side.

SYSTEMS AFFECTED
Skin, Musculoskeletal

DIAGNOSIS

SYMPTOMS AND SIGNS
• May occur any age; however, usually manifest in childhood or early adulthood with history of episodic swelling or drainage.
• Nontender swelling in neck locations (noted above), usually upper-middle third of anterior sternomastoid muscle.
• If first arch, parotid mass or swelling, ear, and temporomandibular joint pain.
• Sinuses and fistulae with clear to mucopurulent drainage that may discharge externally or into pharynx.
• May become infected with associated abscess formation, dysphagia, dyspnea.

LABORATORY
Elevated WBC (if infected)

IMAGING/SPECIAL TESTS
• CT or MR scan for mass locations
• Ultrasound may help delineate solid and cystic components.
• Sinogram (when not infected)
• Thyroid scan when paratracheal presentation to rule out thyroid lobe involvement or thyroglossal duct cysts.
• Cultures (when infected)

Histologic examination
◇ cyst lined with stratified squamous and/or pseudostratified columnar epithelium. Epithelial aspect contains lymphoid elements with well-formed germinal centers. Mature fibrous connective tissue capsule present.

DIFFERENTIAL
• Parotid tumor or infection
• Submandibular tumor, swelling, abscess
• Chronic odontogenic infection
• Vascular malformation, cystic hygroma
• Carotid body tumor
• Dermoid cyst

TREATMENT

MEDICATIONS
• Antibiotics if secondarily infected.

SURGERY
• Definitive treatment is complete surgical excision.
• First arch cyst or tract may require excision to and including some of the external auditory canal. Access via superficial parotidectomy may be necessary.
• Lower arch cysts or tracts require neck incisions along the anterior sternomastoid muscle.
• Prognosis is good unless incomplete tract excision; then recurrence and infection likely.

CONSULTATION SUGGESTIONS
Oral-Maxillofacial Surgeon, Otolaryngologist

REFERRAL SUGGESTIONS
Oral-Maxillofacial Surgeon, Otolaryngologist

PATIENT INSTRUCTIONS
Seek removal prior to pronounced enlargement.

COURSE/PROGNOSIS
If properly excised, recurrence rare.

CODING

ICD-9-CM
744.42 Branchial cleft cyst

CPT
17200 Electrosurgical destruction multiple skin tags
17250 Chemical cauterization granulation tissue
21550 Biopsy, soft tissue neck
21555 Excision tumor, soft tissue neck
21899 Unlisted procedure neck
70360 Radiologic exam, soft tissue neck
76999 Unlisted ultrasound procedure

MISCELLANEOUS

SYNONYMS
Branchial cysts
Cervical lymphoepithelial cyst

SEE ALSO
Thyroglossal duct cyst
Neck mass

REFERENCES
Donegan JO: Congenital Neck Masses. In: Otolaryngology Head & Neck Surgery. 2nd ed. Cummings CW, Frederickson JM, Harker LA, Krause CJ, Shiller DE (eds). St. Louis, Mosby Year Book, 1993, pp. 1554-1559.

Myers EN, Cunningham MJ: Inflammatory presentation of congenital head and neck masses. Pediatr Infect Dis J: S162, 1988.

Hickey SA, et al: Defects of the first branchial cleft. J Laryngol Otol 108: 240-243, 1994.

AUTHOR
Bruce Horswell, DMD, MD

Bronchiectasis

BASICS

DESCRIPTION
Dilatation of one or more segments of the bronchial tree associated with chronic cough, purulent expectoration, recurrent pneumonia, and occasional hemoptysis.

ETIOLOGY

• Recurrent bacterial insults leading to chronic inflammatory changes and necrosis are the usual cause. Bronchial obstruction with resultant severe mucopurulent pneumonia appear to predispose to bronchiectasis.
• Congenital bronchiectasis is rare.
• Mucociliary clearance defects predispose to bronchiectasis, eg, hypogammaglobulinemia, agammaglobulinemia, IgG deficiency.

SYSTEMS AFFECTED
Lungs
◊ dilated airways, air trapping, poor clearance of bacteria. Diseased segments are further predisposed to infection. Airflow obstruction is common and progressive. Hypoxemia and hyperventilation are evident. Recurrent pneumonia, abscesses, and empyema occur.
Heart
◊ cor pulmonale may result due to pulmonary hypertension, right ventricular hypertrophy, and subsequent failure as a direct consequence of pulmonary hypertension.
Extremities
◊ clubbing of digits is common.
Systemic
◊ may rarely predispose to amyloidosis.

DIAGNOSIS

SYMPTOMS AND SIGNS
• Chronic cough
• Extensive, copious purulent expectoration
• Occasional hemoptysis
• Recurrent fevers
• Dyspnea
• Fatigue
• Orthopnea
• Tachycardia
• Weight loss
• Clubbing of digits, cyanosis, rhonchi, wheezing
• Right ventricular hypertrophy, cor pulmonale in advanced cases

LABORATORY
CBC- anemia, leukocytosis
Immunoglobulin studies
◊ check for hypogammaglobulinemia
IgE levels
Sputum stains and cultures

IMAGING/SPECIAL TESTS
CT scan and chest radiograph reveal thickened, dilated bronchi air fluid levels, occasional abscess and fibrosis.
Specific tests: Spirometry demonstrating obstruction to air flow with decreased FEV, FVC.

DIFFERENTIAL
Foreign body obstruction
Bronchial stenosis
Tumor-induced obstruction
Tuberculosis
Fungal disease
Lung abscess
Cystic fibrosis

Bronchiectasis

 TREATMENT

General
◇ Vigorous treatment of childhood infections
• Avoidance of smoking
• Chest physical therapy
• Postural percussion and drainage
• Vibration

MEDICATIONS
• Bronchodilators, expectorants, mucolytics.
• Aggressive antibiotic therapy with broad-spectrum antibiotics.
• Oxygen therapy for hypoxemic patients.
• Diuretics for patients with advanced disease and right sided congestive heart failure secondary to pulmonary hypertension, cor pulmonale.

SURGERY
May be curative if bronchiectasis is localized to a segment or lobe and is treated early. Results are less favorable in diffuse or multilobe disease.

CONSULTATION SUGGESTIONS
Pulmonologist

REFERRAL SUGGESTIONS
Primary Care Physician

PATIENT INSTRUCTIONS
Avoid smoking.
Contact American Lung Association (212)315-8700 for patient literature.

COURSE/PROGNOSIS
• Usually complicated by presence of associated disease eg, hypogammaglobulinemia, cystic fibrosis, amyloidosis, cor pulmonale etc.
• Chronic recurrent pulmonary infections, abscesses, and pneumonia are the usual course.

 CODING

ICD-9-CM
494 Bronchiectasis

 MISCELLANEOUS

SEE ALSO
COPD
Pneumonia

REFERENCES
Baum GL, Hershko EP: In: Textbook of Pulmonary Disease. 5th ed. Vol. 1, Baum GL, Wolinsky E, (eds). Boston, Little Brown & Co., 1994.

Westcott JL. Bronchiectasis: Radiologic Clinics N Am 29(5), 1991.

AUTHOR
André Montazem, DMD, MD

Bronchitis (Acute)

BASICS

DESCRIPTION
Acute inflammatory disease of the trachea and bronchi. Generally self-limited with resolution and return to baseline function. Rarely a cause of hospital admission in children or adults.

ETIOLOGY

• Acute infectious bronchitis shows a consistent January-February peak and an August trough. Illness usually develops following a common cold or other viral infection of the nasopharynx, throat, or tracheobronchial tree. Acute bronchitis is also causally related during epidemics of influenza and measles.
• In the very young, the most frequently isolate viruses are respiratory syncytial virus (RSV), parainfluenza 1 to 3, and coronaviruses. Among those from 1 to 10 years of age, parainfluenze types 1 and 2, enterovirus, RSV, and rhinoviruses predominate. 10 years old and above, influenza A and B, RSV, and adenoviruses are found most frequently.
• Mycoplasma pneumoniae and Chlamydia are reported to cause acute bronchitis in young adults.
• Parainfluenza types 1 and 3 and rhinoviruses are found most frequently in the fall; influenzae, RSV, and coronaviruses cause infections in winter and early spring, while enteroviruses induce infections in summer and early fall.
• In the compromised host and older individuals, Herpes simplex-1 virus as well as Gram-negative infections such as Klebsiella, Serratia, Enterobacter, and Pseudomonas may cause acute bronchitis.
• Common bacterial isolates most often include H. influenzae, S. pneumoniae, Mycobacterium tuberculosis, Branhamella catarrhalis, Salmonella typhosa, S. aureus, and Bordetella pertussis.
• There is increasing evidence that yeasts and fungi may produce bronchitis. This is true of Candida albicans, Candida topicalis, Cryptococcus neoformans, Histoplasma capsulatum, Coccidiodes immitis, and Blastomyces dermatitidis.
• Bronchitis can also occur due to migration of Strongyloides and Ascaris larvae.
• Acute irritative bronchitis may be caused by mineral and vegetable dusts, fumes from strong acids, ammonia, certain volatile organic solvents, chlorine, hydrogen sulfide, sulfur dioxide, or bromine. Ozone and nitrogen dioxide as well as tobacco or other smokes can be causative.
• Allergen inhalation may trigger acute bronchitis is an atopic individual.

SYSTEMS AFFECTED
Tracheo-bronchial tree
◊ hyperemia of the mucous membranes followed by desquamation, edema, leukocytic infiltration of the submucosa, and production of sticky or mucopurulent exudate. Bronchial cilia has disturbed function and there is spasm of bronchial smooth muscle.

DIAGNOSIS

SYMPTOMS AND SIGNS
Cough
◊ initially dry/nonproductive but later becomes mucoid or mucopurulent (does not abate once the original signs and symptoms of the URI/common cold have ended). The sputum occasionally contains streaks of blood for short periods of time.
• Coryza
• Malaise, headache
• Chilliness, slight fever (101 to 102 degrees F. for 3 to 5 days). Persistent fever suggests complicating pneumonia.
• Back and muscle pain
• Sternal discomfort/tightness (sometimes described as "burning").
• Sore throat
• Dyspnea (secondary to airway obstruction).
• Scattered high or low-pitched rhonchi, occasional moist rales at bases (shifts after patient coughs).
• Wheezing
• Acute respiratory failure (in severe cases).

LABORATORY
Arterial blood gas
◊ if hypoxia suspected
• Leukocytosis
• Sputum culture, Gram stain (sputum), Acid-fast stains.
• Serologic analyses of antibody titers against specific viruses.

IMAGING/SPECIAL TESTS
• Bronchoscopy
• Chest radiograph
• Pulmonary function tests

DIFFERENTIAL
• Pneumonia
• Emphysema
• Asthma
• Exacerbation of chronic bronchitis

TREATMENT

General
◊ Rest until fever subsides. Oral hydration (3 to 4 liters/day). Antipyretic analgesics. Children 2 to 16 years old should not receive aspirin because
◊ Reye's syndrome may occur as a complication in a wide range of viral infections.

MEDICATIONS
• When there are numerous neutrophils on the Gram stain in addition to the historical and physical findings suggestive of bacterial etiology, antibiotic therapy should be initiated. If no likely etiologic agent is recovered in culture and there are many neutrophils in the sputum, the possibility of M. pneumonia should be considered and treated with either erythromycin 250 to 500 mg q.i.d. or tetracycline 250 mg q.6h.
• Trimethoprim/sulfamethoxazole (160/800 mg orally b.i.d.) may be given. In children younger than 8 years old give amoxicillin 40 mg/kg/day in divided doses t.i.d. If symptoms persist or recur, then the antibiotic is chosen according to the predominant organism and its sensitivity. In general, antibiotics may reduce the possibility of secondary bacterial infections.
• Amantadine may also be used prophylactically for susceptible individuals, such as the elderly and those with co-existing cardiopulmonary disease. Amantadine need only be taken for 2 weeks if an influenza vaccine is given simultaneously. Rimantadine is currently under investigation as an alternative agent and appears to be less prone to produce side-effects.
• Bronchodilator therapy is used to help ease cough in patients and is of benefit in those who demonstrate a reduction of FEV1.
• Inhaled steroid therapy and other anti-inflammatory agents such as disodium cromolyn may be of benefit in managing this inflammatory condition.

CONSULTATION SUGGESTIONS
Pulmonologist, Infectious Disease Specialist

REFERRAL SUGGESTIONS
Primary Care Physician

FIRST STEPS TO TAKE IN AN EMERGENCY
• If pending respiratory failure suspected, consider endotracheal intubation.

PATIENT INSTRUCTIONS
Although bacterial origin of acute bronchitis possible and merits use of antibiotics, acute bronchitis is usually viral and will resolve with supportive care.

COURSE/PROGNOSIS
Acute bronchitis is a commonly diagnosed condition in general practice during the winter months, approaching a rate of 150 cases per 100,000 population per week. Attack rates are highest in the extremes of life and lowest in the 15 to 44 age group. Most cases have a benign outcome and ordinarily are not life-threatening. It is unclear whether antibiotics truly make a difference in an uncomplicated acute bronchitis, although the literature suggests that upwards of 93% of patients are given antibiotics anyway. The disease may last for up to 6 or 8 weeks. If it persists further, then a careful assessment must be made as to possible pneumonia or a superimposed airway disease.

CODING

ICD-9-CM
466.0 Acute bronchitis

MISCELLANEOUS

SEE ALSO
Chronic bronchitis
Laryngitis

REFERENCES
Gayres J: Seasonal pattern of acute bronchitis in general practice in the United Kingdom 1976-83. Thorax 41:106-110, 1986.

Boldy D, Skidmore S, Ayres J: Acute bronchitis in the community: clinical features, infective factors, changes in pulmonary function and bronchial reactivity to histamine. Resp Med 84:377-385, 1990.

Ayres J, Noah N, Fleming D: Incidence of episodes of acute asthma and acute bronchitis in general practice 1976-87. Brit J General Prac 43:361-364, 1993.

AUTHOR
Jonathan S. Sasportas, DMD, MD

Bruxism

 BASICS

DESCRIPTION
Excessive and repetitive contraction of masticatory muscles with nonfunctional grinding and clenching of the teeth. Nocturnal bruxism occurs in association with REM sleep. Intensity of masseter muscle contraction is more than can be achieved by conscious activity either during the day and/or during sleep. Associated with psychosocial stressors.

 ETIOLOGY

Unknown. May be associated with increased stress and anxiety. Although thought by some to be due to occlusal interferences, little scientific support for that theory.

SYSTEMS AFFECTED
Oral cavity
◊ excess tooth wear, trauma from occlusion, fracture of restoration, temporomandibular dysfunction.
Neuromuscular
◊ masseter muscles.
Neurologic
◊ persistent anxiety, nervousness, disturbed sleep, depression, instability, and restlessness.

 DIAGNOSIS

SYMPTOMS AND SIGNS
• Pain of the temporomandibular joint and the muscles of the face. Chronic clenching of jaws and grinding of teeth either during the day and/or during sleep.
• Tooth abrasion and fractures
• Tooth mobility
• Masseter muscle hypertrophy
• Headaches
• Earaches
• Tenderness of the masticatory muscles and painful spasm of the sterno-mastoid, temporalis, frontalis and masseter muscles.
• Restricted mandibular movements, as well as joint sounds during mastication and mouth opening.

DIFFERENTIAL
• Malocclusion
• Temporomandibular joint disorder
• Panic disorder
• Anxiety disorders
• Myofascial pain disorder
• Excessively abrasive diet

TREATMENT

General
◇ Full arch maxillary occlusal splint (night guard) reduces nocturnal masseter activity in approximately 50% of patients.
◇ Occlusal dental splints for nocturnal bruxers, relaxation techniques, hypnosis, use of warm compresses in jaw area, EMG biofeedback. Evaluate for substance abuse.

MEDICATIONS
• Use of short-term pharmacological treatment can be effective.
• Antianxiety agents
◇ diazepam 5 to 10 mg or alprazolam 0.25 mg q.h.s. for 10 to 14 days maximum.
• Antidepressants
◇ doxepin HCl 25 mg q.h.s.
• Muscle relaxers
◇ methocarbamol 4 to 4.5 g/day in 3 to 6 divided doses.

CONSULTATION SUGGESTIONS
Mental Health Professional

REFERRAL SUGGESTIONS
Referral for psychotherapy to address the patient's psychological stressors may be indicated.

PATIENT INSTRUCTIONS
• Use night guard.
• Take medications as prescribed.
• Try regular aerobic exercise to relieve stress.

COURSE/PROGNOSIS
Highly variable from resolving with no treatment to chronic pain with no successful intervention.

 ## CODING

ICD-9-CM
306.8 Bruxism
524.62 Arthralgia of TMJ

CPT
21085 Impression and custom preparation, oral surgery splint

 ## MISCELLANEOUS

SYNONYMS
Clenching
Grinding of teeth

SEE ALSO
Temporomandibular disorders
Depression

REFERENCES
Scully C, Cawson RA: Medical problems in dentistry. Oxford. Butterworth-Heinemann, 1993.

American Psychiatric Association. Diagnostic and statistical manual of mental disorders, DSM-IV, Washington, DC, 1994.

VanDongen CA: Update and literature review of bruxism. R I Dent J 25(4): 11, 13-14, 16, 1992.

Thompson BA, et al: Treatment approaches to bruxism. Am Fam Physician 49:1617-1622, 1994.

Menapace SE, et al: The dentofacial morphology of bruxers versus non-bruxers. Angle Orthod 64:43-52, 1994.

AUTHORS
Hillary Broder, PhD, MEd
Kani Nicolls, DDS

Bulimia Nervosa

BASICS

DESCRIPTION
Eating disorder characterized by recurrent episodes of binge eating (average 2 episodes/week for at least 3 months); feeling lack of control over eating behavior during the eating binges; self-induced vomiting, use of laxatives, enemas, or diuretics; strict dieting or fasting, or vigorous exercise to prevent weight gain; and persistent overconcern with body shape and weight. Onset typically in adolescence or early adulthood. More frequently seen in females than in males.

ETIOLOGY

Unknown, psychosocial stressors

SYSTEMS AFFECTED
• Nervous
• Gastrointestinal
• Dentition

DIAGNOSIS

SYMPTOMS AND SIGNS
• Most are within a normal weight range though some may be slightly underweight, and others may be overweight.
• Depressed mood and are subject to substance abuse of dependence (ie, sedative, amphetamines, cocaine or alcohol).
• Gastric dilatation
• Impulsivity
• Poor self-esteem
• Ambivalence about independence
• Psychosocial stressors
• Body image distortions
• Abdominal pain
• Parotid swelling
• Ritualistic behaviors
• Electrolyte imbalance
• Dehydration
• Cardiac dysrhythmias
• Sudden death
• Dental erosion
• Repeated vomiting of gastric contents results in typical pattern of erosion of the lingual, palatal, and posterior occlusal surfaces of the teeth. Amalgam restorations may stand above eroded dentition. Attrition resulting from bruxism may accelerate this type of tooth loss.
• Increase in dental caries due to excessive carbohydrate intake during binge-eating.
• Angular cheilitis
• Xerostomia resulting from a decrease in salivary flow, and parotid dysfunction may predispose the anorectic and bulimic to caries development.
• "Sensitive teeth" is a common dental complaint. Dentin hypersensitivity results from the chronic exposure of enamel and dentin to the hydrochloric acid.
• Traumatic palatal lesion or petechia occur from objects used to induce vomiting.
• Poor retention of orthodontic bands and temporary restoration may also occur as temporary cement is dissolved by the acid in vomitus.
• Compulsive behaviors include: excessive tooth brushing, ice chewing, consumption of diet soda, chronic gum chewing, frequent use of mouthwash. Most patients deny such behaviors (ie, vomiting, compulsions) when confronted.

LABORATORY
• Elevated BUN
• Hypokalemia
• Metabolic alkalosis
• Hypochloremia
• Elevated basal serum prolactin

IMAGING/SPECIAL TESTS
• Psychological screening
• Eating Attitudes Test
• ECG
• Thyroid Function Tests
• Positive dexamethasone suppression test
• Gastric motility

DIFFERENTIAL
Anorexia nervosa (less severe weight fluctuations than anorexia) but can have a dual diagnosis. In schizophrenia there may be unusual eating behavior, but rarely the full extreme of anorexia or bulimia nervosa. In certain neurologic diseases such as epileptic equivalent seizures, central nervous system tumors, and Kluver-Bucy-like syndrome and Kleine-Levin syndrome, there are abnormal eating disorders. Binge eating is often observed among females with borderline personality disorder and body dysmorphic disorder.

TREATMENT

General
◇ Fluoride therapy

MEDICATIONS
• Psychopharmacological treatment; frequently heterocyclic antidepressants (HCAs).
• Treatment with HCAs may result in side effects of xerostomia, stomatitis, bad taste, parotid swelling, and/or black tongue.
• MAO inhibitors, serotonin-release inhibitors or lithium may also be effective.
• Metoclopramide (Reglan) useful for abdominal discomfort.

CONSULTATION SUGGESTIONS
• Mental Health Professional
• Nutritional counseling
• Family therapy
• Perceptual training

REFERRAL SUGGESTIONS
Refer patient to eating disorders program and/or work with nutritional counselor and psychotherapist to help create a therapeutic alliance.

PATIENT INSTRUCTIONS
• See mental health professional.
• Rinse mouth with water immediately after vomiting.

COURSE/PROGNOSIS
Highly variable, although spontaneous resolution possible, best success occurs with therapy.

CODING

ICD-9-CM
783.6 Bulimia

CPT
21085 Oral surgical splint (fluoride application)

MISCELLANEOUS

SEE ALSO
Anorexia Nervosa

REFERENCES
Little J, Falace D: Behavioral and psychiatric disorders. In: Dental Management of the Medically Compromised Patient. 4th ed. St. Louis, CV Mosby, 1993, pp. 483-511.

Scully C, Cawson RA: Medical problems in dentistry. Oxford, Butterworth-Heinemann, 1993.

American Psychiatric Association. diagnostic and statistical manual of mental disorders, DSM-IV, Washington, DC, 1994.

Yates A: Bulimia nervosa. In: Griffith's 5 Minute Clinical Consult. Dambro M, Griffith J (eds). Baltimore, Williams and Wilkins, 1995, pp. 156-157.

AUTHORS
Hillary Broder, PhD, MEd
Kani Nicolls, DDS

Burkitt's Lymphoma

BASICS

DESCRIPTION
Burkitt's lymphoma is a type of small, noncleaved non-Hodgkin's lymphoma, and is recognized as the fastest growing malignancy in humans.

ETIOLOGY

Burkitt's lymphoma is endemic in parts of equatorial Africa and is related to the Epstein-Barr virus. Non-endemic forms of the disease, such as occur in North America, have only a 20% association with the virus.
Tumors are invariably B-cell derived.

SYSTEMS AFFECTED
Lymphatic
◇ may be site of origin.
Digestive
◇ abdominal tumors can produce mechanical bowel obstruction.

DIAGNOSIS

SYMPTOMS AND SIGNS
• Rapidly expanding, initially painless mass of abdomen, in American type.
• Rapidly expanding maxillary or mandibular mass, in African type.
• Rapid onset of a mass, most commonly in a male child. The mass is more common in the head and neck among American (endemic) Burkitt's patients, and is more common in the abdomen among American (non-endemic) patients.
• African Burkitt's shows a predilection for the jaws with involvement of the maxilla more common than the mandible.

LABORATORY
CBC
◇ anemia.
• Serum urate often elevated.
• Bone marrow aspirate.
• Serum LDH (lactate dehydrogenase) levels allow clinical monitoring of the disease.

IMAGING/SPECIAL TESTS
• Biopsy of involved node demonstrates histology of "starry sky" pattern of phagocytic lymphocytes, in monotonous sea of cells with round to oval nuclei, prominent nucleoli, frequent mitotic figures, and a pyroninophilic cytoplasm.
• CT scan allows staging.

DIFFERENTIAL
• Hodgkin's disease
• Non-Hodgkin's lymphoma
• Differential includes various inflammatory and infectious disorders as no other neoplastic disease grows at this rate.

Burkitt's Lymphoma

TREATMENT

General
◇ Prompt biopsy is essential to establish the diagnosis and begin treatment.

MEDICATIONS
• Chemotherapy is the primary therapy for Burkitt's lymphoma, although surgery can be required for intestinal obstruction or mass.
  • Cyclophosphamide
  • Vincristine
  • Prednisone
  • Cytosine arabinoside

SURGERY
Surgery may be needed to resect abdominal tumor.

IRRADIATION
Irradiation useful for managing central nervous system spread of lymphoma.

CONSULTATION SUGGESTIONS
Oncologist

REFERRAL SUGGESTIONS
Primary Care Physician

FIRST STEPS TO TAKE IN AN EMERGENCY
• Tumor lysis syndrome may occur as chemotherapy given with resultant renal failure and hyperkalemia, hyperuricemia, and hypocalcemia.

PATIENT INSTRUCTIONS
Jaw involvement may necessitate soft diet. Excellent oral hygiene measures must be practiced.

COURSE/PROGNOSIS
• Two-year survival of Burkitt's lymphoma is around 50%, with a better prognosis for American (non-endemic) forms of the disease that demonstrate an elevated Epstein-Barr virus titers.
• Among non-endemic patients, tumor recurrence following initial response to chemotherapy is almost always fatal.

CODING

ICD-9-CM
  200.2 Lymphoma, Burkitt's type (lymphoblastic) (undifferentiated)

CPT
  20220 Biopsy, bone, superficial
  21085 Oral surgical splint
  21089 Unlisted maxillofacial prosthetic procedure
  21550 Biopsy, neck
  41108 Biopsy, floor of mouth
  99000 Specimen handling and transport

MISCELLANEOUS

SYNONYMS
Small, noncleaved lymphoma
African lymphoma
Maxillary lymphosarcoma

SEE ALSO
Hodgkin's disease (lymphoma)

REFERENCES
Myers EN, Cunningham MJ: Tumors of the neck. In: Pediatric Otolaryngology, 2nd ed. Bluestone CD, Stool SE, Scheetz MO (eds), Philadelphia, WB Saunders Co., 1990, pp. 1346-1347.

Link MP, Donaldson SS: The lymphomas and lymphadenopathy. In: Hematology of Infancy and Childhood, 4th ed. Nathan DG, Oski FA (eds), Philadelphia, WB Saunders Co., 1993, p. 1324.

Eigler JL: Burkitt's lymphoma. N Engl J Med 305: 735-745, 1981.

Hupp JR, Collins F, Ross A, Myall R: A review of Burkitt's lymphoma: importance of radiographic diagnosis. J Maxillofac Surg 10: 240-245, 1982.

Lynch Jr TJ, Harris NL: 41 year old woman with neurologic abnormalities on osteolytic lesion in the mandible CPC. N Engl J Med 331: 107-114, 1994.

AUTHOR
Eric J. Dierks, DMD, MD

Burning Mouth Syndrome

 BASICS

DESCRIPTION
Burning, painful, itching sensation in the oral mucosa, with or without tongue involvement, but without associated physical abnormality or other clinical signs. In instances in which local or systemic findings are associated with burning mouth, the term burning mouth syndrome should not be used.

 ETIOLOGY

- Etiology of idiopathic burning mouth syndrome is unknown. May represent a somatoform (psychogenic) disorder. Women affected by burning mouth syndrome outnumber men 7 to 10:1. Idiopathic burning mouth should be distinguished from painful sensations due to mucosal disorders such as geographic tongue or lichen planus. When there is an associated physical abnormality or clinical sign, the etiology of the sensation is usually related to the abnormality. Although the majority of cases are idiopathic, other causes for burning mouth include:
oral candidiasis
  ◇ usually associated with mucosal erythema, although subclinical candidiasis can occur.
xerostomia
  ◇ mucosal dryness can lead to a burning sensation.
- anemia or vitamin deficiency (B_{12}, iron, folate). Rarely a cause in the absence of other findings such as lingual atrophy and mucosal erythema.
- systemic illnesses such as diabetes, amyloidosis, connective tissue disorders that have neuropathic components.

SYSTEMS AFFECTED
Burning mouth includes sensations arising in or from any oral mucosal surface, including the tongue. Because most patients suffer for months to years with the sensation, secondary depression and a sense of hopelessness may develop.

 DIAGNOSIS

SYMPTOMS AND SIGNS
- Persistent burning or itching of the oral mucosa that does not interrupt sleep. Typically present shortly after waking and is often worsened by prolonged talking and spicy/acidic foods and drinks. Most patients get relief while eating or chewing gum. Sources of psychologic and physiologic stress can often be identified.
- Thorough oral examination fails to reveal any associated physical abnormality and a review of systems fails to identify a possible systemic illness related to the sensation.

LABORATORY
Because some patients with burning mouth exhibit hematologic deficiencies, most patients who suffer enough to seek help merit screening exam. This should include a CBC with a red cell indices, SMA 12, and serum iron, B_{12}, and folate levels. Other less common disorders that may be evaluated include zinc deficiency and progesterone or estrogen deficiency.

IMAGING/SPECIAL TESTS
- When oral atrophic candidiasis is present or subclinical infection is suspected, a simple smear of the mucosa can be obtained and examined for the presence of yeast or hyphae.
- When indicated, diagnostic local anesthetic injections are indicated; symptoms typically persist to some degree after lingual anesthesia is achieved.

DIFFERENTIAL
- Burning mouth due to systemic illness (discussed above)
- Burning mouth due to local abnormality (ie, candidiasis, trauma, mucosal ulceration, geographic tongue)
- Medication induced (look for temporal relationship between onset of symptoms and medication use)
- Xerostomia

Burning Mouth Syndrome

TREATMENT

General
◇ When the diagnosis is idiopathic burning mouth, the patient must be reassured that there is no serious underlying disease. The patient must be periodically re-evaluated so any changes can be detected and evaluated. When the burning mouth is due to some local or systemic factor, successful treatment of the latter usually relieves the burning sensation.

◇ In addition to reassuring the patient, the objective in managing idiopathic burning mouth is to minimize the impact of the sensation on quality of life. For some patients, this is achieved by the reassurance alone. For others, referral to a behavioral psychologist to learn coping and distraction strategies is beneficial. This is particularly beneficial for patients with identified anxiety, depression, or stress.

MEDICATIONS

• Judicious use of psychopharmaceuticals provides significant relief for many patients. Classes of drugs that are most beneficial include tri-cyclic antidepressants (amitriptyline, nortriptyline), benzodiazepines (clonazepam), and serotonin uptake antagonists.

• These medications should only be prescribed by clinicians familiar with their use and in consultation with the patient's physician.

• Other simple measures include avoiding spicy or acidic foods and drinks, sugar-free chewing gum, or, for short-term relief, topical analgesics such as 0.5% aqueous diphenhydramine alone or mixed 1:1 with 0.5% dyclonine.

CONSULTATION SUGGESTIONS
Oral Medicine, Primary Care Physician

REFERRAL SUGGESTIONS
Oral Medicine

PATIENT INSTRUCTIONS
Reassurance that sensation is not indicative of serious disease.

COURSE/PROGNOSIS
Most patients with burning mouth sufficient in magnitude to seek professional help will continue to seek treatment in hopes of finding an undiagnosed problem or a magical cure. If the patient has received a thorough physical examination and a screening laboratory exam, it is unlikely that additional tests will yield meaningful results. The patient should be discouraged from seeing multiple doctors and agree to periodic re-evaluations to monitor progress. Most patients will experience symptoms for years. Patients who improve using the medications mentioned above typically require medications for months to years.

CODING

ICD-9-CM
350.2 Atypical facial pain
354.1 Causalgia
529.0 Glossitis
529.1 Geographic tongue
529.6 Glossodynia
781.1 Altered taste

CPT
64450 Diagnostic Injection
87205 Exfoliative cytology
99000 Specimen Handling

MISCELLANEOUS

SYNONYMS
Glossodynia
Glossopyrosis
Stomatopyrosis

SEE ALSO
Xerostomia
Causalgia
Glossitis

REFERENCES
Grushka M: Clinical features of burning mouth syndrome. Oral Surg Oral Med Oral Path. 63:30-38, 1987.

Gorsky DM, Silverman S, Chinn H: Clinical characteristics and management outcome in burning mouth syndrome. Oral Surg Oral Med Oral Path. 72:192-199, 1991.

Mott AE, Grushka M, Sessle BJ: Diagnosis and management of taste disorders and burning mouth syndrome. In: D'Ambrosio JA, Fotos PG. Topics in Oral diagnosis II. Dent Clin N Am 37:33-45, 1993.

Maresky LS, et al: Burning mouth syndrome. Evaluation of multiple variables among 85 patients. Oral Surg, Oral Med, Oral Path 75(3): 303-307, 1993.

AUTHOR
David A. Sirois, DMD, PhD

Burns

BASICS

DESCRIPTION
Thermic injury to the skin is directly related to time and temperature which then results in degrees of skin hyperemia, ischemia, stasis, and necrosis.

ETIOLOGY

Pathophysiology
  ◇ Skin burn occurs once temperature exceeds 45°C when irreversible protein coagulation occurs.
Three recognized zones of burn injury:
  ◇ Zone of coagulation (irreversible injury)
  ◇ Zone of stasis (burn progression 24 to 48 hours due to microcirculatory failure)
  ◇ Zone of hyperemia (reversible injury)
Immunologic effects of burns:
 • Microcirculatory changes consisting of neutrophil adherence to endothelium, red cell sludging, edema formation, and decreased tissue perfusion
 • Release of oxygen free radicals
 • Decrease in circulating immunoglobulins
 • Alteration in lymphocyte helper/suppressor cell ratio
Inflammatory response in burns:
 • Histamine release initially followed by kinin and serotonin production
 • Leukotriene, thromboxane, prostaglandin production with progressive neutrophil aggregation.
Burn Classification
  ◇ First Degree
 • Outer layer epidermis
 • Erythema, pain
 • Minimal tissue damage
  ◇ Second Degree (partial thickness burn)
 • Epidermis and portion of dermis
 • Tissue edema, blistering, loss of fluids
 • Very painful due to nerve ending involvement
  ◇ Third Degree (full thickness burn)
 • Destruction of all skin elements including nerve endings
Burn Evaluation
  ◇ Factors in patient assessment and outcome
 • Size and depth of injury
 • Location of burn
 • Patient medical status and age (<3 years, >60 years tolerate burns poorly)
 • Associated injuries
 • Body surface area (BSA) involved is critical
Areas requiring specialized care
 • Face, hands, feet, perineum
American Burn Association Categories:
  ◇ Major Burns
 • Second degree burns > 25% BSA
 • Third degree burns > 10% BSA
 • Burns of hands, face, feet, ears, perineum
 • Poor risk patients with burns
 • Inhalation, electrical burns
  ◇ Moderate Burn
 • Second degree burn 15 to 25% BSA in adults
 • Second degree burn 10 to 20% BSA in children
 • Third degree burn <10% BSA
  ◇ Minor Burn
 • Second degree burn <15% BSA in adults
 • Second degree burn <10% BSA in children
 • Third degree burn <2% BSA

SYSTEMS AFFECTED
Skin
Musculoskeletal
Fluid and electrolyte regulation

DIAGNOSIS

SYMPTOMS AND SIGNS
First and second degree burns associated with severe pain. Third degree burn painless.
Dehydration, hypothermia
  1st degree burn skin erythematous and edematous
  2nd degree burn skin erythematous and blistered
  3rd degree burn skin is leathery and charred

LABORATORY
Electrolyte abnormalities
 • Hypoglycemia (especially in children)
 • If associated smoke inhalation, may have arterial blood gas abnormalities and carboxyhemoglobin.
 • If electric burn, may have elevated urine myoglobin and serum creatinine phosphokinase (CPK).

IMAGING/SPECIAL TESTS
ECG in electrical burns
Bronchoscopy if smoke inhalation.

DIFFERENTIAL
Toxic epidermal necrolysis
Scalded skin syndrome

TREATMENT

• Admission to burn center, if available, for large or severe burns.
• Pain Management
• Second degree most painful initially Important in wound debridement, dressing changes
• General anesthesia for extensive debridement, grafting procedures
• Narcotic drips and peak dosing for dressing changes
  Nutritional Support
Metabolic stress great in burns and may increase caloric needs 2 to 3 times baseline
Energy stores depleted early
  ◊ need institution of nutritional support within 48 hours
• Enteral feeding preferred to maintain gut integrity and immunoglobulin production

MEDICATIONS

• Fluid Management
• Rule of nines to guide fluid needs:
• Head and neck
  ◊ Adult 9%, Child 18%
• Anterior trunk
  ◊ 18%
• Posterior trunk
  ◊ 18%
• Upper extremity
  ◊ 9%
• Lower extremity
  ◊ Adult 18%, Child 14%
• Critical when burns >15% BSA
• Individualized toward patients; needs and response
• Monitor pulse, urine output, cardiac output/index, electrolytes, blood gases
• Lactated Ringer's solution most commonly used
• Add dextrose for young children due to depleted sugar stores
• Add colloids (glucose, albumin) after 24 to 36 hours to increase plasma oncotic pressure
• Parkland Formula
  ◊ crystalloid solution
  ◊ 4 ml/kg/BSA%
  ◊ 1/2 first 8 hours
  ◊ 1/2 remainder over next 16 hours
• Antimicrobials
  ◊ IV ineffective unless good vascularity
  ◊ Should reserve for established infection to discourage resistant flora
  ◊ Topical agents, most popular
• Silver sulfadiazine, 1%
  ◊ Painless on application
  ◊ Wound visibility impaired
  ◊ Penetrates eschar poorly
  ◊ Possible marrow suppression
• Mafenide (Sulfamylon)
  ◊ Penetrates well
  ◊ Wound visible
  ◊ Painful on application
  ◊ No resistant gram-negatives
  ◊ Possible postburn hyperventilation syndrome
• Silver Nitrate
  ◊ No hypersensitivity
  ◊ Painless
  ◊ No gram-negative resistance
  ◊ No eschar penetration
• Nitrofurazone (Furacin)
  ◊ Nontoxic to epithelial cells
  ◊ Broad-spectrum coverage
  ◊ Poor penetration
  ◊ Renal-decreased glomerular filtration
• Cover new burn sites with silver sulfadiazine (Silvadene).
• Use narcotics for pain control.
• Consider H-2 blockers to prevent GI stress ulcers for large 2nd and 3rd degree burns.
• Tetanus prophylaxis for large 2nd and 3rd degree burns.

SURGERY

Wound Care
Circumferential limb or chest wounds may require escharotomy to relieve construction
Goal of burn care is wound closure
• Optimize tissue perfusion
• Conservative debridement of marginal tissue; however, early and aggressive removal of dead tissue is important
• Wound cover for protection against infection and desiccation
• Autologous skin grafts:
  Partial thickness split skin
  Sheet grafts for face, neck, hands, antecubital fossa
  Meshed grafts (2 or 3:1) elsewhere
• Allografts for temporary coverage
  Fresh cadaver or fresh frozen grafts
  Porcine xenograft
  Synthetic (Biobrane)

CONSULTATION SUGGESTIONS

Intensivist, General Surgeon, Plastic Reconstructive Surgeon, Burn Specialist

REFERRAL SUGGESTIONS

Intensivist, General Surgeon, Plastic Reconstructive Surgeon, Burn Specialist

FIRST STEPS TO TAKE IN AN EMERGENCY

• Remove all jewelry and clothing from affected areas.
• Cover affected areas with clean dry sheet
• Start intravenous lines

COURSE/PROGNOSIS

First and second degree burns typically not life-threatening. Skin grafting may be needed in 2nd degree burn sites if severe scarring occurs. 3rd degree burns covering significant percentages of skin surface are life-threatening. 50% survival in 62% burns if 0 to 14 years old, 63% burns if 15 to 40 years old, 38% burns in 40 to 65 years old and 25% burns in 65 years old and older patients. Skin grafting mandatory for 3rd degree burn sites. Associated problems such as smoke inhalation or electrical damage to heart also affect prognosis.

CODING

ICD-9-CM
  741.x Burns of face, head, neck
  948.x Burn, % body surface specified
  949.x Burn, degree specified

MISCELLANEOUS

SEE ALSO
Respiratory distress syndrome
Shock, circulatory

REFERENCES
Kucan JO: Burns and Trauma. In: Plastic Surgery. A Core Curriculum, Bugerg RL, Smith DJ. (eds.), St. Louis, CV Mosby Co., 1994, pp. 207-237.

Demling RH, Way LW: Burns and other thermal injuries. In: Current Surgical Diagnosis and Treatment. Way LW, (ed.), Norwalk, CT. Appleton and Lange. 1991, pp. 235-244.

Wellisz T, et al: The role of alloplastic skeletal modification in the reconstruction of facial burns. Ann Plast Surg 30: 531-536, 1993.

Carvajal HF: Fluid resuscitation of pediatric burn victim. Pediatr Nephrol 8: 357-366, 1994.

AUTHOR
Bruce Horswell, DMD, MD

Cancer (General Concepts)

BASICS

DESCRIPTION
A mass of tissue characterized by abnormal cellular growth that will invade surrounding tissues and will, left untreated, ultimately metastasize to regional or distant sites.

ETIOLOGY

Naturally occurring chromosomal abnormalities or those produced by chemical carcinogens, infectious agents (viruses, bacteria), or radiation result in a line of cells with an irreversibly altered genetic structure. If host resistance is unable to control these cells, malignancy results. The vast majority of head and neck carcinomas are caused by chemical carcinogens. Alcohol and tobacco, which seem to act synergistically, are the most common causes. Rarely, malignancies may metastasize to the jaws. The most common carcinomas to do so are breast, kidney, lung, and prostate.

SYSTEMS AFFECTED
All systems may be affected.

DIAGNOSIS

Usually based on the histologic evaluation of the abnormal cell line. Biopsy of the appropriate site (eg, tongue, lung, or bone marrow) provides tissue for histologic evaluation.

SYMPTOMS AND SIGNS
Varies widely from asymptomatic to extremely painful. Numbness, tingling, burning have been described. Patients may complain of anorexia and weight loss. Carcinoma often produces nonhealing skin or mucosal wounds. Intraorally, the most common sites are floor of the mouth, tongue, and lip. These common sites frequently present as white or mixed white and red lesions that are painless until late in the course of the disease. Metastasis to regional lymph nodes can often be palpated. Such nodes will present as hard, painless, and fixed to the surrounding tissues.

LABORATORY
Most common is the histologic evaluation of biopsy tissue. Numerous special laboratory investigations are used for specific tumor types. Fine needle aspiration biopsy cytology can be used when patients refuse biopsy or in whom open biopsy is contraindicated. Non-exfoliative cytology can be used for nonkeratotic ulcerated lesions. The Papanicolaou stain is most often employed.

IMAGING/SPECIAL TESTS
CT scans and MRI are often used to determine location and extent of disease. Endoscopy, bronchoscopy, and laparoscopy are routinely used to help stage the disease. Occasionally, electron microscopy can be useful in the diagnosis of undifferentiated tumors.

DIFFERENTIAL
Cancer must be included in the differential diagnosis of almost any skin or mucosal abnormality that does not respond to conventional therapy. Examples include ulcerative disorders, hyperkeratotic lesions, fungal infections, trauma, etc. Any mucosal swelling may represent an underlying tumor. Any bony lesion of unknown etiology should include malignancy in the differential diagnosis.

TREATMENT

MEDICATIONS
• Chemotherapy
◇ the effects of chemotherapy are systemic and produce several oral complications. These include hemorrhage, poor wound healing, infections, and mucositis. Except for mucositis, these complications occur secondary to the effects of chemotherapy on the bone marrow. Perhaps the most important information obtained in the evaluation of a patient prior to chemotherapy is estimation by the oncologist of the potential effects on the bone marrow. Additionally, it is important to know if the chemotherapy will be a single or multiple course regimen. Multiple course regimens often tend to be additive and produce more significant drops in the patients counts in the later courses. It must also be kept in mind that some malignancies are actually diseases of the bone marrow (eg, leukemia, multiple myeloma) that may produce abnormal blood values prior to chemotherapy.
• Hemorrhage is primarily a function of diminished production of platelets. Bleeding is seldom a problem if levels of 50,000/μL can be maintained (via transfusion if necessary). Primary closure of oral surgical sites (alveolectomy if necessary) should be obtained and black silk sutures placed. Because the patient's neutrophils are also diminished, phagocytosis of resorbable sutures is greatly inhibited. Also, silk sutures are more easily visualized for removal after 7 days. Packing materials should be avoided for the same reasons.
• Infections
◇ pulpal and periodontal infections are typically seen in these patients when their WBC drops below 2000/mm³. Judicious use of periodontal therapy, including chlorhexidine (Peridex), endodontic therapy, and extraction of teeth can prevent most of the infections during chemotherapy when little or no invasive dental treatment is indicated.
• Mucositis
◇ this is a toxic reaction to the chemotherapy that cannot be prevented. It can be treated palliatively in a manner similar to that described in the radiation therapy section.
• In treatment planning for the patient about to receive myelosuppressive chemotherapy, the following guidelines should be considered:
• Prior to chemotherapy:
  1. Dental consult, exam, radiographs, treatment plan: 3 to 7 days before.
  2. Oral surgery: 3 days before.
  3. Periodontal, endodontic restorative care:

- Before myelosuppression
- During Myelosuppression:
  1. Reinforce oral hygiene: Daily
  2. Chlorhexidine rinses if indicated: Thrice daily
- After Chemotherapy:
  1. Routine care as necessary

SURGERY
Effects are local and may require prosthetic repair of the defect caused by surgery.

IRRADIATION
Effects are local and lead to the development of mucositis, xerostomia, radiation caries, altered nutrition, and osteoradionecrosis.

Mucositis
◇ is primarily a short-term toxic reaction to the radiation, producing atrophy, pseudomembrane formation, and frank ulceration. It is treated palliatively with topical anesthetics (5% viscous Xylocaine) and mixtures (50:50 Benadryl elixir and Kaopectate). A tablespoon of anesthetic/mixture is swished in the mouth for 1 minute and expectorated. Can be repeated every 2 to 3 hours. Mucositis can become secondarily infected, most commonly with Candida albicans. Such cases can often be treated topically with nystatin or clotrimazole, or with systemic ketoconazole or amphotericin B.

Xerostomia
◇ results from damage to the salivary glands. This diminished output of saliva results in a more viscous saliva. The rampant caries that may be seen in these patients is largely due to the decreased protection afforded by saliva. Where possible, lead shielding should be used during radiation therapy to protect the parotid glands. Recently, the use of pilocarpine has been reported to increase salivary output following radiation therapy.

Osteoradionecrosis
◇ is the most serious sequela of radiation therapy to the jaws. The vasculature of the jaws, especially the mandible, becomes permanently fibrosed following radiation therapy. Subsequent trauma and infection in the damaged bones produces this specific type of osteomyelitis. While dentoalveolar surgical procedures are the most common cause, pulpal infection, oral ulcers, and trauma from prostheses have also led to the development of osteoradionecrosis. Prevention is therefore most important.

Prior to Radiation Therapy
◇ The following treatment planning considerations are recommended. The patient should be evaluated at least 3 weeks prior to radiation therapy for recommendations to:
1) extract all teeth with large carious lesions,
2) extract all teeth with moderate to severe periodontal disease,
3) extract impacted teeth,
4) remove tori and exostoses,
5) consider extracting all teeth in patients with poor oral hygiene,
6) construction of custom fluoride trays.

Surgical considerations include possible empirical antibiotic coverage, extensive alveolectomies to get primary closure, and close follow-up care.

Following Radiation Therapy
1) Maintain emphasis on oral hygiene.
2) Daily application of topical fluoride for 5 min. (Neutracare, Oral B) (Gelkam, Colgate).
3) Avoid dentoalveolar surgery if at all possible. If surgery becomes necessary, use of hyperbaric oxygen therapy before and after surgery should be considered.

CONSULTATION SUGGESTIONS
Oral-Maxillofacial Surgeon, Radiation Oncologist, Medical Oncologist

REFERRAL SUGGESTIONS
Oral-Maxillofacial Surgeon, Primary Care Physician

COURSE/PROGNOSIS
Prognosis for cancer is extremely variable. Overall, 5-year survival rate for oral cancer is about 51%. In tumors localized to the oral cavity, this increases to 70%, while in those presenting with metastases, survival rate drops to 33%.

CODING

ICD-9-CM
143.0 Malignant neoplasm of upper gingiva
145.2 Malignant neoplasm of hard palate
160.2 Malignant neoplasm of maxillary sinus
170.0 Malignant neoplasm of facial bone
180.9 Squamous cell carcinoma, unspecified site
198.5 Secondary malignant neoplasm of bone and bone marrow
230.0 Carcinoma in situ of lip or oral cavity
526.89 Osteoradionecrosis, jaw
909.2 Late effect of radiation

CPT
21034 Excise malignant tumor of facial bone
21044 Excise malignant tumor of mandible
21079 Preparation of interim obturator
21080 Preparation of definitive obturator
99183 Supervision of hyperbaric oxygen

MISCELLANEOUS

SYNONYMS
Carcinoma

SEE ALSO
Malignant jaw tumors
Salivary gland tumors
Xerostomia
Carcinoma, tongue
Carcinoma, floor of mouth

REFERENCES
Overholser CD: Oral Care for the Cancer Patient. In: Handbook of Supportive Care in Cancer. Klastersky, Schimpff, Hans-Joi Senn, (eds), New York, Dekker, 1994, pp. 125-145.

Overholser CD: Oral complications of cancer therapy. In: Comprehensive Textbook of Oncology. 2nd ed. Moossa AR, Robson MC, Schimpff SC, (eds), Baltimore, Williams & Wilkins, 1991.

Peterson DE, Overholser CD, Beckerman T. Initial detection and evaluation intra-oral neoplasm. In: Head and Neck Management of the Cancer Patient. Peterson DE, Elias EG, Sonis ST (eds), The Hague, Martinus Nijhoff Publ., 1986, pp. 163-177.

Regezi JA, Sciubba J: Oral Pathology, Clinical-Pathologic Correlations, 2nd ed., Philadelphia, WB Saunders Co., 1993.

AUTHOR
C. Daniel Overholser, DDS, MSD

Candidiasis

BASICS

DESCRIPTION
A group of local (mucocutaneous) and systemic infections caused, most commonly, by the yeast-like fungus Candida albicans.

ETIOLOGY

• Candida albicans and other candida species are part of the normal oral and vaginal flora.
• Infection involves surface epithelium, particularly mucous membranes and occurs in healthy patients when normal bacterial flora is decreased, altering the microbial balance allowing candida to overgrow. Also occurs in immunocompromised individuals.
• Candida often associated with broad spectrum antibiotic use.
• Candida may also develop in patients with a compromised immune status caused by leukemia, chronic corticosteroid use, diabetes mellitus or HIV.

SYSTEMS AFFECTED
• Oral mucosa is most commonly affected, but also commonly affects, other parts of the GI tract and female lower genitourinary tract.
• If there is systemic involvement, any organ system may become involved.

DIAGNOSIS

SYMPTOMS AND SIGNS
• Few with the condition being discovered upon examination.
• May complain of a painful, burning mouth, nonhealing sores at angles of the mouth, or white patches intraorally.
• Dependent on the site of involvement and the manner in which the organism interacts with the host tissue.
• Oral candidiasis
  1) Erythematous (atrophic) candidiasis
  Localized form:
  ◇ Red patch in the midline of the posterior dorsal tongue
  ◇ Also termed median rhomboid glossitis or central papillary atrophy
  ◇ Asymptomatic
  Generalized form:
  ◇ Results from broad spectrum antibiotics
  ◇ Loss of filiform papilla
  ◇ Pain (antibiotic sore mouth)
  Angular cheilitis:
  ◇ Candidiasis and Staphylococcus aureus
  ◇ Lesions at the corners of the mouth, seen predominantly in elderly patients and those with overclosure of jaws due to missing teeth or inadequate dental prosthesis.
  2) Pseudomembranous candidiasis
  Also known as thrush
  Creamy white plaques seen primarily in infants.
  3) Chronic hyperplastic candidiasis (candidal leukoplakia)
  White patch located on the anterior buccal mucosa
• Systemic candidiasis
  ◇ Eyes, kidney, skin, meninges, brain, thyroid, liver, and spleen
  ◇ Endocardial infection (chronic drug abuse, indwelling intravenous lines)

LABORATORY
Culture of the organism on Sabouraud's agar, yeast forms visible on fresh slide treated with 10% KOH (KOH prep), but remember organism also part of normal oral flora.
Cytology
  ◇ presence of hyphae signifies infection versus just a carrier state

Candidiasis

IMAGING/SPECIAL TESTS
• Barium swallow may reveal cobblestone pattern of esophageal candidiasis.
• Endoscopy also useful for GI involvement.

DIFFERENTIAL
Lichen planus
Pemphigus
Pemphigoid
Epithelial dysplasia
Epithelial malignancy
Hairy leukoplakia

TREATMENT

• Remove possible causes (antibiotic or corticosteroid) if possible.
• Control diabetes.
• Suspect underlying disease (HIV, malignancy, etc.)
• Sterilize dental prosthesis.
• Assess possibility of overclosure and address as necessary.

MEDICATIONS
• Clotrimazole (Mycelex), 10 mg troche. Slowly dissolved in mouth 5 times per day for 7 to 10 days. Not effective if swallowed.
• Nystatin oral suspension, 5 to 10 mL held in mouth 5 minutes then swallowed 5 times a day for 2 weeks. Works topically and, less effectively, systemically.
• Ketoconazole (Nizoral), 200 to 400 mg tablets once per day for 2 to 3 weeks. Acts systemically, not topically. Idiosyncratic liver toxicity, so not desirable first line drug.
• Fluconazole (Diflucan), 200 mg tablet once, then 100 mg per day for 2 to 3 weeks. Well absorbed and highly effective though expensive. Not associated with liver toxicity.
• Amphotericin B (Fungizone). Dangerous drug best administered by primary care physician or specialist.

SURGERY
Removal of hyperplastic soft tissue of palate.

CONSULTATION SUGGESTIONS
Infectious Disease Specialist if systemic disease or if immunodeficiency suspected. Oral Medicine or Oral-Maxillofacial Surgeon for localized oral involvement.

REFERRAL SUGGESTIONS
Primary Care Physician for systemic disease

PATIENT INSTRUCTIONS
Carefully comply with medication protocol.

COURSE/PROGNOSIS
• Lesions respond well to medication
• Underlying disease must be treated or lesions recur

CODING

ICD-9-CM
112.0 Candidiasis, oral
112.3 Candidiasis, skin
112.5 Candidiasis, disseminated
112.9 Candidiasis, general
771.7 Congenital candidiasis

CPT
40490 Biopsy of lip
40808 Biopsy, vestibule of mouth
41100 Biopsy of tongue, anterior two-thirds
42100 Biopsy of palate
87205 Smear, primary source with interpretation, routine stain for fungi
87220 KOH smear

MISCELLANEOUS

SYNONYMS
Thrush
Moniliasis
Antibiotic sore mouth
Angular cheilitis
Median rhomboid glossitis

SEE ALSO
Immunodeficiency other than AIDS.
HIV

REFERENCES
Allen CM: Diagnosing and managing oral candidiasis. JADA 123:77-82, 1992.

Lynch DP: Oral candidiasis: History, classification and clinical presentation. Oral Surg Oral Med Oral Path 78:189-193, 1994.

AUTHOR
Peter E. Larsen, DDS

Cardiac Arrest

BASICS

DESCRIPTION
Complete cessation of circulation due to absence of all spontaneous cardiac electrical activity or, in spite of electrical activity, cessation of pump activity.

ETIOLOGY

• Ischemic heart disease/myocardial infarction
• Chronic congestive failure
• Electrolyte abnormalities
• Pulmonary disease/respiratory arrest
• Acute blood loss
• Anaphylactic reactions
• Valvular heart disease
• Vagal stimulation
• Hereditary/acquired cardiac conduction abnormality

SYSTEMS AFFECTED
Heart
   ◊ coronary blood flow ceases with global myocardial ischemia.
Brain
   ◊ absent cerebral blood flow with rapid loss of consciousness and global cerebral ischemia.
Other Organs/Tissues
   ◊ multi-system ischemia/failure.

DIAGNOSIS

SYMPTOMS AND SIGNS
• Rarely prodromal symptoms related to underlying disorder eg, chest pain associated with myocardial infarction, palpitations associated with premature ventricular beats preceding degenerating into ventricular tachycardia/fibrillation.
• Pulselessness
• Cyanosis
• Loss of consciousness
• Apnea

IMAGING/SPECIAL TESTS
ECG
   ◊ no cardiac electrical activity. Ventricular tachycardia/fibrillation or other pulseless electrical activity.

DIFFERENTIAL
• Vasovagal syncope
• Myocardial infarction
• Anaphylaxis/drug reaction
• Congestive heart failure
• Electrolyte abnormality
• Congenital cardiac conduction abnormality
• Valvular heart disease
• Electromechanical dissociation

TREATMENT

General
◇ Establish unresponsiveness
◇ If vasovagal syncope suspected, place patient in Trendelenberg (15° head reclining) position. Expect prompt return of pulse and consciousness.
◇ Establish pulselessness
◇ Begin cardiopulmonary resuscitation.
◇ Summon paramedics (advanced cardiac life support).
◇ If monitor reveals ventricular fibrillation, give defibrillation at 200, 300, and 360 joules.

MEDICATIONS
• Epinephrine 0.5 mg IV, IM or SQ q 5 min (can give into bronchi)
• Atropine 0.5 to 1 mg IM or IV
• Lidocaine 1 mg/kg IV
• Bretylium 5 mg/kg (watch for hypotension)

CONSULTATION SUGGESTIONS
Cardiologist

FIRST STEPS TO TAKE IN AN EMERGENCY
• Activate EMS
• Initiate BLS
• Defibrillate

COURSE/PROGNOSIS
Prognosis dismal if advanced cardiac life support measures not instituted within 8 minutes of cardiac arrest. Up to 30 percent survival with rapid availability of rescuers trained in advanced cardiac life support.

CODING

ICD-9-CM
427.41 Ventricular fibrillation
427.5 Myocardial infarction

MISCELLANEOUS

SYNONYMS
Sudden death
Cardiac standstill
Code blue

SEE ALSO
Ventricular tachycardia/fibrillation
Myocardial infarction

REFERENCES
Albarran-Sotelo R, Atkins JM, Bloom RS, et. al: Textbook of Advanced Cardiac Life Support. American Heart Association, 1987, pp. 3-6.

AUTHOR
Samuel J. McKenna, DDS, MD

Cardiac Septal Defects

BASICS

DESCRIPTION
Congenital defects (holes) in atrial septum (ASD) or ventricular septum (VSD).
ASD types -
Ostium primum
  ◊ occur adjacent to A-V values that are themselves abnormal often associated with Down's syndrome
Ostium secondum
  ◊ most frequent type involves fossa ovalis (mid-septal)
Sinus venosus
  ◊ high or low in septum near vena cava often associated with abnormal pulmonary veins

ETIOLOGY

Congenital cardiac anomaly usually discovered soon after birth.
Ostium primum defects often associated with Down's syndrome.
Rare cause of ASD is rheumatic heart disease (Lutembacher's syndrome).

SYSTEMS AFFECTED
Heart
  ◊ cardiac enlargement is common response to both a left and right shunt and from increased pulmonary resistance. This can lead to congestive cardiac failure with impaired cardiac output if severe.
Lungs
  ◊ the left to right shunting causes increased pulmonary blood flow and increased pulmonary vascular resistance

DIAGNOSIS

SYMPTOMS AND SIGNS
Can be asymptomatic, but large defects can produce signs and symptoms. Dyspnea, fatigue weakness, ankle edema, orthopnea, paroxysmal nocturnal dyspnea, cyanosis, clubbing.
ASD
  ◊ Prominent right cardiac impulse
  ◊ S1 normal or split
  ◊ S2 widely split
  ◊ Mid-systolic pulmonary ejection murmur
  ◊ Mid-diastolic rumbling murmur
VSD
  ◊ Loud pansystolic murmur
  ◊ Thrill over precordium
  ◊ Cardiac enlargement

LABORATORY
CBC
  ◊ erythrocytosis
Blood gas
  ◊ hypoxia

IMAGING/SPECIAL TESTS
Chest radiograph
  ◊ cardiomegaly
Echocardiogram
ECG
  ◊ cardiomegaly
Cardiac catheterization
  ◊ best for identifying pressure differences and abnormal flow patterns.

DIFFERENTIAL
• Congestive heart failure due to coronary artery disease, myopathy, or valvular defects.
• Pulmonary diseases that increase vascular resistance.

Cardiac Septal Defects

TREATMENT

A majority of these defects close spontaneously; therefore surgery is limited to symptomatic patients with significant left to right shunt. The risk of bacterial endocarditis requires antibiotic coverage as per the American Heart Association (See endocarditis).

MEDICATIONS
• Medications given to control congestive heart failure (See CHF)

SURGERY
• Common to close in ASD if significant left-to-right shunting at age 3 to 6 years. Patched with pericardium or alloplast.
• Rarely performed to close VSD. Moderate to large left-to-right shunt requires surgery.

CONSULTATION SUGGESTIONS
If in doubt as to need for antibiotic prophylaxis, consult primary care physician or cardiologist.

REFERRAL SUGGESTIONS
Primary Care Physician

FIRST STEPS TO TAKE IN AN EMERGENCY
• If dyspnea suddenly develops, position upright, administer oxygen, and call for emergency assistance.

PATIENT INSTRUCTIONS
Take antibiotic prophylaxis prior to invasive dental procedures if advised to do so by the primary care physician or cardiologist. Usually needed only if murmur present.

COURSE/PROGNOSIS
• Patients commonly asymptomatic early in life. By fourth decade often symptomatic due to shunting and heart failure.
• Small persistent defects, which close spontaneously and those which can be surgically corrected are compatible with a full life. Uncorrected or severe defects lead to increased pulmonary resistance and congestive failure in adulthood.

CODING

ICD-9-CM
ASD
 429.71 Acquired
 745.5 Ostium secundum
 745.61 Ostium primum
VSD
 429.71 Acquired
 745.4 Congenital

MISCELLANEOUS

Dental Implication
 Prophylaxis against endocarditis
 Watch for heart failure
 May be on drugs used for heart failure

SEE ALSO
Congestive heart failure
Endocarditis

REFERENCES
Friedman WF, Child JS: Congenital heart disease in adults. In: Harrison's Principles of Internal Medicine 13th ed. Isselbacher KJ, et al. (eds), New York, McGraw-Hill, Inc., 1994, pp. 1040-1041.

Roberts WC: Congenital Heart Disease in Adults 2nd ed. Philadelphia, FA Davis, 1984.

AUTHOR
Michael J. Buckley, DMD, MS

Cardiomyopathy

BASICS

DESCRIPTION
Diseases characterized by cardiac dysfunction in which the abnormality lies in the myocardium (working heart muscle). Disease can be either primary or secondary.

ETIOLOGY

Primary cardiomyopathies are categorized as restrictive, hypertrophic or dilated, and are often viral related, but may also be idiopathic (pathophysiology not determined). Secondary cardiomyopathies are the result of other diseases in which the myocardium is secondarily affected. These include hypertensive heart disease, glycogen storage disease, amyloidosis, congenital heart defects, aortic stenosis, coarctation of the aortic, sarcoidosis, ischemic heart disease, as well as nutritional and toxic cardiomyopathies. May also occur during or after pregnancy.

SYSTEMS AFFECTED
Heart
Pulmonary
    ◊ secondary pulmonary edema with respiratory difficulties especially while reclined or with exertion.

DIAGNOSIS

SYMPTOMS AND SIGNS
Dyspnea on exertion, at rest, or postprandial fatigue, orthopnea, paroxysmal nocturnal dyspnea, chest pain, productive cough, syncope, tachypnea, pallor, cool extremities, weak peripheral pulses.
Cardiac
    ◊ Enlargement, third and fourth heart sounds, mitral and tricuspid regurgitation, dependent edema, ascites, enlarged liver and spleen, jugular venous distention.
Pulmonary
    ◊ Basilar rales, rhonchi

IMAGING/SPECIAL TESTS
Chest radiograph,
ECG,
echocardiogram,
nuclear multiple gaited acquisition ventriculogram (MUGA),
cardiac biopsy,
cardiac catheterization for assessment of pulmonary wedge pressures,
and cardiac output measurements.

DIFFERENTIAL
• Pulmonary hypertension (cor pulmonale)
• Hypothyroidism
• Pulmonary embolism
• Congestive heart failure

TREATMENT

General
◇ weight loss, sodium restriction, limit activity

MEDICATIONS
• Beta-antagonists, calcium channel antagonists, ACE inhibitors, diuretics such as furosemide (need KCl supplements), digoxin (0.125 to 0.25 mg/d), oxygen, long-acting nitrates such as isosorbide dinitrate.

SURGERY
Cardiac transplant

CONSULTATION SUGGESTIONS
Cardiologist, Primary Care Physician

REFERRAL SUGGESTIONS
Primary Care Physician

FIRST STEPS TO TAKE IN AN EMERGENCY
• Sudden onset of dyspnea during treatment calls for activation of EMS system, elevate upper body above pelvis and legs, monitor vital signs, administer oxygen, transport to emergency facility.

PATIENT INSTRUCTIONS
Take prescribed medications and follow dietary instructions.

COURSE/PROGNOSIS
Variable, commonly a downhill course with poor prognosis. Aggressive medical intervention improves prognosis.

CODING

ICD-9-CM
425.4 Primary cardiomyopathies
425.5 Alcoholic cardiomyopathy
428.1 Acute pulmonary edema
428.0 Chronic heart failure
428.9 Acute heart failure

MISCELLANEOUS

SYNONYMS
End-stage cardiomyopathy

SEE ALSO
Congestive heart failure
Cardiac arrest

REFERENCES
Braunwald E: Heart Failure. In: Harrison's Principles of Internal Medicine, 13th ed., N.Y., McGraw-Hill, Inc., 1994, pp. 998-1009.

Wynne J, Braunwald E: The Cardiomyopathies and Myocarditidies: Toxic, Chemical and Physical Damage to the Heart. In: Heart Disease, 4th ed., Braunwald E. (ed) Philadelphia, WB Saunders, 1992, pp. 1394-1450.

AUTHOR
Michael J. Buckley, DMD, MS

Cat Scratch Disease

BASICS

DESCRIPTION
A benign, self-limiting condition characterized by a primary lesion often accompanied by tender regional lymphadenopathy. Uncommon, cat scratch disease (CSD) may be associated with serious complications, and rarely with life-threatening manifestations.

ETIOLOGY

• A relatively common infectious disorder recently identified with a gram-negative bacillus grown in vitro from nodes of affected individuals and assigned the name Afipia felis.
• Host inoculation by the bacillus can occur via a bite, scratch, defect in skin, puncture wound, or intact mucous membrane.
• Usual mechanism of transmission is exposure to a cat (usually immature) or dog.
• Rare cases have been reported from a thorn, wood splinter or fish bone.
• In immunodeficient patients, related condition affecting liver and/or small arteries can occur due to Rochalimaea henselae.

SYSTEMS AFFECTED
Typical -
Skin
   ◊ 3 to 10 days after exposure a papule or pustule develops. Over the next 2 to 3 days the lesions become vesicular, crust, and then heal without scarring.
Lymph nodes
   ◊ tender regional lymphadenopathy develops within 1 to 2 weeks after exposure.
Atypical -
Eyes
   ◊ Parinaud's oculoglandular syndrome (conjunctivitis, preauricular lymphadenopathy)
CNS
   ◊ encephalitis, polyneuritis, and meningitis
Liver/Spleen
   ◊ granulomatous hepatitis, hepatosplenomegaly, and hepatic and splenic abscesses
Lungs
   ◊ pneumonia and pleural effusion
Bone
   ◊ thrombocytopenia purpura and hemolytic anemia
Renal
   ◊ glomerulonephritis
Skin/Mucosa
   ◊ erythema nodosum and erythema multiforme

DIAGNOSIS

A clinical diagnosis of CSD can be made when three (3) of the following four (4) criteria are met:
   1. Contact with a cat and the presence of a primary dermal or periocular lesion.
   2. Positive CSD skin test
   3. Negative laboratory workup for other causes of lymphadenopathy
   4. Characteristic histologic features of biopsied skin lesion or lymph node (granulomas, central necrosis of germinal centers, neutrophil infiltration).

SYMPTOMS AND SIGNS
Headaches, fever, malaise, chills, lassitude, rash, anorexia, weight-loss, nausea, sore throat, myalgias, and arthralgias.
• Skin or mucosal papulo-pustular lesion
• Lymphadenopathy (cervical)

LABORATORY
• Elevated erythrocyte sedimentation rate
• Other laboratory values usually normal
• Serologic test for Rochalimaea henselae
• Conclusive diagnosis if bacillus is identified with Warthin-Starry silver impregnated stained specimens.

IMAGING/SPECIAL TESTS
• CSD antigen skin test
• Excisional biopsy of infected node

DIFFERENTIAL
• Because lymphadenopathies are the single characteristic presenting symptom, differential diagnosis must include all diseases that result in lymphadenopathy and that have additional signs and symptoms of CSD. Diseases that should be considered include:
   • infectious diseases
   • noninfectious diseases
   • metastatic carcinoma
   • lymphoma, Hodgkin's or non-Hodgkin's
   • sarcoidosis
   • lymphangioma
   • carotid body tumor
   • branchial cleft cyst

Cat Scratch Disease

 TREATMENT

Because CSD is self-limiting, therapy is palliative.
Bedrest during febrile period

MEDICATIONS
- Antipyretics
  ◊ NSAID or acetaminophen
- Analgesics
- Antibiotics are not recommended in immunocompetent patients.
- In severe cases
  ◊ rifampin, ciprofloxacin, trimethoprim-sulfamethoxazole, or gentamicin.

SURGERY
Aspiration or incision and drainage of suppurative lymphadenitis.

CONSULTATION SUGGESTIONS
Infectious Disease Specialist

REFERRAL SUGGESTIONS
Oral-Maxillofacial Surgeon, Otolaryngologist

COURSE/PROGNOSIS
- Inoculated wound followed within 1 to 2 weeks by regional lymphadenopathy.
- Spontaneous resolution of signs and symptoms occurs in 1 to 3 months
- Prognosis is excellent
- Recurrence is rare
- Systemic sequelae are unusual
- Serious complications or life threatening illness is unusual, but can occur.

 CODING

ICD-9-CM
078.3 Cat scratch disease
289.3 Lymphadenitis, unspecified, except mesenteric
372.02 Parinaud's oculoglandular syndrome

CPT
38300 Drainage of lymph node abscess of lymphadenitis; simple
38305 extensive
38500 Biopsy or excision of lymph node(s); superficial (separate procedure)
38505 by needle, superficial

 MISCELLANEOUS

SEE ALSO
Lymphoma
Neck mass

REFERENCES
Burnett JW: Cat-scratch disease. Cutis 48 (6):443-444, 1991.

Elizondo JM, Montgomery MT, Tiner BD, Murrah VA, Fairbanks CE: Painful preauricular mass. J Oral Maxillofac Surg. 52:295-299, 1994.

Lucas SB: Cat-scratch disease diagnosis and treatment. Ear, Nose, Throat J 71:540, 1992.

Roberge R: Cat-scratch disease. Emerg Med Clin N Am 9:327-334, 1991.

Rubin E, Farmer JL: Cat-scratch disease. In: Pathology. Philadelphia, JB Lippincott Co., 1990, p. 392.

AUTHOR
Paul A. Danielson, DMD

Causalgia

 BASICS

DESCRIPTION
• A syndrome of pain and swelling followed by atrophy of an extremity, followed by signs of trophic skin changes (eg, skin atrophy, hyperhidrosis) in the extremity, and signs and symptoms of vasomotor instability.
• Seen following crush or pressure injuries to extremities.
• Begins as unprovoked burning pain arising in days to weeks following injury.
• Pain shows periodic variation and may be intensified by emotion or thermal changes.

 ETIOLOGY

• Crush, pressure, or penetrating injuries to extremities resulting in partial denervation of tissue distal to injury.
• Partial injury of mixed peripheral nerve causes a change in remaining intact sensory neurons. Following partial denervation, cutaneous nociceptors become sensitive to sympathetic stimulation.
• Partial injuries also induce increased adrenergic innervation of dorsal root ganglia.

SYSTEMS AFFECTED
Nervous
◊ chronic, burning pain in affected extremity; abnormal sympathetic tone resulting in edema and decreased temperature in affected extremity.
Skin
◊ bronze discoloration, glossy appearance.
Musculoskeletal
◊ muscle atrophy and osteopenia/osteoporosis may occur as late changes.

 DIAGNOSIS

SYMPTOMS AND SIGNS
• Deep aching or burning pain with superimposed severe, lancinating pain.
• Pain from non-noxious stimuli (allodynia)
• Exaggerated response to painful stimuli (hyperalgesia)
• Joint stiffness
• Hyperhidrosis
• Edema in affected extremity
• Skin cold and discolored
• Nails brittle and curved
• Muscular atrophy
• Osteopenia/osteoporosis

LABORATORY
Bone scan if osteomyelitis suspected.

IMAGING/SPECIAL TESTS
• Radiograph reveals severe, generalized osteopenia in affected extremity.
• Pain relief following intravenous infusion with alpha-adrenergic antagonist (phentolamine) is diagnostic for causalgia.
• Regional intravenous sympathetic blockade (guanethidine, reserpine) may be used in diagnosis as well.
• Local anesthetic blockade of regional sympathetic ganglion less sensitive and more risky diagnostic procedure.

DIFFERENTIAL
• Scleroderma
• Polymyositis
• Infection
• Neuroma
• Herpes zoster

TREATMENT

General
◊ Early physical and/or occupational therapy very important.
◊ Physical/occupational therapy following extremity injuries can play preventive role if initiated prior to onset of signs/symptoms of causalgia.
◊ Serial regional sympathetic ganglion local anesthetic blocks may have therapeutic effect.
◊ Transcutaneous electrical nerve stimulation (TENS) or spinal cord stimulation may be used to control pain.
◊ Early, aggressive analgesia may interfere with progression from acute to chronic pain.
◊ Psychological support essential.

MEDICATIONS
• Regional intravenous sympathetic blockade (guanethidine, reserpine, labetolol) may have therapeutic effect.
• Local application of topical mixed alpha-receptor agonist-antagonists (clonidine) may have therapeutic effect.
• Tricyclic antidepressants and/or anticonvulsants have been useful in some patients.
• Other drugs found useful in some cases include prazosin, nifedipine, and prednisone.
• Avoid use of narcotic analgesics.

CONSULTATION SUGGESTIONS
Seek out dentist or physician with special expertise in facial pain disorders.

REFERRAL SUGGESTIONS
Oral-Maxillofacial Surgeon, Oral Medicine

PATIENT INSTRUCTIONS
Stay physically active and have on-going rehabilitation of affected extremity.

COURSE/PROGNOSIS
Course is chronic and variable. Therapy can be difficult and no one established treatment is consistently effective. Relapses are common.

CODING

ICD-9-CM
354.4 Causalgia

CPT
64400 Anesthetic agent injection, trigeminal nerve
64450 Anesthetic agent injection, peripheral nerve branch
64510 Anesthetic agent injection, stellate ganglion

MISCELLANEOUS

SYNONYMS
Reflex sympathetic dystrophy
Sympathetically maintained pain
Sudeck's atrophy or osteodystrophy
Post-traumatic neuralgia

SEE ALSO
Trigeminal neuralgia
Herpes zoster

REFERENCES
Raja SN, Treede RD, David KD, Campbell JN: Systemic alpha-adrenergic blockade with phentolamine: a diagnostic test for sympathetically maintained pain. Anesthesiology 74:691-698, 1991.

Drummond PD, Finch PM, Smythe GA: Reflex sympathetic dystrophy: the significance of differing plasma catecholamine concentrations in affected and unaffected limbs. Brain 114:2025-2036, 1991.

Bonica JJ: The management of pain. 2nd Ed. Philadelphia, Lea and Febiger, 1990.

AUTHOR
Warren P. Vallerand, DDS

Cavernous Sinus Thrombosis

BASICS

DESCRIPTION
An infection of the cavernous sinus via a septic thrombosis usually associated with chronic bacterial sinusitis. Also can be related to abscesses in the upper lip and nasal labial area.

ETIOLOGY

A sphenoid or episphenoid sinusitis may spread to the cavernous sinus either directly via contiguous anatomy or along vascular structures such as emissary veins. An abscess in mid-face area may spread along vascular structures; this region of the head is supplied with a vast network of interconnecting valveless venous channels and thus bacteria may spread in a retrograde fashion into the cavernous sinus.

SYSTEMS AFFECTED
Ocular
◇ proptosis (protrusion of the eyeball), chemosis (edema of the bulbar conjunctiva, forming a swelling around the cornea), ophthalmoplegia (paralysis of the extraocular muscles), decreased visual acuity. Contralateral eye is frequently also affected.
Face
◇ because the cavernous sinus is secondarily infected, periorbital cellulitis may be present. Cardinal signs of periorbital cellulitis are tenderness, erythema, swelling, and occasionally proptosis. Purulent nasal discharge may be present.
CNS
◇ signs of meningitis may occur (severe headache, decreased level of consciousness, photophobia, and convulsions).

DIAGNOSIS

SYMPTOMS AND SIGNS
• High, spiking fevers, severe headaches, pain in the area of ophthalmic and maxillary branches of V1.
• Drowsiness, confusion.
• Ptosis (upper lid droop), proptosis, chemosis, decreased extraocular muscle function, papillary edema (edema of the optic disc), fever, nasal discharge, decreased visual acuity. Classic case includes palsies of cranial nerves III, IV, V and VI.

LABORATORY
CBC, culture of nasal discharge, blood cultures.

IMAGING/SPECIAL TESTS
• Head MRI or CT scan to include paranasal sinuses, orbit and cavernous sinus.
• Panorex or periapicals of maxillary teeth.

DIFFERENTIAL
• Odontogenic infection
• Meningitis
• Sinusitis
• Acute closed angle glaucoma

TREATMENT

General
◇ hospital admission to intensive care unit

MEDICATIONS
• High-dose intravenous antibiotics to cover beta-lactamase producing organisms (nafcillin 1 gram q 4 hours) and other likely causative organisms. Routine anticoagulation not indicated.

SURGERY
Drainage of cavernous sinus may be necessary but controversial. If any paranasal sinus shows evidence of infection, early surgical drainage important. If odontogenic in origin, immediate removal of involved tooth mandatory.

CONSULTATION SUGGESTIONS
Infectious Disease Specialist, Otolaryngologist, Neurosurgeon

REFERRAL SUGGESTIONS
Primary Care Physician

FIRST STEPS TO TAKE IN AN EMERGENCY
• Hospital admission
• Remove source of infection
• Begin high dose intravenous antibiotics

COURSE/PROGNOSIS
Grave mortality rate (approximately 30%) despite antibiotic therapy.

CODING

ICD-9-CM
325 Cavernous sinus thrombosis

CPT
10060 Incision & drainage of abscess of skin
20000 Incision & drainage superficial abscess
20005 Incision & drainage deep or complicated abscess
31000 Maxillary sinus lavage
31030 Caldwell-Luc without polyp removal
31032 Caldwell-Luc with polyp removal
31233 Nasal/maxillary sinus endoscopy
41899 Unlisted dentoalveolar procedure

MISCELLANEOUS

SYNONYMS
Cavernous sinus thrombophlebitis

SEE ALSO
Sinusitis
Odontogenic infection

REFERENCES
Ballenger JJ: Disease of the Nose, Throat, Ear, Head, and Neck. Philadelphia, Lea & Febiger, 1991, pp. 196-201.

Pararella MM, Shumrick DA, Gluckman JL, Meyerhoff WL: Otolaryngology. Philadelphia, WB Saunders, 1991, pp. 1847-1848.

AUTHOR
Michael J. Buckley, DMD, MS

Cellulitis

BASICS

DESCRIPTION
An acute, rapid progressive, diffuse, septic inflammation of the dermis and subdermal tissues by micro-organisms producing substances that breakdown intercellular proteins resulting in spread of infection.

ETIOLOGY

• Cellulitis of the maxillofacial region commonly results from dental infection, either from an apical abscess, osteomyelitis, pericoronitis, periodontitis, infection following a tooth extraction, needle infection, or following jaw fracture.
• Aerobic microbes are the predominant pathogens, producing hyaluronidase; particularly Streptococci, Staph. aureus.
• Facial cellulitis in children is almost always caused by Haemophilus influenzae Type B, and has high risk of secondary infection such as meningitis.
• Facial cellulitis in adults usually due to Staph., Strep. pyrogenes or H., influenzae Type B.
• Cellulitis in extremities due to Group A Strep. or Staph. aureus.

SYSTEMS AFFECTED
• Soft tissues and fascial spaces of cervico-facial and periorbital tissues.
• Acute cellulitis of bilateral submental, submandibular, sublingual spaces is known as "Ludwig's angina."

DIAGNOSIS

SYMPTOMS AND SIGNS
• Painful swelling
• Malaise
• Chills and sweats
• Difficulty in breathing, swallowing
• Indurated swelling that is brawny on palpation.
• Cutaneous erythema, sometimes purplish skin
• Regional lymphadenopathy
• High fever over 100°F, increased pulse-rate
• Electrolyte imbalance
• Trismus

LABORATORY
• CBC; leukocytosis, shift to the left, Increased ESR
• Blood chemistry
• Blood culture

IMAGING/SPECIAL TESTS
• Computerized tomograph to identify the involved area and to localize suppuration, particularly coronal CT scans in addition to axial views are very useful for the diagnosis of orbital cellulitis.
• Radiographs to find dental foci.
• Aspirates from point of maximum inflammation. 45% positive culture rate compare to 5% from leading edge culture.
• Serological testing with antistreptolysin O, anti-DNAase B and anti-hyaluronidase.

DIFFERENTIAL
• Erysipelas
• Ludwig's angina
• Necrotizing fasciitis
• Cavernous sinus thrombosis
• Orbital abscess

TREATMENT

General
◇ Mild cases may be treated on outpatient basis with oral antibiotic therapy, incision and drainage (if fluctuance present) and removal of the source of the infection.
◇ Severe infections with extensive involvement of fascial spaces require aggressive empiric systemic antibiotic therapy and immediate hospitalization, constant monitoring, and frequent reevaluation.
◇ Secure airway early in the course of Ludwig's angina.
◇ Removal of the cause of the infection
◇ Measure fluid intake and output, provide adequate fluid therapy
◇ Prompt evacuation of suppuration by incision and drainage
◇ Culture and antibiotic sensitivity testing
◇ Moist heat or infra-red lamp to the swollen area

MEDICATIONS
• Initial empiric antibiotic therapy based on site and suspected cause and organisms. Obtain culture and sensitivity and alter antibiotic if indicated.
• Aqueous penicillin G potassium
◇ 1 to 2 million units IV q 4hr
• Cefazolin
◇ 1 gram IV q 6hr
• Clindamycin (if anaerobes suspected)
◇ 300 mg IV q. 8hr, 150 to 450 mg PO q 6hr
• Cefadroxil
◇ 1 gram PO b.i.d.
• Cephalexin
◇ 500 mg PO q 6hr

SURGERY
Not indicated unless collection of pus present or highly suspected, or if Ludwig's angina developing.

CONSULTATION SUGGESTIONS
Infectious Disease Specialist

REFERRAL SUGGESTIONS
Oral-Maxillofacial Surgeon (for facial cellulitis)

FIRST STEPS TO TAKE IN AN EMERGENCY
• If airway compromise of any degree, transport immediately to emergency facility.

COURSE/PROGNOSIS
• Rapid progress by direct extension, or may suppurate involving the maxillary sinus, nose, temporal fossa and brain, as well as deep neck and mediastinum.

• Bacterial virulence, low host resistance, or ineffective antibiotic therapy are aggravating factors that support spread through adjacent tissues and distant areas.
• Possible dissemination of infection into carotid sheath.
• Orbital cellulitis can lead to CNS involvement such as meningitis or cavernous sinus thrombosis via the angular vein.

CODING

ICD-9-CM
326.01 Orbital cellulitis
528.3 Cellulitis of floor of mouth, Ludwig's angina
682.0 Facial cellulitis excluding mouth, orbit
682.1 Cellulitis involving the neck

MISCELLANEOUS

SYNONYMS
Phlegmon

SEE ALSO
Ludwig's angina
Cavernous sinus thrombosis
Meningitis
Erysipelas

REFERENCES
Hanna C:. Cefadroxil in the management of facial cellulitis of odontogenic origin. Oral Surg, Oral Med, Oral Path 71:496-498, 1991.

Quinn PD: Dermatologic infections of the head and neck. Oral Maxillofac Surg Clin N Am. 3:425, 1991.

Goldberg MH, Topazian RG: Odontogenic infections and deep fascial space infections. In: Oral and Maxillofacial Infections, 3rd ed., Philadelphia, WB Saunders Co., 1994, p. 70.

AUTHOR
Myung-Rae Kim, DDS, PhD

Cerebrovascular Accident (CVA, Stroke)

 BASICS

 ETIOLOGY

 DIAGNOSIS

DESCRIPTION
Sudden focal neurologic deficit due to ischemia of the brain; infarction of brain tissue occurs if ischemia is prolonged. Neurologic deficits that result depend on the location of the injury. Transient ischemic attacks (TIAs) are focal neurologic deficits lasting from 5 to 20 minutes, but which may last as long as several hours. They indicate a high likelihood for a frank stroke in future.

• CVAs are due to thrombosis, embolism, or hemorrhage within the cerebral vasculature. Differentiation among these is important because treatment may be significantly different, eg, anticoagulation for thrombosis but not for hemorrhage. Systemic hypotension, such as from cardiac dysrhythmias, may cause syncope, but rarely cerebral ischemia or infarction. It is important to rule out metabolic abnormalities, such as hyponatremia or drug toxicity, that may present with neurologic signs. Consider oral contraceptives, which predispose to stroke in some females. Cerebral atherosclerosis may be the cause of ischemia, possibly manifested as TIAs initially.
• Chronic hypertension is a known risk factor in hypercoagulable states. Cardiac dysrhythmias that allow atrial thrombosis are also a common cause of cerebral embolism.

SYSTEMS AFFECTED
• Neurologic
• Cardiovascular

Evaluation & Work-up:
History:
◊ Onset, duration, level of consciousness; possible predisposing factors such as cardiac disease, hypertension, malignancy, IV drug use, connective tissue disease.
Physical Examination:
◊ Focal neurologic findings (cranial nerves, peripheral motor and sensory exam, deep tendon reflexes, mentation, speech); cardiac evaluation to assess for irregularly, irregular rhythm (eg, atrial fibrillation), new or changing murmurs that may indicate endocarditis; carotid thrill or bruit suggesting stenosis. Evaluate hypertension, which could be cause of hemorrhage.

SYMPTOMS AND SIGNS
• Headache
• Amnesia
• Confusion
• Diplopia
• Vertigo
• Dysarthria
• Decreased level of consciousness
• Visual field defects
• Seizures
• Facial or peripheral paralysis or weakness
• Ataxia
• Aphasia
• Nausea

LABORATORY
Should include clotting studies (PT, PTT, platelets), CBC (rule out polycythemia), sedimentation rate, serum chemistries (rule out metabolic disturbance presenting with neurologic signs), possible urine or blood drug screen.
Lumbar puncture
◊ helps to evaluate for meningitis or septic embolism from bacterial endocarditis.

IMAGING/SPECIAL TESTS

Carotid duplex doppler studies may help to detect source of emboli or obstruction.

Computed tomography (CT)

◊ helps to evaluate for tumors, hematoma, hemorrhage, cerebral edema or infarction. Some of these findings may coexist such as hemorrhage and infarction.

Cerebral angiography

◊ may help to define the vascular anatomy before surgery (eg, aneurysm).

Electrocardiogram and chest radiograph and possible transthoracic or transesophageal echocardiogram

◊ To rule out primary cardiac source of embolism. Holter monitor for suspected dysrhythmias. EEG for seizure evaluation.

DIFFERENTIAL

- Brain tumor
- Focal seizure
- Subdural hematoma
- Hypoglycemia
- Migraine

TREATMENT

- Control blood pressure, correct any clotting abnormalities, control ischemic injury by ventilatory and pharmacologic methods to reduce edema and to reduce metabolic demands of the brain (hyperventilation reduces CO_2 concentrations which will decrease perfusion pressure).
- Hemorrhagic stroke may require neurosurgical intervention to evacuate hematomas which may be causing a mass effect or obstructive hydrocephalus with increased intracranial pressure or to repair an aneurysm.
- Defer elective dental care for about 6 months after serious stroke.
- Aggressive control of hypertension after stroke important.

MEDICATIONS

- Steroids may reduce edema and inflammation; sedative drugs may control cerebral metabolism.
- Infectious causes must be aggressively treated with antimicrobials.
- Treatment of TIAs is preventive and consists of daily aspirin or possibly ticlopidine. As 2% of patients on ticlopidine (Ticlid) develop neutropenia, monitor neutrophil counts.

SURGERY

Carotid endarterectomy (effective in high-grade stenosis) indicated for symptomatic patients with 70% or more stenosis on angiography, and possibly chronic anticoagulant therapy (controversial because of increased risk for hemorrhage).

CONSULTATION SUGGESTIONS

Neurosurgeon, Neurologist

REFERRAL SUGGESTIONS

Neurologist, Primary Care Physician

FIRST STEPS TO TAKE IN AN EMERGENCY

- Supine position
- Administer oxygen
- Monitor vital signs
- Transport to emergency facility quickly

PATIENT INSTRUCTIONS

Comply with antihypertensive therapy.

COURSE/PROGNOSIS

Permanence of neurologic deficits, response to rehabilitation, and mortality highly dependent on degree and site of brain injury.

CODING

ICD-9-CM

435.9 Evolving stroke
436 Stroke

MISCELLANEOUS

SYNONYMS

Stroke
Reversible ischemic neurologic accident

SEE ALSO

Transient ischemic attack
Atrial fibrillation

REFERENCES

Bonita R: Epidemiology of stroke. Lancet 339:342-347, 1992.

Iso H, Jacobs DR, Wentworth D, Neaton JD, Cohen JD: Serum cholesterol levels and six-year mortality from stoke in 350,977 men screened for multiple risk factor intervention trial. N Engl J Med 320:904-910, 1989.

Kistler JP, Ropper AH, Martin JB: Cerebrovascular diseases. In: Harrison's Principles of Internal Medicine 13th ed. Isselbacher KJ,et al (eds), New York, McGraw-Hill Inc., 1994, pp. 2233-2256.

AUTHOR

Robert Chuong, MD, DMD

Cervical Caries

BASICS

DESCRIPTION
A soft, progressive lesion of the tooth, at or near the cemento-enamel junction (CEJ), characterized by destruction of cementum and enamel, with penetration of the underlying dentin allowing continued microbial invasion.

ETIOLOGY

• Multifactorial disease involving four factors: the host (the saliva and teeth), the microflora, diet, and time.
• Dental plaque, a soft, nonmineralized, bacterial deposit formed on the teeth that are not adequately cleansed, is a major contributing factor. Organic acids formed in the plaque contribute to caries development.
• Organisms most commonly found in cervical caries are Streptococcus mutans, Actinomyces viscosus, A. naeslundi, A. odontolyticus, A. eriksonii, as well as Rothis dentocariosa, and Nocardia. The predominance of these bacterial types may vary depending on the location of the lesion in relation to the CEJ.
• Saliva protects the tooth surface by regulating the quantity and species distribution of oral microbes and by interfering with the attachment of cariogenic bacteria to teeth. Saliva also buffers plaque acids and elevates plaque pH. Salivary nonimmunological factors are lysozyme and salivary peroxidase. Salivary immunological factors are the immunoglobulin, secretory IgA, and IgA and IgG antibodies.
• Xerostomia, especially that caused by radiation therapy of the mouth, contributes to an increase rate of cervical caries and rapid tooth destruction.
• Increased amount and frequency of ingestion of sucrose is a major contributing factor.
• An industrial risk exists for those workers in bakeries and candy factories whose teeth are exposed daily to air polluted with sugar dust.
• Risk factors for high cervical caries index include older age, lower salivary buffering capacity, prolonged sugar clearance time, exposed root surfaces, unmet periodontal-treatment needs, previous caries experience, taking xerostomic medications, frequent fermentable carbohydrate intake, infrequent dental care, insufficient personal dental hygiene, use of tobacco, and time lived in low-fluoride area.

SYSTEMS AFFECTED
Teeth
◇ preferentially occurs in premolars, mainly in areas exposed by gingival recession.
• In radiation caries or rampant caries, all teeth may be affected by cervical lesions.
• When considering root caries only, mandibular molars are most frequently involved, followed by mandibular premolars and maxillary canines. Mandibular incisors are least frequently involved.

DIAGNOSIS

SYMPTOMS AND SIGNS
• Pain
• Hypersensitivity to thermal extremes, mechanical stimulation, air, or osmotic fluid shifts (that occur with exposure to refined sugar).
• Sensitivity to percussion.
• Brown discolored cavitation with a softening of the tooth structure at or near the CEJ.
• Usually seen as a shallow (less than 2 mm), ill-defined, softened area.
• Usually occurs on the facial tooth surfaces with extensions into the proximal surfaces, but it may also occur on the lingual.
• Cervical caries caused by radiation will be more extensive at times to the point of causing amputation of the crown.
• Clinical
◇ penetration and sticking of the explorer when pressed into the lesion.

LABORATORY
Caries-activity tests can be used to determine susceptibility for caries
◇ reductase test, buffer capacity test, mutans group of streptococci screening tests.

IMAGING/SPECIAL TESTS
Periapical or bitewing radiographs show radiolucent area at or near the CEJ.

DIFFERENTIAL
• Erosion
• Abrasion
• External idiopathic resorption Abfraction [loss of cervical enamel] due to chronic, repetitive bending of teeth (controversial)].

TREATMENT

General
◇ Total removal of carious dentin and cementum with excavators and dental burs and replacement of tooth structure with a dental restorative material.
◇ A variety of restorative techniques are clinically acceptable:
- Amalgam restoration with mechanical retention created in the tooth (less common treatment modality).
- Composite resin (microfill); acid etching enamel, and using a dentin bonding system prior to applying composite resin. The dentin bonding system involves pretreating the dentin with a conditioner (etchant) and primer (impregnator), and applying dentin bonding agent (bridge to composite). In newer systems, all three stages can occur in one step.
- Glass ionomer; pretreating the dentin with citric acid or polyacrylic acid conditioner.
- Complete crown may be indicated if the lesion is extensive.
- Historically, direct gold, cast gold inlays, and ceramic inlays have been treatment options.
- Incipient cervical lesions have been successfully treated by excavation, polishing, and applying a layer of fluoride varnish containing 5.0% NaFl. Home care includes brushing with a fluoride gel and rinsing with a remineralization solution (Moi-Stir).

MEDICATIONS
- Chlorhexidine gluconate (0.12%) mouthrinse, used twice a day to reduce plaque concentration, S. mutans activity, acid production, and thus caries activity.
- OTC sodium fluoride (0.05%) rinses (Fluoroguard).
- Fluoride gel (0.4% stannous fluoride, 1.1% neutral sodium fluoride, or 0.5% acidulated phosphate fluoride) applied for 6 minutes in a custom soft mouth tray at home at bedtime.
- Patients receiving radiation to the oral cavity are placed prophylactically on the above fluoride tray therapy, preferably twice a day to continue for their lifetime.
- Patients experiencing xerostomia can be placed prophylactically on fluoride mouth trays.
- Prevention -
- In addition to the above medications, other measures are necessary for prevention:
- Effective oral hygiene, including daily brushing with a fluoridated tooth paste and flossing.

- Diet modification to decrease intake of refined sugars and fermentable carbohydrates.
- Lasers are being experimentally used on enamel to cause a 70 to 80% increase in resistance to organic acids produced by bacteria.

CONSULTATION SUGGESTIONS
Prosthodontist

REFERRAL SUGGESTIONS
Family (General) Dentist

PATIENT INSTRUCTIONS
Modify type and use of toothbrush if evidence of cervical wear may be partly attributable to or exacerbated by improper brushing.

COURSE/PROGNOSIS
Location of the lesion in relation to the CEJ is important in treatment strategy and long-term success of the restoration. Lesions completely surrounded by enamel are more cervical, the cavosurface margin is increasingly bound by cementum, treatment becomes difficult and threatens root structure and the dental pulp. Often in these situations after restoration, the patient is left with postoperative hypersensitivity and experiences recurrent caries around the restoration due to microleakage.

CODING

ICD-9-CM
521.0 Dental caries (all sites)

CPT
21085 Oral surgical splint (fluoride application)
70300 Periapical, one
70310 Periapicals, less than full mouth
70320 Full mouth series radiographs
70355 Panorex

MISCELLANEOUS

SYNONYMS
Smooth surface caries
Root caries

SEE ALSO
Cancer (General considerations)
Osteoradionecrosis
Discoloration of teeth
Xerostomia

REFERENCES
Bayne SC, Heyman HO, Swift EJ: Update on dental composite restorations. J Am Dent Assoc 125:687-701, 1994.

Cox CF: Etiology and treatment of root hypersensitivity. Amer J Dent 7:266-270, 1994.

Ellen RP: Ecological determinants of dental root caries. In: Cariology for the Nineties. Bowen WH, Tabak LA (eds), Rochester, New York, University of Rochester Press, 1993, pp. 319-332.

Heyman HO, Bayne SC: Current concepts in dentin bonding: focusing on dentinal adhesion factors. J Am Dent Assoc 124:27-36, 1993.

Jacob JA: Looking at the future of lasers. J Am Dent Assoc 126:414, 1995.

Johnson BT: Uses of chlorhexidine in dentistry. Gen Dent 43:129-140, 1995.

Knibbs PJ: A clinical report on the use of a glass ionomer cement to restore cervical margin lesions. J Oral Rehab 14:105-109, 1987.

Markitziu A, Rajstein J, Deutch D, Rahamin E, Gedalia I. Arrest of incipient cervical caries by topical chemotherapy. Geriodontics 4:293-298, 1988.

Newbrun E: Microflora in Cariology. 3rd ed. Chicago, Quintessence Publishing Co., Inc., 1989, pp. 66-70.

Mandel ID: Nature vs. nurture in dental caries. J Am Dent Assoc 125:1345-1351, 1994.

Westerman GH, Hicks MJ, Flaitz CM, et al: Argon laser irradiation in root surface caries: an in vitro study. JADA 125:401-407, 1994.

AUTHOR
Sharon C. Siegel, DDS, MS

Cervical Lymphadenitis

BASICS

DESCRIPTION
Lymph nodes of the neck may become clinically evident and palpable from an infectious (eg, Staphylococcus), inflammatory (eg, drug reactions), neoplastic (eg, lymphoma), or infiltrative (eg, amyloidosis) processes.
Depending on the etiology and pathogenesis, the lymph nodes may be tender or nontender, movable or fixed, and soft or hard; the overlying skin may be inflamed or normal.

ETIOLOGY

• Except for diseases of unknown cause with prominent lymphadenopathy (eg, mucocutaneous lymph node syndrome) or a primary neoplasm of lymph nodes (eg, lymphoma), lymph nodes are enlarged secondarily as a response related to another system or micro-organism.
• Bacterial or viral infections of the oral cavity, sinuses, ears, eyes, scalp or pharynx.
• Rubella
• Tuberculosis (pulmonary, oral)
• Head and neck malignancy

SYSTEMS AFFECTED
Neck, submandibular, and supraclavicular areas

DIAGNOSIS

SYMPTOMS AND SIGNS
• When of infectious etiology, lymph nodes are usually movable, tender and initially soft; the patient may be febrile and toxic; usually younger age.
• When of neoplastic etiology, lymph nodes are most often nontender and fixed with possible other constitutional symptoms of weight loss, night sweats, and low grade fever; usually older age.
• Nodes may be suppurative, especially when involved with a pyogenic bacterium such as Staphylococcus or by mycobacterium; overlying skin may be red and tender.

LABORATORY
CBC with differential, biopsy (excision or needle aspiration), culture and sensitivity.

IMAGING/SPECIAL TESTS
• Ultrasonography
• CT scan
• MR imaging

DIFFERENTIAL
• Infections of skin, sinuses, ears, eyes, scalp, or pharynx.
• Tuberculosis
• Epstein-Barr virus
• Cytomegalovirus
• Toxoplasmosis
• Rubella
• Cat-scratch disease
• Lymphoma
• Metastatic disease
• Leukemia
• Medication reaction
• Systemic lymphadenopathy syndrome

TREATMENT

General
◇ If infection suspected, treat with appropriate antibiotic and eliminate etiology, if known, eg, abscessed tooth.
• If malignancy suspected, biopsy should be performed on the node immediately.
• Workup and treatment as indicated by the primary disease process.

SURGERY
Persistent unexplained adenopathy warrants nodal biopsy.

CONSULTATION SUGGESTIONS
Oral-Maxillofacial Surgeon, Infectious Disease Specialist, Otolaryngologist

REFERRAL SUGGESTIONS
Primary Care Physician, Oral-Maxillofacial Surgeon

PATIENT INSTRUCTIONS
Cervical node enlargement warrants investigation if no clear acute etiology present. Thus, patients with persistently enlarged lymph node in neck should be advised to have a biopsy.

COURSE/PROGNOSIS
Varies, depending upon the primary disease.

CODING

ICD-9-CM
017.2 Tuberculosis cervical lymph gland
289.1 Chronic or subacute cervical adenitis
289.3 Cervical adenitis
683   Acute cervical adenitis
785.6 Adenopathy

CPT
38300 Drainage of lymph node abscess or lymphadenitis; simple
38305 extensive
38500 Biopsy or excision of lymph node(s); superficial (separate procedure)
38505 By needle, superficial (eg, cervical, inguinal, axillary)
38510 Deep cervical node(s)

MISCELLANEOUS

SYNONYMS
Lymphadenopathy

SEE ALSO
Leukemia
Cat-scratch disease
HIV infection
Infectious mononucleosis
Toxoplasmosis
Squamous cell carcinoma
Tuberculosis
Herpes simplex virus
Lymphoma

REFERENCES
Elizondo MJ, Montgomery MT, Tiner BD, Murrah VA, Fairbanks CE: Painful preauricular mass. J Oral Maxillofac Surg 52:295-299, 1994.

Sanders BJ, Wu-Ng SL, Hennon DK: Cervical adenitis: Report of two cases. J Dent Children 61:62-64, 1994.

Regezzi JA, Sciubba J: Oral Pathology Clinical Pathologic Correlations, 2nd ed. Philadelphia, WB Saunders, 1993, pp. 60-65, 87-88.

Margileth AM: Cat Scratch disease. In: Current Diagnosis. 8th ed. Conn RB (ed). Philadelphia, WB Saunders Co., 1991, pp. 188-190.

Faller DV: Disease of the lymph nodes and spleen. In: Cecil Textbook of Medicine, 19th ed. Philadelphia, WB Saunders Co., 1992, pp. 978-981.

AUTHOR
Dennis L. Johnson, DDS, MS

Cherubism

DESCRIPTION
• More commonly and appropriately termed "familial fibrous dysplasia," cherubism is a benign, hereditary giant cell lesion of the jaws. Expansion of the maxilla and mandible begins in childhood, progresses through puberty, and then regresses as the individual reaches adulthood.
• Affected children appear normal at birth, but begin to show manifestations of the disorder before five years of age. The earlier the disorder presents, the faster the growth progresses.

The disorder is transmitted genetically in an autosomal dominant route with variable expressivity. Penetrance in males is 100%, and in females 50 to 75%. Spontaneous mutations occur in approximately 20% of cases.

SYSTEMS AFFECTED
• The most common site of occurrence is the mandible, particularly the molar region and ascending rami. The condyles are usually spared, although condylar involvement has been reported. The lesion usually presents as unilateral painless swelling, but eventually bilateral enlargement is produced.
• The maxilla is less commonly involved. The tuberosity regions manifest initially with extension involving the anterior maxilla and maxillary sinuses. Should extension progress to involve the orbital floor, the eyes will be directed superiorly and demonstrate increased scleral show, thus giving the patient the appearance of a cherub. Maxillary involvement usually results in more disfigurement than mandibular.
• Due to reticuloendothelial hyperplasia and fibrosis, lymphadenopathy of the submandibular and upper cervical lymph nodes is common.
• Dental anomalies include agenesis of the second and third molars in the affected regions. As the lesions enlarge, displaced teeth with delayed eruption is seen. Tooth resorption may also occur.
• Rarely, the zygomas and palatal bones become involved. Rib and long bone lesions have been reported.

SYMPTOMS AND SIGNS
• The patient reports swelling of the buccal regions that is most often bilateral and painless in nature. The swelling occurs in childhood before the age of five. Steady enlargement is experienced; however, periods of rapid enlargement and quiescence are also noticed.
• Displacement of the tongue may result in difficulties with mastication, speech, deglutition, and respiration.
• The most obvious feature is the characteristic fullness of the cheeks. Orbital involvement will result in an upturned gaze and an increase in scleral display. Benign cervical lymphadenopathy can be appreciated.
• Intraorally, the alveolar processes in the affected regions will be enlarged and are hard and painless to palpation. As the maxillary lesions progress medially, the palate may become V-shaped. Should cortical erosion occur, the mucosa will present with a blue-gray coloration. The molars will show displacement and delayed eruption.

LABORATORY
Disease does not alter laboratory tests.

IMAGING/SPECIAL TESTS
The disorder is first detected radiographically, and when bilateral is pathognomic for cherubism. The characteristic appearance is multiple multilocular osteolytic spaces with rather distinct borders divided by bony trabeculae, and expansion of the cortical plates associated with thinning. The teeth may be unerupted, displaced, or appear as if they are floating in cyst-like spaces. As the patients enter their teens, the trabeculae increase in number and thickness, and the overall appearance may become ground glass in nature. By adulthood, the cyst-like spaces become diminutive and bony ingress occurs from the periphery.
Histologic
◇ characterized by numerous multinucleated giant cells in a collagenous stroma with large numbers of spindle shaped fibroblasts.

DIFFERENTIAL
• Cherubism familial fibrous dysplasia
• Ameloblastic fibroma
• Giant cell granulomas secondary to hyperparathyroidism

TREATMENT

<u>General</u>
◊ The entity is self-limiting by the time the patient reaches adulthood. Therefore, recognition, observation, and routine dental care are the only treatments necessary.

SURGERY
On occasion, the swelling may result in severe facial disfigurement which can cause psychosocial problems, or may result in difficulties with respiration or swallowing. Under these circumstances, surgery would be warranted. As opposed to resection or curettage, re-contouring of the osseous tissues is most often advocated. This must be undertaken with caution because the lesions are very vascular and significant bleeding may result. Furthermore, it should be performed during a quiescent period in the growth process or surgical intervention may exacerbate the growth process.

CONSULTATION SUGGESTIONS
Endocrinologist

REFERRAL SUGGESTIONS
Primary Care Physician

PATIENT INSTRUCTIONS
Assure parents and patient that process is almost always self-limiting.

COURSE/PROGNOSIS
The disease process is usually self-limiting by adulthood (20 to 30 years of age). Any residual facial asymmetries or deformities can usually be managed by recontouring at this time.

CODING

ICD-9-CM
520.0	Partial agenesis of teeth
520.6	Delayed tooth eruption
521.4	Pathologic resorption of teeth
524.3	Displacement of teeth
526.89	Cherubism
784.5	Speech disturbance
785.6	Lymphadenopathy
787.2	Dysphagia

CPT
20240	Biopsy bone, excisional; superficial
21029	Removal by contouring of benign tumor of facial bone
41899	Extraction of teeth
70100	Radiologic exam, mandible; partial, less than four views
70355	Panorex

MISCELLANEOUS

SYNONYMS
Familial fibrous dysplasia of the jaws
Disseminated juvenile fibrous dysplasia
Familial multilocular cystic disease of the jaws

SEE ALSO
Hyperparathyroidism

REFERENCES
Zachariades N, Papanicolaou S, Xypolyta A, Constantinidis I: Cherubism. Intl J Oral Surg 14:138-145, 1985.

Kaugars GE, Niamtu J, Suirsky JA: Cherubism: diagnosis, treatment and comparison with central giant cell granulomas and giant cell tumors. Oral Surg Oral Med Oral Path 73:369-374, 1992.

Koury ME, Stella JP, Epker BN: Vascular transformation in cherubism. Oral Surg Oral Med Oral Path 76:20-27, 1993.

AUTHOR
Robert Rudman, DDS

Child Abuse and Neglect

 BASICS

 ETIOLOGY

 DIAGNOSIS

DESCRIPTION
• Child maltreatment involves intentional physical or psychologic harm or threat of such harm to a child by a parent or caretaker. Maltreatment is commonly divided into four types: physical abuse, emotional abuse, sexual abuse, neglect.
Physical abuse
◇ Includes the application of excessive force, forcing the child to engage in dangerous activity or actual battery of a child.
Emotional abuse
◇ Includes verbal statements to a child that demean them, or overly distant behavior from a parent or caregiver.
Sexual abuse
◇ Includes actual sexual contact between a parent or caregiver and a child, exposure of a child to sexual material or acts, or use of a child as sexual stimuli for adults.
Neglect
◇ Involves failure of parent or caregiver to provide shelter, food, medical care, or supervision.
• Occurs in all economic strata, particularly sexual abuse. Neglect and physical abuse are more frequent in lower socioeconomic groups.
1988 statistics show 1.4 million U.S. children subject to some form of maltreatment. Eighty percent of deaths due to abuse occur under age 5, 40% under age 1. Teens twice as likely to be abused as are children under age 3.

ETIOLOGY
• Economic or emotional problems of parents or caregivers.
• Parents who were victims of abuse during their own childhood often are abusers.
• Substance abuse (ethanol, illicit drugs) often leads to child abuse.

SYSTEMS AFFECTED
General
◇ malnutrition, poor hygiene, poor growth.
Skin
◇ burns, bruising, bite marks.
Bones
◇ fractures
GU
◇ injury to genitals or anus, venereal disease.
Head/CNS
◇ closed head injury, skull or facial fractures.
Mental
◇ anxiety, withdrawal, extreme fear, behavioral problems.

SYMPTOMS AND SIGNS
Frequent clandestine nature of maltreatment can make diagnosis difficult. Need to carefully approach children with direct but empathetic questioning if abuse suspected.
Physical abuse
◇ Multiple skin, facial, rib or long bone injuries at various stages of healing. Various explanations for injuries that seem implausible.
◇ "Shaken-baby syndrome" acute brain injuries despite no external signs of head trauma.
◇ Burns in shapes of glove or stocking (scald) or shape of an object.
◇ Bruises in shape of an object or in various states of resolution.
◇ Oral-torn labial frenum, dental injuries to anterior teeth.
◇ Periorbital ecchymosis, retinal hemorrhage.
Sexual abuse
◇ Genital or anal/rectal injury with bleeding, laceration, pain, diarrhea.
◇ Venereal disease at any site.
◇ Distortion of genitals
Neglect
◇ Slow growth (less than 5th percentile)
◇ Decreased velocity of growth
◇ Signs of nutritional deficiency
◇ Missed school days
◇ Poor general hygiene (dental and body)

LABORATORY
• Evidence of syphilis, gonococcal disease, or chlamydia.
• Positive toxicology tests
• Bloody CSF in infant with altered mental status.

IMAGING/SPECIAL TESTS
• Rib and long bone fractures at various stages of healing (large calluses).
• Skull fractures, facial bone fractures

DIFFERENTIAL
• Accidental injuries
• Incoordination due to visual, neuromuscular, or other problems leading to injuries.
• Emotional problems causing self-inflicted injuries.
• Anorexia (in teens)
• Consensual sexual activity (teens)
• Abuse by siblings or other children (seen in young children or mentally handicapped older children or teens).
• Platelet disorders (bruising)
• Endocrine disorder (growth disturbance).
• Unexpected fractures (various bone diseases).

TREATMENT

General
◇ Injuries managed as warranted.
◇ Once child abuse or neglect diagnosed, governmental authorities must be notified in most jurisdictions. In many jurisdictions, even a suspicion of child abuse mandates that doctors notify authorities or social services.
◇ Recent sexual abuse may require careful gynecologic or pediatric examination for treatment and collection of evidence.
◇ Photographic documentation important.
◇ Many communities offer child abuse management teams that will coordinate care of abused child.
◇ Treatment may require removal of child from abusive environment, and counseling or criminal management of abusers.

CONSULTATION SUGGESTIONS
Primary Care Physician, Social Service, Attorney, Police

REFERRAL SUGGESTIONS
Primary Care Physician, Child Abuse Management Team, Social Services

COURSE/PROGNOSIS
• Study has shown that 1/3 of abusive adults continue to abuse even during treatment, and 1/2 unlikely to stop abuse.
• Prognosis for perpetrators of incest is better than for unrelated molesters.

CODING

ICD-9-CM
995.5 Child abuse

CPT
99080 Extended medical report preparation

MISCELLANEOUS

SEE ALSO
Anorexia
Platelet disorders

REFERENCES
Reece RM (ed): Child abuse: medical diagnosis and management. Philadelphia, Lea & Febiger, 1994.

Ludwig S, Kornberg AE (eds): Child abuse: a medical reference. 2nd ed. New York, Churchill Livingstone, 1992.

Wissow LS: Child advocacy for the clinician. Baltimore, Williams & Wilkins, 1990.

Dahaime AC, Alario AJ, Lewander WJ, et. al: Head injury in very young children. Pediatrics 90:179-185, 1992.

Alexander R, Sato Y, Smith W, Bennett T: Incidence of impact trauma with cranial injuries ascribed to shaking. Am J Dis Child 144:724-726, 1990.

Wissow LS: Child abuse and neglect. N Engl J Med 332:1425-1431, 1995.

Carter-Lourensy JH, Johnson-Powell G: Physical abuse, sexual abuse and neglect of child. In: Comprehensive Textbook of Psychiatry, 6th ed. Kaplan HI, Sadock BJ (eds), Baltimore, Williams & Wilkins, 1995, pp. 2455-2469.

AUTHOR
James R. Hupp, DMD, MD, JD

Chronic Obstructive Pulmonary Disease (COPD)

BASICS

DESCRIPTION
Irreversible forms of progressive obstructive airway disease, including, among others, chronic bronchitis and emphysema.

Chronic Bronchitis
◇ Excessive mucous and recurrent cough for at least 3 months in each of last two years.

Emphysema
◇ Destruction of interalveolar septae of terminal airways and alveoli.

ETIOLOGY

• Cigarette smoking is the major antecedent factor in emphysema and chronic bronchitis.
• Serum alpha-1-antitrypsin deficiency causes a special form of emphysema in young adults or children.

Bullous lung disease
◇ Bullae in normal lungs can cause compression of normal lung and obstructive disease.

Environmental pollutants
◇ Serve some small role in the development of chronic bronchitis. Exposure to cadmium fumes associated with development of emphysema.
• Recurrent bronchial infections play important role in non-smokers with chronic bronchitis.

SYSTEMS AFFECTED
Lung
◇ In emphysema, diminished elastic recoil leading to air trapping and functional obstruction. In chronic bronchitis, decreased airway caliber due to enlargement of mucous glands, inflammation, and fibrosis of airway.

Heart
◇ Cor pulmonale (right and to lesser extent left ventricular failure) from chronically elevated pulmonary vascular pressures. Frequently occurs in chronic bronchitis.
-Coexisting coronary artery disease from smoking.

Liver
◇ Cirrhosis can occur in some with serum alpha-1-antitrypsin deficiency.

Pancreas
◇ Pulmonary and pancreatic abnormalities in cystic fibrosis cause obstructive pulmonary disease and pancreatic insufficiency.

DIAGNOSIS

SYMPTOMS & SIGNS
• Dyspnea, shortness of breath (often severe in emphysema)
• Cough, sputum production
• Wheezing, orthopnea (dyspnea while recumbent in severe COPD)
• Barrel chest, distant breath sounds on auscultation, prolonged expiratory phase of respirations.
• Right-sided S3 gallop heart rhythm
• Peripheral edema
• Frequent infections
• Cyanosis
• Plethora

LABORATORY
Arterial blood gas
◇ Compensated respiratory acidosis. Elevated pCO_2, depressed pO_2, especially in chronic bronchitis. Occurs late in emphysema.

Sweat
◇ Cl^-, Na^+
◇ Elevated in cystic fibrosis.

CBC
◇ Increased eosinophil count

IMAGING/SPECIAL TESTS
Chest radiograph
◇ Hyperinflation, low, flat diaphragm, small heart more evident in chronic emphysema.

ECG
◇ Enlarged right ventricle in COPD and hypertrophic right ventricle when cor pulmonale exists.

Pulmonary function tests
◇ Total lung capacity increased especially with chronic emphysema. Decreased expiratory flow in both emphysema and chronic bronchitis.

DIFFERENTIAL
• Chronic emphysema
• Chronic bronchitis
• Reversible obstructive disease (asthma)
• Heart failure
• Respiratory infection
• Special forms of bronchial disease (cystic fibrosis)
• Sleep apnea
• Chronic sinusitis

Chronic Obstructive Pulmonary Disease (COPD)

 TREATMENT

General
◇ Cessation of smoking
◇ Aggressive treatment of respiratory infections
◇ Chest physiotherapy to mobilize secretions
◇ Avoid sedatives
◇ Maximize nutritional status
◇ Moderate exercise program

MEDICATIONS
• Oxygen
◇ Either nocturnal or continuous
• Antimicrobials
◇ Empirically for pulmonary infections.
• Sympathomimetics (albuterol or metaproterenol) 1 to 2 puffs from inhaler every 4 to 6 hrs for bronchodilatory effect.
• Anticholinergic (ipratropium) 2 puffs q.i.d. for bronchodilatory effect.
• Bronchodilators
◇ May be useful in chronic bronchitis. Obstruction largely irreversible in emphysema.
• Methylxanthines (Theophylline) 400 mg/d.
• Corticosteroids
◇ Occasional response in bronchitis with eosinophilia. Prednisone 7.5 to 15 mg/d or q.o.d.

CONSULTATION SUGGESTIONS
Pulmonologist, Primary Care Physician

REFERRAL SUGGESTIONS
Primary Care Physician

FIRST STEPS TO TAKE IN AN EMERGENCY
• Activate EMS for acute respiratory distress.
• Treat pulmonary infections aggressively
• Administer oxygen cautiously

PATIENT INSTRUCTIONS
• Stop smoking and exposure to other respiratory irritants.
• Maintain good nutrition.
• Receive vaccines against influenza.

COURSE/PROGNOSIS
Good prognosis with emphysema. Low 5-year survival with severe respiratory failure in chronic bronchitis.

 CODING

ICD-9-CM
492.8 Emphysema
496 COPD

 MISCELLANEOUS

SYNONYMS
Chronic obstructive lung disease (COLD)
Chronic airflow obstruction.
Bronchitis
Emphysema

SEE ALSO
Cor pulmonale
Asthma
Cystic fibrosis

REFERENCES
Robin ED, Snow CF: Obstructive lung diseases. In: Rubenstein E, Federman DD. (eds). Scientific American Medicine Section 14, Subsection IV, New York, Scientific American, Inc., 1986, pp. 1-14.

Hancock WE: Pulmonary Vascular Disease and Cor Pulmonale. In: Rubenstein E, Federman DD. (eds). Scientific American Medicine, Section 1, Subsection XIX, Scientific American, Inc., 1993, pp 1-7.

McKenna SJ, Roser SM, Werther JR: Management of the Medically Compromised Patient. In: Alling CC, Helfrick JF, Alling BD (eds). Impacted Teeth, Philadelphia, WB Saunders, Co., 1993, p. 76.

Burrows B: Airways obstructive disease: pathogenetic mechanisms and natural histories of disorders. Med Clin N Am. 74:547-559, 1990.

AUTHOR
Samuel J. McKenna, DDS, MD

Cleft Lip with or without Cleft Palate

 BASICS

DESCRIPTION

• A congenital orofacial deformity that consists of clefting of the lip with or without clefts of the palate (CL/P), and isolated clefts of the hard and soft palate (CP). Because of different embryologic, etiologic, and epidemiologic factors, CL/P and CP are often associated with an orocraniofacial deformity or syndrome, and deformities in other areas of the body.

• Incidence - CL/P, the most common craniofacial deformity, 1:700, most common in Asians (3.6 per 1000), moderately common in Whites (1 per 1000), least common in Blacks (0.3 per 1000); CP (1 per 2500) about the same in all ethnic groups.

• In CL/P, male preponderance, in severe or complete and bilateral clefts; in CP, female preponderance. CL/P 1.5 to 3.0 times as frequent as isolated CL.

• Syndromes that may cause either CL/P or CP include: Van der Woude syndrome, fetal alcohol syndrome, facioauriculovertebral spectrum, holoprosencephaly sequence, deletion (4p) syndrome (Wolf-Hischhorn syndrome).

• Syndromes associated with CP include: Velocardiofacial syndrome, Pierre Robin sequence, Stickler syndrome, Treacher Collins syndrome, Trisomy 18, retinoic acid embryopathy.

• Syndromes associated with CL/P include: Amniotic deformity and mutilation sequence, Trisomy 13, fetal hydantoin syndrome.

• Syndromes with other significant craniofacial anomalies such as frontonasal dysplasia sequence.

 ETIOLOGY

Syndromal etiologic factors classified into three categories:
• Major mutant genes usually with a known Mendelian inheritance pattern such as Treacher Collins, Stickler, or Van der Woude syndrome.
• Chromosomal aberrations such as the more common trisomies and other associated chromosomal deletion or duplication syndromes.
• Teratologic syndromes secondary to drug and alcohol ingestion, eg, corticosteroids and dilantin.

SYSTEMS AFFECTED

• Primary palate (premaxilla, anterior septum, lip, and dentoalveolar ridge), unilateral and bilateral, complete or incomplete.
• Secondary palate (posterior of the incisive foramen or incisive papilla: hard and soft palate and uvula), unilateral and bilateral, complete or incomplete. Also submucous cleft (not visible on oral inspection).
• Teeth
  ◇ congenital absence of teeth, particularly the maxillary lateral incisors in the cleft, also the maxillary and/or mandibular second premolars. The presence of supernumerary teeth usually adjacent to the cleft, labially or palatally, erupted or unerupted. Fused teeth and variations in tooth size and location. Rotated central incisors.
• Maxilla
  ◇ deformed maxillary dentoalveolar arch and possible deficiency in vertical and anteroposterior dimensions. Oronasal fistula after posterior palate repair.
• Mandible
  ◇ sometimes in a relative prognathic relationship.
• Congenital cardiac defects, genito-urinary anomalies, including horseshoe kidneys, and other associated spinal anomalies.

 DIAGNOSIS

SYMPTOMS AND SIGNS
Infants
  ◇ difficult feeding, recurrent ear infections.
Children
  ◇ hypernasal speech, missing teeth, rotated teeth, collapsed dental arch, poorly supported alar rim, deviated nasal septum, abnormal lip movement during speech.

IMAGING/SPECIAL TESTS
• Echocardiograms for heart, ultrasound screening for genito-urinary anomalies, extremity and spinal radiographs for syndromic work-up, panoramic and periapical radiographs, lateral cephalograms.
• Audiograms for hearing loss due to recurrent infections.
• Chromosomal analysis.

TREATMENT

General
◊ Orthodontic treatment from infancy through adulthood: in the infant, to provide symmetry in the dental arch and the bony support for the definitive nasal repair; to align the distorted and constricted palatal segments of the maxilla; and to maintain the gains made by expansion and dental alignment procedures.

• Newborn period:
◊ Presurgical orthopaedic appliance therapy such as a molding plate or a pinned Latham appliance to reposition the severely malpositioned maxillary segments. Feeding training for parents, special nipples for bottle feeding.

• Primary dentition period: Expansion of the constricted and distorted maxillary arch.

• Mixed dentition period:
◊ Full-banded orthodontic therapy. Speech therapy. Before eruption of the permanent canines in unilateral or bilateral clefts, autogenous bone grafting procedures.

• Permanent dentition period:
◊ Full-banded orthodontic therapy. Possible secondary bone grafting procedures. If maxillary and mandibular skeletal discrepancy is great, a full orthodontic/orthognathic work-up, and presurgical orthodontic treatment and orthognathic correction (maxillary advancement, possible mandibular set-back).

• Retention considerations during all phases of treatment.

SURGERY
• Early soft tissue reconstruction repairing the cleft lip and nasal deformity, typically done when infant has achieved about 10 grams of hemoglobin, 10 weeks of age, and 10 pounds of weight.

• Cleft palate repair.

• Possible subsequent palatal lengthening procedures ie, pharyngeal flap or posterior pharyngealplasty only if speech hypernasal.

• Possible otolaryngologic procedures: myringotomies and P-E tubes placement when otitis media becomes chronic or recurs frequently.

• Missing lateral incisors and alveolar cleft present and need management. Alveolar cleft bone grafting at time of central incisor eruption or when canine root half-formed. Replace lateral incisor with implant or bonded bridge.

CONSULTATION SUGGESTIONS
Orthodontist, Oral-Maxillofacial Surgeon, Plastic-Reconstructive Surgeon, Speech Pathologist, Otolaryngologist

REFERRAL SUGGESTIONS
Orthodontist

PATIENT INSTRUCTIONS
Parents need great amount of support to overcome common feeling of guilt and helplessness. Most clefted individuals lead productive, happy lives.

COURSE/PROGNOSIS
Structural cleft deformities correctable with surgery and dental care. Important to bone graft alveolar cleft before adjacent teeth lose periodontal support.

CODING

ICD-9-CM
525.8   Alveolar cleft
749.0   Cleft palate
749.02 Cleft uvula
749.1   Cleft lip
749.14 Bilateral cleft lip
749.2   Cleft lip and palate

CPT
21082 Palatal augmentation prosthesis
21083 Palatal lift prosthesis
21084 Speech aid prosthesis
21085 Oral surgical splint
21146 LeFort I, two pieces requiring bone grafts
21147 LeFort I, three pieces requiring bone grafts
21210 Bone graft maxilla
40700 Repair cleft lip, unilateral
40701 Repair cleft lip, bilateral, one stage
40702 Repair cleft lip, bilateral two stages
40720 Secondary cleft lip repair
42999 Unlisted procedure, pharynx
42200 Palatoplasty for cleft palate
42205 Palatoplasty with closure of alveolar ridge, soft tissue
42210 Palatoplasty with closure of alveolar ridge, bone graft
42226 Lengthening of palate, pharyngeal flap
42260 Repair of nasolabial fistula
42280 Maxillary impression for palatal prosthesis
42281 Insertion of pin-retained prosthesis
42999 Unlisted procedure, pharynx
70350 Cephalogram
70355 Panorex

MISCELLANEOUS

SYNONYMS
Harelip

REFERENCES
Dufresne CR, So IHS: Facial clefting malformation. In: Dufresne CR, et al (eds). Complex Craniofacial Problems, London, Churchill Livingstone, 1992, pp. 195-226.

McPherson E: Genetic Function in Craniofacial syndromes. In: Dufresne CR et al, (eds). Complex Craniofacial Problems, London, Churchill Livingstone, 1992, pp. 97-130.

McCarthy JG, Cutting CB, Hogan VM: Introduction to Facial Clefts In: McCarthy JG (ed). Plastic Surgery, Vol.4, Cleft lip and palate and craniofacial anomalies. Philadelphia, WB Saunders, 1990, pp. 2437-2450.

Grayson BH, Coccaro PJ, Valauri AJ: Orthodontics in Cleft Lip and Palate Children. In: McCarthy JG (ed). Plastic Surgery, Vol. 4, Cleft lip and palate and craniofacial anomalies. Philadelphia, WB Saunders, 1990, pp. 2878-2902.

AUTHOR
Irene H.S. So, DMD

Cleidocranial Dysplasia (Dysostosis)

 BASICS

DESCRIPTION
A disorder associated with characteristic facial features, significant oral manifestations, and varying degrees of pan-skeletal abnormalities. Also known as mutational dysostosis and Marie and Sainton's disease.

 ETIOLOGY

Unknown. Most plausible theory is spontaneous mutation causing pan-skeletal abnormalities. Both dominant and recessive patterns of inheritance seen. No gender or race predilection.

SYSTEMS AFFECTED
• Pathognomonic hypoplasia or complete absence of one or both clavicles with dysplastic muscle attachments.
• Brachycephalic skull exhibiting a sunken midline sagittal suture, with prominent parietal, frontal, and occipital bossing.
• Characteristic facial appearance: face appears small, hypoplastic midface (maxillary, lacrimal, zygomatic bones, and underdeveloped paranasal sinuses), relative or true mandibular prognathism, broad-based nose with depressed bridge, ocular hypertelorism, and mild exophthalmus.
• Oral:
  ◇ supernumerary teeth, impacted permanent teeth, high palatal vault, submucous or complete palatal clefting, nonfusion of mandibular symphysis.
• Deformities of spine, pelvis, phalanges.

 DIAGNOSIS

SYMPTOMS AND SIGNS
Ears
  ◇ conduction deafness.
Oral
  ◇ potential for infection associated with impacted teeth and potential for pathological fracture of the jaw.
Teeth
  ◇ hypoplastic enamel, dilacerated roots, absence of cementum.

IMAGING/SPECIAL TESTS
Panoramic and periapical radiographs, skull films.

DIFFERENTIAL
Primary failure of tooth eruption

Cleidocranial Dysplasia (Dysostosis)

 TREATMENT

<u>General</u>
◊ Removal of primary teeth and the bone over the permanent teeth and any supernumeraries as early as age 8.
◊ Orthodontic consultation for maxillary underdevelopment.

SURGERY
May require orthognathic and/or implant surgery.
Expose or remove unerupted teeth when indicated.

CONSULTATION SUGGESTIONS
Oral-Maxillofacial Surgeon, Orthodontist, Prosthodontist

REFERRAL SUGGESTIONS
Oral-Maxillofacial Surgeon, Orthodontist

COURSE/PROGNOSIS
Excellent, most problems related to disease can be resolved with well-proven dental procedures.

 CODING

ICD-9-CM
520.6   Impacted teeth
755.59 Cleidocranial dysostosis

CPT
21079 Impression and fabricate, interim obturator
21085 Oral surgical splint
21144 LeFort I osteotomy
21206 Osteotomy, maxilla, segmental
21208 Osteoplasty, facial bones, augmentation
21248 Endosteal implant, partial
21249 Endosteal implant, complete
21299 Unlisted maxillofacial procedure
70300 Radiologic exam, teeth, single
70310 Radiologic exam, less than full mouth
70320 Radiologic exam, full mouth
70350 Cephalometric radiograph
70355 Panorex

 MISCELLANEOUS

SYNONYMS
Marie and Sainton's disease

SEE ALSO
Failure of tooth eruption

REFERENCES
Nebgen D, et al: Management of a mandibular fracture in a patient with cleidocranial dysplasia. J Oral Maxillofac Surg 48:405-409, 1991.

Eppley BL, et al: Developmental significance of delayed closure of the mandibular symphysis. J Oral Maxillofac Surg 50:677-680, 1992.

Hitchin AD: Dental treatment strategy in cleidocranial dysplasia. Br Dent J 172:366, 1992.

AUTHOR
Irene H.S. So, DMD

Coagulopathies (Clotting Factor Problems)

 BASICS

DESCRIPTION
• Proper coagulation of blood requires the presence of a series of coagulant proteins (clotting factors) to interact with initiating factors, propagate factor activation, and cause the formation of fibrin and fibrin stabilization proteins. The polymerization of fibrin, combined with adhesive platelets, forms a coagulum that stops blood flow in low pressure vessels or in extravascular blood. Depletion or underproduction of clotting factors lead to coagulation disorders.
• Most common inherited factor deficiencies are factor VIII, causing hemophilia A, and factor IX, causing hemophilia B. The four most common acquired coagulation disorders are those due to: (1) disseminated intravascular coagulation, (2) hemorrhagic diathesis due to liver disease, (3) vitamin K deficiency, and (4) complications of anticoagulant therapy.

 ETIOLOGY

• Hemophilia A and B are X-linked hereditary disorders. Factor VIII is synthesized in the liver and circulates complexed to von Willebrand protein. Although normal hemostasis requires at least 25% factor VIII activity, patients showing symptoms and signs usually have less than 5% activity. Spontaneous bleeding occurs when there is no factor VIII activity (severe disease), patients with 1 to 5% activity have moderate disease with only occasional bleeding problems. Factor activity between 5 to 25% (mild disease), usually only presents with prolonged bleeding after significant trauma (ie, tooth extraction).
• Factor IX is one of the factors requiring vitamin K for biologic activity.
• Factor XI deficiency is inherited as an autosomal recessive trait. It is especially common in Ashkenazi Jews.
• Deficiencies of factors V, VII, X, and II are rare, and are due to autosomal recessive disorders.
• Von Willebrand's disease represents a group of disorders (Types I, II, and III) in which the factor involved with platelet adhesion, von Willebrand's factor, is abnormal. Types I, IIA, and IIB are autosomal dominant traits, while types IIC and III are autosomal recessive.
• Vitamin K deficiency causes decreases in all the prothrombin complex proteins (V, VII, IX, X, proteins C and S). Vitamin K is obtained from the diet and from synthesis by the endogenous bacterial flora. Causes of Vitamin K deficiency are inadequate dietary intake, intestinal malabsorption, and loss of storage sites due to liver disease. Antibiotics that disrupt gut bacteria have potential to cause Vitamin K deficiency.
• Disseminated intravascular coagulation (DIC) causes bleeding problems due to rapid consumption of clotting factors. Although a large number of diseases may cause DIC, the most common are obstetric catastrophies, massive trauma, bacterial sepsis, and metastatic malignancy.
• Liver disease can cause coagulopathies by underproduction of factors V, VII, IX, X, XI, proteins C and S, or by portal hypertension, which causes splenic sequestration of platelets.

SYSTEMS AFFECTED
Primary
◊ hematologic
Secondary to bleeding
◊ joints, large muscles, stroke, GI or GU bleeding, epistaxis.
Any site of trauma or surgery.

 DIAGNOSIS

SYMPTOMS AND SIGNS
• Prolonged bleeding from minor wounds or extraction sites, frequent epistaxis, pain and swelling of weight-bearing joints due to hemarthrosis, prolonged bleeding after circumcision, headache and central nervous system disorders due to cerebral bleeding, hematuria, gastrointestinal bleeding, menorrhagia.
• DIC presents with bleeding from sites of recent trauma or surgery including, venapuncture sites, peripheral acrocyanosis with pregangrenous changes in the digits, genitalia, and nose.

LABORATORY
• Prothrombin time (PT) and partial thromboplastin time (PTT) used to detect factor deficiencies. Platelet count and bleeding time used to detect platelet abnormalities.
• Factor VIII, IX, XI, XII deficient patients have abnormal PTT, normal PT.
• Fibrinogen deficient patients have a slightly prolonged PT and PTT, a prolonged thrombin time (TT), and abnormal fibrinogen levels.
• Von Willebrand's disease revealed by prolonged bleeding time, impaired platelet adhesion in presence of ristocetin, and decreased factor VIII activity.
• Vitamin K deficiency can present with normal PTT and prolonged PT early in deficiency state, but later both are prolonged.
• DIC causes a prolonged PT, PTT, TT, reduced fibrinogen level and elevated level of fibrin split products.
• Coumadin use causes PT to prolong.
• Heparin use causes PTT to prolong.

IMAGING/SPECIAL TESTS
Each specific factor can be measured from serum.

DIFFERENTIAL
Hemophilia A
Hemophilia B
Other clotting factor deficiencies
Qualitative or quantitative platelet disorders
Disseminated intravascular coagulation
Severe liver disease
Circulating anticoagulants
◊ natural or administered

TREATMENT

General
◇ Although factor deficiencies are correctable with cryoprecipitate or fresh frozen plasma, in some cases more purified preparations are available. Factor VIII concentrates are available, but because they are prepared from a large number of donors they carry a significant risk of transmitting viral hepatitis or HIV. Partially purified factor VIII is available in which processing inactivates the HIV. Also recombinant factor VIII is becoming available, which eliminates disease transmission.

MEDICATIONS
• Desmopressin (DDAVP) transiently increases factor VIII levels 2 to 3 times. Can also cause hyponatremia or thrombosis in elderly patients.
• Genetic counseling useful for all patients having genetic basis for coagulopathy.
• Von Willebrand's disease treated with fresh frozen plasma, cryoprecipitate, and DDAVP if bleeding occurs or is expected.
• Vitamin K deficiency managed by parenteral administration of 10 mg of Vitamin K. If cause of deficiency cannot be eliminated, monthly injections will be necessary.
• DIC
◇ need to treat underlying cause. If bleeding present, administer fresh frozen plasma. Patients showing acrocyanosis or sequelae of thrombosis need to be heparinized.
• Patients using anticoagulants therapeutically should be switched to heparin while the PT falls close to control, have heparin stopped just before the procedure, have coumadin restarted just after the procedure and be monitored with PTs until they are again therapeutic. Surgical site should be closely monitored, with primary closure of wound if possible.

SURGERY
Prior to dental procedures that may cause bleeding, patients with factor VIII deficiency should receive an infusion of factor VIII concentrate, and then 4 to 6 g of epsilon-aminocaproic acid (EACA) 4 times daily for 96 hours.

CONSULTATION SUGGESTIONS
Hematologist, Oral Medicine, Oral-Maxillofacial Surgeon

REFERRAL SUGGESTIONS
Oral-Maxillofacial Surgeon (for dental procedures)

FIRST STEPS TO TAKE IN AN EMERGENCY
Severe bleeding in known hemophiliac requires immediate transport to site where fresh frozen plasma or specific factor replacement can be done. Direct pressure, and when necessary, tourniquets can be applied to area of bleeding.

PATIENT INSTRUCTIONS
Patients with known coagulopathies should wear medic alert jewelry and, when possible, have factor concentrates available at home and when traveling out of town.

COURSE/PROGNOSIS
Availability of factor replacements and Vitamin K make treatment of coagulopathy usually successful. Patients having received blood products from others may contract hepatitis or HIV. Poorly controlled hemophilia may leave residual defects at sites of abnormal internal bleeding.

CODING

ICD-9-CM
286.0 Classical hemophilic
286.1 Hemophilia B
286.6 Consumption coagulopathy
286.7 Non-familial hemophilia
286.9 Coagulopathy

CPT
30901 Control nasal hemorrhage, simple
30903 anterior, complex
30905 posterior

MISCELLANEOUS

SYNONYMS
Hemophilia A (Factor VIII deficiency) (Classic hemophilia).
Hemophilia B (Factor IX deficiency) (Christmas disease).
Von Willebrand's disease
Disseminated intravascular coagulation, (DIC), (consumptive coagulopathy).

SEE ALSO
Platelet disorders
Bleeding, post extraction

REFERENCES
Handin RI: Disorders of coagulation and thrombosis. In: Harrison's Principles of Internal Medicine, 13th ed. Isselbacher KJ, et al (eds). New York, McGraw Hill, 1994, pp. 1804-1810.

Little JW, Falace DA: Bleeding Disorders. In: Dental Management of the Medically Compromised Patients. 4th ed. St. Louis, CV Mosby, 1993, pp. 413-438.

AUTHOR
James R. Hupp, DMD, MD, JD

Coarctation of the Aorta

 BASICS

DESCRIPTION
Congenital anomaly characterized by an infolding of the aortic wall that constricts the aortic lumen most common distal to the origin of the left subclavian artery near the insertion of the ligamentum arteriosum. Often leads to hypertension and limits blood flow distal to the constriction.

 ETIOLOGY

• A congenital anomaly more common in males than females (3 to 4:1) and in patients with Turner's syndrome.
• Fifty percent of all coarctation is associated with such other anomalies such bicuspid aortic valve, aortic stenosis, ventricular septal defects, and mitral valve anomalies.

SYSTEMS AFFECTED
Cardiovascular
  ◇ hypertension possibly secondary to increased renin levels, systolic murmur, endocarditis, aortic rupture, and heart failure. Preductal coarctation manifests early in life and is rapidly fatal with associated right heart failure. Postductal coarctation is generally asymptomatic unless very severe.
Upper and lower extremities
  ◇ hypertension is common in the arms and fatigue, claudication, and underdevelopment may be present in the legs.
Kidneys
  ◇ perfused at subnormal blood pressure.
Cerebral
  ◇ hemorrhage, aneurysm of the circle of Willis.

 DIAGNOSIS

General
  ◇ If the coarctation of the aorta does not cause heart failure due to pressure overload in childhood, it may not be detected until it presents as hypertension in the adult.

SYMPTOMS AND SIGNS
• Headache secondary to cerebral overload, aneurysmal arterial dilatation of the circle of Willis with a high risk of sudden rupture and death.
• Claudication, leg fatigue, and underdevelopment of the lower extremities.
• Epistaxis.
• Upper extremity hypertension (brachial artery)
  ◇ an estimate of the gradient and severity of the coarctation can be made by comparing the difference of the systolic pressure in the arm and leg.
• Disparity in arterial pulse amplitude between upper and lower extremity, usually with delayed or absent femoral pulse.
• Mid-systolic murmur best heard in the back between the scapulae. If stenosis is severe, a continuous murmur may be heard over the chest cavity due to increased flow through collateral vessels.

IMAGING/SPECIAL TESTS
• Chest radiograph
  ◇ aortic constriction and silhouettes of the pre- and post-stenotic vascular dilatations that are referred to as the "3" sign, ventricular enlargement, and notching of the inferior border of the ribs due to the effects of collateral vessels.
• MRI or echocardiogram can delineate the anatomy of the coarctation.
• Transesophageal echocardiography allows localization of the length and severity of the obstruction as well as the associated collateral arteries.
• ECG is usually normal except in the case of significant left ventricular hypertrophy.
• Doppler provides a noninvasive measure of the gradient.
• Cardiac catheterization permits an invasive measurement of the gradient across the coarctation.

DIFFERENTIAL
• Aortic stenosis
• Takayasu's arteritis
• Neurofibromatosis
• Pseudocoarctation

TREATMENT

MEDICATIONS
Hypertension may persist despite relief of the obstruction as well as the risk of endocarditis. Therefore, pharmacologic means of controlling hypertension are essential along with lifelong prophylaxis for endocarditis.

SURGERY
Surgical correction of the luminal defect is standard therapy. Resection and end-to-end anastomosis or subclavian flap angioplasty are commonly employed. Percutaneous balloon aortoplasty appears effective in some cases.

CONSULTATION SUGGESTIONS
Primary Care Physician, Thoracic Surgeon

REFERRAL SUGGESTIONS
Primary Care Physician, Thoracic Surgeon

PATIENT INSTRUCTIONS
Contact American Heart Association (214) 373-6300 for educational materials.

COURSE/PROGNOSIS
The long-term prognosis is fair. Untreated, the mean life span is 40 years with death secondary to CHF, the effects of hypertension, cerebrovascular disease, aortic rupture, and the risk of endocarditis.

CODING

ICD-9-CM
747.1 Coarctation

MISCELLANEOUS

SEE ALSO
Endocarditis
Hypertension

REFERENCES
Friedman WF, Child JS: Coarction of the aorta. In: Harrison's Principles of Internal Medicine, 13th ed., Isselbacher KJ, et al (eds.), New York, McGraw-Hill, Inc., 1994, pp. 1043-1044.

AUTHOR
Jonathan S. Sasportas, DMD, MD

Common Cold

BASICS

DESCRIPTION
An acute, self-limited, viral infection of the upper respiratory tract, commonly affecting the nasal passages, lasting 5 to 10 days.

ETIOLOGY

• Rhinoviruses are the most common cause, coronoviruses second most common.
• Spread via the aerosol route
• Most common illness in humans

SYSTEMS AFFECTED
Respiratory system

DIAGNOSIS

SYMPTOMS AND SIGNS
• Sore throat (pharyngitis)
• Coryza [sneezing and nasal discharge (rhinorrhea)]
• Hearing loss
• Headache
• Malaise, lethargy
• Nasal congestion
• Sinus pressure
• Watery eyes
• Muscular aches (myalgia)
• Hoarseness
• Fever and chills

LABORATORY
Generally not indicated unless Streptococcal or Mycoplasma suspected, in which in-offices testing available, or other nonviral micro-organism suspected requiring culturing.

IMAGING/SPECIAL TESTS
None
◇ diagnosis is usually clinical, unless bacterial sinusitis suspected in which Water's film may be helpful.
Culture and sensitivity in chronic cases.

DIFFERENTIAL
• Allergic rhinitis
• Bacterial sinusitis
• Vasomotor rhinitis
• Epidemic viral disease prodrome (rubeola, rubella)
• Streptococcal pharyngitis
• Influenza
• Pneumonia (particularly Mycoplasma)

TREATMENT

- General-bedrest or only limited activity for 2-3 days.
- Hydration
- Humidification of air
- Symptomatic treatment
- Avoid smoking and secondary smoke

MEDICATIONS

- Analgesics such as acetaminophen or aspirin. But avoid aspirin in children due to possible development of Reye's syndrome (rapidly progressive liver failure).
- Decongestants such as pseudoephedrine. Topical oxymetazoline (Afrin) useful for severe nasal congestion but avoid frequent or prolonged use.
- Antihistamines such as diphenhydramine (Benedryl) useful for sedation.
- Antitussives such as hydrocodone or dextromethorphan.
- Antibiotics not indicated unless bacterial infection documented. If Haemophilus influenzae suspected in children, use amoxicillin or second generation cephalosporins. In adults, amoxicillin, erythromycin, or sulfamethoxazole-trimethoprim useful empiric drugs.

CONSULTATION SUGGESTIONS
Primary Care Physician

REFERRAL SUGGESTIONS
Primary Care Physician

PATIENT INSTRUCTIONS
Rest, hydration, use medications as directed.

COURSE/PROGNOSIS
Usually lasts approximately 5 to 10 days, with or without treatment.

CODING

ICD-9-CM
460   Cold (common)
477.9   Allergic rhinitis
487.1   Cold with influenza

CPT
87060   Throat/nose culture
99000   Transport of specimen to outside laboratory.

MISCELLANEOUS

SYNONYMS
Upper respiratory infection
Head cold
Coryza

SEE ALSO
Influenza
Bronchopneumonia
Allergic rhinitis
Bronchitis (acute)
Laryngitis

REFERENCES
Dambro MR: Common cold. In: Griffith's 5 Minute Clinical Consult. Dambro MR, Griffith JA (eds). Baltimore, Williams and Wilkins, 1995, pp. 242-243.

Tierney LM, et al (eds): Current Medical Diagnosis & Treatment. Norwalk, CT, Appleton and Lange, 1994.

AUTHOR
Alan L. Felsenfeld, DDS

Condyloma Acuminatum

BASICS

DESCRIPTION
Related to other warts; condyloma acuminata or anogenital warts represent an infectious disease caused by a common human virus capable of affecting a wide range of dermal and mucosal sites.

ETIOLOGY

• Condyloma acuminata is clinically evident as an exophytic neoplastic process, generally considered to be benign, due to one of a number of human papilloma virus (HPV) strains (6, 10, 11, 40-45, 51).
• HPV is a small non-enveloped, double-stranded DNA virus (55 nm) that is capable of producing latent, transformative or replicative infections of basal epithelial cells.
• Close personal contact is the major means of viral transmission. Unfortunately, HPV cannot be grown in laboratory culture, and highly variable periods of time exist between viral inoculation to the appearance of clinical lesions. This complicates the tracking of infection sources.
• Condyloma acuminata also is described as a sexually transmitted disease that has a rapidly increasing incidence with 1500 new cases reported annually in the U.S.
• Strong circumstantial evidence has implicated genital HPV infections with human cervical carcinoma. In addition, HPV genes can be demonstrated in several oral malignancies, leading to the suspicion that these viruses are capable of producing benign and malignant neoplastic disease.

SYSTEMS AFFECTED
• Anogenital dermal and mucosal surfaces.
• Oral mucosa and perioral regions.
• Laryngeal and respiratory mucosal sites.

DIAGNOSIS

SYMPTOMS AND SIGNS
• Classically, condyloma acuminata appears as solitary or a collective coalescent mass of soft pink, exophytic lesions (papillomatous clusters) that occur at a site of previous inoculation.
• Lesions are typically nontender, occurring most frequently in warm, moist intertriginous areas of the skin.
• Growth is generally slow over periods of months, occasionally with periods of growth cessation only to be followed by a continuation later.

LABORATORY
• Koilocytes (cells with pyknotic nuclei surrounded by optically clear zone) can be demonstrated on cytologic specimens (Pap smear).
• Histologic exam
  ◇ papillary shaped process covered by stratified squamous epithelium. Hyperplasia without dysplasia and koilocytic cells may be present. No inflammatory cells in underlying stroma.
• HPV nucleic acids can be detected using DNA hybridization procedures and specific probes from biopsy tissues.
• Electron microscope (EM) examination may demonstrate intranuclear inclusions in basal epithelial cells.
• HPV common-antigen can be detected in biopsy specimens using peroxidase-antiperoxidase immunochemical staining.

DIFFERENTIAL
• Chancroid
• Molluscum contangiosum
• Epidermoid cysts
• Seborrheic keratoses
• Nodular scabies

Condyloma Acuminatum

 TREATMENT

 MISCELLANEOUS

 CODING

MEDICATIONS
• Podophyllin, a resin extract, has been used topically as a 10% solution in benzoin. Application should be over a 10 to 14 day period directly onto the wart surface.

5-fluorouracil can also be applied as a 5% cream to lesions and has been reported to present a 30 to 95% cure rate.

• A variety of caustic chemical applications such as trichloracetic acid also has been shown to be effective. Chemical cautery, however, often results in incomplete removal and subsequent relapse.

• Immunotherapy represents the newest approach for the treatment of condyloma acuminata. Compounds, including the interferons, have been studied most, and are generally administered by injection directly into the lesion three times weekly for a month. Side-effects have included cytopenias and flu-like symptoms.

SURGERY
• Cryotherapy, using liquid nitrogen combined with podophyllin, is currently the most accepted (CDC recommended) for staged removal of extensive lesions with cure rates ranging from 50 to 100%.

• Surgical removal provides immediate cosmetic improvement although postsurgical scarring and a 30% recurrence rate should be considered in such treatment approaches.

• CO_2 lasers and electrocautery have also been applied to the removal of condyloma acuminata lesions, but their use is accompanied by significant discomfort that requires anesthesia, and holds no real benefit over surgery from the standpoint of postprocedural scarring.

CONSULTATION SUGGESTIONS
Oral Pathologist

REFERRAL SUGGESTIONS
Oral-Maxillofacial Surgeon, Primary Care Physician

PATIENT INSTRUCTIONS
Notify past sexual partners of disease

COURSE/PROGNOSIS
Lesions persist and continue to enlarge until removed.
Although definitive proof is still lacking due to extreme difficulty in finding a suitable culturing system for HPV, this virus has been strongly implicated in malignant disease through epidermiologic and genetic studies.

SYNONYMS
Venereal warts
Papillomas
Verruca acuminata

ICD-9-CM
078.10 Viral warts
078.11 Condyloma acuminatum

CPT
11100 Biopsy of skin, simple closure
11440 Excision benign lesion, lips 0.5 cm or less
17110 Destruction by any method, warts
40490 Biopsy of lip
41110 Excision of lesion of tongue
41116 Excision, lesion floor of mouth
41825 Excision of lesion, dentoalveolar structures

REFERENCES
Mandell GL, Douglas RG, Bennett JE: Principles and Practices of Infectious Diseases. 3rd ed. New York, Churchill Livingstone, 1990, pp. 1819-1827.

Holms KK, Mardh PA, Sparling PF, Stamm WE: Sexually Transmitted Diseases. 2nd ed., New York, McGraw-Hill, 1990, pp. 213-263.

Habif TP: Clinical Dermatology. 2nd ed. St. Louis, C.V. Mosby, 1990, pp. 242-299.

AUTHOR
Peter G. Fotos, DDS, MS, PhD

Congenital Defects of Enamel

BASICS

DESCRIPTION
Heritable disorder of tooth enamel unassociated with known changes elsewhere in body. These disorders are known as amelogenesis imperfectae. Three types: (1) Hypoplastic, characterized by insufficient enamel formation. Can be found in deciduous and permanent dentition. Teeth appear small with open contacts and thin or non-existent enamel. Teeth are sensitive to thermal stimuli. (2) Hypomaturation, characterized by normal enamel thickness but low mineral content and poor calcification. Enamel becomes pitted and stained. The defect is in the enamel matrix apposition. (3) Hypocalcification, defect is in the calcification stage. Enamel has normal quantity but poor quality and is easily fractured. Enamel is soft and fragile with the underlying dentin often exposed.
Amelogenesis imperfecta
◇ a heritable enamel defect, is distinguished from other enamel defects in that its occurrence is separate from any systemic metabolic condition or syndrome, and in that it follows distinct patterns of inheritance. Four major categories are described according to the suspected stage of tooth development affected: hypoplastic, hypomaturation, hypocalcified, and hypomaturation
◇ hypoplastic with taurodontism.
Environmental enamel hypoplasia
◇ includes defects caused by metabolic, systemic, and syndromic conditions. An example: prenatal syphilis infection, presents with Hutchinson's incisors and mulberry molars.
Localized enamel hypoplasia
◇ when individual teeth are affected due to local infection, local trauma
◇ as of trauma to the primary precursor, iatrogenic surgery, and primary teeth over-retention.
Enamel hypocalcification
◇ results from faults in the mineralization of the organic matrix in enamel formation. Usually, these occur subsequent to localized infection and trauma.

ETIOLOGY

Multiple inheritance patterns depending upon type of amelogenesis imperfecta and the 14 subgroups. These patterns may be either autosomal dominant or recessive, and in some cases X-linked dominant or recessive. In the hypoplastic type, the enamel organ has areas that lack inner epithelium, thereby causing an absence of cell differentiation into ameloblasts. This condition is inherited as an autosomal dominant trait. Hypomaturation occurs due to the presence of organic material remaining after enamel matrix apposition. Hypocalcification occurs when the enamel matrix is disturbed during the calcification stage.

SYSTEMS AFFECTED
Affected teeth are fragile and subject to fracture, thermal sensitivity, poor oral hygiene, unattractive appearance, and, in children, emotional problems associated with persistent pain and unsightly appearance. The hypocalcification type may also show increased incidence of anterior open bite and delay in eruption.

DIAGNOSIS

SYMPTOMS AND SIGNS
Patients present with generalized defects in enamel. The quality and quantity of enamel can determine the specific type of amelogenesis and due to the hereditary factor, a familial pattern can be derived. Signs can include thin to nonexistent enamel on all teeth, pitted and discolored enamel, and areas of exposed dentin with cheesy enamel that can be scraped off tooth. Secondary symptoms include thermal sensitivity, calculus formation, poor oral hygiene, guarded or reluctance to smile.

IMAGING/SPECIAL TESTS
Radiographic evidence reveals teeth with thin enamel or fractured enamel.

DIFFERENTIAL
A number of other disturbances may produce enamel hypoplasias. Of those that are heritable there is involvement with other systems that differentiate them from amelogenesis imperfecta. Examples include tricho-dento-osseous syndrome, Morquio's syndrome. Other causes of enamel hypoplasias can be environmental, as in vitamin deficiencies (particularly A,C, and D), neurologic injury, cleft palate repair, nephrosis, local infection or trauma, lead poisoning, and dental fluorosis.

TREATMENT

General
◇ Management of generalized enamel hypoplasia is multi-phasic. In the primary dentition, restoration will depend on nature and size of defect and may range from simple amalgam of composite repair to full stainless steel crown for severely affected teeth. In the permanent dentition, the severity of the defect will dictate choice of restoration. For discoloration or minor pitting, microabrasion or simple composite restoration may suffice. For more involved defects, veneers to full crown restoration will be needed.

MEDICATIONS
• When restoration is delayed due to patient management or partial eruption, topical fluoride is indicated as a desensitizing treatment.

SURGERY
Teeth may require removal and replacement with conventional or implant borne prostheses.

CONSULTATION SUGGESTIONS
Pediatric Dentist, Prosthodontist

REFERRAL SUGGESTIONS
Family Dentist, Pediatric Dentist

PATIENT INSTRUCTIONS
Genetic counseling as to familial pattern. Use of desensitizing toothpastes, and fluoride topical home rinses and/or gels. Avoid foods and habits that tend to abrade teeth. Consider use of nightguard if bruxism suspected.

COURSE/PROGNOSIS
Untreated hypoplasias may increase likelihood of fracture, caries attack, and chronic pain. With treatment and effective restoration and oral hygiene, a normal function and aesthetic appearance can be maintained.

CODING

ICD-9-CM
520.2 Enameloma
520.4 Hypocalcification of teeth
520.5 Amelogenesis imperfecta

CPT
21085 Oral surgical splint (as nightguard or for fluoride applications)
21248 Endosteal-implant, partial edentulism
21249 Endosteal-implant, edentulous
41899 Unlisted dentoalveolar structures
70300 Periapical film, simple
70310 Periapical film, less than full mouth
70320 Periapical film, full mouth
70355 Panorex

MISCELLANEOUS

SYNONYMS
Amelogenesis imperfecta

SEE ALSO
Congenital defects of dentin
Fluorosis
Discoloration of teeth

REFERENCES
Levin LS: Genetic Disease in Children. Pediatric Dental Medicine. Forrester DJ, Wagner ML, Fleming J (eds). Philadelphia, Lea & Febiger, 1981, pp. 108-110.

Dummett CO, Jr: Anomalies of the Developing Dentition. Pediatric Dentistry Infancy through Adolescence. 2nd ed. Pinkham JR (ed). Philadelphia, WB Saunders Co. 1994, pp. 61-64.

AUTHORS
Mark Wagner, DMD
Maria Rosa Watson, DDS, MS, MPH

Congenital Defects of Dentin

BASICS

DESCRIPTION
Disturbances in dentin development and formation may be isolated or associated with other heritable conditions. Dentinogenesis imperfecta has been described by Shields as Type I, II, or III. Type I is associated with osteogenesis imperfecta. Primary teeth are more affected than permanent teeth. Characterized by amber to blue opalescent appearance and inherited as an autosomal dominant trait. Type II is also known as hereditary opalescent dentin. This condition occurs separately from the osteogenesis imperfecta, and both the primary and permanent dentitions are equally affected. The teeth are similar in appearance to the Type I. Type III is rare and the severest form. Multiple pulp exposures, periapical radiolucencies, and shell-like crowns (limited to Brandywine population). Another congenital dentin defect is dentin dysplasia characterized by normal crown morphology with amber translucency and short, spike-shaped roots with pulp obliteration.

ETIOLOGY

Autosomal dominant inherited trait. Originates during histodifferentiation. Disturbance of predentin matrix.

SYSTEMS AFFECTED
The Type I form of dentinogenesis imperfecta is found in conjunction with osteogenesis imperfecta which is a collagen formation defect resulting in osteoporosis, brittle bones, curvature of limbs, blue sclera, and temporal bossing.

DIAGNOSIS

SYMPTOMS AND SIGNS
Patient presents with bulbous shaped crowns, reddish-brown to blue gray translucent color. Primary teeth may be more severely involved and enamel may be chipped, and dentin worn and abraded.

IMAGING/SPECIAL TESTS
Radiographic evidence of multiple periapical radiolucencies, pulpal constriction or obliteration, and root fractures.

DIFFERENTIAL
Intrinsic discolored teeth due to prolonged antibiotic therapy, for example, tetracycline staining. Amelogenesis imperfecta in which enamel may be worn and chipped, but dentin is sound.

Congenital Defects of Dentin

 TREATMENT

General
◊ Management of this disorder is difficult in both permanent and primary dentitions. Stainless steel crowns on the primary molars to prevent abrasion and exposure is often the treatment of choice. The permanent teeth usually require full coverage restoration from cast gold to metal ceramic. Laminate veneer on anteriors has been successful when full coverage of anterior teeth has not been necessary.

SURGERY
Teeth with periapical radiolucencies require extraction due to pulpal constriction and/or obliteration. Implants may be helpful to replace teeth due to unsuitability of other teeth for use as abutments. Caution during tooth removal due to brittleness of dentin.

CONSULTATION SUGGESTIONS
Pediatric Dentist, Prosthodontist, Oral-Maxillofacial Surgeon

REFERRAL SUGGESTIONS
Pediatric Dentist, Family Dentist

PATIENT INSTRUCTIONS
Complex restorative care will usually be indicated, requiring careful self-administered oral hygiene.

COURSE/PROGNOSIS
With proper sequenced restoration, a reasonable esthetic and functional form can be realized. With severe forms resulting in root fracture and multiple periapical infections, extraction and prosthetic replacement will be required.

 CODING

ICD-9-CM
520.5 Dentinogenesis imperfecta
522.3 Secondary dentin in pulp
756.51 Osteogenesis imperfecta

CPT
21085 Oral surgical splint (for fluoride applications)
21248 Endosteal-implant, partial edentulism
21249 Endosteal-implant, edentulous
41899 Unlisted dentoalveolar structures
70300 Periapical film, simple
70310 Periapical film, less than full mouth
70320 Periapical film, full mouth
70355 Panorex

 MISCELLANEOUS

SYNONYMS
Dentinogenesis imperfecta

SEE ALSO
Congenital defects of enamel
Discolorations of teeth

REFERENCES
McDonald RE, Avery DR: Acquired and developmental disturbances of the teeth and associated oral structures. Dentistry for the Child and Adolescent. 4th ed. St. Louis, CV Mosby Co., 1983, pp. 70-79.

Levin LS: Genetic Disease in Children. Pediatric Dental Medicine. Forrester DJ, Wagner ML, Fleming J (eds). Philadelphia, Lea & Febiger, 1981, pp. 111-113.

AUTHOR
Mark Wagner, DMD

Congestive Heart Failure

BASICS

DESCRIPTION
Syndrome resulting from the inability of the heart to adequately perfuse organs and peripheral tissues. Left heart failure causes inadequate systolic emptying, while right heart failure causes poor diastolic filling of left ventricle.

ETIOLOGY

Intracardiac
◇ acute myocarditis from infection or toxic agent, amyloidosis, sarcoidosis, rheumatic fever, collagen-vascular diseases, cardiomyopathies, degenerative valvular disease, and pericardial inflammation.
Extracardiac
◇ systemic hypertension, pulmonary hypertension from parenchymal disease or pulmonary embolism, anemia, hyperthyroidism, alcoholic liver disease.

SYSTEMS AFFECTED
Heart
◇ increases in size but decreases in function due to thinning of myocardium.
Lungs
◇ inefficient systolic ejection causes pulmonary hypertension and fluid accumulation in the lungs.
Liver/spleen
◇ enlargement due to venous congestion.
Skin
◇ pitting edema due to venous congestion.

DIAGNOSIS

SYMPTOMS AND SIGNS
• Dyspnea at rest or on exertion, fatigue, weakness, decreasing exercise tolerance, paroxysmal nocturnal dyspnea, edema, orthopnea, tachypnea, cool extremities.
• Peripheral pitting edema, basilar rales, ascites, jugular venous distension, cardiomegaly, congestive hepatomegaly, gallop rhythm, cyanosis, nocturnal wheezing.

LABORATORY
• CBC (polycythemia), liver function tests, (elevated SGOT, hyperbilirubinemia), renal function tests (proteinuria elevated creatinine), arterial blood gases (resp. alkalosis). Monitor digoxin levels and potassium.

IMAGING/SPECIAL TESTS
Chest radiograph (pulmonary edema, Kerley B lines, enlarged cardiac silhouette), electrocardiogram (increased heart size), echocardiogram, Swan-Ganz catheterization (measure pulmonary artery wedge pressures), cardiac catherization to evaluate coronary artery potency.

DIFFERENTIAL
• Right heart versus left heart failure
• Pulmonary disease
• Sepsis
• Pulmonary embolism
• Hypoadrenalism
• Hypothyroidism
• Hypovolemia
• Nephrotic syndrome
• Primary pulmonary hypertension

Congestive Heart Failure

TREATMENT

General
◇ reduce activities, sodium restriction, control hypertension, weight loss, eliminate smoking, reduce fat intake, use antiembolism support hose, supplemental oxygen.

MEDICATIONS
• Diuretics to reduce preload, digoxin to increase cardiac output (positive inotropic agent), and treat atrial fibrillation. Vasodilators to reduce afterload (nitrates, calcium channel antagonists, hydralazine). Angiotension-converting enzyme inhibitors to decrease water retention and vasoconstriction. Dopamine or dobutamine used to increase contractility and for other effects.

SURGERY
Heart valve surgery as indicated. Mechanical circulatory assistance. Cardiac transplant feasible, particularly in patients less than age 55 and without other severe systemic diseases.

CONSULTATION SUGGESTIONS
Cardiologist

REFERRAL SUGGESTIONS
Cardiologist, Primary Care Physician

FIRST STEPS TO TAKE IN AN EMERGENCY
• Semi-erect sitting position
• Oxygen
• Monitor vital signs
• Quickly transport to emergency facility

PATIENT INSTRUCTIONS
• Avoid excessive sodium, smoking, and fluid intake
• Take prescribed medications
• Contact American Heart Association (214)373-6300 for helpful literature.

COURSE/PROGNOSIS
Variable, from mild symptoms to severe failure requiring complete bed rest or mechanical assistance. Mortality rate with mild symptoms 10%, with severe symptoms 50%.

CODING

ICD-9-CM
428 Congestive heart failure

MISCELLANEOUS

SYNONYMS
Heart failure
Congestive cardiomyopathy
Dropsy
Cardiac asthma

SEE ALSO
Cardiac arrest
Cardiomyopathy
Atrial fibrillation
Myocardial infarction
Pulmonary edema

REFERENCES
Braunwald E. Heart Failure: In: Harrison's Principles of Internal Medicine, 13th ed. Isselbacher KJ, et. al. (eds.), New York, McGraw-Hill Inc., 1994, pp. 890-900.

Goodman LS, Gilman A. (eds): Cardiovascular Drugs. In: The Pharmacological Basis of Therapeutics, 7th ed., New York, Macmillan, 1985, pp. 716, 887.

AUTHOR
Michael J. Buckley, DMD, MS

Conjunctivitis

BASICS

DESCRIPTION
Inflamed conjunctiva of eye with marked erythema characterized by pain or irritation, discharge and/or eyelid stickiness.

ETIOLOGY

Most common etiology is infectious, including bacterial (Staph. aureus, Strep. pneumoniae, and Haemophilus influenzae), viral (adenovirus, herpes simplex) or chlamydial. Other causes or noninfectious sources include chemical burns and hypersensitivities. Hypersensitivities are associated with contact dermatitis, keratoconjunctivitis, and hay fever.

SYSTEMS AFFECTED
Eye
◇ this is limited to the periorbital bulbar and vestibular conjunctiva.

DIAGNOSIS

SYMPTOMS AND SIGNS
• Tearing, photosensitivity, red eye, eye pain or burning sensation, eye pruritus.
• Watery, mucous discharge; eyelid edema; pinpoint subconjunctival hemorrhage; chemosis; periauricular adenopathy, blurred vision.

LABORATORY
Conjunctival scrapings for cultures, sensitivities, and Gram stains.

IMAGING/SPECIAL TESTS
• Slit-lamp examination of cornea. Immunofluorescence for chlamydia.
• Viral and Pap smear for herpes simplex.
Culture

DIFFERENTIAL
• Dactrocystitis
• Acute glaucoma
• Corneal ulceration
• Acute allergic reactions
• Uveitis
• Canaliculitis
• Dry eye syndrome (sicca syndrome)
• Nonspecific conjunctivitis (measles, mumps, influenza)

TREATMENT

<u>General</u>
◊ artificial tears 4 to 8 times per day for 1 to 3 weeks.
Cold compresses several times a day for 1 to 2 weeks for allergic etiology. Warm compresses for infection.

MEDICATIONS
• Topic vasoconstrictors/oral antihistamine q.i.d if itching is severe. Topical antibiotic therapy for infectious conjunctivitis (tobramycin or gentamicin, erythromycin).
• If viral etiology suspected, topical trifluridine or acyclovir.

CONSULTATION SUGGESTIONS
Ophthalmologist

REFERRAL SUGGESTIONS
Ophthalmologist, Primary Care Physician

FIRST STEPS TO TAKE IN AN EMERGENCY
• Avoid rubbing eye.
• Seek medical treatment immediately.
• Wash hands before coming in contact with others.

PATIENT INSTRUCTIONS
Avoid rubbing eye.

COURSE/PROGNOSIS
Excellent if treated early. Expected resolution in 2 to 4 days after starting treatment. Scarring can occur if severe viral infection.

 CODING

ICD-9-CM
372.0   Acute conjunctivitis
372.05 Chemical conjunctivitis
372.14 Allergic conjunctivitis

 MISCELLANEOUS

SYNONYMS
Pink eye (non-Neisserial bacterial conjunctivitis)
Keratoconjunctivitis

SEE ALSO
Corneal ulceration

REFERENCES
Lam S, Rapuano C, Krachmer J: Cornea and External Disease. In: Vrabec M, Florakis G, (eds). Ophthalmic Essentials. Oxford. Blackwell Scientific, 1992, pp. 54-63.

Cullom R, Chang B: In: The Willis Eye Manual, Philadelphia, JB Lippincott Co. 1994, pp. 109-115.

AUTHOR
Michael J. Buckley, DMD, MS

Contact Allergy

BASICS

DESCRIPTION
• An acute or chronic inflammatory reaction produced by an immunologic response directed against substances in contact with epithelium.
• Reaction occurs 24 to 48 hours after contactant exposure.
• On the skin, contact allergy also called contact allergic dermatitis, while on the oral mucosa, it is referred to as stomatitis venata.
• Only rarely affects the oral mucosa or the lips.

ETIOLOGY
• Represents a form of delayed-type hypersensitivity reaction (cellular immune reaction).
• Inducing agents (antigens) are usually low molecular-weight substances that can combine covalently with host proteins. Examples are metal compounds (nickel, chromate), plant products (poison ivy, oak, sumac), cosmetics (hair dye, preservatives, perfumes), processing agents (free formaldehyde in durable-press finishes, rubber accelerators, anti-oxidants, foods), and topical drugs (topical anesthetics, antibiotics).
• Contact dermatitis can be a serious problem for medical, dental, and health care workers because of repetitive exposure to potential allergens as:
    latex gloves, methylmethacrylate, chromic acid, chlorhexidine, guteraldehyde, oil of cloves, epoxy resins, acrylic, eugenol, and impression materials.
• Stomatitis venata can be caused by a wide variety of substances, such as:
    chrome cobalt dentures, gold crowns, denture soft-lining material, acrylic dentures, benzocaine, impression materials, chlorhexidine, orthodontic wires, latex (gloves of practitioner and orthodontic bands), tooth-paste, and chewing gum (flavoring oils).

SYSTEMS AFFECTED
Oral mucosa
  ◇ ulcerations and erosions may predispose patient to secondary infection.
Skin
  ◇ may have severe swelling with bulla formation; possibly secondary infection.

DIAGNOSIS

SYMPTOMS AND SIGNS
Mouth
  ◇ initial symptom may be burning or itching at the site of contact. Later symptoms include burning and pain.
Skin
  ◇ itching and pain.
Mouth
  ◇ erythema, vesicles, and later ulceration and erosions. Lesions may appear as lichenoid.
Skin
  ◇ usually erythematous, itchy with vesicles. Usually begin 24 to 48 hours after contactant exposure.

LABORATORY
Patch testing with a standard group of contact allergens may be helpful. A specialist should be consulted because the testing allergen may worsen the eruption and patch testing may yield ambiguous results. Patch testing is not always a good indicator of sensitization of the oral cavity. As a result, when such tests are negative, testing of the oral mucosa may be indicated.

IMAGING/SPECIAL TESTS
Biopsy may be helpful to confirm a diagnosis and rule out other diseases. It is especially helpful in lichenoid reactions.

DIFFERENTIAL
Mucosa
    Plasma cell gingivitis
    Trauma
    Atrophic candidiasis
    Lichen planus
    Recurrent Herpes Simplex
    Apthous ulcers
    Erythema multiforme
    Vesiculobullous diseases
Skin
    Atopic dermatitis
    Vesiculobullous diseases

TREATMENT

General
Mucosa
    Removal of causative agent
    Sucking on ice cubes to reduce
      edema and pain
    Erosions and ulcers may be covered
      with protective pastes (Orabase or
      Zilactin)
Skin
    Removal of offending agent
    Use wet compresses in early stages

MEDICATIONS
• Mucosa
• If erosions or ulcers are severe, use a topical steroid ointment (clobetasol propionate or betamethasone).
• If widespread, use steroid rinse (Decadron elixir), topical anesthetics (lidocaine (viscous) 4% or Dyclonine .05%).
• Topical steroid cream or an ointment if lesions are dry (not helpful in blister stage)
• Oral antihistamines may also be of benefit.
• In severe cases, oral prednisone (60 mg/day). This can be increased by 10 mg after 3 to 4 days. Total steroid therapy for 7 to 14 days is effective.
• Watch for secondary infection.

CONSULTATION SUGGESTIONS
Allergist, Dermatologist, Oral Medicine

REFERRAL SUGGESTIONS
Sensitivity testing is best carried out by an allergist.

FIRST STEPS TO TAKE IN AN EMERGENCY
• Stop contact with all potential allergens.
• Administer epinephrine and steroids if airway compromise or anaphylactic reaction imminent.

PATIENT INSTRUCTIONS
Avoid contact with offending agents.
• Seek skin testing to clarify antigenic substance.

COURSE/PROGNOSIS
In mild cases, removal of the allergen will suffice. In uncomplicated cases, the lesions will heal in 1 to 2 weeks.

CODING

ICD-9-CM
  692.9 Contact dermatitis
  995.3 Allergic reaction

CPT
  11100 Biopsy of skin, subcutaneous tissue and/or mucous membrane
  99000 Transport specimen to outside laboratory.

MISCELLANEOUS

SYNONYMS
Contact dermatitis
Stomatitis venata

SEE ALSO
Allergic reactions

REFERENCES
Duxbury AJ: Systemic pharmacotherapy. In: Jones JH, Mason DK (eds). Oral Manifestations of Systemic Disease, 2nd ed. London, Balliere Tindal, 1990, pp. 420-424.

Porter PR, Scully C: Immunologically mediated disease. In: Jones JH, Mason DK (eds). Oral Manifestations of Systemic Disease, 2nd ed. London, Balliere Tindal, 1990, p. 186.

Lockey RF, Bukantz C. Principles of Immunology and Allergy. Philadelphia, WB Saunders Co., 1987.

Kirkpatrick CH: Delayed Hypersensitivity. In: Santer M, et. al. (eds). Immunologic Disease, Boston, Little, Brown and Co., 1988, pp. 261-277.

AUTHOR
John Jandinski, DMD

Cor Pulmonale

BASICS

DESCRIPTION
Enlargement of the right ventricle secondary to diseases of the lung, thorax, or pulmonary circulation. Right ventricular failure results from the lung disease. Twenty percent of hospital admissions for heart failure are due to associated cor pulmonale. More than 50% of patients with chronic obstructive pulmonary disease (COPD) have cor pulmonale.

ETIOLOGY

Severity of right ventricular enlargement (cor pulmonale) is function of the magnitude of the increase in pulmonary arterial afterload. Afterload increases secondary to pulmonary vascular diseases or parenchymal pulmonary diseases. Reasons for increased right ventricular afterload:
• When lung volume is enlarged (COPD), secondary to lengthening of pulmonary vessels and compression of alveolar capillaries.
• When lung volume is reduced (pulmonary resection) or with compressed and distorted vessels (restrictive lung disease).
• Hypoxic pulmonary vasoconstriction (hyperventilation), as seen with obstructive sleep apnea and is made worse by hypercarbia.
• Polycythemia or increase in hematocrit associated with chronic hypoxemia will increase blood viscosity and increase the pulmonary hypertension.
Pulmonary Vascular Diseases:
• Right ventricular afterload is elevated secondary to restriction to pulmonary blood flow.
• Chronic cor pulmonale may result from repeated pulmonary emboli, pulmonary vasculitis, pulmonary vasoconstriction secondary to high altitude and pulmonary venocclusive disease.
• When the course of elevated pulmonary resistance is unknown, the condition is referred to as primary pulmonary hypertension.

SYSTEMS AFFECTED
Pulmonary
Right heart

DIAGNOSIS

SYMPTOMS AND SIGNS
Acute Cor Pulmonale:
◇ History of sudden onset of dyspnea and cardiovascular collapse in a patient predisposed to venous thrombosis.
◇ Low cardiac output with pallor, sweating, hypotension, and tachycardia.
◇ Neck veins are distended with prominent V waves of tricuspid regurgitation.
◇ Liver may be pulsatile, distended and tender.
◇ May see a murmur of tricuspid regurgitation at left sternal border and a presystolic gallop (S4).
◇ Blood gases show hypoxemia and decreased $PaCO_2$ due to hyperventilation.
Chronic cor pulmonale secondary to pulmonary vascular disease:
◇ Breathlessness is a characteristic feature.
◇ Anterior chest pain due to dilation of root of the pulmonary artery or right ventricular ischemia may occur.
◇ Hepatomegaly and ankle edema may be seen.
◇ Right ventricular heave along left sternal border.
◇ Fixed splitting of the second heart sound with protodiastolic gallop (S3) heard on inspiration.
• Prominent A and V waves in the jugular pulse are seen.
Chronic obstructive pulmonary disease (COPD)
◇ History of productive cough, dyspnea, and wheezing.
◇ Hypoxia secondary to hypoventilation is usually worse at night and may be associated with obstructive sleep apnea.
◇ Increased in chest diameter.
◇ May see peripheral edema and hepatojugular reflux.

LABORATORY
Elevated hematocrit

IMAGING/SPECIAL TESTS
Radiologic
◇ the pulmonary trunk and hilar vessels are enlarged on chest radiograph. In COPD may see hyperinflation and increased A-P dimension. Ventilation/perfusion lung scans and systemic venography revealing thrombosis may reveal embolic disease.
ECG
◇ reveals P pulmonale (right axis deviation and right ventricular hypertrophy).
Echocardiography
◇ shows increased thickness of right ventricular wall, interventricular septum may be displaced leftward.
MRI
◇ useful to measure right ventricular mass, wall thickness, cavity volume, and ejection fraction.
Cardiac catheterization
◇ used to measure pulmonary vascular pressures and confirm vascular obstruction.
Lung biopsy
◇ may demonstrate vasculitis in diseases such as collagen vascular disease, rheumatoid arthritis, and Wegener's granulomatosis.
Pulmonary function studies
◇ reveal airflow obstruction with hypoxemia and hypercarbia. $FEV_1 < 1.0L$ and $PaO_2 < 60$ mm Hg.

TREATMENT

DIFFERENTIAL
General
◇ stop smoking, moderate sodium restriction, phlebotomy sometimes useful.

MEDICATIONS
• Improve alveolar ventilation by increasing inspired O_2.
• Bronchodilators and antibiotics lessen the airflow obstruction and diuretics relieve the edema.
• Digitalis may be used in presence of ventricular failure, and phlebotomy should be considered when the hematocrit exceeds 55 percent.
• Acute cor pulmonale treated with thrombolytic agents and/or heparinization.

CONSULTATION SUGGESTIONS
Pulmonologist

REFERRAL SUGGESTIONS
Primary Care Physician

FIRST STEPS TO TAKE IN AN EMERGENCY
• Sudden appearance of respiratory distress, administer oxygen and activate EMS. Administer BLS as necessary.

PATIENT INSTRUCTIONS
Confer with physician if symptoms develop or worsen. Avoid smoking and high altitudes.

COURSE/PROGNOSIS
• If etiology determined, prognosis depends on its control.
• Presence of cor pulmonale confers poor prognosis with 3-year survival rate at approximately 40 percent.

CODING

ICD-9-CM
415.0 Cor pulmonale (acute)
416.9 Cor pulmonale (chronic)

MISCELLANEOUS

SYNONYMS
Pulmonary hypertension

SEE ALSO
Valvular heart diseases
Heart failure

REFERENCES
Internal Medicine for Dentistry, 2nd ed. Rose LF, Kaye D (eds), St. Louis, CV Mosby Co. 1990.

Butler J, Braunwald E: Cor Pulmonale. In: Harrison's Principles of Internal Medicine 13th ed. Isselbacher et al (eds), New York, McGraw-Hill, Inc., 1994, pp. 1085-1088.

AUTHOR
Jerry L. Jones, DDS, MD

Corneal Ulceration

BASICS

DESCRIPTION
A defect in the cornea with absence of epithelium and underlying stromal loss. Ulceration may be central and/or marginal in location and frequently is or becomes (secondarily) infected.

ETIOLOGY

Infectious
◇ bacterial is the most common infectious etiology (Staphylococcus, Pseudomonas, Haemophilus); fungal (Candida); viral (herpes simplex).
Noninfectious
◇ traumatic abrasion, collagen vascular disease.

SYSTEMS AFFECTED
Limited to globe and periorbital tissue.

DIAGNOSIS

SYMPTOMS AND SIGNS
• Red eye, mild to severe ocular pain, photophobia, blurred vision, excessive tearing.
• Focal opacities in corneal stroma, conjunctival injection, corneal thinning, stromal edema and inflammation, mucopurulent discharge, upper eyelid edema.

IMAGING/SPECIAL TESTS
Slit-lamp examination using fluorescein, corneal scrapings for Gram stain, smears, and cultures.

DIFFERENTIAL
• Dry eye syndrome (Sicca syndrome)
• Rheumatoid arthritis or other collagen vascular diseases
• Keratoconjunctivitis
• Neurotrophic keratopathy
• Vitamin A deficiency
• Foreign body

TREATMENT

Medications

Noninfectious

◇ a cycloplegic eye solution, and prophylactic antibiotic ointment, such as erythromycin or tobramycin, then patch eye.

Infectious

◇ broad spectrum topical antibiotic (polymyxin B/Bacitracin ointment), ciprofloxacin, cephalosporins with or without aminoglycoside such as gentamicin or tobramycin.

Fungal infections
◇ systemic antifungal agents such as ketoconazole or amphotericin B, then patch eye.

CONSULTATION SUGGESTIONS

Ophthalmologist

REFERRAL SUGGESTIONS

Ophthalmologist

FIRST STEPS TO TAKE IN AN EMERGENCY

• Cover affected eye
• Remove foreign body from inside of eyelid by everting lid.

PATIENT INSTRUCTIONS

Keep eye patched while corneal heals.

COURSE/PROGNOSIS

Good if diagnosed early and treatment instituted

 CODING

ICD-9-CM

370.0 Corneal ulcer

 MISCELLANEOUS

SEE ALSO

Conjunctivitis

REFERENCES

Lam S, Rapuano C, Krachmer J: Cornea and External Disease. In: Ophthalmic Essentials. Vrabec M. Florakis G. (eds), Oxford: Blackwell Scientific 1992, pp. 106-109.

Cullom R, Chang B: In: The Willis Eye Manual, Philadelphia, JB Lippincott Co., 1994, pp. 69-73.

AUTHOR

Michael J. Buckley, DMD, MS

Coronoid Hyperplasia

 ## BASICS

DESCRIPTION
A disorder that results in the limitation of mandibular opening due to the impingement of the coronoid process on the medial and anteromedial surface of the zygomatic arch. The condition may result from unilateral or bilateral enlargement.

 ## ETIOLOGY

• The etiology of this disorder is unknown, although many theories exist. Most hypotheses characterize the disorder as being hyperplastic in nature.
• A history of trauma is present in many cases, but a definite relationship between the traumatic event and the onset of the coronoid growth is unreliable.
• Most cases have been reported to occur in males in their late teens, and x-linked transmission is suspected by some. The condition has also been reported in females, casting discredit on the hereditary etiology.
• Patients with loss of condylar support have demonstrated coronoid enlargement secondary to increased pull of the temporalis muscle.
• An osteochondroma of the coronoid process may result in impingement on the zygomatic arch and mimic coronoid hyperplasia.

SYSTEMS AFFECTED
The manifestations of coronoid hyperplasia are limited to restriction of movement of the mandible. Mandibular opening, lateral excursive, and protrusive movements are decreased.

 ## DIAGNOSIS

SYMPTOMS AND SIGNS
• A painless limitation in mandibular opening and excursion of the mandible. A positive "end-stop" can be appreciated, and forcing further opening is unsuccessful. In cases of bilateral hyperplasia, all excursions are diminished. In unilateral cases, excursions are diminished but the patient may have a normal lateral movement toward the affected side.
• When the condition occurs in males, it is often first noticed when the patient reaches puberty and becomes progressively worse with time, and reaches the maximum restriction in the teenage years. Normal occlusion typically present.

IMAGING/SPECIAL TESTS
• A panorex is the most useful radiograph, showing elongation of the coronoid processes, which will often appear longer than the condyle. Superimposition of the zygomatic arch onto the coronoid process is evident.
• The temporomandibular joints will show normal architecture on imaging.

DIFFERENTIAL
• Internal derangements of the temporomandibular joint
• Osteochondroma
• Scleroderma
• Tetanus
• Myositis ossificans

Coronoid Hyperplasia

 TREATMENT

SURGERY
• Surgical removal of the coronoid process (coronoidectomy) is the recommended treatment. Following stripping of the insertion of the temporalis muscle, the superior portion of the coronoid is removed. Some surgeons maintain the muscle insertion and allow the coronoid process to retract superiorly following an osteotomy; however, reattachment or fusion to the zygomatic arch may occur. The procedure is most commonly performed through a transoral approach.
• Aggressive postoperative physical therapy with active range of motion exercises is mandatory.

CONSULTATION SUGGESTIONS
Oral-Maxillofacial Surgeon

REFERRAL SUGGESTIONS
Oral-Maxillofacial Surgeon

COURSE/PROGNOSIS
Following coronoidectomy and physical therapy, a significant increase in the mandibular range of motion is noticed. Rarely, the coronoid may redevelop to an elongated form, and the procedure may have to be repeated.

 CODING

ICD-9-CM
213.1 Mandible, benign neoplasm
524.0 Unspecified anomaly coronoid hyperplasia
524.5 Abnormal jaw closure
715.9 Osteoarthrosis; degenerate joint disease; mandibular condyle

CPT
21041 Excision of benign tumor of mandible; complex
21070 Coronoidectomy
70100 Radiologic exam, mandible; partial, less than four views
70355 Panorex
97265 Physical therapy; joint mobilization

 MISCELLANEOUS

SEE ALSO
TMJ intracapsular and extracapsular disorders

REFERENCES
Kreutz RW, Sanders B: Bilateral coronoid hyperplasia resulting in severe limitation of mandibular movement. Oral Surg Oral Med Oral Path 60:482-484, 1985.

Marra LM: Bilateral coronoid hyperplasia: A developmental defect. Oral Surg Oral Med Oral Path 55:10-13, 1983.

Hecker R, Corwin JO: Bilateral coronoid hyperplasia: Review of the literature and report of case. J Oral Maxillofac Surg 38:606-608, 1980.

AUTHOR
Robert Rudman, DDS

Costochondritis

BASICS

DESCRIPTION
An inflammatory condition resulting in pain localized to the costosternal cartilaginous junctions. Occurs in patients ages 20 to 40, and most commonly affects females.

ETIOLOGY

Idiopathic
◇ in most cases, no definite cause can be identified.
Coughing
◇ violent coughing may precede the onset.
Trauma
◇ compression of the thoracic cage can precipitate or result in subluxation/separation of the costosternal joints.
Overuse
◇ overstrenuous exercise, sport injury.

SYSTEMS AFFECTED
Costosternal joint
◇ overlying skin appears normal and no obvious abnormality is noticeable. A single costal cartilage is affected in 80% of patients (the second and third being the most common).
Tietze's syndrome
◇ firm swellings of the costochondral junctions that are tender and reddened, but not warm. Affects both males and females equally, and the age of onset is usually under 40.

DIAGNOSIS

SYMPTOMS AND SIGNS
• Sharp pain that is unilateral and paramidline to the sternum. May be most noticeable when lying in bed. Deep breathing and coughing may also elicit pain.
• Tenderness to palpation that is clearly localized to one or more of the costal cartilages.

LABORATORY
Leukocytosis may occur.

IMAGING/SPECIAL TESTS
Chest radiograph and ECG in patients over 40 years of age.

DIFFERENTIAL
• Angina pectoris
• Pericarditis
• Upper abdominal disorder
• Pulmonary infarction
• Metastatic tumor
• Rheumatoid arthritis
• Ankylosing spondylitis
• Reiter's syndrome
• Xyphoidynia
• Rib trauma
• Herpes zoster
• Anxiety disorder
Hyperventilation

TREATMENT

MEDICATIONS
• Nonsteroidal anti-inflammatory medications are often effective.
• Refractory cases may respond to local anesthetic or corticosteroid injections.

CONSULTATION SUGGESTIONS
Rheumatologist

REFERRAL SUGGESTIONS
Primary Care Physician

PATIENT INSTRUCTIONS
Advise patient disease self-limited and to avoid overuse trauma.

COURSE/PROGNOSIS
The onset can be acute or insidious. Spontaneous remission may occur, or the pain can last for years.

 CODING

ICD-9-CM
733.6   Tietze's syndrome
733.99 Costochondritis
756.3   Costosternal subluxation

CPT
64450 Introduction/injection of anesthetic agent, diagnostic or therapeutic
71010 Radiologic examination, chest, single view, frontal
90782 Therapeutic or diagnostic injection (corticosteroid)
93000 Electrocardiogram, with at least 12 leads; with interpretation and report.

 MISCELLANEOUS

SYNONYMS
Costosternal syndrome
Tietze's disease

SEE ALSO
Angina pectoris
Herpes zoster
Pericarditis

REFERENCES
Gilliland BC: Relapsing polychondritis and miscellaneous arthritides. In: Harrison's Principles of Internal Medicine, 13th ed. Isselbacher KJ, et al (eds). New York, McGraw-Hill, Inc., 1994, p. 1708.

Hazelman BL: Other Inflammatory Arthritides. In: Oxford Textbook of Medicine, 2nd ed. Weatherall DJ, Ledingham JG, Warrell DA (eds). Oxford, Oxford University Press, 1987, p. 1660.

Murray JF: Respiratory Diseases. In: Cecil Textbook of Medicine, 12th ed. Wyngaarden JB, Smith LH (eds). Philadelphia, WB Saunders, Co., 1985, p. 378.

AUTHOR
Robert Rudman, DDS

Craniopharyngioma

BASICS

DESCRIPTION
• Neoplasm usually found in the region of the pituitary gland whose anterior lobe is derived from embryologic Rathke's pouch. Histologically, lesion is almost identical to the calcifying odontogenic cyst (Gorlin's cyst). It has also been compared to ameloblastomas. Clinical behavior and recurrence/persistence rates relate better to the calcifying odontogenic cyst.
• Usually manifested in childhood, but 45% present in patients over age 20, and 20% are over age 40 at time of diagnosis.

ETIOLOGY

• Acenohypophysis, the glandular secretory anterior lobe of the pituitary, is embryologically derived from Rathke's pouch. Epithelial remnants can form neoplasms, cysts, or cystic neoplasms.
• Lesion can form anywhere along craniopharyngeal duct or location of Rathke's pouch remnants.
• The infundibulum is also derived from Rathke's pouch.

SYSTEMS AFFECTED
• Parasella
  ◇ location the most common site, with suprasellar location the most common.
• Nasopharyngeal lesions have been reported.
• Third ventricle and hypothalamic regions can be involved.
• Widespread secondary effects can be seen due to mass effect on endocrine function of the pituitary.
• Suprasellar location can lead to optic chiasm involvement with resultant visual field disturbances.

DIAGNOSIS

SYMPTOMS AND SIGNS
• Mass effect at site of tumor growth including:
• Hypothyroid-induced cold intolerance, weight gain, and myxedema
• Hypoadrenal-induced fatigability and orthostatic hypotension
• Visual field defects
• Headaches
• Mental status abnormalities
• Diabetics insipidus symptoms of thirst, frequent urination, and decreased urine-specific gravity.
• Gait disturbances
• Galactorrhea
• Papilledema
• Growth retardation in children
• Fifty percent of suprasellar childhood neoplasms are craniopharyngiomas
• Optic atrophy (visual changes in 80% of adults)
• Children usually present with hydrocephalus and associated headache, vomiting, and papilledema.

LABORATORY
Preliminary endocrine studies possibly indicated include
• Luteinizing hormone level
• TSH level
• Fasting cortisol level
• Cortisol 30 and 60 minutes after ACTH
• Free T3 uptake
• Prolactin level

IMAGING/SPECIAL TESTS
• Calcifications can be seen, and lesion is most often suprasellar.
• Sellar enlargement present about 30% of the time. Simple way to examine cephalographic film for sellar enlargement is to place a dime over the sella; if it does not completely cover the sella, then sella is enlarged. Normal sella size anterior-posteriorly is 17 mm (dimes are 18 mm in diameter).
• Computed tomography is test of choice for maximum lesion delineation. Contrast is helpful in enhancing the lesion.
• MRI and/or angiography may be helpful in surgical access work-up.
• Biopsy often possible.

DIFFERENTIAL
Pituitary adenoma
Rathke's cleft cyst

TREATMENT

MEDICATIONS
• Intracystic radioactive colloid has been used.
• Both pre- and postsurgical hormonal therapy may be necessary.

SURGERY
• Visual disturbances may benefit from simple fluid aspiration.
• Surgical approach depends on exact location of the lesion and the proximity to other structures. Obstruction of the foramen of Monro or the third ventricle may also be a complicating factor.
• Typically, most difficult decision is whether to attempt complete removal or to attempt a sub-total removal.
• Recurrence rate is approximately 71% when sub-total removal and 25% when lesion supposedly totally removed.

IRRADIATION
Sub-total removal with combined radiotherapy has a reported 21% recurrence rate.

CONSULTATION SUGGESTIONS
Endocrinologist

REFERRAL SUGGESTIONS
Otolaryngologist, Neurosurgeon

PATIENT INSTRUCTIONS
Seek treatment immediately

COURSE/PROGNOSIS
• Most commonly seen in children but can be seen in all age groups.
• Craniopharyngiomas comprised 2 to 4% of all brain tumors.
• Postsurgical and postradiation quality of life issues continue to be major problems.
• Tumors less than 3 cm in diameter have better prognosis.

CODING

ICD-9-CM
237.0 Craniopharyngioma

CPT
70450 CT, head or brain
70451 CT, head or brain, with contrast
70480 CT, sella
70481 CT, sella with contrast
70350 Cephalogram, orthodontic
70240 Radiographic exam, sella turcica

MISCELLANEOUS

SYNONYMS
Pituitary ameloblastoma
Rathke's pouch tumor
Adamaminoma craniopharyngoma
Suprasellar cyst

REFERENCES
Tindall GT, Barrow DI, Martin JB: Disorder of the pituitary. St. Louis, CV Mosby, 1986, pp.321-348.

Sanford RA, Muhlbauer MS: Craniopharyngioma in children. Neurologic Clin 9:453-463, 1991.

Bryne MN, Sessions DG: Nasopharyngeal craniopharyngioma. Case report and literature review Ann Otol Rhin Laryngol 99:633-639, 1990.

Crane TB, Yee RD, Hepler RS, Hallinan JM: Clinical manifestations and radiologic findings in craniopharyngiomas in adults. Am J Ophthalmol 94:220-228, 1982.

AUTHOR
John W. Hellstein, DDS

Crohn's Disease

BASICS

DESCRIPTION
Chronic granulomatous disease may occur anywhere in the gastrointestinal tract from the mouth to the anus. The ileum is most often involved. Patients typically present with mild diarrhea, abdominal pain, lassitude, and weight loss. Usual onset is ages 15 to 25, with second, smaller peak at ages 55 to 65.

ETIOLOGY

• Genetic factors appear to play a role. Increased incidence of disease noted in monozygotic twins and siblings. Whites of North American and European decent, especially Ashkenazi Jews, are much more likely to have Crohn's disease than are those of African or Middle-Eastern descent.
• An HLA correlation within the general population has not been found to-date. Even within families, patients do not necessarily share the same HLA type.
• Infectious agents have been theorized, but to-date never identified. Injected extract of Crohn's disease tissue in mice induces an inflammatory response and may reflect a transmissible agent such as an RNA virus or a cell wall-defective bacterium, possibly mycobacterium.
• An immunologic mechanism is the most prominent theory. Bacterial cell products and toxins may be involved in the proinflammatory response. Once the inflammatory process has begun, a host of destructive inflammatory mediators are released that include leukotrienes, prostaglandins, platelet activating thromboxanes, oxygen radicals, and proteases.

SYSTEMS AFFECTED
Oral:
  ◇ buccal aphthous ulcers, angular stomatitis, or glossitis.
Lower G.I. tract:
  ◇ Transmural involvement of colon and/ or small bowel and formation of adhesions between adjacent loops of bowel and between bowel and other abdominal organs such as the bladder. Fistulas may form from bowel segment to bowel segment, and sometimes to skin. The inflamed areas may occur in "skip" areas separated by segments of relatively nonaffected bowel. Perianal fistulae are common.
• Megaloblastic, hemolytic, and Fe^{++} deficiency anemia.
• Growth or sexual retardation probably due to reduced caloric intake.
• Hepatobiliary disorders including gallstones, percholangitis, fatty liver, nonspecific hepatitis, cirrhosis, and sclerosing cholangitis.
• Renal involvement can include right ureteral obstruction secondary to contiguous bowel involvement and nephrolithiasis. Also an increase in calcium oxalate and uric acid stones.
• Episcleritis, corneal infiltrations and uveitis may occur in 3 to 10% of patients.
• Articular manifestations occur in 10 to 20% of patients and include anklylosing spondylitis, which is associated with HLA-B27, and a peripheral, migratory, nondeforming arthritis involving the large joints.

• Skin problems include erythema nodosum, which parallels disease activity.

DIAGNOSIS

SYMPTOMS AND SIGNS
• Small intestine involvement characterized by colicky pain, often postprandial, that is localized to the periumbilical areas or the lower quadrants. Most patients have low-grade fever and weight loss. Diarrhea is common but usually not severe or bloody. Malabsorption and nutritional deficiencies. May mimic peptic ulcer disease.
• Thin, ill-appearing, pale patient, with muscle wasting.
• Low-grade fever
• Buccal aphthous ulcers, angular stomatitis, or glossitis.
• Abdominal exam may reveal a mass in the right lower quadrant.
• Occult or gross blood in the stool and possibly perianal disease such as scarring, abscess, sinus tracts, fissures, and fistulas.

LABORATORY
CBC
◇ anemia due to folate, B12, or Fe^{++} deficiency from blood loss. Leukocytosis and elevated sedimentation rates.
• Hypoalbuminemia resulting from mucosal protein loss.
• Send stool for culture and sensitivity, rule out ova and parasites.

IMAGING/SPECIAL TESTS
• Barium swallow studies demonstrate the presence of strictures, narrowings, and fistulas. Inflamed bowel may have a "cobblestone" appearance and a "string" sign in the transverse colon.
• Endoscopic examination may show deep ulcerations, stricturing, patchy or symmetric involvement.
• Mucosa biopsy
◇ submucosal inflammation, thickening, and fibrosis. Noncaseating granulomas found in serosa.

DIFFERENTIAL
• Intestinal tuberculosis
• Lymphoma
• Enteric pathogens (Yersinia, Amebiasis, C. difficile, Campylobacter)
• Carcinoid tumor
• Radiation enteritis
• Ulcerative colitis

TREATMENT

General
◇ Supportive measures and use of anti-inflammatory and immunosuppressant agents.
◇ Bowel rest.
◇ Normal diet with low residue if there are strictures.

MEDICATIONS
• Supplemental Fe^{++}, calcium, folate, and B_{12} as needed.
• Symptomatic agents
◇ including anti-diarrheals and antispasmodics.
• 5-ASA compounds
◇ sulfasalazine (2 to 4 g daily), olsalazine, oral 5-ASA (mesalamine), topical 5-ASA & 4-ASA.
• Corticoids
◇ oral corticosteroids (40 to 60 mg of prednisone), parenteral corticosteroids, parenteral ACTH, and topical steroids.
• Immunosuppressants
◇ azathioprine, 6-mercaptopurine, cyclosporine.
• Antibiotics
◇ metronidazole up to 750 mg t.i.d.

SURGERY
Surgery may be necessary for recurrent intestinal obstruction, enterocutaneous fistulae, and/or intra-abdominal abscesses.

CONSULTATION SUGGESTIONS
Primary Care Physician, Gastroenterologist, Infectious Disease Specialist

REFERRAL SUGGESTIONS
Primary Care Physician

PATIENT INSTRUCTIONS
Contact Crohn's and Colitis Foundation for useful patient information, (800)343-3637.

COURSE/PROGNOSIS
• Crohn's disease is marked by exacerbations followed by relative periods of remission. Flareups are characterized by anorexia, vomiting, weight loss, abdominal pain, and dehydration. As a result of small bowel resection, patients can be plagued by bacterial overgrowth and malabsorption sequellae. Decreased bile salt absorption, for example, increases the incidence of gallstones. Additionally, calcium becomes saponified and is unavailable to react with oxalate. This eventually leads to an abnormally high amount of oxalate absorption. The result of this high amount of absorption is the formation of oxalate stones and, finally, chronic renal failure.

• Patients with Crohn's disease have a higher incidence of small bowel carcinoma.

CODING

ICD-9-CM
555.9 Regional enteritis (site unspecified)

MISCELLANEOUS

SYNONYMS
Granulomatous colitis
Regional enteritis

SEE ALSO
Ulcerative colitis
Diarrhea

REFERENCES
Fishman M: Medicine, 3rd ed., Philadelphia, JB Lippincott Co., 1991.
Geier D: New therapeutic agents in the treatment of inflammatory bowel disease. Am J Med 93, Aug. 1992.

AUTHOR
Jonathan S. Sasportas, DMD, MD

Cystic Fibrosis

BASICS

DESCRIPTION
An autosomal recessive disease characterized by abnormally thick secretion from mucous glands, pancreatic insufficiency, and an increase in the concentration of sodium and chloride in the exocrine glands.

ETIOLOGY

A genetic defect that encodes for a membrane protein that functions as an ion channel. This protein, cystic fibrosis transmembrane conductance regulator (CFTR), does not function as ion channel in CF patients thereby reducing epithelial salt and water secretion that leads to dehydration of epithelial surfaces, which initiates the pathology of the disease.

SYSTEMS AFFECTED
Multisystems involved at various times during the progression of the disease.
Gastrointestinal System:
Initially, the newborn may have an intestinal obstruction (meconium ileus).
• Pancreatic enzyme insufficiency.
• Large frequent stools. Steatorrhea and creatorrhea, and malabsorption.
• Manifestations, including failure to grow, vitamin deficiency.
• Liver changes, including focal biliary cirrhosis, fatty infiltration.
Pulmonary System:
Viscous secretions
• Rapid respiratory rate
• Faint, hacking cough (may be paroxysmal)
• Nasal polyposis
• Frequent infections with bronchial obstruction (Pseudomonas has been implicated).
• Pulmonary hypertension
Reproductive System:
Male sterility
• Female sterility, and increase in viscosity of vaginal secretions
General:
Salt depletion and heat exhaustion
Dental:
Enamel hypoplasia, anterior open bite (apertognathia), salivary gland involvement, and mouth breathing have been associated with CF.

DIAGNOSIS

SYMPTOMS AND SIGNS
• Hacking cough
• Wheezing
• Dyspnea
• Frequent and large bowel movements
• Excessive appetite
• Failure to grow (or thrive)
• "Salty sweat"
• Intestinal obstruction (meconium ileus)
• High content of albumin in meconium
• Increase in lactase activity
• Steatorrhea/creatorrhea/fat soluble vitamin deficiency
• Increased respiratory rate
• Signs related to pulmonary infection, including, atelectasis, emphysema, bronchitis, pneumonia, hemoptysis, respiratory failure
• Nasal polyposis

LABORATORY
Hypoproteinemia
Anemia
Hypoprothrombinemia

IMAGING/SPECIAL TESTS
• 72-hour fecal fat excretion test
• Test stool for trypsin and chymotrypsin
• Properly performed and interpreted sweat test (quantitative pilocarpine iontophoresis).
• Secretion of LCK-P2 tests demonstration, severe bicarbonate output impairment, and pancreatic enzymes.
• Chest radiograph will reveal patchy atelectasis and air trapping
• Pulmonary function tests
• Sputum culture and sensitivity
• Genetic testing

DIFFERENTIAL
• Immunodeficiency
• Chronic pulmonary diseases
  ◊ bronchitis, pneumonias (recurrent), asthma.
• Dyskinetic cilia
• Because of the implications of a diagnosis of CF, care must be taken in arriving at this diagnosis. Clinical suspicion must correlated with the various special tests.

TREATMENT

General
◇ High fat, high protein diet
◇ High caloric diet (150% of normal caloric requirements)
◇ Prevention of pulmonary infection
◇ Education and cooperation of all involved healthcare workers

MEDICATIONS
• Pancreatic enzyme supplements (Pancrease, Creon)
• Multivitamins (double RDA)
• Salt tablets to decrease incidence of heat exhaustion
• Bronchodilators/aerosols
• Antibiotics for pulmonary infection
• Clinical trials include antiproteases amiloride, a sodium channel blocker, and DNASE
• Gene therapy is also being explored.

CONSULTATION SUGGESTIONS
Primary Care Physician, Pulmonologist, Endocrinologist.

REFERRAL SUGGESTIONS
Primary Care Physician

PATIENT INSTRUCTIONS
Contact Cystic Fibrosis Foundation (800)344-4823 for patient information.

COURSE/PROGNOSIS
In recent years great strides have been made in understanding and treating CF. However, significant morbidity and mortality do prevail. The survival rate seems to be increasing each year, with the mean survival rate at approximately 25 years.

CODING

ICD-9-CM
277.0 Cystic Fibrosis

MISCELLANEOUS

SYNONYMS
Mucoviscoidosis disease

SEE ALSO
Pancreatitis

REFERENCES
Boucher RC: Cystic fibrosis. In: Harrison's Principles of Internal Medicine, 13th ed., New York, McGraw-Hill, Co. 1994. pp. 1194-1197.

Harris A, Argent BE: The cystic fibrosis gene and its product CFTR. Sem Cell Biol 4:37-44, 1993.

Abrons HL: Cystic fibrosis current concepts. W Va Med J 89:236-240, 1993.

Althen ML, Fiel SB: Cystic fibrosis. Disease-a-Month Jan. 391-452, 1993.

Femald GW, Roberts MW, Boat TF: Cystic fibrosis: a current review. Pediatr Dent 12:72-78, 1994.

AUTHOR
Thomas P. Sollecito, DMD

Deep Vein Thrombosis (Thrombophlebitis)

 BASICS

 ETIOLOGY

 DIAGNOSIS

DESCRIPTION
Thrombosis of veins usually occurs in the lower extremity and generally in the prolonged recumbent or bedridden patient. Inflammation (phlebitis) may become a component. Deep vein thrombosis (DVT) is a common condition of postoperative and hospitalized patients. DVTs may progress to a very serious or fatal event of pulmonary embolism.

Virchow postulated three mechanisms:
• Endothelial cell damage (wall abnormalities)
  • Vasculitides, e.g., in Buerger's disease
  • Vein wall trauma (IV catheters)
• Hypercoagulability
  • Pregnancy (oral contraceptives)
  • Antithrombin III, Protein C and S deficiencies
  • Cancer
• Stasis
  • Hospitalized, traumatic or bedridden patient
  • Hypotension (sepsis)
  • Polycythemia (sludging effect 2° hyperviscosity)
  • History of phlebitis (incompetent veins) with venous stasis

Risk Factors
  ◇ Cancer
  ◇ Obesity
  ◇ Varicose veins
  ◇ Previous venous thrombosis
  ◇ Pregnancy (postpartum)
  ◇ Trauma, or surgery, especially pelvis, lower extremities
  ◇ Immobility
  ◇ Age > 60 yrs.
  ◇ High altitude (>14,000 feet)
  ◇ Oral contraceptive use (risk proportional to estrogen content)
  ◇ Indwelling catheters

SYSTEMS AFFECTED
• Lower extremity veins
  - Calf muscle veins (deep veins/ sinuses)
  - Extension into saphenous or femoral veins
• Extension to iliofemoral veins
• Upper extremity thrombosis (usually associated with central IV line placement)
• Thromboembolism with clots to lungs (pulmonary embolism)

SYMPTOMS AND SIGNS
• Aching, tightness in calf or thigh
• Pain increases on walking or movement
• Swelling of ankle, calf or thigh, depending upon position of clot
Clots to lungs
  ◇ dyspnea, palpitations, chest pain
• 40% of patients with DVT have signs of tender, swollen extremity
  • circumference larger than unaffected leg
  • usually warm; if cool, then artery also affected (see phlegmasia alba dolens)
• Fever, leukocytosis (if phlebitic)
• Palpable "cord" (superficial thrombophlebitis)
• Iliofemoral clot
  • Phlegmasia alba dolens; pale, cool leg with pitting edema; may also be associated with arterial spasm
  • Phlegmasia cerulea dolens; severe thrombosis with secondary arterial insufficiency, decreased sensory/ motor function and gangrene.

LABORATORY
CBC/differential
  ◇ leukocytosis if phlebitis
Coagulation profile
  ◇ PT, PTT, bleeding time
• Arterial blood gas if suspect pulmonary embolism
• Protein C and S, antithrombin III, antiphospholipid levels

IMAGING/SPECIAL TESTS
• Doppler ultrasound
  • Sensitivity > 90%; specificity low
  • Better for proximal (thigh) than distal (calf)
• Duplex ultrasound
  • Real time B-mode ultrasound plus doppler flow analysis
  • Blood flow direction and turbulence
  • Sensitivity/Specificity > 95%
• Impedance plethysmography
  • Outflow obstruction detected
  • Better for proximal clots
• Radio-labeled fibrinogen
  • Uptake by clot
  • Better for distal clots
  • Not accurate in infected, fractured or healing extremities
• Contrast venography (gold standard)

DIFFERENTIAL
• Lymphatic obstruction (lymphedema)
• Baker's (synovial) cysts compressing vein
• Cellulitis (acutely inflamed)
• Arterial clot or occlusion (absent pulse, cool, decreased sensory/motor)
• Vascular malformation (venous or arterio-venous)

• Pulled, strained or torn muscle/ligament

TREATMENT

• Prophylaxis
• Reduce venous stasis
  • Early ambulation
  • Pneumatic leg compression until ambulatory
• Prophylactic anticoagulation
  • Mini-heparin administration
  • 5000 u s.q. 2 hrs preop and b.i.d. postop

MEDICATIONS
• Anticoagulation
• Heparin infusion (to increase PTT 1 1/2 to 2 times baseline PTT) for 7 to 10 days.
• Dextran; allergic reactions, bleeding, exacerbation of heart failure may occur
• Oral coumadin therapy (increase PT to 1 1/2 times baseline PT) usually reserved for prophylaxis in long-term treatment
• Fibrinolysis
• Streptokinase, urokinase, recombinant human tissue plasminogen activator (tPA)
• Bleeding common
• Reserved for extensive clots
• Contra-indicated in postop, stroke, or trauma patient

SURGERY
• Venous thrombectomy
  • For iliofemoral or massive clots
  • Must be performed early (within 24 hours)
  • Anticoagulation necessary to prevent re-clotting
• Venous (caval) interruption
  • Indicated for patients who cannot be anticoagulated or who have had recurrent pulmonary embolism
  • Inferior vena cava filter to entrap clots
  • Caval ligation or partial clipping to prevent thromboembolism

CONSULTATION SUGGESTIONS
• Primary Care Physician, Vascular Surgeon

REFERRAL SUGGESTIONS
• Primary Care Physician, Vascular Surgeon

FIRST STEPS TO TAKE IN AN EMERGENCY
• Heparinize

PATIENT INSTRUCTIONS
Avoid prolonged immobility

COURSE/PROGNOSIS
• Most patients with no risk factors will resolve DVT without sequelae. Patients with risk factors (especially recurrences) will require long-term anticoagulation measures.
• The mortality rate is significant for hospitalized patients who have DVT complicated by massive pulmonary embolism.
• Recurrent DVT and development of venous insufficiency (through destruction of venous valves) may develop chronic stasis ulcers, lymphedema, and increased pigmentation of the affected lower extremity (usually below knee).

CODING

ICD-9-CM
451.19 Deep vein thrombosis

MISCELLANEOUS

SYNONYMS
DVT

SEE ALSO
Cellulitis
Pulmonary embolism

REFERENCES
Litin SC, Gastineau DA: Current concepts in anticoagulant therapy. Mayo Clinic Proc 70:266-272, 1995.

Shattil SJ: Diagnosis and treatment of recurrent venous thromboembolism. Med Clin N Am 68:577-601, 1984.

Hyers TM, et al: Antithrombotic therapy for venous thromboembolic disease. Chest 89 (Suppl): 265, 1986.

Coon WWL: Venous thromboembolism: prevalence, risk factors, and prevention. Clin Chest Med 5:391-405, 1984.

Moser KM: Pulmonary thromboembolism. In: Harrison's Principles of Internal Medicine, 13th ed. Isselbacher KJ, et. al. (eds) New York, McGraw-Hill Co., 1994, pp. 1218-1220.

AUTHOR
Bruce Horswell, DMD, MD

Delirium Tremens

BASICS

DESCRIPTION
A phenomenon characterized by hallucinatory episodes, severe agitation, insomnia, muscle cramps, and fever that may occur during withdrawal from chronic alcohol abuse.

ETIOLOGY

Withdrawal or abstinence from chronic alcohol consumption is the precipitating factor. Alcohol and many other drugs may directly interfere with central nervous system synaptic transmission. In delirium following alcohol withdrawal, the excited state may result from the sudden overactivity of a previously depressed transmitter system that has developed the equivalent of denervation hypersensitivity.

SYSTEMS AFFECTED
Neurologic
 ◊ excited state resulting in severe agitation, tremors, hallucinations, and generalized tonic-clonic seizures.
Cardiovascular
 ◊ sympathetic autonomic hyperactivity causes tachycardia and hypertension.
Gastrointestinal
 ◊ nausea and vomiting may result secondary to the excited state.
Muscles
 ◊ become cramped and sore due to tremors, shakes, and seizures; also electrolyte derangements may contribute to spasms.
Skin
 ◊ flushing and sweating are common secondary to sympathetic hyperactivity.

DIAGNOSIS

SYMPTOMS AND SIGNS
Neurologic
 ◊ hallucinations, agitation, anxiety, jitters and shakes (tremors), headache, tonic-clonic seizures.
 • Cardiac tachycardia, palpitations, hypertension.
Skin
 ◊ sweating, flushing, warm (from fever).
Gastrointestinal
 ◊ abdominal cramping, nausea, vomiting, hepatomegaly.
Muscles
 ◊ cramps and soreness

LABORATORY
• Electrolytes and glucose
• Liver function tests

IMAGING/SPECIAL TESTS
• ECG (if cardiac disease is suspected or present).
• Chest radiograph (if pulmonary disease is suspected or present).

DIFFERENTIAL
• Drug withdrawal (eg, heroin, barbiturates, etc.)
• Epilepsy
• CNS infection (meningitis, encephalitis)
• Metabolic encephalopathies (diabetic ketoacidosis, renal failure, liver failure).
• Psychiatric disorder

TREATMENT

General
◇ Hospitalization may be necessary but as a general rule, outpatient detoxification can be considered for mild abstinence syndromes.
◇ Thorough physical examination to evaluate organ systems likely to be impaired by heavy drinking, including looking for evidence of cardiac dysrhythmia, liver failure, gastrointestinal bleeding, head trauma, and glucose/electrolyte imbalance.
◇ Adequate nutrition including multiple B vitamins.
◇ Bedrest
◇ Psychiatric counseling

MEDICATIONS
• Benzodiazepines
◇ (eg, diazepam 10 to 20 mg or chlordiazepoxide 25 to 50 mg every 6 hours given orally on the first day). The dose is then decreased by approximately 20% on successive days over the next 3 to 5 days.
• Anticonvulsants
◇ such as phenytoin are reserved for seizures if they are prolonged or recurrent.
• Beta adrenergic blockers
◇ propranolol.
• Alpha adrenergic blockers
◇ clonidine.
• Vitamin B
◇ especially thiamine 50 to 100 mg, should be given orally every day for a week or more.

CONSULTATION SUGGESTIONS
Neurologist, Psychiatrist

REFERRAL SUGGESTIONS
Primary Care Physician

FIRST STEPS TO TAKE IN AN EMERGENCY
• Begin administration of diazepam or librium, titrating IV until tremor or extreme anxiety improves.

PATIENT INSTRUCTIONS
Withdrawal from chronic ethanol best done under physician's care.

COURSE/PROGNOSIS
A true medical emergency that is usually resolved in 3 to 5 days with proper treatment. Patients with the greatest morbidity and mortality are those with high fever, tachycardia, dehydration, and associated illness such as pneumonia, cardiac disease, pancreatitis, or hepatitis.

CODING

ICD-9-CM
291.0 Delirium tremens
291.1 Korsakoff's psychosis
291.3 Hallucinosis
303.9 Alcoholism
909.1 Late effect nonmedical substance (facial fractures)

MISCELLANEOUS

SYNONYMS
Alcohol withdrawal syndrome
Alcohol withdrawal delirium
DTs

SEE ALSO
Seizure disorders
Alcohol abuse

REFERENCES
Thompson WL: Management of alcohol withdrawal seizures. Arch Intern Med 138:278-283, 1978.

Rubino FA: Neurologic complications of alcoholism. Psychiatric Clinics N Am 15:359-372, 1992.

Brown CG: The alcohol-withdrawal syndrome. Western J Med 138:579-581, 1983.

Liskow BI, Goodwin DW: Pharmacological treatment of alcohol intoxication, withdrawal and dependence. J Stud Alcohol 48:356, 1987.

AUTHOR
Joseph J. Sansevere, DMD

Dementia

BASICS

DESCRIPTION
• Characterized by the development of multiple cognitive deficits (including memory impairment) that are due to the direct effects of a general medical condition, to the persisting effects of a substance, or to multiple etiologies. Dementias share a common symptom presentation but different etiologies.
• Prevalence over age 65 is ten percent.
• Types of dementia include: Alzheimer's type, vascular dementia, dementia due to HIV disease, Parkinson's disease, Huntington's disease, Pick's disease, other general medical conditions, substance-induced persisting dementia, and dementia due to multiple etiologies. Primary degenerative dementia of the Alzheimer type is the most common type of dementia. Other causes include: vascular disease (multi-infarct dementia); central nervous system infections (including tertiary neurosyphilis, tuberculosis and fungal meningitis, viral encephalitis, human immunodeficiency virus [HIV]-related disorders, {AIDS, AIDS-related complex-[ARC]}, and Jakob-Creutzfeldt disease); brain trauma (especially chronic subdural hematoma); toxic metabolic disturbances; neurologic degeneration, progressive supranuclear palsy, and postanoxic or posthypoglycemic degeneration.

ETIOLOGY

Organic brain disorder; associated with aging and cerebral atherosclerosis, but may have other causes. Before age 70 frequently of unknown and untreatable causes. See description under basics.

SYSTEMS AFFECTED
Central Nervous System

DIAGNOSIS

SYMPTOMS AND SIGNS
• Memory impairment (short- and long-term) prominent initial symptom – usually moderate short-term memory loss; impaired abstract thinking is variable.
• Impaired judgment and impulse control
• Aphasia [language disturbance (ie, difficulty naming objects)]
• Agnosia (failure to recognize or identify objects despite intact sensory functions)
• Apraxia (inability to carry out motor activities despite intact comprehension and motor function)
• Disturbance in executive function (ie, planning, organizing, sequencing); personality change
• May be accompanied with delirium, paranoia, delusions, or depression
• Weight loss
• Tremors
• Oral injuries common from falls. Be alert to signs of elder abuse. Poor oral hygiene is typical; dentures commonly misplaced.

LABORATORY
Thyroid, syphilis, serum B_{12}, CBC, metabolic profile

IMAGING/SPECIAL TESTS
Mental status exam, depression test, neuropsychological testing.

DIFFERENTIAL
• Delirium
• Depression
• Schizophrenia
• Alcoholism
• Normal aging

TREATMENT

General
◊ Treat secondary causes with medications.

Outpatient
◊ socialization
◊ adult care; family therapy
◊ support and education; behavior modification
◊ written and visual cues, schedules, sensory stimulation (eg, prominent clocks), pharmacotherapy
◊ treating secondary causes (ie, specific behaviors or conditions).

MEDICATIONS
• Sundowning, aggressive behaviors
◊ antipsychotics
◊ haloperidol (Haldol);
• Depression
◊ desipramine (Norpramin), fluoretine (Prozac)
• Sleep disturbances
◊ lorazepam (Ativan), triazolam (Halcion)
• Neuroleptic medications may induce agranulocytosis, leukopenia, and thrombocytopenia (rule-out with CBC) with secondary ulceration, infection, bleeding, candida or stomatitis. Elective dental treatment should not be undertaken if there is significant bone marrow suppression (WBC < 3000 per mm or granulocyte count < 1500 per mm).
• Neuroleptics also induce extrapyramidal side effects including xerostomia and movement disorders (tardive dyskinesia, mandibular tics, spasm of perioral and jaw muscles, and dysphagia with secondary drooling). High-dose or long-term use of neuroleptics may cause tachycardia, orthostatic hypotension, or blood pressure fluctuations. Anticholinergics, antihistamines, and beta-blockers may be used to control these side effects. Anticholinergic properties may contribute to sedation, hypotension, and body temperature elevations.
• Drug interactions in dentistry with neuroleptics
◊ epinephrine
◊ severe hypertension; CNS depressants
◊ additive sedation; atropine
◊ increased anticholinergic effect.
Use local anesthetics without vasoconstrictor whenever possible, and never more than 3 cartridges. Aspirate before injecting. Avoid topical epinephrine in retraction cord. Avoid use of atropine. Decrease dosage of sedative, hypnotics, or narcotics.

• Potential long life expectancy (>10 yrs)
◊ complete restorative and prosthetics early in disease while patient can adapt to new situations and express dental concerns. Begin fluoride and frequent recall so patient becomes accustomed to program as patient will be unable to tolerate change of usual routine later in disease. Always reintroduce yourself and staff. Use concrete expressions and short phrases to communicate. Simplify tasks for patients.

CONSULTATION SUGGESTIONS
Mental Health Professional

REFERRAL SUGGESTIONS
Primary Care Physician

FIRST STEPS TO TAKE IN AN EMERGENCY
• If extrapyramidal reaction occurs give cogentin or diphenhydramine (Benedryl).

PATIENT INSTRUCTIONS
If Alzheimer's diagnosed, call Alzheimer's Association (800)621-0379 for helpful literature.

COURSE/PROGNOSIS
May be progressive, static, or remitting. Reversibility a function of the underlying pathology, and of the availability and timely application of effective treatment.

CODING

ICD-9-CM
290.0 Senile dementia, uncomplicated
290.10 Dementia, Alzheimer's type
290.40 Multiple infarct dementia
331.0 Alzheimer's disease

MISCELLANEOUS

SYNONYMS
Senility

SEE ALSO
Alzheimer's disease

REFERENCES
Papas A, Niessen L, Chauncey H: Geriatric Dentistry: Aging and Oral Health. St. Louis, CV Mosby, 1991, pp. 34-36.

Hazzard W, et al: Principles of Geriatric Medicine and Gerontology. 2nd ed. New York, McGraw Hill, 1990, pp. 934-1096.

Scully C, Cawson RA: Medical Problems in Dentistry. Oxford. Butterworth Heinemann, 1993.

American Psychiatric Association. Diagnostic and Statistical Manual of Mental Disorders, DSM-IV, Washington, DC, 1994.

AUTHORS
Hillary Broder, PhD, MEd
Kani Nicolls, DDS

Dental Fluorosis

BASICS

DESCRIPTION
Generalized enamel defects due to excessive fluoride intake that may be mild to severe. Mild fluorosis is manifested as a defect in the calcification of the teeth. Severe fluorosis includes significant pigmentation and ameloblast impairment.

ETIOLOGY

Dental fluorosis occurs during the later pre-eruptive phase of tooth formation. Therefore, regardless of the amount of fluoride exposure, no fluorosis occurs before the infant is 11 months of age. Ingestion of systemic fluoride that is above 1.8 parts per million per day is deemed excessive, and is likely to produce enamel defects. The critical period of exposure for the dental incisors for teeth perceived as aesthetically important, as well as for the first molars, occurs between 24 to 27 months of age.

SYSTEMS AFFECTED
Disruption of enamel formation during the later pre-eruptive stage of mineralization.

DIAGNOSIS

SYMPTOMS AND SIGNS
Discoloration of dental enamel, mild brown to dark brown-black coloration.

DIFFERENTIAL
Amelogenesis imperfecta
Extrinsic staining

Dental Fluorosis

TREATMENT

General
◇ Aesthetical restorative treatment may be indicated in certain patients with bonding or placement of crowns.
Prevention
◇ Fluorosis has been associated with the fluoride concentration of drinking water, use of dietary fluoride supplements, early use of fluoride-containing dentifrices, and prolonged use of infant formula. The risk of fluorosis is increased among young children who ingest higher dosages of supplement than are indicated, or ingest them while receiving optimally fluoridated water.
• Often, fluoride supplements are prescribed based on insufficient information regarding the fluoride concentration in the patient's water supply. As of 1994, the Council on Dental Therapeutics adopted a revised fluoride supplement dosage schedule, which should be observed by pediatricians and dentists prescribing fluoride supplements (Table below).
• Dentists should inquire their patients about fluoride and/or vitamin dietary supplements that may contain fluoride that are prescribed by physicians, to ensure optimal daily ingestion of fluoride.
• Certain parts of the U.S., particular areas of the Southwest (New Mexico, Arizona) have local water supplies with excessive fluoride concentrations. In those areas, parents should have water tested for fluoride concentration. Concentration above 1.8 ppm should trigger use of alternative drinking water source for children during dental development.

MEDICATIONS
• Revised Fluoride Dosage Schedule
• Fluoride concentration in drinking water (ppm) /Fluoride supplement per day (mg).
• Age: 0 to 6 months
  <0.3 ppm/0 mg
  0.3 to 0.6 ppm/0 mg
  >0.6 ppm/0 mg
• Age: 6 months to 3 years
  <0.3 ppm/0.25 mg
  0.3 to 0.6 ppm/0 mg
  >0.6 ppm/0 mg
• Age: 3 to 6 years
  <0.3 ppm/0.50 mg
  0.3 to 0.6 ppm/0.25 mg
  >0.6 ppm/0 mg
• Age: 6 to 16 years
  <0.3 ppm/1.00 mg
  0.3 to 0.6 ppm/0.50 mg
  >0.6 ppm/0 mg

SURGERY
Dental esthetic bonding, or, less desirable, crowns.

CONSULTATION SUGGESTIONS
Fluoride Testing Agency (available at many dental schools), Pediatric Dentist

REFERRAL SUGGESTIONS
Family Dentist, Pediatric Dentist

PATIENT INSTRUCTIONS
Follow supplemental fluoride instructions carefully. Test water for fluoride concentration.

COURSE/PROGNOSIS
Prevention best method of management. Once problem occurs, it can only be managed by esthetic dentistry. Fluoride changes of enamel assist in caries prevention.

CODING

ICD-9-CM
520.3 Dental fluorosis

CPT
41899 Unlisted dentoalveolar procedure
82735 Testing water for fluoride concentration

MISCELLANEOUS

SEE ALSO
Congenital defects of enamel
Discolorizations of teeth

REFERENCES
Burt BA, Eklund SA: Dentistry, dental practice, and the community. Philadelphia, WB Saunders Co., 1992, pp. 137-156.

AUTHOR
Maria Rosa Watson, DDS, MS, MPH

Dermatitis - Perioral Dermatitis

BASICS

DESCRIPTION
A persistent erythematous eruption composed of tiny papules and papulopustules.

ETIOLOGY

• Most frequently associated with overuse of potent topical corticosteroids such as clotrimazole/betamethasone dipropionate, fluocinoinide, and desoximethasone.
• Often a pre-existing mild facial eruption was present for which topical corticosteroids were used.
• Fluoride-containing and tartar control toothpastes, as well as toothpaste flavoring and preservatives have been implicated for both acneiform eruption and contact dermatitis.
• Pathophysiologically related to acne rosacea.

SYSTEMS AFFECTED
Skin
  ◇ perioral dermatitis with relation to cosmetics may include involvement of forehead, periorbital skin, cheeks, and nasolabial folds.
Nose/Eyes
  ◇ frequent perinasal and periocular lesions.

DIAGNOSIS

SYMPTOMS AND SIGNS
• Itching, burning, and rash
• Small, grouped, erythematous papules, vesicles, or pustules located periorally and infraorbitally.
• Diffuse scaling and pruritic perioral patches of erythema separated by normal skin.

LABORATORY
Histologic findings are nondiagnostic

DIFFERENTIAL
• Contact or allergic dermatitis
• Atopic dermatitis
• Seborrheic dermatitis
• Acne rosacea
• Psoriasis
• Thermal or chemical burn

TREATMENT

General
◇ Prompt discontinuation of topical corticosteroids.
◇ Avoid long-term prescriptions for potent topical corticosteroids.
◇ Discontinuation of any agent that may be implicated in a contact dermatitis.

MEDICATIONS
• Systemic and topical antibiotics such as tetracycline (contraindicated in children) or erythromycin, if felt to be secondarily infected. If contact dermatitis suspected, use high potency topical steroid such as fluocinonide 0.05% ointment (Lidex) 3 to 4 times daily in all areas except skin folds where use should be minimal. Continue only as long as required due to risks of prolonged use such as atrophy or production of telangiectasias.
• Corticosteroid-free antipruritic such as benzocaine, if due to chronic steroid applications.

CONSULTATION SUGGESTIONS
Dermatologist

REFERRAL SUGGESTIONS
Oral medicine

PATIENT INSTRUCTIONS
• Use medications as prescribed.
• Avoid frequent licking of lips.
• Keep perioral area free of excessive moisture.

COURSE/PROGNOSIS
Following a 1 to 2 month course of oral tetracycline, treatment is usually effective and recurrence is rare.

CODING

ICD-9-CM
690 Seborrheic dermatitis
691.8 Atopic dermatitis
692.9 Dermatitis (allergic) (contact)
692.9 Acneiform dermatitis
696.2 Psoriasis nodularis dermatitis

MISCELLANEOUS

SEE ALSO
Contact dermatitis
Thermal or chemical burns

REFERENCES
Regezi JA, Sciubba JJ: Oral Pathology Clinical Pathologic Correlations. 2nd ed. Philadelphia, WB Saunders Co., 1993, pp. 24-26.

Wells K, Brodell RT: Topical corticosteroids "addiction." A cause of perioral dermatitis. Postgrad Med 93:225-230, 1993.

Veien NK, et al: Topical metronidazole in the treatment of perioral dermatitis. J Am Acad Derm 24:688-692, 1992.

Beacham BE, Kurgan D, Gould WM: Circumoral dermatitis and cheilitis caused by tartar control dentifrices. J Amer Acad Derm 22:1029-1032, 1990.

AUTHOR
Paul A. Danielson, DMD

Dermoid Cyst

 BASICS

DESCRIPTION
• Cystic lesion that can be found in many areas of the body. About 2% of cystic lesions are found on the head and neck region and, when in the oral cavity, usually occur in the anterior floor of the mouth with division into three types: epidermoid, dermoid, and teratoid.
• Distinction is made by the lining and contents of the cyst. The epidermoid form has a squamous epithelium with a fibrous wall and no adnexal structures; the dermoid with an epithelial wall and skin appendages (ie, hair follicles and sebaceous glands); and the teratoid form has stratified squamous to respiratory epithelium and multiple structures derived from mesoderm and endoderm in the cyst wall. All configurations may contain a cheesy, keratin material.

 ETIOLOGY

Dermoid cyst in the head and neck region is said to be related to implantation of epithelium with subsequent cystic breakdown or to developmental entrapment of multipotential cells. Traumatic implantation of cells has also been suggested. Dermoids can be classified as median or lateral, depending on location. The median occurs between the genioglossus and geniohyoid muscles and close to the floor of the mouth, with the lateral type located between the mylohyoid, genioglossus, and geniohyoid muscles involving the floor of the mouth. The lesion can grow to several centimeters in size with a "doughlike" feel to palpation. These lesions are often seen in young adults.

SYSTEMS AFFECTED
Oral mucosa and skin
◊ often seen as raised or swollen secondary to cyst development
Epithelium, mesoderm, endoderm
◊ all of these tissues can be involved presenting as: epithelial lining, hair, hair follicles, sebaceous glands, muscle, cartilage, and alimentary tissues.
Tongue
◊ can be raised or deflected depending upon the size and location of the lesion.

 DIAGNOSIS

SYMPTOMS AND SIGNS
Mouth
◊ pain or discomfort affecting floor of mouth or tongue. Elevation in floor of mouth with deflection of tongue. Speech may be affected.
Face
◊ pain, swelling, or discomfort in submental region.

IMAGING/SPECIAL TESTS
MRI
◊ study of choice to properly evaluate the extent and position of the lesion.

DIFFERENTIAL
• Dermoid cyst
• Salivary gland tumor
• Cystic hygroma
• Branchial cyst
• Thyroglossal duct cyst
• Neurofibroma
• Hemangioma
• Infectious (actinomycosis, cat-scratch disease)

TREATMENT

SURGERY
Complete surgical excision via an intraoral approach. Recurrence is rare.

CONSULTATION SUGGESTIONS
Oral-Maxillofacial Surgeon

REFERRAL SUGGESTIONS
Oral-Maxillofacial Surgeon

PATIENT INSTRUCTIONS
Lesions tend to continue to enlarge if not removed.

COURSE/PROGNOSIS
Lesions can grow to very large size with interference of oral activities. Prognosis is excellent for complete cure following removal.

CODING

ICD-9-CM
528.4 Dermoid cyst

CPT
10160 Puncture aspiration of abscess, hematoma, bulla, or cysts
40800 Drainage of abscess, cyst, hematoma, vestibule of mouth; simple
40801 Drainage of abscess, cyst, hematoma, vestibule of mouth; complicated
41000 Intraoral incision and drainage of abscess, cyst, or hematoma of tongue or floor of mouth; lingual
41005 Intraoral incision and drainage of abscess, cyst, or hematoma of tongue or floor of mouth; sublingual, superficial
41006 Intraoral incision and drainage of abscess, cyst, or hematoma of tongue or floor of mouth; sublingual, deep, supramylohyoid
41007 Intraoral incision and drainage of abscess, cyst, or hematoma of tongue or floor of mouth; submental space
41008 Intraoral incision and drainage of abscess, cyst, or hematoma of tongue or floor of mouth; submandibular space
41009 Intraoral incision and drainage of abscess, cyst, or hematoma of tongue or floor of mouth; masticator space
41015 Extraoral incision and drainage of abscess, cyst, or hematoma of floor of mouth; sublingual
41016 Extraoral incision and drainage of abscess, cyst, or hematoma of floor of mouth; submental
41017 Extraoral incision and drainage of abscess, cyst, or hematoma of floor of mouth; submandibular
41018 Extraoral incision and drainage of abscess, cyst, or hematoma of floor of mouth; masticator space
41800 Drainage of abscess, cyst, hematoma from dentoalveolar structures
41825 Excision of lesion or tumor (except listed above), dentoalveolar structures; without repair
41826 Excision of lesion or tumor (except listed above), dentoalveolar structures; with simple repair

MISCELLANEOUS

SYNONYMS
Cyst (mouth)

SEE ALSO
Neck mass

REFERENCES
Sciubba J, Regezi JA: Oral Pathology. 2nd ed. Philadelphia, WB Saunders Co., 1993, pp. 353-356.

Black EE, et al: Dermoid cyst of the floor of the mouth. Oral Surg Oral Med Oral Path. 74:556-558, 1992.

Reddy VS, et al: Lingual dermoid. J Pediatr Surg. 26:1389-1390, 1991.

Clark MJ, et al: Review of the literature and report of a case of a dermoid cyst. Texas Dent J. 108:15-18, 1991.

AUTHOR
Lawrence T. Herman, DMD

Diabetes Insipidus

 BASICS

DESCRIPTION

A condition characterized by excessive water intake and hypotonic polyuria, usually due to the failure of vasopressin (AVP) release in response to normal physiologic stimuli (central or neurogenic diabetes insipidus), or the failure of the kidney to respond to AVP (nephrogenic diabetes insipidus).

 ETIOLOGY

• The antidiuretic hormone, vasopressin, is required to maintain the normal osmotic pressure of plasma. Increased plasma osmolality associated with dehydration stimulates neurohypophyseal terminals in the supraopticohypophyseal tract to release vasopressin. In the kidney, AVP acts on the distal renal tubules and collecting ducts to increase reabsorption of water. Deficiency of AVP or lack of kidney response is characterized by water diuresis and secondary polydipsia.
• Vasopressin deficiency or failure of renal response to vasopressin is rarely genetically based, and is usually due to secondary causes.
Major causes include:
  • Neoplasms or infiltrative lesions of the hypothalamus or pituitary
  • Pituitary or hypothalamic surgery
  • Trauma or head injuries usually associated with skull fractures in which the pituitary stalk is injured or is compromising its vascular supply.
  • Idiopathic diabetes insipidus can begin in childhood, and is usually not associated with anterior pituitary dysfunction.
  • Lithium and the antibiotic demeclocycline may produce a type of nephrogenic diabetes insipidus.
  • May appear during pregnancy and cease after delivery or commence after parturition in women with Sheehan's syndrome

SYSTEMS AFFECTED
Endocrine

 DIAGNOSIS

SYMPTOMS AND SIGNS
Polyuria, excessive thirst, and polydipsia almost invariably present. Also may have nocturia, headache, visual disturbance and dehydration.

LABORATORY
• Serum and urine glucose usually normal.
• Hypernatremia common in younger patients.

IMAGING/SPECIAL TESTS
• Chest and bone radiographs may reveal sarcoid or eosinophilic granuloma, which are important causes of diabetes insipidus.
• Brain MRI
• Dehydration test
  ◊ urinary and serum osmolality are measured after fluid deprivation and then after vasopressin is administered. A significant rise in urine osmolality is a positive test result.
• Administer desmopressin (DDAVP) to test renal responsiveness to vasopressin.

DIFFERENTIAL
• Psychogenic polydipsia.
• Nephrogenic diabetes insipidus.
• Other states of osmotic diuresis (diabetes mellitus, renal disease, use of various diuretics, excessive salt intake).
• Drug-induced polydipsia (chlorpromazine or anticholinergic drugs).

TREATMENT

General
◇ Hormonal replacement for deficiency
◇ Nephrogenic or neurogenic diabetes insipidus is treated by sodium restriction and use of thiazide diuretics.

MEDICATIONS
• Oral administration is ineffective; drug is given either intranasally or subcutaneously.
• -Arginine vasopressin is used by subcutaneous route
• -Desmopressin (DDAVP) is most common drug used, and is given intranasally (10 to 25 ug) or subcutaneously (2 to 4 ug) b.i.d.

CONSULTATION SUGGESTIONS
Endocrinologist

REFERRAL SUGGESTIONS
Endocrinologist, Primary Care Physician

FIRST STEPS TO TAKE IN AN EMERGENCY
• Water restriction

PATIENT INSTRUCTIONS
Compliance with water restriction instructions critical to recovery.

COURSE/PROGNOSIS
• Deficiency of vasopressin usually permanent and requires lifetime replacement therapy.
• Prognosis of other forms of diabetes insipidus dependent upon treatment of underlying condition.
• Symptoms and normalization of urine/plasma osmolality occur with use of hormone replacement. Long-term course dependent on underlying diagnosis

CODING

ICD-9-CM
253.5 Diabetes insipidus

MISCELLANEOUS

REFERENCES
Rose LF, Kay D: Internal Medicine for Dentistry. St. Louis, C.V. Mosby Co. 1990, p. 996.

Robinson AG: DDAVP in the treatment of central diabetes insipidus. N Engl J Med 294:507, 1976.

Moses AM, Streeten DH: Disorders of the neurohypophysis. In: Harrison's Principles of Internal Medicine, 13th ed. Isselbacher KJ, et al (eds). New York, McGraw-Hill, 1994, pp. 1923-1928.

AUTHOR
Jerry L. Jones, DDS, MD

Diabetes Mellitus

 BASICS

DESCRIPTION
A genetically and clinically heterogeneous group of disorders that are characterized by hyperglycemia resulting from decreased insulin secretion and/or effectiveness. Diabetes mellitus (DM) is classified as either insulin dependent diabetes mellitus (IDDM) or non-insulin dependent diabetes mellitus (NIDDM). Complications arising from DM include diabetic ketoacidosis (DKA) or non-ketotic hyperglycemic hyperosmolar coma (NKHHC), and also late stage complications such as microvascular disease (retinopathy and nephropathy), macrovascular disease (coronary artery, cerebrovascular and peripheral vascular diseases), neuropathic disease, foot ulcers, dermopathies and infections (periodontal and vulvovaginal).

Incidence
◊ DM is a common disorder with an estimated prevalence of 2 to 4% in the USA, of which 10 to 15% are insulin-dependent diabetics. Approximately 25% of all end-stage renal failure patients are diabetics, as are 50% of all lower extremities amputees. Diabetes is also the leading cause of blindness in the USA.

 ETIOLOGY

The etiology of IDDM is unknown; however, it is thought that following an initial insult to the beta cells of the pancreas, there is a slow auto-immune destruction of the beta cells. This is borne out by the presence of serum islet cytoplasmic antibodies or islet cell surface antibodies in approximately 90% of all IDDM patients at time of diagnosis, although this drops to being evident in only 5 to 10% after 20 years of the disease. Presentation of these antibodies is followed by a decrease in insulin production, deterioration in glucose tolerance, and the onset of the clinical disease. Because of the decreased or nonexistent insulin production, IDDM patients are more prone to present with acute complications of the disease (polyuria, polydipsia, polyphagia, and ketoacidosis) and require chronic insulin therapy. Onset of IDDM most commonly occurs during childhood or early adolescence coinciding with puberty. Patients with this disorder are usually of normal weight or thin. There is thought to be less of a genetic link to IDDM than NIIDM, with IDDM showing less than 50% concordance rate amongst twins as compared to an almost 100% concordance rate in NIIDM twins.

SYSTEMS AFFECTED
Endocrine/Metabolic
◊ insulin insufficiency versus resistance
Eyes
◊ deterioration of vision
Immune
◊ cellular immunodeficiency (lymphocytes, neutrophils) with poor handling of bacterial and fungal infections.
Vascular
◊ premature atherosclerotic changes
Neurologic
◊ peripheral neuropathies

 DIAGNOSIS

SYMPTOMS AND SIGNS
• Hypoglycemia can result in the presentations of many symptoms. Polyuria and nocturia occur when the plasma glucose concentration exceeds the renal threshold for reabsorption (180 mg/dL plasma glucose) causing a glucosuria and resultant osmotic diuresis. This osmotic diuresis leads to dehydration and hyperosmality causing thirst and polydipsia. This spillage of glucose in the urine can result in significant weight loss and stimulation of the appetite (polyphagia). Candida of the oral and vaginal cavities that appears resistant to therapy is highly suspicious of DM, and will be difficult to control until the plasma glucose levels are brought under control. Hyperglycemia will also lead to complaints of general fatigue.
• Diagnosis of diabetes mellitus is confirmed by the presence of any of the following:
  1. Presence of the classic symptoms of diabetes together with a gross and unequivocal elevation of plasma glucose.
  2. Elevated fasting glucose concentration on more than one occasion of greater than 140 mg/dL.
  3. Fasting glucose concentration less than 140 mg/dL, but sustained elevated glucose concentration during the glucose tolerance test on at least two trials.
• The purpose of monitoring patients with DM is to identify those at risk of symptomatic hyperglycemia, DKA or NKHHC, and late complications.

LABORATORY
• Serum glucose, electrolytes, creatinine (fasting)
• CBC
• Urine glucose and ketones

IMAGING/SPECIAL TESTS
• Glucose tolerance test
• Hemoglobin A_1C
  ◊ tests amount of chronic hyperglycemia
• C-peptide insulin levels
• Islet-cell and thyroid antibodies
• HLA typing
• ECG in adults

DIFFERENTIAL
• Cushing's disease or steroid use
• Renal glucosuria
• Pancreatic disease (pancreatitis, cystic fibrosis)
• Salicylate poisoning
• Glycogen storage disease
• Multiple endocrine adenomatosis
• Pheochromocytoma
• Stress hyperglycemia

TREATMENT

General
◇ Normalize serum glucose as much as is feasible
◇ Regular exercise of similar intensity
◇ Appropriate diabetes exchange diet [American Diabetes Association (ADA)]
◇ ADA support groups
◇ Foot care

MEDICATIONS
• Insulin
◇ human or pure pork.
• Types
◇ NPH, lente, regular, ultralente
• Given in daily 1, 2, 3 or 4 dose patterns or by infusion pump
• Common 2 dose pattern -
• NPH/Lente and regular in 2:1 ratio before breakfast and supper. Morning dose 1/2 to 2/3 of total daily dose.

SURGERY
When surgery contemplated, consider effects of diabetes on vasculature and wound healing. Also, although well-controlled diabetics seem able to resist infection, they handle invasive infections relatively poorly. Prophylactic antibiotics for invasive surgery but not routine extractions.

IRRADIATION
Oral hypoglycemics
First generation
◇ tolbutamide, tolazamide, chlorpropamide
Second generation
◇ glyburide, glipizide
Oral agents and insulin sometimes both used in NIDDM.

CONSULTATION SUGGESTIONS
Primary Care Physician, Endocrinologist

REFERRAL SUGGESTIONS
Primary Care Physician, Endocrinologist

FIRST STEPS TO TAKE IN AN EMERGENCY
• If hypoglycemic (insulin shock) suspected, give glucose source orally or intravenously. Parenteral glucagon or epinephrine alternatives.
• If hyperglycemic, administer insulin and/or summon EMTs.

PATIENT INSTRUCTIONS
• Contact local Diabetes Association for literature.
• Monitor blood glucose as recommended by Primary Care Physician or Endocrinologist.

COURSE/PROGNOSIS
IDDM
◇ initial remission (honeymoon) phase with no supplemental insulin needs followed by progressively increased insulin needs. With good glucose control, complications minimized or delayed. Eye, vascular, neurologic problems occur later in life and life expectancy may be shortened.
NIDDM
◇ complications may occur with poor control of serum glucose, weight, and diet.

CODING

ICD-9-CM
250.0 Diabetes mellitus
250.01 Diabetes mellitus without complications (juvenile)
250.11 Diabetes mellitus with complications (juvenile)
250.2 Diabetes mellitus with hyperomolarity
250.4 Diabetes mellitus with renal manifestations
250.5 Diabetes mellitus with eye manifestations
250.6 Diabetes mellitus with neurologic manifestations
250.7 Diabetes mellitus with peripheral vascular disease
250.8 Diabetes mellitus with other specified manifestations
250.9 Diabetes mellitus with unspecified manifestations

CPT
90780 IV infusion

MISCELLANEOUS

SYNONYMS
IDDM = Childhood (Juvenile) diabetes
Brittle diabetes
NIDDM = Adult onset diabetes
Nonketotic diabetes

SEE ALSO
Diabetes insipidus

REFERENCES
Davidson MB: Diabetes mellitus. 3rd ed. New York, Churchill Livingstone, 1991.

Foster DW: Diabetes mellitus. In: Harrison's Principles of Internal Medicine. 13th ed. Isselbacher KJ, et. al (eds). New York, McGraw-Hill, 1994 pp. 1979-2000.

Diabetes. In: Dental Management of the Medically Compromised Patient. 4th ed. Little JW, Falace DA (eds). St. Louis, CV Mosby. 1993, pp. 341-360.

AUTHOR
Janet Leigh, BDS, DDS

Diarrhea

BASICS

DESCRIPTION
Increase in stool liquidity, weight, and frequency (chronic diarrhea defined as greater than 200 g/day stool for more than 1 month).

ETIOLOGY

Secretory
- Increased secretion or decreased absorption of Na^+ and Cl^-, (eg, in cholera, salmonella enterotoxin).

Osmotic
- Nonabsorbable substances in gut, (eg, lactose intolerance, laxative abuse, enteral tube feeds).

Inflammatory
- Intestinal mucosa inflammation with loss of solute, fluids, blood, eg, in ulcerative colitis, amebiasis, chemo/radiation enteritis

Decreased Absorption
- Due to reduced intestine after resection
- Enteric fistulae (Crohn's disease; diverticulitis)

Motility Disorder
- Increased motility, (eg, in irritable bowel syndrome), when fast transit allows poor absorption.
- Decreased motility with subsequent bacterial overgrowth, (eg, in diabetes or scleroderma, resulting in malabsorption).

SYSTEMS AFFECTED
Acute Diarrhea
Usually due to inflammatory conditions, toxins, or infections.
- Localized bowel involvement, portions of colon, or extension to all bowel.

Chronic Diarrhea
Often a mixed osmotic and secretory diarrhea.
- Secondary to underlying illness or gastrointestinal disease.
- Lactose intolerance (lactose deficiency).
- Anorectal involvement with fissuring, bloody stools; common in radiation for colorectal cancer.

Multiple small stools
◊ distal colon obstruction or after total colectomy.

Large volumes
◊ small bowel or proximal colon, eg, in celiac disease or bacterial overgrowth.

DIAGNOSIS

SYMPTOMS AND SIGNS
Frequent, loose stools
Cramping, nausea, vomiting, anorexia
◊ inflammatory bowel disease; amebic dysentery; viral illness in children.
Timing, duration
Alternating with constipation
◊ obstruction by tumor, diverticulitis, fecal impaction
Recurrent
◊ ulcerative colitis, irritable bowel
Seasonal
◊ Summer (giardiasis); Winter (Rotavirus)
- Pain often in inflammatory bowel disease or diverticulitis
Tenesmus
◊ (urgency to defecate) carcinoma, ulcerative colitis
Mucous
◊ villous adenoma, ulcerative colitis
Large, pale bulky stools
◊ pancreatic insufficiency
- Fever, weight loss, malaise, arthritis-inflammatory bowel disease; malabsorption
Tenderness
◊ infectious or inflammatory; toxins
Abdominal mass
◊ carcinoma; diverticulitis
Rectal exam
◊ polyps; granuloma; fecal impaction
Proctosigmoidoscopy
◊ friable mucosa; blood; polyps; villous adenomas, carcinoma
- Flushing-carcinoid syndromes
Neuropathy
◊ diabetic diarrhea

LABORATORY
Blood
◊ CBC with differential, electrolytes, folate/B_{12}, ESR
Stool
- WBC; Wright's stain (infectious or inflammatory)
- C. difficile toxin
- Blood, pus (colitis, infectious)
- Quantitative fat (steatorrhea)
Microbiology
◊ stool ova and parasites

IMAGING/SPECIAL TESTS
Radiographs
◊ Upper GI, small bowel (enterocolysis), barium enema
- Abdominal CT (tumor, chronic pancreatitis)
- Colonoscopy/Signoidoscopy, Upper Endoscopy
- Small bowel biopsy
- Examine pancreatic function
- D-xylose absorption tests

DIFFERENTIAL
- Celiac Disease
- Inflammatory bowel disease
- Irritable bowel syndrome

- Gastroenteritis
  - Viral illness
  - Bacterial (enterotoxins)
  - Parasitic infection
  - AIDS (venereal and nonvenereal infections)
- Pseudomembranous colitis (Clostridium difficile)
- Laxative abuse
- Chronic pancreatitis

TREATMENT

Address underlying disorder is key
Acute diarrhea
- Rehydration
- Avoid caffeine, ethanol, dairy products, fruits, red meats, vegetable fiber.
- Encourage water, clear soups, starches, sherbets
- Monitor electrolytes
- Antibiotics reserved for disabling infection in compromised patients or culture confirmed amebiasis, giardiasis, C. difficile.

MEDICATIONS
- Inflammatory bowel disease
  ◇ Prednisone
  ◇ systemic or enema
  ◇ Sulfasalazine
- Pseudomembraneous colitis
  ◇ (C. difficile toxin)
  ◇ Metronidazole (Flagyl) 250 mg t.i.d.
- Chronic diarrhea
  ◇ Cholestyramine to bind bile acids
  ◇ Bismuth (Pepto-Bismol) 2 to 16 tbsp q.d.
  ◇ Kaolin/pectin(Kaopectate) 1 to 8 tbsp q.d.
  ◇ Diphenoxylate (Lomotil) 5 to 20 mg
- Inhibits GI motility
  ◇ Loperamide (Imodium) 4 to 16 mg q.d.
  ◇ Synthetic opioid

SURGERY
Carcinoma (colo-rectal)
  ◇ bowel resection and radiation.
Blind loop (small bowel)
  ◇ resection; ileostomy; reanastomosis.
Polyposes
  ◇ resection of familial adenomatous or diffuse juvenile types.
  • Close follow-up
Diverticulitis
  • Antibiotics
    • Resection if recurrent or severe
Ulcerative colitis
  • Surgery reserved for severe, intractable colitis or dysplastic/malignant changes

CONSULTATION SUGGESTIONS
Gastroenterologist, Infectious Disease Specialist

REFERRAL SUGGESTIONS
Gastroenterologist, Primary Care Physician

FIRST STEPS TO TAKE IN AN EMERGENCY
• Ensure adequate hydration

PATIENT INSTRUCTIONS
Follow dietary and medication instructions

COURSE/PROGNOSIS
Acute diarrhea will usually resolve with supportive medical management and rehydration. Chronic diarrhea due to malabsorption, ulcerative colitis/Crohn's, irritable bowel, pancreatic insufficiency, etc., will have an involved, protracted course that will require careful, long-term surveillance and management.

CODING

ICD-9-CM
  558.9 Diarrhea

CPT
  99000 Transport specimen to outside laboratory

MISCELLANEOUS

SEE ALSO
Ulcerative colitis
Gastroenteritis
Pancreatitis
Diabetes mellitus
AIDS
Cancer, in general

REFERENCES
Gastro-Intestinal Diseases. In: Cecil Essential of Medicine. Anreoli TE, et. al. (eds.) Philadelphia, WB Saunders Co., 1990. pp. 269-275.

Jewell DP: Medical management of ulcerative colitis. Intl J Colonorect Dis 3:186-197, 1988.

Dobbins JW, Binder HJ: Pathophysiology of diarrhea. Clin Gastroenterol 10:605-620, 1981.

AUTHOR
Bruce Horswell, DDS, MD

Dilantin Hyperplasia

BASICS

DESCRIPTION
Fibrous hyperplasia of the gingival tissues. Usually observed 2 to 3 months after dilantin therapy is instituted and presents as a painless enlargement of the interdental papilla. Dilantin (phenytoin) has been used as an anticonvulsant drug that has side effects ranging from hepatic impairment to skin eruptions and erythema.

ETIOLOGY

The reason for the gingival proliferation is not well understood, although it has been suggested that there is a specific subpopulation of gingival fibroblasts that may be sensitive to the drug. The interrelationship between plaque, gingival inflammation, dosage and concentration of dilantin has been investigated extensively. Widely felt that a direct relationship exists between the soft tissue overgrowth and the level of oral hygiene. The incidence of this condition is about 50% of patients taking the drug and is reduced to 10% by meticulous oral hygiene. This would indicate that there is more involved in the etiology than local irritants alone. Dilantin does appear to have a regulating effect on fibroblast metabolism, and all fibroblasts are thought to be influenced by the drug to some extent.

SYSTEMS AFFECTED
Gingiva
◊ a painless enlargement of the interdental papilla usually seen 2 to 3 months after drug therapy begins.
Oral mucosa
◊ hypertrophic enlargement only rarely seen in edentulous patients or children prior to tooth eruption. When ill-fitting dentures are remade and excess tissue removed, recurrence is rare.

DIAGNOSIS

SYMPTOMS AND SIGNS
Mouth
◊ nonpainful enlargement of the attached gingival tissues.
Gingival hyperplasia seen 2 to 3 months after the use of the drug has commenced. Initially, surface of the gingiva shows increased stippling, and as enlargement progresses, it takes on a lobulated appearance. Degree of the enlargement may be excessive, completely covering the teeth.

LABORATORY
• Plasma and salivary concentrations of dilantin have been suggested by investigators to have correlation with the degree of gingival hyperplasia.
• Histologic inspection of tissue excised should be performed to rule out concomitant pathology.

IMAGING/SPECIAL TESTS
Panoramic or dental radiographs
◊ to assess the level of concomitant periodontal disease and rule out other pathology.
Soft tissue biopsy
◊ to confirm the diagnosis and rule out other disease.
Microscopic
◊ abundant collagen with numerous fibroblasts and varying degrees of inflammatory cells. Overlying epithelium may be hyperplastic. Capillaries may be prominent.

DIFFERENTIAL
• Hormonal (ie, pregnancy) hyperplasia
• Cyclosporine-induced gingiva hyperplasia
• Nifedipine-induced gingival hyperplasia
• Leukemia
• Hereditary gingival fibromatosis (idiopathic hyperplasia)
• Local factors (poor oral hygiene, mouth breathing) in physically or mentally compromised patients.

TREATMENT

General
<u>Oral hygiene</u>
◊ essential in the management of this condition. Can often control the process without the need for surgery.
• Psychological counseling
• Possible switch to other anticonvulsant medications if condition difficult to control

MEDICATIONS
• Chlorhexidine may help reduce plaque.

SURGERY
<u>Gingivoplasty or gingivectomy</u>
◊ often necessary to debulk the overgrowth but should always be done in conjunction with heroic oral hygiene efforts.

CONSULTATION SUGGESTIONS
Periodontist, Oral-Maxillofacial Surgeon, Oral Medicine, Neurologist

REFERRAL SUGGESTIONS
Periodontist, Oral-Maxillofacial Surgeon

PATIENT INSTRUCTIONS
Maintain strict oral hygiene.
Regular visits to dentist and hygienist for monitoring and hygiene assistance.

COURSE/PROGNOSIS
Most patients can be managed with good oral hygiene and surgical debulking. Cessation of dilantin usage results in gradual reduction in the bulk of the gingival tissue. However, patients must be managed with other drugs for their underlying seizure problem.

CODING

ICD-9-CM
523.1 Gingivitis chronic

CPT
41820 Gingivectomy, excision gingiva, each quadrant
41821 Operculectomy, excision pericoronal tissues
41872 Gingivoplasty
70355 Panorex

MISCELLANEOUS

SYNONYMS
Gingival hyperplasia

SEE ALSO
Seizure disorders

REFERENCES
Regezi JA, Sciubba J: Oral Pathology, 2nd ed. 1993, pp. 198-202.

Chee WL, Jansen CE: Phenytoin hyperplasia occurring in relation to titanium implants: A clinical report. Intl J Oral Maxillofac Implants, 9:107-109, 1994.

Thomason JF, Seymour, Rawlins MD: Incidence and severity of phenytoin-induced gingival overgrowth in epileptic patients in general medical practice. Comm Dent Oral Epidemiol, 20:288-291, 1992.

AUTHOR
Lawrence T. Herman, DMD

Discoid Lupus Erythematosus

 BASICS

DESCRIPTION
A chronic autoimmune disease involving skin and oral mucosa. It is more common in women, with peak incidence in fourth decade.

 ETIOLOGY

Autoantibodies are deposited in basement membrane of skin and mucosa.
Sun exposure exacerbates skin lesions.

SYSTEMS AFFECTED
Skin
   ◇ face, scalp, and other sun-exposed areas most commonly involved.
Oral mucosa
   ◇ white lesions, erythema, and ulcers; usually accompanied by skin lesions.

 DIAGNOSIS

SYMPTOMS AND SIGNS
Skin
   ◇ facial lesions and alopecia may be a cosmetic problem, but are asymptomatic. Early lesion is raised, red to purple plaque covered by scale. Follicular plugging is common. Older lesions may have central atrophic scarring and hyperkeratosis at periphery. Hyper- or hypopigmentation and telangiectasia may occur. Alopecia is common.
Oral mucosa
   ◇ painful ulcers and erosions. Ulcers and erosions have white rough epithelial thickening or white striae similar to lichen planus at periphery.

LABORATORY
• Incisional biopsy of skin and/or oral mucosa for histopathology and immunopathology.
• To exclude systemic lupus: antinuclear antibodies, serum complement, CBC and differential, platelet count, rheumatoid factor, sedimentation rate, VDRL for syphilis and urinalysis.

DIFFERENTIAL
Oral lichen planus
Oral carcinoma in situ
Early squamous cell carcinoma

TREATMENT

General
◇ lesions cannot be cured, but can usually be controlled with medications. Minimize UV exposure, use sunscreens

MEDICATIONS
• Skin lesions- topical steroids, intralesional injection of steroids, antimalarial drugs.
• Oral mucosal lesions
◇ topical and/or systemic steroids. Topical corticosteroids may be used as initial treatment, as an adjunct to systemic corticosteroids, or to maintain remissions. Triamcinolone acetonide 0.1% aqueous suspension, rinse with 5 ml and expectorate, four times a day, nothing by mouth for 1 hour. (Directions to pharmacist: Dilute injectible triamcinolone 40 into 200 ml of water for irrigation, add 5 ml of 95% ethanol).
• Systemic: Prednisone 40 to 60 mg 1 hour after arising for 5 days followed by 10 to 20 mg every other day. Systemic corticosteroids are contraindicated for patients with peptic ulcer, active infections, tuberculosis incompletely treated, and other conditions. Confer with the patient's primary physician before initiating treatment.

CONSULTATION SUGGESTIONS
Dermatologist, Oral Medicine

REFERRAL SUGGESTIONS
Dermatologist, Oral Medicine, Primary Care Physician

PATIENT INSTRUCTIONS
Advise patient that no cure exists but that typically lesion can be controlled with medications. Use potent sunscreens when skin is exposed to sunlight. If steroids used, patient should warn doctors prior to surgery in case steroid supplementation indicated. May also need to wear medical alert jewelry.

COURSE/PROGNOSIS
Lesions may have exacerbations and remissions, but can usually be managed with medications.
A small percentage of patients develop systemic lupus erythematosus.

CODING

ICD-9-CM
695.4 Lupus erythematosus (discoid)

CPT
11100 Biopsy of skin, subcutaneous tissue and/or mucous membrane.
40808 Biopsy, vestibule of mouth
41108 Biopsy of floor of mouth
99000 Transport of specimen to outside laboratory.

MISCELLANEOUS

SYNONYMS
Chronic cutaneous lupus erythematosus
Discoid lupus

SEE ALSO
Lichen planus
Systemic lupus erythematosus

REFERENCES
Brown RS, Flaitz CM, Hays GL, Trejo PM: The diagnosis and treatment of discoid lupus erythematosus with oral manifestations only: A case report. Compend Contin Educ Dent 15:724-734, 1994.

Fotos PG, Finkelstein MW: Discoid lupus erythematosus of the lip and face. J Oral Maxillofac Surg 50:642-645, 1992.

Habif TP: Clinical Dermatology. A Color Guide to Diagnosis and Therapy, 2nd ed. St. Louis, CV Mosby Co., 1990, pp. 425-435.

AUTHOR
Michael W. Finkelstein, DDS, MS

Discoloration of Teeth

BASICS

DESCRIPTION
The normal whitish yellow color of teeth can be altered by numerous intrinsic and extrinsic factors.

ETIOLOGY

- Intrinsic

  Enamel hypoplasia
  ◊ occurs when ameloblasts are adversely affected by local (trauma, infection) or systemic (childhood infectious diseases) injury during the time of enamel deposition. Depending on the insult, single, multiple, or all teeth may be affected.

  Amelogenesis imperfecta
  ◊ a group of three hereditary enamel defects.

  Dentinogenesis imperfecta
  ◊ a group of three hereditary dentinal defects.

  Endogenous stains
  ◊ pulpal trauma, tetracycline, fluorosis, erythroblastosis fetalis, and other congenital diseases that result in circulating substances that are deposited during tooth development.

- Extrinsic

  Exogenous stains occur on the surface of teeth and can be caused by dietary factors (eg, coffee, tea, tobacco), by-products of chromogenic bacteria, caries, and chlorhexidine.

SYSTEMS AFFECTED
Intrinsic
◊ Amelogenesis and dentinogenesis imperfecta render the teeth more susceptible to fracture. All intrinsic discolorations are cosmetically objectionable.

Extrinsic
◊ Systemic effects are related to the causative agent (eg, coffee, tea, tobacco).

DIAGNOSIS

SYMPTOMS AND SIGNS
• Patient may complain of esthetic problems.
• Intrinsic defects are seen when teeth erupt.

Enamel hypoplasia
◊ may produce white, hypocalcified area or actual pits and irregularities in the enamel.

Amelogenesis imperfecta
◊ may present as white, yellow or brown discoloration, which may darken with time due to tendency to acquire further staining. Enamel fracture is common. Hereditary pattern depends on type.

Dentinogenesis imperfecta
◊ dentitions exhibit both a yellow brown to gray opalescent appearance. Hereditary pattern and association with osteogenesis imperfecta help to distinguish among the three types.

Endogenous stains
  Pulpal trauma
  ◊ deposition of hemoglobin breakdown-products resulting in a dark discoloration.

  Tetracycline
  ◊ produces yellow to gray colors that often fluoresce when UV light is applied.

  Fluorosis
  ◊ ranges from white enamel spots to mottled, brown, pitted enamel and results from the ingestion of greater than 1 ppm fluoride drinking water during tooth development.

  Erythroblastosis fetalis
  ◊ results in green to brown primary teeth.

Extrinsic
◊ appear after eruption and can usually be removed with abrasives.

IMAGING/SPECIAL TESTS
Ultraviolet light helpful in identifying tetracycline and congenital porphyria staining.

DIFFERENTIAL
Other congenital disorders, including congenital porphyria, neonatal liver disease (biliary atresia, hepatitis).

TREATMENT

General
Intrinsic discoloration
  Enamel hypoplasia
  ◇ primarily cosmetic, but in severe
      forms restorative procedures are
      needed to prevent gross caries.
  Amelogenesis imperfecta
  ◇ cosmetic restorations.
  Dentinogenesis imperfecta
  ◇ treatment is aimed at prevention
      of wear as well as cosmetic.
      Single crowns are often required
      to prevent crown loss.
  Endogenous staining
  ◇ treatment is primarily cosmetic.
  Bleaching of teeth can be
      accomplished in the dental office
      by the dentist. This requires
      several appointments. As an
      alternative, patients can be fitted
      with customized mouthguards.
      Bleach is placed in these and the
      patient wears them for one to
      several hours a day for a few
      weeks.
  Bonding of composite materials to
      teeth can change the color and
      shape of teeth to improve
      esthetics.
  Veneers can be constructed to mask
      these defects, but some tooth
      structure must be removed to
      accommodate them when they are
      bonded to the teeth.
  Crowns can be made if necessary.
Extrinsic discoloration
  Most can be removed with dental
      abrasives.

SURGERY
Implants may be alternative to crowns in
dentinogenesis imperfecta.

CONSULTATION SUGGESTIONS
Prosthodontist, Endodontist

REFERRAL SUGGESTIONS
General Dentist, Prosthodontist

PATIENT INSTRUCTIONS
Avoid use of any tetracycline during
ages of tooth development or in
pregnant patients. Regular oral hygiene
at home can mitigate degree of extrinsic
staining.

COURSE/PROGNOSIS
Prognosis depends on etiology of
discoloration and capabilities of dentist
treating condition.

CODING

ICD-9-CM
  277.1 Porphyria
  520.3 Fluorosis
  520.5 Amelogenesis imperfecta,
dentinogenesis imperfecta
  520.8 Tooth discoloration during
formation
  521.7 Tooth discoloration due to
drugs, metals, pulp bleed, tobacco.
  773.2 Erythroblastosis fetalis

CPT
  41899 Unlisted procedure,
dentoalveolar structures

MISCELLANEOUS

SYNONYMS
Staining of teeth
Dental stains
Tooth discoloration

SEE ALSO
Amelogenesis imperfecta
Dentinogenesis imperfecta

REFERENCES
Esthetic considerations in operative
dentistry: In: Textbook of Operative
Dentistry, 3rd ed. Baum L, Phillips RW,
Lund MR (eds), Philadelphia, WB
Saunders Co., 1995, pp. 270-290.

Crispin BJ, et al: Nonrestorative esthetic
procedures. In: Contemporary Esthetic
Dentistry. Tokyo, Quintessence Publ. Co.
1994, pp. 33-56.

AUTHOR
C. Daniel Overholser, DDS, MSD

Dissociative Identity Disorder (formerly Multiple Personality Disorder)

BASICS

DESCRIPTION
Two or more distinct personalities or personality states within the same person. Personalities have relatively enduring patterning of perceiving, relating to, and thinking about the environment and self. At least two of these personalities or personality states recurrently take full control of the person's behavior. Onset usually in childhood, but most cases do not come to clinical attention until much later. Three to nine times more frequently diagnosed in females than in males.

ETIOLOGY
Often preceded by abuse (often sexual) or another form of severe emotional trauma in childhood.

SYSTEMS AFFECTED
Nervous
◊ mental disorder

DIAGNOSIS

SYMPTOMS AND SIGNS
• In classic cases, personalities and personality states have unique memories, behavior patterns, and social relationships; in other cases, there may be varying degrees of sharing of memories and commonalities in behavior or social relationships.
• In children and adolescents, classic cases with two or more fully developed personalities are not as common as they are in adults.
• In adults, the number of personalities varies from 2 to over 100.
• Transition from one personality to another is usually sudden (within seconds to minutes) and is often triggered by psychosocial stress of idiosyncratically meaningful social or environmental cues.
• Some patients are aware of the other personalities, lost periods of time, or time distortion, and periods of amnesia or confusion. Some may admit to these experiences, yet others may be unaware, or confabulate memories to cover the amnestic periods.
• Different personalities with various levels of dental awareness or oral hygiene may present at dental appointments. Personality may change suddenly during a procedure, especially if the procedure is perceived as threatening.
• Blunted perception of pain; patient may not express any discomfort. Adaptation could be for the other personality to become dominant. Personalities are often extremely different (ie, immature voice, seductive, impulsive, and explosive).
• Various personalities in the same person may respond differently to IQ tests, the same medication, and may report being a different sex, age, or race.
• Variations in pain tolerance and sensitivity to allergens may be found across identity states.
• Each personality displays behaviors characteristic of its sense of its specific age. Frequently, these personalities have distinctive proper names and should be referred to as that individual.

LABORATORY
Toxicology screening to rule out the influence of alcohol or other psychotropic drug abuse.

IMAGING/SPECIAL TESTS
CT and MRI to rule out multiple infarct dementia, brain tumors.
Psychological interview
◊ diary analysis
Neuropsychological testing
◊ to rule out cognitive deficits

Dissociative Identity Disorder (formerly Multiple Personality Disorder)

DIFFERENTIAL
- Borderline personality disorder
- Malingering
- Post-traumatic stress disorder
- Sleep disorder
- Brain tumors
- Eating disorders
- Early dementia
- Endocrinopathies
- Depression
- Identity disorder

TREATMENT

General
◇ In-patient: regular (daily) psychotherapy; out-patient: at least weekly psychotherapy.
• Examine for self-inflicted violence, drug/ alcohol abuse, suicide ideation.
Psychotherapy
◇ in-patient (especially, if suicidal) or out-patient.
• Support groups
• Relaxation therapy/self-hypnosis
At times, dental treatment may need to be postponed
◇ avoid personalizing the episode or becoming angry. Avoid using restraints. Hypnosis not recommended for dental treatment. Should be followed for psychiatric disturbance; consultation with treating psychiatric/psychologist is critical. Contacting former dentists to ascertain dental history is also highly recommended.
• Xerostomia is common because of medications. Alternative medications may be indicated. Additionally, because of the patient's history, he or she may have poor oral hygiene associated with their avoidance of the oral area. May view dental examination and treatment as invasive; may prefer dentist of different gender from his/her sexual abuser.

MEDICATIONS
• No medications are specifically curative.
• Benzodiazepines for anxiety and insomnia.
• Neuroleptics in low doses for patients with self abusive behavior.
• Antidepressants when depression is present.

CONSULTATION SUGGESTIONS
Mental Health Professional, Former Dentist

REFERRAL SUGGESTIONS
Mental Health Professional

COURSE/PROGNOSIS
Chronic
◇ from mild to severe impairment.

CODING

ICD-9-CM
300.15 Dissociative disorder or reaction unspecified

MISCELLANEOUS

Associated Conditions
Substance abuse, depression, suicide attempts, eating disorders, and substance dependence are possible complications of this disorder.

SYNONYMS
Split personality

SEE ALSO
Psychosis
Dementia

REFERENCES
Scully C, Cawson RA: Medical problems in dentistry. Oxford, Butterworth-Heinemann, 1993.

American Psychiatric Association. Diagnostic and statistical manual of mental disorders, DSM-IV, Washington, DC, 1994.

AUTHORS
Hillary Broder, PhD, MEd
Kani Nicolls, DDS

Dry Socket (Osteitis Sicca)

BASICS

DESCRIPTION
• A painful complication that involves premature disintegration or loss of the blood clot from the extraction site after tooth removal.
• Incidence: 2 to 3 % for all extractions, 10 to 30% after surgical removal of impacted mandibular third molars. More prevalent in females (4.1%) than males (0.5% in incidence).

ETIOLOGY

• Trauma and/or infection in the bone marrow surrounding the extraction socket results in inflammation with releasing of tissue activators, which produce plasmin that cause lysis of the fibrin in the clot and the formation of kinins.
• Risk factors (contributing factors; not clear yet due to poorly controlled studies) include excessive trauma to the alveolar bone, curettage of the socket, smoking, inadequate irrigation, oral contraceptives, corticosteroids, vasoconstrictor in the local anesthetics, increased bacterial activity, foreign bodies or tissue in the socket, salivary factors, reactivated herpes simplex-type 1, excessive use of mouthwashes.
• Micro-biologic isolation; aerobic micro-organisms such as Streptococcus viridans, Str. lactitis, Staphylococcus aureus and significance of anaerobic organisms exhibiting higher fibrinolytic activity such as Actinomyces viscosus, Treponema denticola, Str. mutans, which are the predominant organisms in pericoronitis.

SYSTEMS AFFECTED
Extraction socket

DIAGNOSIS

SYMPTOMS AND SIGNS
• Severe throbbing pain with radiation to the ear usually begins 2 to 5 days after extraction and persists for days.
• Pain is frequently refractory to the usual postoperative analgesics and may last for weeks.
• Unpleasant odor from the extraction socket.
• Bare alveolar socket bone that is extremely sensitive and socket has no clot, or a minimal, necrotic clot at the base.

LABORATORY
No changes in the normal red or white blood cell indices.

IMAGING/SPECIAL TESTS
• Radiographs to find any foreign bodies, root tips, alveolar fragments or residual lesions in the extraction socket.
• Hot spot in the bone scan using radioisotopes. Not typically indicated.

DIFFERENTIAL
• Traumatic neuropathy
• Trigeminal neuralgia
• Early postsurgical infection
• Causalgia

Dry Socket (Osteitis Sicca)

 TREATMENT

General
◇ Decreasing the symptoms and allowing better environment for healing; Irrigate with warm sterile saline, place sedative dressings, and prescribe analgesics.
◇ Doughy mixture of zinc-oxide-eugenol in petrolatum gauze pad is placed over the socket opening to prevent food impaction to suppress or eliminate pain.
◇ Remove, irrigate with sterile saline, and repack every second or third day until healing apparent and pain absent.

MEDICATIONS
• Local block anesthesia with long-acting anesthetics (bupivacaine, etiodocaine)

CONSULTATION SUGGESTIONS
Oral-Maxillofacial Surgeon

REFERRAL SUGGESTIONS
Oral-Maxillofacial Surgeon

PATIENT INSTRUCTIONS
Maintain oral hygiene in remainder of mouth.
Call if fever or swelling arises.

COURSE/PROGNOSIS
• Pain lasts to 7 to 14 days.
• Alveolar socket covered with new granulation tissues, and gradual sequestration of the exposed alveolar walls delineated from the slowly formed granular beds.
• No permanent sequelae.

 CODING

ICD-9-CM
526.5 Dry socket, tooth
906.0 Late effect of open wound of head

CPT
41821 Operculectomy, excision pericoronal tissue
41899 Unlisted procedure, dentoalveolar structures

 MISCELLANEOUS

Prevention
◇ Local application of antibiotics (particularly tetracyclines) decrease the incidence.
◇ Prophylaxis by preoperative mouthrinse with chlorohexidine to reduce the concentration of bacterial flora.

SYNONYMS
• Alveolalgia
• Alveolar osteitis
• Alveolitis sicca dolorosa
• Fibrinolytic alveolitis
• Localized alveolar osteomyelitis
• Necrotic socket
• Postextraction osteitis
• Postextraction osteomyelitic syndrome

SEE ALSO
Osteomyelitis

REFERENCES
Larsen PE: Alveolar osteitis after surgical removal of impacted mandibular third molars. Oral Surg, Oral Med, Oral Path 73:393-397, 1992.

Swanson AE: Prevention of dry socket. Oral Surg, Oral Med, Oral Path 70:131-136, 1990.

Birn H: Etiology and pathogenesis of fibrinolytic alveolitis. Intl J Oral Surg 2:211-263, 1973.

Awang MN: The aetiology of dry socket. Intl Dent J 39:236-240, 1989.

AUTHOR
Myron-Rae Kim, DDS, PhD

Dysphagia

BASICS

DESCRIPTION
Difficulty in swallowing. May represent subjective sensation of obstruction or inability to swallow or objective difficulty of swallowing.

ETIOLOGY

• May result from mechanical obstruction or a neurologic disorder. Causes of mechanical obstruction include tumors or swelling from infection involving the oropharynx or esophagus, foreign bodies, macroglossia, trauma, stylohyoid (Eagle's) syndrome, or scleroderma. Xerostomia can also result in dysphagia. Patients who have undergone surgical removal of tumors involving the oropharynx will experience dysphagia to varying degrees depending on the structures involved and the reconstruction performed. Similarly, patients who have received radiation in the head and neck may experience dysphagia due to xerostomia and/or radiation fibrosis.
• Neurologic disorders may involve cranial nerves V, VII, IX, X or XI because all are involved in coordinated swallowing. Neurologic diseases of the central nervous system that can affect these nerves and swallowing include poliomyositis, multiple sclerosis, myasthenia gravis, muscular dystrophy, and neuropathies related to connective tissue disorders such as lupus erythematosus.
• Esophageal motility disorders such as achalasia will produce dysphagia, as will congenital or acquired disorders of esophageal architecture.

SYSTEMS AFFECTED
Oropharynx, esophagus, gastrointestinal tract. The consequences of impaired swallowing include aspiration while swallowing, regurgitation of oral contents into the nose, and pain.

DIAGNOSIS

SYMPTOMS AND SIGNS
• Pain while swallowing is the cardinal symptom, accompanied by a feeling of fullness or choking. Aspiration or regurgitation also suggest a swallowing disorder. Changes in voice such as hoarseness suggest mechanical obstruction at or above the larynx.
• Difficulty swallowing solids usually develops before difficulty with fluids in mechanical but not neurologic disorders.
• Tongue size is increased (macroglossia) in disorders such as muscular dystrophy, amyloidosis, and several congenital defects.
• Cranial nerve examination may reveal motor abnormalities such as asymmetric soft palate, loss of gag reflex, deviation of the tongue, and other mild deficits involving the lips, tongue, and palate.

LABORATORY
No specific test. When a connective tissue disorder such as scleroderma or lupus is suspected based on clinical findings, appropriate serology is indicated. Dysphagia due to Sjögren's syndrome-related xerostomia should also be investigated by serologic examination, minor salivary gland biopsy, and Schirmer Test (see Xerostomia).

IMAGING/SPECIAL TESTS
CT scan of the head and neck may be necessary to identify associated masses or dilation of the pyriform recess and pharynx due to muscle atony. A panoramic radiograph may reveal a calcified stylohyoid ligament in Eagle's syndrome. Videofluoroscopy can be used to evaluate to study swallowing function. Endoscopic examination of the oropharynx, larynx, and esophagus will identify abnormalities involving these structures.
Esophageal manometry.

DIFFERENTIAL
While the term dysphagia accurately describes the condition, further investigation into the cause is essential:
Mechanical:
    Tumor   Swelling
    Foreign body Trauma
    Macroglossia Eagle's syndrome
Neurologic:
    Focal neuropathy due to local disease (tumor)
    Myasthenia   Muscular dystrophy
    gravis
    Multiple scle- Poliomyositis
    rosis
Brainstem infarction
Psychogenic
    Globus hystericus

Dysphagia

TREATMENT

General
◇ Treatment is directed at the underlying cause. Mechanical dysphagia due to tumors, foreign bodies, trauma, and Eagle's syndrome can be treated surgically.
◇ Neurologic dysphagia is more difficult to manage. Most of the neuro-degenerative disorders that result in dysphagia are progressive. Ingesting smaller pieces of food may relieve symptoms. Patients with dysphagia due to postsurgical defects may benefit from an orthotic that supports intraoral tissue or an obturator that prevents regurgitation.
◇ Patients with dysphagia due to neuro-degenerative disorders often require special considerations for routine dentistry, especially when significant weakness, tremor, or dyskinesia occur.
◇ Some considerations include short appointments, assisted opening, or treatment under general anesthesia.

MEDICATIONS
• Esophageal spasm
◇ attempt therapy with calcium channel antagonists or glucagon.
• Esophagitis treated with antacids, H-2 antagonist, proton-pump inhibitors.

CONSULTATION SUGGESTIONS
Neurologist, Otolaryngologist

REFERRAL SUGGESTIONS
Any patient who develops unexplained dysphagia should be referred to a neurologist or otolaryngologist.

FIRST STEPS TO TAKE IN AN EMERGENCY
• Nothing by mouth.

PATIENT INSTRUCTIONS
Follow physician's instructions.

COURSE/PROGNOSIS
• Surgical correction of mechanical dysphagia has a good prognosis. However, when radical surgery or radiation therapy is performed to remove a tumor responsible for the dysphagia, the post-treatment outcome may be worse than the original complaint.
• The prognosis for neurologic dysphagia is poor and usually progressively worsens.

CODING

ICD-9-CM
787.2 Dysphagia

CPT
21079 Custom preparation interim obturator
21080 Custom preparation definitive obturator
21082 Custom preparation, palatal augmentation prosthesis
70355 Panoramic x-ray

MISCELLANEOUS

SEE ALSO
Esophageal tumors
Scleroderma
Styloid process hyperplasia

REFERENCES
Duranceau A, Lafontaine ER, Taillefer R, Jamieson GG: Oropharyngeal dysphagia and operations on the upper esophageal sphincter. Surg Ann 19:317-321, 1987.

Bennet MR: Eagle's syndrome: a review of the literature and implications for craniomandibular disorders. J Craniomand Pract 4:323-328, 1986.

Goyal RK. Dysphagia: In: Harrison's Principles of Internal Medicine. 13th ed. Isselbacher KJ, et. al. (eds.) New York, McGraw-Hill, Inc., 1994, pp. 206-207.

AUTHOR
David A. Sirois, DMD, PhD

Elongated Styloid Process (Eagle's Syndrome)

 BASICS

DESCRIPTION
A calcified, elongated styloid process of the temporal bone.

 ETIOLOGY

Elongated styloid process. Underlying calcinosis may contribute to the calcification of the stylohyoid ligament.

SYSTEMS AFFECTED
Mouth
  ◊ painful swallowing
Throat
  ◊ painful swallowing
Neck
  ◊ occasional pain on head turning

 DIAGNOSIS

SYMPTOMS AND SIGNS
• Dull, nagging pain in the oropharynx that radiates to the ear.
• Dysphagia
• Pain is brought on by swallowing or turning the head.
• Palpated styloid process through the tonsillar area.
• Unilateral pain in the oropharynx that increased upon swallowing or turning of one's head.

IMAGING/SPECIAL TESTS
CT Scan or radiographic imaging (panoramic radiograph) will show an elongated styloid process.

DIFFERENTIAL
• Temporomandibular dysfunction
    (Myofascial pain dysfunction)
Atypical facial pain
• Facial neuralgias
    (Vagoglossopharyngeal)

Elongated Styloid Process (Eagle's Syndrome)

 TREATMENT

General
◊ If symptoms mild or infrequent, reassurance may be adequate therapy.

SURGERY
Treatment of choice is surgical shortening of the process
◊ may be performed via either extraoral or intraoral (pharyngeal) approach.

CONSULTATION SUGGESTIONS
Oral-Maxillofacial Surgeon

REFERRAL SUGGESTIONS
Oral-Maxillofacial Surgeon

COURSE/PROGNOSIS
Excellent
◊ treatment provides 100% relief.

 CODING

ICD-9-CM
350.2   Atypical facial pain
733.99 Styloid process hyperplasia
784.10 Throat pain
787.2   Dysphagia

CPT
25230 Styloidectomy
70355 Panorex

 MISCELLANEOUS

SYNONYMS
Stylagia
Eagle's Syndrome

SEE ALSO
Glossopharyngeal neuralgia
Dysphagia

REFERENCES
Murthy PS, Hazarika P, Mathal M, Kumar A, Kamath MP: Elongated styloid process: an overview. Intl J Oral Maxillofac Surg 19:230-231, 1990.

Breault MR: Eagle's syndrome. Review of the literature. J Craniomand Prac 4:323-337, 1986.

Eagle WW: Elongated styloid process: symptoms and treatment. Arch Otolaryngol 67:172-176, 1958.

AUTHOR
Thomas P. Sollecito, DMD

Endocarditis (Infective)

BASICS

DESCRIPTION
Infective endocarditis results from microbial colonization of previously damaged cardiac valve or wall endothelium. Acute and subacute forms exist.

ETIOLOGY

1) Damage to cardiac endothelium caused by
   Congenital lesions:
   Ventricular septal defect
   Patent ductus arteriosus
   Bicuspid aortic valve
   Tetralogy of Fallot
   Atrial septal defect
   Mitral valve prolapse
   Acquired
   Rheumatic heart disease
   Syphilis
   Atherosclerotic aortic lesion
   Mural thrombosis
   Atrial fibrillation
   Tricuspid infection by IV illicit drug use
   Foreign Body
   Prosthetic valve
   Indwelling catheter
   Vascular prosthesis
   Pacing wires (short term)
2) Circulating platelets adhere to exposed collagen
3) Fibrin is incorporated into the clot
4) Clot grows by further adherence of platelets
5) Organisms are released into the circulation by
   dental, pulmonary, GI, or GU manipulation
6) Organisms adhere to the clot:
   Native valve-Streptococcus viridans
   Prosthetic valve-Staphylococcus
7) Vegetations grow
   Damage to cardiac tissue
   Embolic phenomena occur

SYSTEMS AFFECTED
- Heart
- Pulmonary (emboli)
- Systemic (emboli)
   brain, retina, spleen, kidney, GI, skin, extremities, bone

DIAGNOSIS

SYMPTOMS AND SIGNS
Must have at least one of the following for diagnosis:
   1) Histopathologic evidence of infective endocarditis
   2) Multiple positive blood cultures associated with
      fever (no chill) or
      new or changing murmur
General
   ◇ night sweat, myalgia, joint pain, pallor, weakness, anorexia, weight loss, back pain.
Neurologic
   ◇ headache, delirium, hemiparesis.
Eye
   ◇ conjunctival hemorrhage, Roth spot (white-centered hemorrhagic spots on retina).
Cardiac
   ◇ signs of heart failure, pericardial friction rub, heart murmur, dysrhythmias.
Pulmonary
   ◇ cough, shortness of breath, bloody sputum, pleural friction rub.
Skin
   ◇ petechiae, splinter hemorrhages, Osler's nodes (transient painful erythematous nodules on finger or toe tips), Janeway's lesions (nonpainful erythematous lesions on palms or soles).

LABORATORY
- Elevated WBC
- Normochromic/normocytic anemia
- Elevated ESR
- Proteinuria/hematuria
- Positive blood cultures

IMAGING/SPECIAL TESTS
- 2D Echocardiogram
- Esophageal cardiogram

DIFFERENTIAL
- Pulmonary infection
- Other cardiac disease
- Occult infection from another source

TREATMENT

Wait for identification of organism unless septic, new murmur, aortic valve or prosthetic value involved.

MEDICATIONS
• Choice of antibiotic should be guided by culture and sensitivities (C & S).
• If must proceed without C&S, empirical therapy is as follows:
• Penicillin G or ampicillin; plus an aminoglycoside

SURGERY
May be necessary if valve needs replacement.

CONSULTATION SUGGESTIONS
Cardiologist

REFERRAL SUGGESTIONS
Cardiologist, Primary Care Physician

FIRST STEPS TO TAKE IN AN EMERGENCY
• Transport to emergency facility

PATIENT INSTRUCTIONS
Prevention
    Prophylaxis for procedures likely to
        cause bacteremia
Follow American Heart Association guidelines
Regular risk patients:
    Amoxicillin 3 g orally 1 hour before,
        and 1.5 g orally 6 hours after
        procedure.
    Penicillin allergic patients use either:
    Erythromycin ethylsuccinate 800 mg
        or
    Erythromycin stearate 1 g 2 hr
        before and 1/2 dose 6 hours after
        procedure
High risk patients:
    Ampicillin 2 g IV or IM plus
        gentamicin 1.5 mg/kg IV or IM
        (not to exceed 80 mg) 30 minutes
        prior to procedure, then
        amoxicillin 1.5 g orally 6 hours
        later or parenteral regimen 8
        hours later.
    Penicillin-allergic patients should
        receive vancomycin 1 g IV infused
        over 1 hour prior to procedure.
        No follow-up drug.

COURSE/PROGNOSIS
Untreated
    ◊ 100% fatal
Treated
    ◊ overall 70% survival
        penicillin-susceptible Streptococcus
        90% survival
Prosthetic Valve
    ◊ 50% survival
Poor prognosis associated with:
    CHF, resistant organisms, prosthetic
        valves, delayed treatment

CODING

ICD-9-CM
    421.0   Infective endocarditis
    996.61   Prosthetic valve endocarditis

CPT
    90780 IV infusion for therapy up to
one hour
    90782 Therapeutic injection, sub Q
or IM
    90788 Intramuscular injection of
antibiotic

MISCELLANEOUS

SYNONYMS
Subacute bacterial endocarditis (SBE)
Bacterial endocarditis

SEE ALSO
Rheumatic Fever/rheumatic heart disease
Prosthetic heart valves

REFERENCES
Terpenning MS: Infective endocarditis. Clin Geriatr Med 8:903, 1992.

Barco CT: Prevention of infective endocarditis: a review of the medical and dental literature. J Periodontol 62:510, 1991.

Lukes AS, Bright DK, Durack MB: Diagnosis of infective endocarditis. Infect Dis Clin N Am 7:1, 1993.

Hupp JR: Changing methods of preventing infective endocarditis following dental procedures. J Oral Maxillofac Surg 51:616-623, 1993.

AUTHOR
Peter E. Larsen, DDS

Epiglottitis

BASICS

DESCRIPTION
A rapidly progressive, potentially lethal upper respiratory track infection of the epiglottis, vallecula, aryepiglottic folds, and arytenoids affecting primarily children (ages 2 to 8) and occasionally adults.

ETIOLOGY

• Most common pathogen is Haemophilus influenzae type B, although introduction of vaccine for this organism causing incidence to fall.
• Other pathogens include Streptococci, Staphylococci, and Klebsiella pneumoniae.

SYSTEMS AFFECTED
Pharynx
◊ edematous/enlarged epiglottis can compromise airway, especially in children.

DIAGNOSIS

SYMPTOMS AND SIGNS
General
◊ malaise, fever, cervical adenopathy, ill-appearing, "tripod" position (on hands and knees with head down).
Pharynx
◊ rapidly progressive sore throat, dysphagia, drooling. Possible respiratory obstruction with respiratory distress. Erythematous, edematous epiglottis. Retention of secretions. Muffled voice, soft stridor, possible impending airway obstruction.

LABORATORY
CBC
◊ possible elevated WBC count with "left shift."
Blood culture
◊ frequently diagnostic.

IMAGING/SPECIAL TESTS
Lateral neck radiograph
◊ enlargement of epiglottis, narrowing of posterior airway space.
Indirect/direct laryngoscopy
◊ carefully performed will reveal enlargement.
Epiglottic swab culture.

DIFFERENTIAL
• Croup (laryngotracheobronchitis)
• Peritonsillar abscess (or retropharyngeal abscess)
• Tracheitis
• Foreign body (aspirated)
• Diphtheria
• Angioneurotic edema
• Sepsis

Epiglottitis

 TREATMENT

General
Avoid manipulation of upper airway structures such as using tongue depressor
◊ may precipitate total obstruction.
• Requires hospitalization, consider intensive care unit.
• Humidification of inspired air.
• Nasoendotracheal intubation or tracheostomy selectively to protect airway.
• Culture throat after securing airway.
• Monitor airway patency frequently if not intubated.

MEDICATIONS
• Empiric antimicrobial therapy directed towards H. influenzae, other gram negative bacilli and Staphylococci (cefuroxine, ampicillin-sulbactam, chloramphenicol, etc.).
• Steroids
◊ may decrease edema but role not critically tested.
• Antipyretics
• H. influenzae vaccine may be protective.

CONSULTATION SUGGESTIONS
Otolaryngologist, Infectious Disease Specialist

REFERRAL SUGGESTIONS
Otolaryngologist, Primary Care Physician

FIRST STEPS TO TAKE IN AN EMERGENCY
• Immediate transport to facility that can secure airway.
• Keep patient calm and sitting erect.
• Avoid unnecessary manipulation of airway.

COURSE/PROGNOSIS
Excellent with protection of airway and use of appropriate antimicrobials.

 CODING

ICD-9-CM
464.3 Acute epiglottitis without obstruction
464.31 Acute epiglottitis with obstruction

CPT
31500 Intubation, endotracheal, emergency
31600 Tracheostomy, planned
31601 Tracheostomy, under 2 yrs.
31603 Tracheostomy, emergency
31605 Cricothyrotomy, emergency
70350 Cephalogram
70360 Radiographic exam, neck, soft tissue

 MISCELLANEOUS

SYNONYMS
Supraglottitis

SEE ALSO
Pharyngitis

REFERENCES
Simon HB: Infections of the upper respiratory tract. In: Scientific American Medicine Section 7, Subsection XIX, Rubenstein E, Federman DD (eds). Scientific American Inc, 1989, pp. 9-10.

Leonary G, Lafreniere DC: Infections of the Ear, Nose and Throat. In: Management of Infections of the Oral and Maxillofacial Regions. 3rd ed., Topazian RG, Goldberg MH (eds), Philadelphia, WB Saunders Co., 1994, pp. 370-371.

Schuller DE, Schleuning AJ: Deweese and Saunders' Otolaryngology Head and Neck Surgery, 8th ed. St. Louis, CV Mosby Co, 1994, pp. 265-266.

AUTHOR
Samuel J. McKenna, DDS, MD

Epistaxis (Nosebleed)

 BASICS

DESCRIPTION
• Usually a spontaneous and acute episode of hemorrhage from the nasal cavity.
• Anterior bleeds are from the anterior, inferior nasal septal area (Kiesselbach's plexus).
• Posterior bleeds are from the roof of the nasal cavity or the inferior posterior area of the turbinate.
• Epistaxis may be a sign or symptom of another disease process rather than a disease in itself.
• Nosebleeds tend to be frequent in young patients, but usually are not significant.
• Nosebleeds in older patients tend to be more severe and are more likely to have an underlying pathology.

 ETIOLOGY

• Idiopathic
• Trauma (nose picking)
• Inflammation
• Infection
• Chemical (cocaine use)
• Hypertension
• Blood dyscrasias
• Vascular fragility or abnormalities

SYSTEMS AFFECTED
Vascular
   ◊ vessels in nasal mucosa and their sources
Respiratory
   ◊ nasal airway

 DIAGNOSIS

SYMPTOMS AND SIGNS
• Recurrent nasal bleeding
• Hemoptysis (coughed up blood)
• Hematemesis (vomited blood)

LABORATORY
• CBC for chronic or high volume bleeding
• PT, PTT, bleeding time, liver function tests in suspected coagulopathies

IMAGING/SPECIAL TESTS
Carotid angiogram in extreme cases

DIFFERENTIAL
• Hypertension, malignant
• Vascular anomalies
• Neoplasia
• Coagulopathies
• Trauma (zygomatic, ethmoid fractures)

TREATMENT

General
◇ Debridement of blood clots
◇ Pressure to the anterior, inferior nasal septum
◇ Chemical or electrical cauterization of specific bleeding points
◇ Anterior and posterior nasal packs as needed
◇ Management of underlying causes such as coagulopathy or malignant hypertension.

MEDICATIONS
• Topical vasoconstrictors
• Medical management of underlying causes

SURGERY
Ligation of vessels supplying the areas of hemorrhage in extreme cases. Typically must ligate anterior ethmoidal artery.

CONSULTATION SUGGESTIONS
Oral-Maxillofacial Surgeon, Otolaryngologist

REFERRAL SUGGESTIONS
Oral-Maxillofacial Surgeon, Otolaryngologist, Primary Care Physician

FIRST STEPS TO TAKE IN AN EMERGENCY
• Elevate head
• Squeeze nose
• Place anterior and, if trained, posterior nasal packs.

PATIENT INSTRUCTIONS
• Avoid traumatizing nasal mucosa.
• Use humidifiers when humidity low.

COURSE/PROGNOSIS
• Most nosebleeds are readily treated with simple measures.
• If a nosebleed is not easily controlled, or is significantly recurrent, the patient should be referred for additional evaluation.

CODING

ICD-9-CM
448.0 Hereditary epistaxis
784.7 Epistaxis

CPT
30901 Cauterization and/or packing anterior nose
30905 Cauterization and/or packing posterior nose
30915 Ligation of arteries ethmoidal
30920 Ligation of arteries internal maxillary transantral
37600 Ligation of external carotid artery

MISCELLANEOUS

SYNONYMS
Nosebleed

SEE ALSO
Hypertension
Liver disease
Coagulopathy

REFERENCES
Myerhoff WL, Rise DH: Otolaryngology Head and Neck Surgery. Philadelphia, WB Saunders Co., 1992.

Rosen P, Barkin RM: Emergency Medicine: Concepts and Clinical Practice. St. Louis, Mosby, 1992.

Tierney LM, et al: (eds). Current Medical Diagnosis & Treatment. Norwalk, CT, Appleton and Lange, 1994.

AUTHOR
Alan L. Felsenfeld, DDS

Erysipelas

BASICS

DESCRIPTION
A distinct type of dermal cellulitis with significant lymphatic involvement almost always due to group A Streptococci. Face most common area affected.

ETIOLOGY

• Most common in neonates, young children and geriatric patients, erysipelas usually affects the face or extremities.
• The causative micro-organism is generally Streptococcus pyrogenes (Lancefield Group A), but can also be due to Group B, C or G. These bacteria can usually be cultured from mature skin lesions. In many cases, erysipelas can result from an initiating respiratory infection, but usually attributable to break in epithelial barrier (wound, fissures, ulceration).

SYSTEMS AFFECTED
• Skin
• Erysipelas has a propensity to involve regional lymphatics and will recur in such sites where lymphatic flow is compromised (ie, diabetes, previous trauma, alcohol abuse, venous stasis).

DIAGNOSIS

SYMPTOMS AND SIGNS
• Painful, edematous, erythematous, indurated-appearing dermal lesion with a slightly raised, advancing edge, well-demarcated from normal tissue.
• Vesicles may occur and desquamation follows.
• Fever, malaise, headache.

LABORATORY
• Leukocytosis
• Gram stain and speciation of Streptococci may be possible from the advancing edge of the skin lesion.
• Blood culture may be positive.

DIFFERENTIAL
• Herpes Zoster
• Insect bite (early)
• Allergic dermatitis
• Contact dermatitis
• Erythema chronicum migrans
• Erysipeloid
• Lupus erythematosus

TREATMENT

General
◊ Bed rest and good fluid intake initially.

MEDICATIONS
• The standard for treating proven early Streptococcal infections includes an initial injection with aqueous penicillin G (600,000 units) followed by procaine penicillin (600,000 units) every 8 to 12 hours for 7 to 10 days. If evidence for mixed infection is found, then treatment with penicillinase-resistant drugs such as nafcillin should be considered.
• In penicillin-allergic patients, Vancomycin 1.0 to 1.5 gm/day can be substituted.
• Because recurrence is not uncommon, maintenance dosing with PO Penicillin V or Erythromycin (1 gm/day) may be indicated.

SURGERY
Drainage necessary only if deep spaces involved or if abscesses form.

CONSULTATION SUGGESTIONS
Infectious Disease Specialist

REFERRAL SUGGESTIONS
Primary Care Physician

FIRST STEPS TO TAKE IN AN EMERGENCY
Initiate antibiotic therapy.

PATIENT INSTRUCTIONS
• Comply with antibiotic regimen.
• Avoid shaving affected areas.

COURSE/PROGNOSIS
• Adequate treatment usually results in full recovery.
• Deep cellulitis and extension of bacteria to infect visceral organs.
• Subcutaneous abscess may occur that requires drainage.
• Necrotizing fasciitis rare complication.

CODING

ICD-9-CM
035 Erysipelas

CPT
90780 IV infusion for therapy up to one hour, doctor supervised
90782 Therapeutic injection, sub Q or IM
90788 Intramuscular injection of antibiotic

MISCELLANEOUS

SYNONYMS
Saint Anthony's Fire
Streptococcal superficial cellulitis

SEE ALSO
Cellulitis

REFERENCES
Mandell GL, Douglas RG, Bennett JE: Principles and Practices of Infectious Diseases. 4th ed. New York, Churchill Livingstone, 1995, pp. 913-916.

Habif TP: Clinical Dermatology. 2nd ed. St. Louis, CV Mosby, 1990, pp. 184-188.

Stein JH: Internal Medicine. 2nd ed. Boston, Little, Brown and Co., 1987, pp. 1719-1724.

AUTHOR
Peter G. Fotos, DDS, MS, PhD

Erythema Multiforme

BASICS

DESCRIPTION
An acute dermatologic and mucosal disorder that displays variation in types of lesions as well as clinical presentation. Often a disease of exclusion due to an often nondescript histopathologic picture as well. Most commonly seen in adolescents and young adults. Usually skin and oral lesions are both present, though only one or the other may be seen. Male:female = 3:2.

ETIOLOGY

• Thought most likely to be an antigen-antibody response that reacts preferentially at submucosal and subepidermal blood vessels. IgM and C3, which are a part of many early antibody responses, have been detected by immunofluorescent studies in early lesions.
• Cytotoxic CD8 lymphocytes have also been seen to be associated with the individual cell necrolysis of keratinocytes. This association would point to a cellular rather than humoral immune response.
• Erythema multiforme and Stevens-Johnson syndrome are most likely a result of a complex overzealous immune response, possibly involving both cellular and humeral immune systems.
• Scores of possible antecedent infectious and predisposing medicaments/ substances have been reported to cause erythema multiforme. The most common antecedents are recurrent herpes simplex infections and Mycoplasma pneumoniae for minor reactions. Drugs are the most commonly reported cause for major cases.

SYSTEMS AFFECTED
Oral mucosa
◊ all mucosal surfaces may be affected. Lips, buccal mucosa, palate, and tongue are the most commonly involved. Mucosal lesions are most often ulcerative.
Skin
◊ classic lesion is called a target lesion. These lesions have areas of erythematous skin alternating with normal colored (centrally healed) skin. Joints can be painful.
Systemic
◊ low-grade fever

DIAGNOSIS

SYMPTOMS AND SIGNS
• Low-grade febrile complaints.
• Acute onset usually helps rule out autoimmune vesiculo-bullous diseases such as pemphigus and pemphigoid.
• Vague joint pain.
• Acutely painful ulcerations.
• Concomitant skin and oral ulcers, though this is not found in all instances.
Oral
◊ ulcerations that can range from a few aphthae-form lesions to large 2 to 3 cm lesions.
Lips
◊ can be extensively involved with crusting and necrosis.
Skin
◊ target lesion is the classic lesion though macular, papular, vesicular, and bullous lesions can all be seen in the same patient or as the presenting lesion. Most common areas of involvement are the extremities (with more severe involvement in the more distal areas) and face.

LABORATORY
CBC, culture or cytologic exam for Herpes simplex, serologic tests if pemphigus highly suspected, toxicologic tests if drug history dictates, liver panel if hepatitis symptoms were/are present, glucose level if steroid therapy anticipated and diabetes suspected.

IMAGING/SPECIAL TESTS
• Biopsy to rule out other possibilities in differential diagnosis. Biopsy may need to be divided into two pieces, with one-half in 10% formalin and the other half fresh frozen or placed in Michel's solution. This is needed for immunofluorescent study if autoimmune disease is high in the differential.
• Histologic exam
◊ epidermal necrolysis.

DIFFERENTIAL
Primary herpetic gingivostomatitis if lesions are confined to oral cavity and no history of secondary herpetic events.
Acute drug reaction
Pemphigus vulgaris
Pemphigoid
Lichen planus
Reiter's syndrome
Behcet's syndrome
Contact dermatitis
Pityriasis rosea
Dermatitis herpetiformis
Rocky Mountain Spotted fever
Meningococcemia

TREATMENT

General

◇ Must rule out or take into account the possibility of other disease processes, especially infectious causes.

◇ Dehydration is a major complication that may necessitate hospital admission.

◇ Check for skin turgor and do blood pressure "Tilts." Patients need to be checked daily if not admitted.

◇ Lesions can become secondarily infected.

MEDICATIONS

• Glucocorticosteroids are the therapy of choice with high-dose burst therapy being necessary. IV or oral dosing is necessary as topical preparations will not address the systemic nature of the process. Tapering or maintenance dosing of oral glucocorticosteroids may be necessary depending on disease course.

• Steroids almost absolutely contraindicated in the presence of active infection. Consult physician/infectious disease specialist in face of this possibility.

• Steroids lower immune response, the immunocompetency of the patient must be taken into account.

• Steroids will elevate glucose levels in diabetics. IV fluids for dehydration.

CONSULTATION SUGGESTIONS

Oral Medicine, Primary Care Physician

REFERRAL SUGGESTIONS

Oral Medicine

PATIENT INSTRUCTIONS

• Take medications as prescribed.
• Reassure that disease is self-limited.

COURSE/PROGNOSIS

Self-limiting disease but it may last for 4 to 6 weeks. It is usually of acute onset with the patient being very uncomfortable due to oral/palmar/plantar involvement and the fact that these areas are routinely traumatized in everyday activities. Disease is most commonly seen in young adults and adolescents.

CODING

ICD-9-CM

695.1 Erythema multiforme

CPT

11100 Biopsy, skin
40808 Biopsy, mouth intraoral
99000 Transport specimen to outside laboratory

MISCELLANEOUS

SYNONYMS

Stevens-Johnson is an extreme variant.

SEE ALSO

Pemphigus
Urticaria

REFERENCES

Regezi JA, Sciubba J: Oral Pathology 2nd ed. Philadelphia, WB Saunders, 1992, pp. 61-65.

Patterson R, Dydewicz MS, Gonzales A, et al: Erythema multiforme and Stevens-Johnson syndrome: Descriptive and therapeutic controversy. Chest 98:331-336, 1990.

Moschella SL, Hurley HJ: Dermatology 3rd ed. Philadelphia, WB Saunders, 1993, pp. 580-585.

AUTHOR

John W. Hellstein, DDS

Erythema Nodosum

BASICS

DESCRIPTION
Exquisitely painful, erythematous nodules, usually on pretibial portion of the lower extremities and occasionally developing on the arms, hands, fingers, or other areas of the body.

ETIOLOGY

Considered to be a reaction pattern of skin occurring as a response to a wide variety of etiologic factors including:
drugs (especially, oral contraceptives and sulfonamides)
endocrine-hormonal conditions (thyroid disorders, pregnancy)
inflammatory bowel disease (seen in 2% of patients with Crohn's disease)
sarcoidosis
streptococcal infections (including oropharyngeal)
Yersinia enterocolitis (diarrhea history)
deep fungal infections
tuberculosis (especially in children and young adults)
malignant disease

SYSTEMS AFFECTED
Subcutaneous tissues
◊ especially in the lower extremities.

DIAGNOSIS

SYMPTOMS AND SIGNS
• Weakness, malaise, headache, and moderate fever (38° to 39°C) can be seen with acute onset of the disease. Headache and arthralgia can become severe and the nodules themselves extremely painful.
Skin
◊ acute bilateral bright-red, 1 to 10 cm, firm, tender nodules on shins, knees, and ankles with poorly demarcated boundaries. Nodules may be cutaneous or subcutaneous and palpable with elevation above the skin level. They are warm, nonulcerated, and very painful on palpation.
• In erythema nodosum migrans, the lesions are unilateral and migrate slowly over the front or lateral parts of the lower legs.
• Regional phlebitis may also occur.

LABORATORY
Tests chosen depend upon the clinical situation suspected. For example, a CBC, chest radiograph and TB skin test will help screen for lymphoma, leukemia, tuberculosis, and sarcoidosis. A thorough physical examination is essential.

IMAGING/SPECIAL TESTS
Biopsy
◊ a deep elliptical skin biopsy with adequate portion of subcutaneous fat must be obtained. Early neutrophil infiltration with later mononuclear and histiocytic infiltration.
Chest radiograph
◊ for changes seen in tuberculosis and sarcoidosis, etc.

DIFFERENTIAL
Erythema nodosum (the various etiologies for this must be considered individually in the differential)
Erythema induatum
Panniculitis (any type of this may clinically resemble erythema nodosum)
• Nodular vasculitis
• Periarteritis nodosa cutanea
• Syphilitic gummas
• Cellulitis
• Septal emboli
• Lymphoma

Erythema Nodosum

TREATMENT

General
◊ Treat underlying condition.
◊ Discontinue causative drugs.
◊ Bed rest and supportive care are indicated in most cases.
◊ Rubber support (ACE) bandages and wet dressings are often helpful.
◊ Keep legs elevated as much as possible.

MEDICATIONS
• Salicylates and other nonsteroidal anti-inflammatory agents can be used for management of the pain.
• Potassium iodide can be used (300 to 600 mg daily for up to 8 weeks)
• Corticosteroids
◊ when not contraindicated, can be used topically or systemically.

CONSULTATION SUGGESTIONS
Primary Care Physician, Rheumatologist

REFERRAL SUGGESTIONS
Primary Care Physician, Rheumatologist

COURSE/PROGNOSIS
The nodules are originally bright-red in color, becoming yellowish or greenish as hemoglobin destruction takes place. Dark blue or brown nodules can occur on the forearms and gluteal region, especially during the later course of the disease. It is important to note that the nodules never ulcerate. Regression is rapid with the total disease process running from 3-6 weeks. Recurrences are rare, and it should be noted that erythema multiforme lesions are seen in 10% of erythema nodosum cases.

CODING

ICD-9-CM
695.2 Erythema Nodosum

CPT
11100 Biopsy of skin, subcutaneous tissue and/or mucous membrane

MISCELLANEOUS

SYNONYMS
Erythema contusiforme
Dermatitis contusiformis

SEE ALSO
Sarcoidosis
Tuberculosis
Streptococcal infection
Deep fungal infections
Crohn's disease
Erythema multiforme

REFERENCES
Kirch W, Duhrsen U: Erythema nodosum of dental origin. Clin Investigator, 70:1073-1078, 1992.

Fox MD, Schwartz RA: Erythema nodosum. Am Fam Phys 46:818-821, 1992.

AUTHOR
Lawrence T. Herman, DMD

Esophageal Tumors

 BASICS

DESCRIPTION
Benign or malignant neoplasms. The most common benign tumor is the leiomyoma; the most common malignancy, squamous cell carcinoma. Benign tumors are readily managed surgically; however, malignant esophageal tumors are often advanced at the time of diagnosis and the prognosis is generally poor. Peak incidence 50 to 60 years of age. Male> Female.
Location
◇ 20% upper third, 30% middle third, 50% lower third.

 ETIOLOGY

• Tobacco and alcohol abuse are etiologic factors.
• Lye stricture may predispose.
• Patients with Plummer-Vinson syndrome or achalasia have higher incidence than general population.
• Adenocarcinoma usually arises from Barrett's esophagus (reflux problem).

SYSTEMS AFFECTED
Digestive
◇ esophageal obstruction rapidly leads to cachexia.
Pulmonary
◇ invasion of trachea leads to airway compromise.
Lymphatic
◇ metastasize to mediastinal and cervical lymph nodes.

 DIAGNOSIS

SYMPTOMS AND SIGNS
Neck
◇ painless cervical lymphadenopathy
Throat
◇ progressive dysphagia is usually first symptom, followed shortly by weight loss. Weight loss is often found at the time of diagnosis and may progress on to cachexia. Progressive hoarseness connotes invasion of recurrent laryngeal nerve(s). Stidor occurs when laryngeal nerve invasion is severe due to vocal cord paralysis.
Chest
◇ chronic cough, aspiration
GI
◇ regurgitation

LABORATORY
There is no specific laboratory test or marker for esophageal cancer

IMAGING/SPECIAL TESTS
• Barium contrast esophagram ("barium swallow") is generally first screening test.
• CT scan demonstrates extramural extension and regional lymphadenopathy.
• Esophagoscopy is performed for biopsy/brushing.
• Endoscopic ultrasound

DIFFERENTIAL
• Zenker's diverticulum
• Cricopharyngeal dysfunction
• Achalasia of esophagus
• Other benign disorder of swallowing

Esophageal Tumors

TREATMENT

General
◇ Liquid nutritional supplements orally or through gastrostomy tube.

MEDICATIONS
• Chemotherapy
◇ Cis-platinum and 5-fluorouracil (Antiemetics also then needed)
• Narcotic analgesics
• Liquid nutritional supplements

SURGERY
• Benign lesions are effectively treated by local excision.
• Early malignant tumors can be resected with reconstruction either by free jejunal interposition or gastric pull-up.
• Malignant tumors in the cervical esophagus can require concurrent laryngopharyngectomy.
• Advanced malignant tumors are best palliated with chemotherapy and radiation.
• For palliation or as adjunct to surgery for malignancy.

CONSULTATION SUGGESTIONS
Gastroenterologist, General Surgeon, Dietician, Radiation Oncologist

REFERRAL SUGGESTIONS
Primary Care Physician, Gastroenterologist, General Surgeon

PATIENT INSTRUCTIONS
Those with malignant disease can contact National Cancer Institute for information (301)496-5583.

COURSE/PROGNOSIS
• Benign tumors are almost always controlled by surgery.
• Malignant tumors usually require chemotherapy + surgery + radiation therapy.
• Surgery for malignant tumors is extensive, requiring transposition of stomach or small bowel for reconstruction.
• Radiation fields for esophageal malignancies rarely include the oral region; however, communication with radiation oncologist is advisable prior to oral surgical, endodontic, or periodontal procedures.

CODING

ICD-9-CM
150.0 Neoplasm, cervical esophagus, malignant
150.1 Neoplasm, thoracic esophagus, malignant
150.2 Neoplasm, abdominal esophagus, malignant
150.9 Neoplasm, esophagus, malignant
211.0 Neoplasm, esophagus, benign

CPT
20185 Oral surgical splint
21089 Unlisted maxillofacial prosthetic procedure

MISCELLANEOUS

SYNONYMS
Squamous cell carcinoma of esophagus
Leiomyoma of esophagus

REFERENCES
Ellis FH, et al: Cancer of the Esophagus. In: American Cancer Society Textbook of Clinical Oncology, Atlanta, American Cancer Society, 1991.

Peters JH, DeMeester TR: Esophagus and diaphragmatic hernia. In: Principles of Surgery, Schwartz SI, Shires GT, Spencer FC (eds), 6th ed, New York, McGraw-Hill Co., 1994.

Herrera JL: Benign and metastatic tumors of the esophagus. Gastroenterol Clin N Am 20:775-789, 1991.

AUTHOR
Eric J. Dierks, DMD, MD

Failure of Tooth Development

BASICS

DESCRIPTION
Conditions in which there is failure to form one or more teeth are described as hypodontia, oligodontia, and anodontia. Hypodontia is the absence of one or a few teeth; oligodontia the absence of many teeth associated with syndromes or systemic abnormalities; and anodontia the complete failure of tooth formation as seen in the severest form of hereditary ectodermal dysplasia (HED). In hypodontia, the most frequently occurring absent tooth is the third molar, followed by the mandibular second premolar and maxillary lateral incisor. In American populations, the incidence has been reported to range from 1.5 to 10%. Oligodontia is a finding in forms of HED, and permanent anterior teeth may also exhibit conical shape. Anodontia is rare and is one of the manifestations of ectodermal dysplasia along with anhidrosis, asteatosis, and hypotrichosis.

ETIOLOGY

The factors that play a role in the failure of teeth to develop are disruption of the dental lamina, space limitation causing tooth germ regression as in the absence of third molars, and functional abnormalities of the dental epithelium. Familial hereditary patterns are the most common etiologic factor.

SYSTEMS AFFECTED
Anodontia may cause lack of growth of the alveolar process thereby complicating future prosthetic management. Oligodontia anterior permanent teeth may have abnormalities in shape (ie, conical). Primary molars may be ankylosed in the absence of permanent premolar.

DIAGNOSIS

SYMPTOMS AND SIGNS
Clinical observation of absence of teeth, delayed exfoliation of primary molar or lateral incisor. Signs and symptoms of associated syndrome of hereditary ectodermal dysplasia (ie, thin sparse hair, aplasia of sweat glands). Other syndromes that may exhibit hypodontia include chondroectodermal dysplasia, achondroplasia, Reiger's incontinentia pigmenti, and Seckel syndrome.

IMAGING/SPECIAL TESTS
Periapical or panoramic imaging to detect presence or absence of unerupted teeth.

DIFFERENTIAL
• Chondroectodermal dysplasia
• Impaction of teeth
• Achondroplasia
• Seckel syndrome

Failure of Tooth Development

 TREATMENT

General
Generally prosthetic management. Anodontia requires complete denture. In young children, denture fabrication is difficult and must be periodically adjusted. In cases of absent permanent lateral incisors, orthodontic movement of the permanent canines mesially and reshaping to mimic the lateral incisor is necessary when there is inadequate space for lateral pontic placement. Partial dentures are employed in primary dentition and adjusted as permanent teeth erupt. Bonding or porcelain veneered crowns may be indicated in instances of conical shaped permanent anterior teeth.
Placement of implants when feasible.

CONSULTATION SUGGESTIONS
Pediatric Dentist, Prosthodontist, Orthodontist, Oral-Maxillofacial Surgeon

REFERRAL SUGGESTIONS
Pediatric Dentist, Family Dentist, Prosthodontist

PATIENT INSTRUCTIONS
Proper dental care can usually ameliorate problems of missing teeth.

COURSE/PROGNOSIS
Condition is throughout life. May require tooth replacement to achieve oral-facial form and function.

 CODING

ICD-9-CM
520.0 Hypodontia

CPT
41899 Unlisted dentoalveolar procedure
70355 Panorex

 MISCELLANEOUS

SYNONYMS
Hypodontia

SEE ALSO
Failure of tooth eruption

REFERENCES
MacDonald R, Avery D: Dentistry for the Child and Adolescent. 5th ed. St. Louis, CV Mosby Co., 1987. pp. 80-83.

AUTHOR
Mark Wagner, DMD

Failure of Tooth Eruption

BASICS

DESCRIPTION
Delayed eruption and/or failure of eruption is a characteristic of several congenital disorders. These would include Down's syndrome or trisomy 21, cleidocranial dysplasia, hypothyroidism (cretinism) achondroplasia (dwarfism), and ankylosis of primary or permanent teeth in which failure to erupt or to complete eruption is observed.

ETIOLOGY

• Cause of ankylosis in primary molars is unknown; however, it has been seen as following a familial pattern that is a nonsex-linked trait. Some have suggested that the congenital absence of permanent successor may correlate with ankylosed primary molars. This has not been confirmed.
• Trisomy 21 (Down's syndrome) is a condition in which delays in eruption may occur and primary teeth may be delayed up to 2 years in eruption and be retained until age 14 or 15.
Cleidocranial dysostosis
  ◇ Transmission of trait from mother or father, true Mendelian dominant pattern. Development of dentition is delayed as is primary root resorption, and thus a delay in permanent tooth eruption.
• Hypothyroidism causes delay in dentition in all stages. Juvenile hypothyroidism and hypopituitarism have as their sequelae delays in eruption.

SYSTEMS AFFECTED
Down's syndrome (trisomy 21). Oral-facial disturbances include underdevelopment and delays in development of mandible and maxilla along with smaller upper facial height. Small jaws may account for large tongue and dental crowding. Periodontal disease has increased incidence. Cleidocranial dysplasia exhibits supernumerary teeth.

DIAGNOSIS

SYMPTOMS AND SIGNS
Unerupted primary or permanent teeth, exfoliation of primary teeth delayed. Presence of multiple supernumerary teeth.

IMAGING/SPECIAL TESTS
Periapical or panoramic imaging to disclose status of unerupted (missing) teeth.

DIFFERENTIAL
• Tooth ankylosis usually not associated with another syndrome.
• Simple, slow or delayed eruption pattern. Dental impaction (eg, maxillary canines). Diagnosis of existing congenital syndromes with the specific characteristics such as seen in Down's, cleidocranial dysplasia, hypothyroidism (cretinism).

TREATMENT

<u>General</u>
Extraction of retained primary teeth and uncovering unerupted permanent teeth. Supernumerary tooth removal, as with cleidocranial dysplasia, has been followed up with orthodontic therapy with some success. In older patients, tooth and/or impaction removal followed by prosthesis, with or without prior implant placement, may be necessary. Oral hygiene and soft tissue management to prevent caries and development of periodontal disease.

SURGERY
Supernumerary tooth removal, uncovering of unerupted teeth.

CONSULTATION SUGGESTIONS
Orthodontist, Pediatric Dentist, Oral-Maxillofacial Surgeon

REFERRAL SUGGESTIONS
Pediatric Dentist, Oral-Maxillofacial Surgeon

PATIENT INSTRUCTIONS
Advise parents that careful monitoring of dental eruption necessary if delays or other abnormalities of dental eruption occur.

COURSE/PROGNOSIS
<u>If delayed eruption due to dental interferences or thick overlying bone, treatment likely to be successful</u>
◊ if root development still occurring. Ankylosed or severely malpositioned unerupted teeth have poor prognosis for eventual eruption.

CODING

ICD-9-CM
520.6 Impacted teeth, delayed tooth eruption, or natal teeth
521.6 Ankylosis of teeth
524.3 Impacted, malpositioned tooth

CPT
41899 Unlisted dentoalveolar procedure
70355 Panorex

MISCELLANEOUS

SYNONYMS
Impacted teeth

SEE ALSO
Cleidocranial dysostosis
Failure of tooth development
Hypothyroidism

REFERENCES
McDonald RE, Avery DR: Eruption of Teeth, Local Systemic and Congenital Factors. Dentistry for the Child and Adolescent. 6th ed. St. Louis, CV Mosby, 1994, pp. 205-214.

AUTHOR
Mark Wagner, DMD

Fever of Unknown Origin (FUO)

BASICS

DESCRIPTION

<u>Fever of unknown origin (FUO)</u>
◇ defined as presence of fever as the dominant sign or symptom in a patient's illness with temperatures >101 degrees F (38.3° C) for a prolonged period (2 to 3 weeks), the cause of which is undetermined after intensive studies over at least 1 week. Excludes fever secondary to another known illness.

ETIOLOGY

Various possible causes of prolonged fever. Usually is not secondary to bacterial or viral infections that typically follow a more acute course.

<u>Granulomatous infections</u>
◇ eg, tuberculosis and deep mycoses. In TB, FUO more likely with miliary or extrapulmonary disease, ie, with involvement of bone, liver, lymph nodes, peritoneum.

<u>Pyogenic infections</u>
◇ FUO may be due to intra-abdominal, renal, or retroperitoneal infections, particularly if they have been walled off by adhesions and reactive tissues, such as in the perforated appendix in the elderly or debilitated; intrarenal or perinephric abscess; renal papillary necrosis with ureteral obstruction; aortic aneurysm with organizing infected clot.

<u>Bacterial endocarditis</u>
◇ usually associated with a heart murmur; secondary effects may include constitutional symptoms or cerebral embolus, which may be misdiagnosed as a thrombotic or hemorrhagic stroke; consider acute forms. Diagnosed by blood cultures and cardiac imaging.

<u>Parasitic infection</u>
◇ liver abscess due to amebiasis; malaria is possible if there has been travel to endemic areas.

<u>Neoplasms</u>
◇ various malignancies may produce prolonged fevers, especially lymphomas, sarcomas of bone or lymphoid tissue, carcinoma of the stomach or pancreas, and primary or metastatic hepatic malignancy, leukemias, and atrial myxoma. Atrial myxoma may be confused with bacterial endocarditis because of associated heart murmurs, fever, peripheral embolic effects and arthralgias.

<u>Drug fever</u>
◇ any drug may cause allergies or side-effects manifested as fever. Even drugs that have been tolerated for extended periods must be considered and possibly discontinued. Protracted fever as an allergic reaction may occur without rash or other sign.

<u>Connective tissue diseases</u>
◇ consider temporal arteritis, rheumatoid arthritis, rheumatic fever, systemic lupus erythematosus. Consider constitutional, ocular, joint, and skin signs or symptoms.

<u>Gastrointestinal disease</u>
◇ consider regional enteritis, ulcerative colitis, Whipple's disease, cholecystitis, pancreatitis. FUO may be initial manifestation without frank changes in bowel function or abdominal pain.

<u>Pulmonary embolism</u>
◇ multiple small pulmonary emboli from asymptomatic deep venous thrombosis (calves or pelvis) may cause fever. Consider signs or symptoms of hemoptysis, shortness of breath, pleuritic pain, cough, poorly-defined chest discomfort, or leg discomfort.

<u>Hyperthyroidism</u>
◇ fever may be the primary manifestation.

<u>Malingering</u>
◇ psychiatric problems with purposeful alteration of thermometer readings. Look for lack of correlation of high temperature with pulse, absence of chills, sweats, and dehydration.

DIAGNOSIS

SYSTEMS AFFECTED
Evaluation and Treatment
◇ Fever work-up must be done after a thorough history and physical examination, including consideration of possible environmental and occupational exposures. Also consider age, because neoplastic disease is more likely in the older population. Be aware of all medications, including over-the-counter agents, which patients may not consider to be medications.
Physical examination
◇ particular emphasis on skin lesions, lymph nodes, fundoscopic findings, heart murmur, abdominal masses or organomegaly, petechiae of the oral mucosa, genital and rectal examination. Thyroid evaluation (nodules, asymmetry).

SYMPTOMS AND SIGNS
Variable, based on etiology.

LABORATORY
Complete blood count (CBC)
◇ with differential, sedimentation rate (ESR), peripheral smear to help in differential diagnosis of possible viral, bacterial or parasitic causes, possible chronic inflammation (eg, osteomyelitis, temporal arteritis), possible hemolysis.
Cultures
◇ blood (Brucellosis) (not to exceed 6) and urine
Chemistries
◇ particularly liver function studies, electrolytes, amylase. Urinalysis
Rheumatology work-up
◇ ANA, rheumatoid factor, LE prep, febrile agglutinins, Lyme's disease, HIV.
Bone marrow analysis
◇ to rule out abnormal hematopoiesis, tumor cells, granulomas.
Thyroid function studies
◇ TSH, T3, T4.

IMAGING/SPECIAL TESTS
Radiographic Studies
◇ common screening radiographs include chest radiograph, possibly paranasal sinus studies. CT or MRI scans of chest, abdomen, cranium, pelvis, etc. may be considered. Echocardiogram for endocarditis. Ventilation/perfusion scanning for pulmonary emboli. Nuclear scanning of bone or soft tissue possible to evaluate for osteomyelitis, chronic abscesses, or gallbladder disease. Barium enema or upper GI series may reveal ulcers, tumors, or diverticulae. Abdominal, renal, and pelvic ultrasound may help to locate masses, stones, or abscesses. Tuberculin skin testing.

Biopsy
◇ suspicious tissues should be considered, including any pulmonary, hepatic, bowel, sinus, or skin lesion. Elevated ESR, particularly if there is facial pain or headache, should prompt temporal artery biopsy.
Therapeutic trials
◇ if no cause of fever is found and the criteria for FUO are fulfilled, consider elimination of all medications. Reluctant consideration can be given to antibiotic or steroid trials after repetitive cultures of blood, urine, and sputum have proven negative.

DIFFERENTIAL
See etiology section.

TREATMENT

General
Based on discovering etiology.

MEDICATIONS
• Antipyretics if degree of temperature elevation threatens seizures or metabolic well-being.

SURGERY
Only as indicated by circumstances. Exploratory surgery occasionally needed.

CONSULTATION SUGGESTIONS
Infectious Disease Specialist, General Surgeon, Endocrinologist, Neurologist.

REFERRAL SUGGESTIONS
Primary Care Physician

COURSE/PROGNOSIS
Depends entirely on nature of fever.

CODING

ICD-9-CM
780.6 Fever of unknown etiology

CPT
70355 Panorex
99000 Transport of specimen to outside laboratory

MISCELLANEOUS

SYNONYMS
FUO

SEE ALSO
Actinomycosis
Brain abscess
Cavernous sinus thrombosis
Crohn's disease
Endocarditis
Fungal disease (deep)
Giant cell arteritis (temporal arteritis)
Hepatitis
Histoplasmosis
Hyperthyroidism
Rheumatic fever
Rheumatoid arthritis
Serum sickness
Thrombosis, deep vein (DVT)
Toxoplasmosis
Ulcerative colitis
Urinary tract infection

REFERENCES
Atkins E: Fever. In: Signs and Symptoms, 5th ed., McBryde, Blacklow, (eds), Philadelphia, JB Lippincott, 1972.

Brusch J. Weinstein L: Fever of unknown origin. Med Clin N Am 72:1247-1261, 1988.

Knockaert DC, et al: Fever of unknown origin in the 1980s. Arch Int Med 152:511-515, 1992.

AUTHOR
Robert Chuong, MD, DMD

Fibrous Dysplasia

BASICS

DESCRIPTION
• A condition in which fibrous connective tissue gradually replaces normal medullary bone. Two completely separate forms of the disease exist: monostotic and polyostotic. In the monostotic form, the disease process is limited to one bone. Polyostotic fibrous dysplasia represents a systemic disorder, and is further subdivided into two types: Jaffe's and Albright's. Both Jaffe's and Albright's types demonstrate the dysplastic process involving a variable number of bones, and cutaneous melanotic pigmentation. Albright's syndrome is also associated with endocrine abnormalities.
• Initially presents in the first or second decade of life.
• The monostotic form of the disease is much more common and accounts for approximately 80% of the reported cases.

ETIOLOGY

• The etiology of fibrous dysplasia remains unknown. Theories of the origin include hamartomatous growth of abnormal mesenchymal response to infection or trauma, or an arrest in the maturation of mesenchymal tissue.
• The monostotic form is clinically distinct from the polyostotic form, and the former will not progress into the latter.

SYSTEMS AFFECTED
Mandible
◊ presents as a hard, painless swelling almost always on the buccal surface. The body region is the most common site of occurrence in mandible. Pathologic fracture may occur if the lesion is large.
Maxilla
◊ most frequently affected bone in the skull. Presents as a hard swelling on the buccal surface, and will often spare the palate. Lesions may extend to involve the maxillary sinus, zygoma, sphenoid bone, and floor of the orbit. Severe facial disfigurement may result. When the maxilla and adjacent bones are involved, the condition is referred to as craniofacial fibrous dysplasia.
Teeth
◊ displacement of teeth is common, which may result in a malocclusion. Normal eruption patterns can be altered.

DIAGNOSIS

SYMPTOMS AND SIGNS
Face
◊ painless, hard swelling of the maxilla or mandible is usually the reason for seeking treatment.
Teeth
◊ may present with tipping, displacement, or a malocclusion.
Skin
◊ melanotic pigmentation, termed "café-au-lait" macules may present in the polyostotic form.
Endocrine
◊ precocious puberty is the most frequently reported endocrine disturbance in Albright's syndrome.

LABORATORY
Serum values are normal, and no specific test will confirm the diagnosis.

IMAGING/SPECIAL TESTS
Radiographic
◊ traditionally has been described as a "ground glass" appearance. Also may present as unilocular or multilocular radiolucencies. The borders of the lesion are poorly defined and appear to be blending into the surrounding normal bone.
Bone scans can be used to show location and level of activity of disease process.

DIFFERENTIAL
• Ossifying fibroma
• Paget's disease
• Chronic osteomyelitis
• Malignant tumors of bone

TREATMENT

General
◇ Treatment is based on the extent of the disease process. Small lesions may only require observation, biopsy to confirm the presumptive diagnosis, or an en bloc resection.

SURGERY
Large lesions that demonstrate cortical expansion or extensive midfacial involvement could result in severe disfigurement if resection attempted. Therefore, large lesions are generally treated with recontouring. Fibrous dysplasia demonstrates periods of rapid growth and remission. Recontouring should be performed when the disease process is stable.

CONSULTATION SUGGESTIONS
Oral-Maxillofacial Surgeon

REFERRAL SUGGESTIONS
Oral-Maxillofacial Surgeon

PATIENT INSTRUCTIONS
Reassure younger patients that process typically abates during latter part of puberty.

COURSE/PROGNOSIS
Fibrous dysplasia is characterized as a disease of childhood and will often stabilize after puberty. The affected area is inherently weaker than the normal bone and is at increased risk for pathologic fracture. If it does occur, the healing process is suspect. Malignant transformation has been reported to occur approximately 1% of the time; therefore, close follow-up is mandatory.

CODING

ICD-9-CM
520.6 Delayed tooth eruption
524.3 Displacement of teeth
525.8 Enlargement of alveolar ridge
526.89 Fibrous dysplasia

CPT
20240 Biopsy, excisional; superficial
21029 Removal by contouring of benign tumor of facial bone
70100 Radiologic exam, mandible; partial, less than four views
70355 Panorex

MISCELLANEOUS

SYNONYMS
Jaffe-Lichtenstein syndrome
McCune-Albright syndrome

SEE ALSO
Cherubism
Diabetes insipidus

REFERENCES
Regezi JA, Sciubba JJ: Benign Non-Odontogenic Tumors. In: Oral Pathology Clinical

Pathologic Correlations, 2nd ed. Philadelphia, WB Saunders, Co., 1993, pp. 372-375.

AUTHOR
Robert Rudman, DDS

Food Allergy

BASICS

DESCRIPTION
Perioral manifestations of food allergy can include urticaria, angioedema, aphthous stomatitis, and rhinitis. The symptoms usually appear within minutes of ingesting the offending food and last minutes to hours.

ETIOLOGY

• True food allergy is an IgE-mediated type 1 hypersensitivity reaction. Patients typically have elevated serum IgE and eosinophilia. Muco-cutaneous lesions develop due to mast cell degranulation. Additionally, some food allergies may lead to intestinal mucosal atrophy, malabsorption, and secondary oral ulceration, as in gluten sensitive enteropathy. However, in the latter case, the lesions are delayed and chronic.
• Common agents include milk, seeds, eggs, wheat, fish, nuts, chocolate, and foods with dyes and other additives.

SYSTEMS AFFECTED
Oral mucosa
  ◇ erythema, edema, ulceration, burning (mucositis); angioedema
Skin
  ◇ erythema, urticaria
Airway
  ◇ mucosal edema, bronchial constriction and asthma, rhinitis.
Gastrointestinal
  ◇ edema, ulceration, malabsorption, colitis.

DIAGNOSIS

SYMPTOMS AND SIGNS
• Itching, edema, erythema, rhinitis, wheezing all occurring within minutes of ingesting the offending food. GI symptoms include nausea, vomiting, diarrhea, abdominal pain, bloating. The key to diagnosis is the temporal association of food ingestion with lesion eruption.
• Anaphylaxis can occur such as with allergy to shellfish.

LABORATORY
Elevated IgE and peripheral eosinophilia.

IMAGING/SPECIAL TESTS
• Skin puncture or patch test, radioallergosorbent test (RAST), elimination diet.
• Examine stool or mucous for eosinophilia.
• Proctologic examination for rectal inflammation.

DIFFERENTIAL
• Angioedema
• Possibly contact mucositis

TREATMENT

General
◇ Patients should be tested for and avoid offending foods.
◇ No evidence desensitization effective.

MEDICATIONS
• Type I hypersensitivity can be life-threatening when there is prominent airway involvement. Intramuscular or subcutaneous epinephrine (0.5 ml, 1:1000) should be given immediately. Aerosolized corticosteroid and beta-adrenergic agonists will reduce airway inflammation and constriction.

CONSULTATION SUGGESTIONS
Allergist, Dietician

REFERRAL SUGGESTIONS
Primary Care Physician, Allergist

FIRST STEPS TO TAKE IN AN EMERGENCY
• Epinephrine (1 mL of 1:1000) s.q. or IM for anaphylaxis.

PATIENT INSTRUCTIONS
Carry self-administered epinephrine for anaphylaxis.

COURSE/PROGNOSIS
Symptoms and signs limited to the mucocutaneous surfaces are not long-lasting and have limited significance. However, airway involvement is life-threatening. Identified foods should be strictly avoided. Children sensitive to certain foods commonly outgrow problem. Adults with food allergy tend to always be sensitive.

CODING

ICD-9-CM
693.1 Allergy, food

CPT
99000 Specimen handling, transport to outside laboratory

MISCELLANEOUS

SYNONYMS
Anaphylaxis
Allergic bowel disease
Contact allergy
Dietary protein sensitivity syndrome

SEE ALSO
Epiglottitis
Anaphylaxis
Contact allergy

REFERENCES
Sampson HA: Adverse reactions to foods. In: Allergy Principles and Practice. 4th ed., St. Louis. CV Mosby Co., 1993.

AUTHOR
David A. Sirois, DMD, PhD

Gastroenteritis

BASICS

DESCRIPTION
A spectrum of infectious diseases affecting the gastrointestinal tract resulting in fever, malaise, nausea/vomiting, diarrhea, abdominal cramping, and pain. These enteric infections are very common and worldwide.

ETIOLOGY

Invasive organisms
Shigella: person-to-person transmission
- Salmonella: zoonosis-poultry, meat
- Campylobacter: zoonosis-dairy products
- Vibrio p.: seafood
- Yersinia: zoonosis
  ◇ dairy products
- Clostridia difficile: after antibiosis
- Viruses: Rotaviruses
  ◇ children (in winter)
Norwalk virus
◇ all ages
- Entamoeba histolytica: person-to-person
Noninvasive organisms
E. coli: must be ingested in large numbers to survive low pH of stomach
- Vibrio cholerae: contaminated water, food
Enteric toxins
Staphylococci: ingested with food
- Bacillus cereus: similar to staphylococcal food poisoning
- Vibrio, E. coli: similar enterotoxins
- Clostridia perfringens
  ◇ small bowel colonization
- Clostridia difficile
  ◇ large bowel colonization
Some organisms possess ability to adhere to (Vibrio) or invade (Shigella) gut mucosa
Protozoan organisms
- Giardia lamblia: small bowel colonization; chronic diarrhea
- Entamoeba histolytica: rare in U.S.
- Cryptosporidium: life-threatening disease in AIDS patients.

SYSTEMS AFFECTED
Stomach rarely affected due to low pH.
Small bowel
- common site of colonization; invasive organism
- usually terminal ileum
- enterotoxins site of action
- hemorrhagic strain of E. coli produces bloody stool
- viruses attack villi cells
Colon
- Shigella: invasive mechanism
- Campylobacter: generalized enterocolitis
- result in voluminous, watery diarrhea
CNS may be affected by toxins
- seizures, nausea/vomiting from Staphylococci
Myalgias and fever accompany mucosal invasion by organisms as a result from bacteremia
- Yersinia in children
Hepatic abscess in amebiasis

DIAGNOSIS

History
◇ epidemiology more important than identifying agent
Endemic regions
- Traveler's diarrhea; E. coli strains
Outbreaks regionally
- Food poisoning; S. aureus, B. cereus, C. perfringens, Salmonella, Shigella
Antibiotic usage: Clostridia difficile
Outbreaks in child care centers; viruses

SYMPTOMS AND SIGNS
Fever, malaise, nausea, vomiting, anorexia, abdominal cramping
Diarrhea
- Watery; "rice water" of V. cholerae
- Bloody; E. coli, amebiasis
- Dark-colored; C. difficile
Appendicitis-like syndrome of Yersinia
Chronic (>10 days)
◇ consider giardiasis or cryptosporidiosis
Abdominal pain; "acute abdomen," but diffuse in characterization
Sigmoidoscopy
- Mucosal damage; C. difficile plaques/pseudomembranes
- Frank blood
- Ulceration; typhoid enteritis
Early
◇ active or hyperactive bowel sounds
Late
◇ quiet abdomen (particularly with toxic megacolon)

LABORATORY
CBC/differential
Electrolytes
- acute loss in diarrhea may be life-threatening

IMAGING/SPECIAL TESTS
Stool cultures
◇ Shigella, Salmonella, Campylobacter
- Stool exam for WBC/pus, blood
- C. difficile toxin assay

DIFFERENTIAL
- Inflammatory bowel disease
- Other viral illnesses, especially children
- Diverticulitis
- Appendicitis
- Mittelschmerz syndrome (young women)

TREATMENT

<u>General</u>
◇ Fluid/electrolytes most important
  • Na⁺, K⁺, Cl⁻ all lost
  • Lactated Ringer's sufficient
  • Monitor glucose
If bloody, monitor hemoglobin
Stop antibiotics that predate onset

MEDICATIONS
• <u>Culture</u>
  ◇ directed antibiotics in:
• Cholera; tetracycline
• Shigellosis; ampicillin; TMP/SMZ
• Typhoid (Salmonella typhi)
• Ampicillin or TMP/SMZ for 3 to 4 weeks
• Eliminate carrier state (reservoir), especially those with gall bladder disease.
• E. coli; TMP/SMZ or ciprofloxacin
• Pseudomembranous colitis (C. difficile); metronidazole or oral vancomycin.
• Giardias; metronidazole; quinacrine or furazolidone.
• Amebiasis, metronidazole or rodoquinol;
• Antidiarrheals generally not indicated; may exacerbate shigellosis.

CONSULTATION SUGGESTIONS
Primary Care Physician, Gastroenterologist, Infectious Disease Specialist

REFERRAL SUGGESTIONS
Primary Care Physician, Gastroenterologist

FIRST STEPS TO TAKE IN AN EMERGENCY
• Administer intravenous fluids and electrolytes.

PATIENT INSTRUCTIONS
Try to keep well hydrated with electrolyte-containing fluids orally.

COURSE/PROGNOSIS
Most acute infections have a self-limiting course which resolves after several days; supportive fluid therapy is important. Children, elderly, and immunocompromised persons may require antibiotics and/or hospitalization if symptoms are severe. Monitoring fluid and electrolyte status is mainstay of treatment.

CODING

ICD-9-CM
005.9 Enteritis due to food poisoning
008.45 Pseudomembranous colitis
558.9 Gastroenteritis (Colitis)

MISCELLANEOUS

SYNONYMS
Enteritis
Colitis

SEE ALSO
Diarrhea
Pseudomembranous colitis
Inflammatory bowel disease
AIDS

REFERENCES
Donowitz M, Kokke FT, Saidi R: Evaluation of patients with chronic diarrhea. N Engl J Med 332:725-729, 1995.

Acute Infectious Diarrhea. In: Cecil's Essentials of Medicine. Andreoli TE, et al (eds). Philadelphia, WB Saunders Co., 1990, pp. 548-603.

Guerrant RE, Shields DS, et al: Evaluation and diagnosis of acute infectious diarrhea. Am J Med 78:91-98, 1985.

Hamilton JR: Treatment of acute diarrhea. Pediatr Clin N Am 32:418-428, 1985.

AUTHOR
Bruce Horswell, DMD, MD

Gastroesophageal Reflux Disease

BASICS

DESCRIPTION
• Reflux of gastroduodenal contents into esophagus.
• Occurs when normal or increased levels of reflux produce symptoms such as heartburn or result in esophagitis or tracheal aspiration. At least 10% of the population suffers from daily heartburn and as much as one-third of these people suffer from gastroesophageal reflux disease (GERD).

ETIOLOGY

• Patients with GERD have lower esophageal sphincter pressures for a variety of reasons: diseases that damage the esophageal sphincter (ES) muscle or from agents that antagonize stimulatory pathways; transient ES relaxation resulting from gastric distension; dietary constituents such as fat, chocolate, ethanol, peppermint, spearmint, coffee; tobacco products, anticholinergic medications, calcium channel antagonists, beta-agonists, alpha-adrenergic antagonists, dopamine, sedatives, and analgesics.
• Delayed gastric emptying and ineffective clearance of refluxed acid due to weak esophageal peristaltic contractions may worsen GERD.
• Esophageal mucosa irritants: stomach acid; bile acids and pepsin; citrus juices, tomato products, and coffee. All increase esophageal discomfort with a pH-dependent irritant effect on inflamed esophageal mucosa.
• Acid reflux in recumbent position (such as during sleep).
• Increased intra-abdominal pressure produced by tight clothing, obesity, or pregnancy.
• Scleroderma weakens the esophageal smooth muscle and the ES region.
• Surgical vagotomy.

SYSTEMS AFFECTED
Upper gastrointestinal tract
◇ esophageal ulceration, Barrett's esophagitis, esophageal stricture formation, dysphagia, reflux-induced laryngitis, and erosion of tooth enamel.
Pulmonary
◇ asthma, pneumonia, or pulmonary fibrosis due to tracheal aspiration.
Hematologic
◇ anemia from esophageal blood loss.

DIAGNOSIS

SYMPTOMS AND SIGNS
• Heartburn
• Dysphagia
◇ particularly for solids, which may indicate developing strictures.
• Weight loss
• Hoarseness, choking, coughing
• Wheezing, pneumonia
• Pallor from anemia
• Melena or hematemesis resulting from esophageal ulcers.
• Atypical noncardiac chest pain relieved by sitting up.
• Enamel erosion.

LABORATORY
CBC
◇ check for Fe^{++} deficiency anemia from chronic blood loss.

IMAGING/SPECIAL TESTS
Barium swallow
◇ evaluate the structure of the esophagus. Can identify peptic stricture or a deep ulceration. The presence of reflux on this study is not that sensitive except for severe gastroesophageal reflux with a very weakened ES.
Acid reflux test
◇ involves monitoring intraesophageal pH after instilling 300 mL of 0.1N hydrochloric acid into the stomach.
Acid perfusion test (Bernstein test)
◇ intended to reproduce the pain associated with reflux and involves esophageal perfusion of 0.1N HCl alternately with normal saline.
Twenty-four hour pH monitoring
Scintigraphy
◇ Technetium 99 introduction into the stomach followed by abdominal compression and radiographic counting over the esophagus. Can demonstrate reflux as well as provide quantitative measure.
Endoscopy with biopsy
◇ direct visualization and biopsy of lesions. Can diagnose esophagitis due to Candida albicans or viruses.
Manometric studies
◇ measure pressure in the esophageal body and at the ES. Can be used to evaluate competency of ES before surgical tightening techniques.

DIFFERENTIAL
• Carcinoma
• Barrett's esophagitis
• Candida albicans esophagitis
• Angina pectoris
• Achalasia
• Peptic ulcer disease
• Gastritis
• Crohn's disease

TREATMENT

General
◊ Elevate head of bed.
◊ Lose excessive weight.
◊ Avoid repeated stooping or bending over.
◊ Avoid acid or high fat foods, coffee, tobacco.

MEDICATIONS
• Antacids
◊ used for intermittent mild symptoms.
• Histamine-2 receptor antagonists
◊ binds receptor on gastric parietal cells. Cimetidine, ranitidine, famotidine, and nizatidine all markedly inhibit basal and stimulated gastric-acid production.
• Hydrogen/potassium adenosine triphosphatase (ATPase) blockers
◊ Omeprazole provides more potent and prolonged protection from the damaging effects of acid reflux.
• Prokinetics
◊ metoclopramide and cisapride increase ES pressure and enhance gastric emptying. They act by stimulating cholinergic nerves and inhibit dopaminergic pathways.

SURGERY
Antireflux surgery such as the Nissen fundoplication
◊ a segment of esophagus is maintained below the diaphragm and the distal esophagus is wrapped with the gastric fundus to increase ES pressure.

CONSULTATION SUGGESTIONS
Primary Care Physician, Gastroenterologist

REFERRAL SUGGESTIONS
Primary Care Physician, Gastroenterologist, General Surgeon

PATIENT INSTRUCTIONS
• Antireflux instructions that include reducing body weight, elevating the head of the bed 2 to 4 inches, and avoidance of eating 3 hours before bedtime.
• Exclude dietary agents that reduce ES pressure (ie, caffeine, peppermint, spearmint, ethanol, high-fat foods, and chocolate).
• Cease tobacco use.
• Avoid tight clothing.
• Avoid anticholinergics, beta-antagonists, calcium channel antagonists, dopamine, and alpha-adrenergic medications.

COURSE/PROGNOSIS
In most patients with mild symptoms, anti-reflux instruction and a trial of medications may prove helpful. When more severe symptoms or complications arise such as strictures or hemorrhage, structural and functional studies should be performed. Persistent bleeds can be treated endoscopically with cautery. Peptic strictures should be dilated to relieve dysphagia. And Barrett's esophagitis needs to have periodic endoscopy and biopsy because of the risk of adenocarcinoma.

CODING

ICD-9-CM
530.1 Esophagitis
750.6 Hiatal hernia
787.1 Heartburn

MISCELLANEOUS

SYNONYMS
Heartburn
Reflux esophagitis
Barrett's esophagitis
Symptomatic hiatal hernia

SEE ALSO
Peptic ulcer disease

REFERENCES
Koufman JA: Otolaryngologic manifestations of gastroesophageal reflux disease. Laryngoscope 101 (Suppl. 53) 1-78, 1991.

AUTHOR
Jonathan S. Sasportas, DMD, MD

Geographic Tongue

BASICS

DESCRIPTION
• A benign migratory inflammation of the tongue characterized by multiple areas of desquamation of the filiform papillae in an irregular coiled or patchy pattern.
• Incidence of 1.4 to 2.4%, with a 1:2 male:female ratio. No racial predilection.

ETIOLOGY

Unknown etiology, although it has been suggested that it is brought on by emotional stress.

SYSTEMS AFFECTED
Tongue
◇ the only site for appearance of these lesions.
• Often seen with other minor variations in tongue structure such as fissured tongue, irregularities at the dorsal/ventral epithelial junction, and isolated patches of keratinized epithelium on the ventral mucosa.
• Lesions appearing in other sites of the oral cavity (buccal mucosa, gingiva, palate, lips, and floor of the mouth), though clinically and histologically similar, are not related.

DIAGNOSIS

SYMPTOMS AND SIGNS
• Mouth
◇ usually lesions are asymptomatic and are an incidental finding on routine examination. A painful, burning sensation of the tongue is occasionally reported affecting speech, swallowing, and mastication, and is worsened by spicy foods or citrus fruits.
• The central portion of the lesion is red and appears inflamed with a thin, yellowish-white border. Filiform papillae may persist in affected areas as small, elevated red dots.

IMAGING/SPECIAL TESTS
Tongue biopsy revealing peripheral hyperkeratosis and acanthosis. The center of the lesion is absent of parakeratin with migration of PMNs and lymphocytes into the epithelium resulting in microabscesses. The underlying connective tissue has a diffuse inflammatory infiltrate.

DIFFERENTIAL
• Thermal or chemical burn of the tongue
• Pernicious anemia (vitamin B_{12} deficiency)
• Pustular psoriatic dermatitis
• Reiter's syndrome
• Lichen planus
• Dermatitis herpiformis

TREATMENT

General
◇ No one treatment has been proven to alleviate symptoms or to alter the course of the lesions regularly.

MEDICATIONS
• Heavy therapeutic doses of vitamins have been used empirically.
• Topical anesthetics (ie, benzocaine or lidocaine), aqueous antihistamines, or topical steroids have variable efficacy on the subjective complaints of the patients.
• Topical applications of salicylic acid and tretinion (Retin-A) have recently been recommended as a way to eliminate lesions.

SURGERY
Removal not indicated.

CONSULTATION SUGGESTIONS
Oral Medicine, Oral-Maxillofacial Surgeon

REFERRAL SUGGESTIONS
Oral Medicine, Oral-Maxillofacial Surgeon

PATIENT INSTRUCTIONS
Reassurance lesions are not malignant.

COURSE/PROGNOSIS
• The duration of attacks are variable lasting from weeks to months.
• Generally, once one is affected, the attacks are recurrent.

CODING

ICD-9-CM
529.1 Geographic tongue

CPT
41100 Biopsy, tongue, anterior 2/3
44105 Biopsy, tongue, posterior 1/3
99000 Transport of specimen to outside laboratory

M MISCELLANEOUS

SYNONYMS
Erythema migrans
Glossitis areata migrans
Glossitis areata exfoliativa
Wandering rash of the tongue
Benign migratory glossitis
Erythema circinata migrans
Annulus migrans

SEE ALSO
Lichen planus
Anemia
Glossitis

REFERENCES
Halperin V, Kolas S, Jefferies KR, Huddleston SO, Robinson HBG: The occurrence of Fordyce spots, benign migratory glossitis, medium rhomboid glossitis, and fissured tongue in 2478 dental patients. Oral Surg Oral Med Oral Path, 6:1072-1077, 1953.

Burket's Oral Medicine Diagnosis and Treatment, 9th ed. Lynch MA, Brightman BJ, Greenberg MS (eds), Philadelphia, JB Lippincott Co., 1994, pp. 258-260.

Geographic tongue. Oral Pathology: Clinical-Pathologic Correlations. 2nd ed. Regezi JA, Scuibba J. (eds), Philadelphia, WB Saunders Co. 1993, pp. 113-114.

AUTHOR
Dale J. Misiek, DMD

Giant Cell (Temporal) Arteritis

BASICS

DESCRIPTION
• A granulomatous vasculitis of large- and medium-sized arteries (with a prominent internal elastic lamina) occurring in the aortic arch and its branches. It can present as headache, painful inflamed temporal arteries, jaw claudication, polymyalgia rheumatica, and elevated erythrocyte sedimentation rate.
• This disease occurs in the 50 to 80 years of age group and has a slight female preponderance. There is an annual incidence of approximately 12 cases in 100,000 individuals. Takayasu arteritis (pulseless disease) is a similar disease, affecting the carotid and subclavian arteries in young oriental women.

ETIOLOGY

• Etiology unknown.
• There is a genetic preponderance with 60% of patients showing a variant of HLA DR1 associated with rheumatoid arthritis.

DIAGNOSIS

SYSTEMS AFFECTED
The importance of early diagnosis and treatment of giant cell arteritis (GCA) cannot be overemphasized due to the danger of irreversible blindness. A 3 cm biopsy of the superficial temporal artery is required to observe the "skip" lesions of GCA. Temporal arteriography is of limited value; however, claudication of an extremity or vasculitis of a large vessel merits confirmation by angiography.

SYMPTOMS AND SIGNS
Severe headache and/or temporal pain, scalp tenderness, and visual disturbances (amaurosis fugax, diplopia, visual blurring, ptosis, and scomata) can be the initial complaints depending on the site of the arteritis. Scalp tenderness makes combing hair painful and is frequently described as tender red cords in the temples. Claudication with associated pain of the tongue and also the masseter and temporalis muscles has been recorded. Anterior ischemic optic nerve neuropathy leading to blindness occurs in approximately 20% of patients. Systemic symptoms are the same as those in polymyalgia rheumatica, which in some patients can present as a manifestation of an underlying giant cell arteritis. Physical examination may reveal swelling, tenderness, and warmth of the temporal arteries.

LABORATORY
Elevated ESRs of greater than 60 mm/hour occur in 97% of patients, but is not specific for GCA. Anemia (normocytic and normochromic) is present in many of these patients, as is an elevated alkaline phosphatase, but there are currently no non-invasive tests for diagnosis of this disease process. Elevated plasma proteins occur as the result of a response to the inflammation.

IMAGING/SPECIAL TESTS
Pathology
◇ Giant cell arteritis affects the aortic arch and all its branches, but does not cause a widespread intracranial cerebral vasculitis. Superficial temporal artery involvement occurs in most patients. Microscopically, it appears as granulomatous inflammatory reaction with lymphocytes and multinucleated giant cells in contact with the internal elastic lamina. This thickening of the intima causes narrowing and closure of the vessel lumen. This reaction can, however, "skip" areas and a biopsy of such an area can lead to a false negative reading.

DIFFERENTIAL
• Headache due to tumor, muscle contraction, migraine, or other non-vasculitis etiology.
• Cerebral vascular insufficiency
• Sinusitis
• Myofascial pain dysfunction

TREATMENT

General
◊ Corticosteroid therapy should be instituted immediately after the likelihood of GCA is suspected to prevent the possibility of blindness even prior to the biopsy. The characteristic histologic appearance will be present up to 1 week after the institution of steroid therapy.

MEDICATIONS
• An initial daily dose of 60 mg of prednisone that should be continued until symptoms resolve and the ESR shows signs of returning to normal. The steroids should then be tapered gradually by 5 mg/week to 40 mg/day, then by 2 mg/week to 20 mg/day, then by 1 mg/week until the patient is weaned. Any evidence of a flare of symptoms will require an increase in the steroids until the symptoms are controlled. Many patients require steroid therapy for years following the occurrence of GCA.

SURGERY
Temporal artery biopsy. Need at least 2.5 cm. If negative, consider biopsy from other side.

CONSULTATION SUGGESTIONS
Oral-Maxillofacial Surgeon, Oral Medicine, Rheumatologist

REFERRAL SUGGESTIONS
Primary Care Physician

FIRST STEPS TO TAKE IN AN EMERGENCY
• Initiate steroid therapy immediately if visual disturbances appear.

PATIENT INSTRUCTIONS
Patients on chronic steroids should receive calcium supplements. Because steroid therapy causes adrenal suppression, patients should obtain medical alert identification jewelry.

COURSE/PROGNOSIS
With steroid therapy, symptoms and potential for visual disturbance should resolve. Without therapy, high risk of permanent blindness.

CODING

ICD-9-CM
446.5 Giant cell arteritis
446.7 Takayasu's disease

CPT
37609 Temporal artery biopsy
90780 IV infusion
99000 Transport specimen to outside laboratory

MISCELLANEOUS

SYNONYMS
Temporal arteritis

SEE ALSO
Polymyalgia rheumatica
Headache (Migraine, Tension)
Temporomandibular disorder (extracapsular)

REFERENCES
Hunter GG: Giant cell arteritis and polymyalgia rheumatica. In: Textbook of Rheumatology, 3rd ed. Kelly WN, et al, (eds), Philadelphia, WB Saunders Co. 1989.

Fauci AS, Leavitt RY: Vasculitis. In: Arthritis & Allied Conditions, 12th ed. McCarty DJ, Koopman WJ (eds), Philadelphia, Lea & Febiger, 1993, pp. 1301-1322.

AUTHOR
Janet Leigh, BDS, DMD

Glaucoma

BASICS

DESCRIPTION
• Increased intraocular pressure from blockage of aqueous humor, due to decreased outflow of fluid into the Canal of Schlemm located in anterior chamber of the eye.
• Incidence 1:1000, Female >Male, Predominant age 55 to 70.

ETIOLOGY

There are two major types of glaucoma: open angle (chronic) and closed-angle (acute). In closed-angle glaucoma, which constitutes 5% of glaucomas, the passageway for aqueous outflow is abruptly blocked by closure of the angle and the iris becomes pressed up against the cornea. With closed-angle attack, the intraocular pressure raises up to 60 mm Hg, causing the eye to become hard. In open angle glaucoma, blockage of the aqueous outflow is more subtle, involving a microscopic blockage of the aqueous outflow in the Canal of Schlemm. The findings in chronic open-angle glaucoma are less severe, being the product of only modest intraocular pressure elevations over a longer period.

SYSTEMS AFFECTED
Eye
◊ permanent visual changes are possible if left untreated.

DIAGNOSIS

SYMPTOMS AND SIGNS
• Decreased vision, painful eye, nausea, vomiting;
• Increased intraocular pressure, corneal edema, visual field defects, conjunctival injection, enlarged and/or fixed pupil, increased lacrimation.

IMAGING/SPECIAL TESTS
• Complete ophthalmology examination, gonioscopic evaluation, slit-lamp examination.
• Normal intraocular pressure (10 to 23 mm Hg). Shallow anterior chamber on slit lamp exam.

DIFFERENTIAL
• Pigmentary glaucoma
Corticosteroid
◊ induced glaucoma
• Optic Atrophy
• Miotic administration

TREATMENT

MEDICATIONS
• Beta-blockers (levobunolol 0.25 to 0.5%, timolol 0.25 to 0.5%); miotics (pilocarpine); carbonic anhydrase inhibitors (acetazolamide (Diamox)), corticosteroids (prednisolone), hyperosmotics (mannitol, glycerin).

SURGERY
Laser trabeculoplasty, glaucoma filter surgery, shunt tube procedure

CONSULTATION SUGGESTIONS
Ophthalmologist

REFERRAL SUGGESTIONS
Ophthalmologist

FIRST STEPS TO TAKE IN AN EMERGENCY
• Immediate referral to ophthalmology through hospital emergency department.

PATIENT INSTRUCTIONS
• Seek care by ophthalmologist.
• Comply with instructions relating to medications for glaucoma control.

COURSE/PROGNOSIS
Usually progressive leading to blindness if not treated. Acute glaucoma is medical emergency.

 ## CODING

ICD-9-CM
364.41 Glaucoma associated with hyphema
365.11 Chronic glaucoma
365.20 Acute angle closure
365.22 Acute glaucoma

 ## MISCELLANEOUS

SYNONYMS
Narrow angle glaucoma
Angle closure glaucoma

SEE ALSO
Conjunctivitis

REFERENCES
Lam S, Rapuano C, Krachmer J: Cornea and External Disease. In: Vrabec M, Florakis G. (eds), Ophthalmic Essentials. Oxford. Blackwell Scientific, 1992, pp. 126-128.

Cullom R, Chang B: The Willis Eye Manual, Philadelphia, JB Lippincott Co., 1994, pp. 209-216.

AUTHOR
Michael J. Buckley, DMD, MS

Glomerulonephritis

BASICS

DESCRIPTION
• Glomerular disease includes all renal conditions in which functional and structural abnormalities of the glomeruli are involved. The kidneys may be involved in multiple system diseases of known cause, but in most cases, the cause is unknown. Predominant age range is 2 to 12 years.
• Acute Glomerulonephritis
  • The acute nephritic syndrome consists of the abrupt onset of hematuria and proteinuria and azotemia (reduced GFR), and renal salt and water retention. Decreased urinary output may be marked, and circulatory congestion, hypertension, and edema may follow.
• Both intracellular and extracellular fluid volumes are expanded by salt and fluid retention. The edema may appear initially in areas of lower pressure (ie, periorbital areas), and progress to dependent areas and lead to ascites and/or pleural effusions. Pulmonary edema and arterial diastolic hypertension may occur.
  • Hematuria may be secondary to migration of erythrocytes across damaged glomeruli. Gross hematuria is common and can be described as smoky, coffee, or cola-colored urine. May be accompanied by red cell casts. Red blood cells are small, distorted, fragmented, and hypochromic.
  • Proteinuria is a consequence of a loss of anionic charges of the capillary wall, or increase in the capillary pore radius, permitting large plasma protein molecules to cross the glomerular filter. The loss of protein may vary with the nature and severity of the underlying glomerular disease. Protein excretion rates may be between 0.5 and 3g/d. If proteinuria is marked and sustained, the nephrotic syndrome will appear.

• Acute Poststreptococcal Glomerulonephritis:
  • Follows a pharyngeal or cutaneous infection with a number of "nephritogenic" strains of group A, beta-hemolytic streptococci. The streptococci may be identified by serotyping of a cell wall antigen (M-Protein).
  • Immunity to M-Protein is type-specific, long-lasting, and protective; therefore, repeated episodes are rare.
  • Most common in children aged 6 to 10, mostly male. The latent period for pharyngeal infections is usually 6 to 10 days. Cutaneous infections are associated with longer latent periods, about 2 weeks.
• Rapidly Progressive Glomerulonephritis: Clinical syndrome characterized by rapid deterioration of renal function leading to uremia. Proliferation of extracapillary cells of Bowman's capsule or crescentic glomerulonephritis may occur.
  • The cause may be unknown, or associated with other diseases such as poststreptococcal glomerulonephritis, hypersensitivity angiitis, systemic lupus, Goodpasture's syndrome, thrombotic thrombocytopenia purpura, hemolytic-uremic syndrome, and membranoproliferative glomerulonephritis.
• Chronic Glomerulonephritis: Describes persistent glomerular dysfunction after apparent clinical healing of acute disease, generally poststreptococcal glomerulonephritis.

MISCELLANEOUS
Guillain-Barré syndrome, diphtheria-pertussis-tetanus vaccine, serum sickness.

ETIOLOGY

• Immunologically, two mechanisms are generally involved:
  • Antiglomerular basement membrane antibodies.
  • Deposition of circulating antigen-antibody complexes in the glomeruli with resultant inflammatory reaction leading to glomerular damage.
• Primarily an antecedent of group A beta-hemolytic streptococcus infection.
• Proliferation of extracapillary cells and formation of crescents in Bowman's capsule in greater than 60% of the glomeruli.
• Antigens are usually found in the crescents and there may be linear deposits of immunoglobulins in antiglomerular basement membrane (anti-GBM) disease.
• Immune-complex disease may occur when immunoglobulin and complement are deposited along glomerular capillaries.
• Nonimmune disease with no deposits of immunoglobulins can be seen, but are not common.
• Causes of acute glomerulonephritis.
• Infectious diseases
• Poststreptococcal glomerulonephritis
  ◇ most common
    • Nonstreptococcal postinfectious glomerulonephritis
    Bacterial: infective endocarditis, "shunt nephritis," sepsis, pneumococcal pneumonia, typhoid fever, meningococcemia.
    Viral: hepatitis B, infectious mononucleosis, mumps, measles, varicella, echovirus, coxsackievirus.
• Multisystem diseases
  • Systemic lupus erythematosus, vasculitis, Henoch-Schönlein purpura, Goodpasture's disease.
• Primary glomerular diseases
  • Membranoproliferative glomerulonephritis, Berger's disease (IgA nephropathy), mesangial proliferative glomerulonephritis.

SYSTEMS AFFECTED
Renal
  ◇ impaired renal function
Skin
  ◇ edema
Cardiovascular
  ◇ circulatory congestion

Glomerulonephritis

DIAGNOSIS

SYMPTOMS AND SIGNS
• Gross hematuria, described as smoky or cola-colored urine. All patients have gross or microscopic hematuria.
• Dull, aching abdominal or flask pain may be present.
• Some degree of edema develops, usually in the face and eyelids in morning, feet and ankles by evening.
• May have mild to moderate hypertension, circulatory congestion or pulmonary edema. Weight gain due to water retention.
• History of pharyngitis, scarlet fever, impetigo, rheumatic fever, or erysipelas.
• Usually oliguria or anuria is present.

LABORATORY
• Proteinuria, hematuria, and red blood cell casts are almost always found.
• CBC
  ◊ anemia
• Decreased calcium.
• ANA
  ◊ to rule out lupus

IMAGING/SPECIAL TESTS
• Hypocomplementemia (C3)
• Throat culture positive for group A beta-hemolytic streptococcus.
• Measurements of changing antibody titers to streptococcal antigens (antistreptolysin O (ASO), antistreptokinase (ASU), anti-NADase, or streptozyme).
• Renal biopsy with histopathology, electron microscopy, immunofluorescene (C3).
• Secondary hyperparathyroidism may cause solitary or multiple giant cell (Brown) tumors in jaws. Appear as radiolucencies with poorly corticated borders. May also see decreased opacity of lamina dura.

DIFFERENTIAL
• Differential diagnosis for poststreptococcal glomerulonephritis includes other infectious or primary renal diseases, including systemic lupus erythematosus, Henoch-Schönlein purpura, and vasculitis. All may present with acute nephritis.
• Also IgA nephropathy.

TREATMENT

General
◊ After glomerulonephritis develops, no treatment modality changes the clinical course, and treatment is supportive.
◊ Complications such as circulatory congestion, hypertension, and metabolic abnormalities are prevented or treated with diet, fluid, and sodium restriction, diuretics, and anti-hypertensives. Dialysis as indicated.

MEDICATIONS
• Streptococcal infection should be treated with antibiotics for 7 to 10 days.
• Steroids, cytotoxic agents, or anticoagulants are of no benefit except for rapidly progressive glomerulonephritis. In 90% of these patients, end-stage renal failure develops within a short time. Large doses of steroids may be beneficial in cases not induced by anti-GBM antibodies.
• Plasmapheresis to decrease levels of anti-GBM antibodies along with steroids and immunosuppressive drugs may be helpful in reducing mortality and morbidity.
• Avoid potassium in IV fluids. Monitor K^+ closely. Correct hypocalcemia.

SURGERY
• Renal biopsy.
• May require renal transplantation.
• Biopsy of jaw radiolucencies reveals multinucleated giant cells.

CONSULTATION SUGGESTIONS
Primary Care Physician, Nephrologist

REFERRAL SUGGESTIONS
Primary Care Physician

FIRST STEPS TO TAKE IN AN EMERGENCY
• If hyperkalemia occurs, use Kayexalate resin 1 gm/kg in 10% sorbitol per rectum or orally.

PATIENT INSTRUCTIONS
Contact National Kidney Foundation for helpful literature (212)889-2210.

COURSE/PROGNOSIS
Mild proteinuria and microscopic hematuria may persist for up to 2 years. Five percent of patients may die in acute phase in spite of dialysis. Otherwise, most patients recover completely.

CODING

ICD-9-CM
580.0 Glomerulonephritis, acute
588.8 Hyperparathyroidism, renal origin

CPT
20220 Bone biopsy
99000 Transport of specimen to outside laboratory

MISCELLANEOUS

SYNONYMS
Acute nephritic syndrome
Postinfectious glomerulonephritis
Acute poststreptococcal glomerulonephritis

SEE ALSO
Rheumatic fever
Erysipelas
Renal failure
Potassium disorders
Hyperparathyroidism

REFERENCES
Glassock RJ, Brenner BM: The Major Glomerulopathies. In: Harrison's Principles of Internal Medicine, 13th ed. Isselbacher KJ, et al (eds), New York, McGraw-Hill, 1994, pp. 1295-1306.

AUTHOR
Jerry L. Jones, DDS, MD

Glossitis

BASICS

DESCRIPTION
• Local or widespread inflammation of the mucosa of the tongue. May occur alone or as a component of a more widespread oral inflammatory disease (stomatitis) and may be the result of several specific diseases.
• Inflammation of the dorsal tongue mucosa characteristically results in atrophy of the filiform papillae, focally or uniformly, giving involved areas a relatively smooth, erythematous appearance. If the inflammation persists or is more profound, focal areas of the mucosa can ulcerate, producing the . characteristic white, fibrin clot.

ETIOLOGY

• Trauma, acute or chronic, mechanical or chemical.
Infectious agents
   ◊ viral, bacterial, fungal (candidiasis).
Idiopathic diseases
   ◊ lichen planus, aphthous, drug reactions.
Autoimmune disease
   ◊ pemphigoid, pemphigus, lupus.
• Vitamin B or zinc deficiencies.
• Anemias.

SYSTEMS AFFECTED
Oral mucosa rendered more susceptible to infection or further inflammation by topical agents, including hot beverages and spicy foods. Taste can be reduced or otherwise altered.

DIAGNOSIS

• Genera
   ◊ Biopsy may be indicated for glossitis, which cannot be diagnosed based on its clinical features alone, such as:
Benign migratory glossitis (geographic tongue)
   ◊ an idiopathic, usually asymptomatic condition characterized by one or more areas of glossal mucosal erythema (atrophy) bordered by incomplete white (hyperkeratotic) rims. These foci heal and reform in different locations on an unpredictable time scale.
Median rhomboid glossitis
   ◊ an erythematous (atrophic), roughly rhomboid patch of mucosa just anterior to the circumvallate papillae in the midline of the dorsal tongue. The lesion is usually asymptomatic and thought by most to be a localized form of candidiasis.
• Cytologic preparations may be indicated if candidiasis is suspected for a generalized or localized glossitis.

SYMPTOMS AND SIGNS
• Usually patients report pain, sometimes characterized as a burning sensation of the tongue, exacerbated by hot and spicy foods and beverages. Sometimes patients report altered taste.
• Focal areas of filiform papillae atrophy, erythema, and sometimes ulceration.

LABORATORY
No clinical laboratory tests are of significant value unless a vitamin or mineral deficiency is suspected, or a systemic disease such as lupus is in differential.

IMAGING/SPECIAL TESTS
• A biopsy may be necessary to diagnose one of the more specific diseases listed above.
• An exfoliative cytology can be used if candidiasis is suspected.

DIFFERENTIAL
See etiology.

TREATMENT

General
◇ Based on the cause (disease) identified.

MEDICATIONS
• Clotrimazole troches 5 to 6 times/day for candida.
• Prednisone (topical or systemic) for autoimmune disease.
• Vitamin supplements for deficiency states.

CONSULTATION SUGGESTIONS
Oral Medicine

REFERRAL SUGGESTIONS
Oral Medicine, Oral-Maxillofacial Surgeon

COURSE/PROGNOSIS
Dependent on the primary disease identified.

CODING

ICD-9-CM
054.2 Primary herpes
054.9 Recurrent herpes
079.9 Viral infection
112.9 Candidiasis
136.9 Bacterial infection
400.0 Burn
528.0 Stomatitis
528.2 Aphthous
529.1 Glossitis
694.4 Pemphigus
694.6 Cicatricial pemphigoid
695.1 Erythema multiforme
695.4 Lupus
697.0 Lichen planus

CPT
11900 Intralesional injection
40812 Incisional biopsy
87252 Culture isolation
88160 Cytologic preparation

MISCELLANEOUS

SEE ALSO
Pemphigoid
Lichen planus
Pemphigus
Erythema multiforme

REFERENCES
Coleman GC: Differential diagnosis of dark mucosal lesions. In: Principles of Oral Diagnosis. Coleman G, Nelson J. (eds.), Mosby Year-Book, 1993, pp. 300-327.

Vincent SD: Clinical management of idiopathic and autoimmune diseases involving oral mucous membrane. In: Oral and Maxillofacial Surgery Clinics of North America. Vol. 5. Gold L. (ed.), Philadelphia, WB Saunders Co., 1993.

Van Dis ML, Vincent SD: Diagnosis and management of autoimmune and idiopathic mucosal disease. Dental Clinics N Am. Vol. 36 Philadelphia, WB Saunders, Co. 1992, pp. 897-919.

Vincent SD, Finkelstein MW: Differential diagnosis of oral ulcers. In: Principles of Oral Diagnosis. Coleman GC, Nelson JF. (eds.), Mosby-Year Book Co., 1993, pp. 328-351.

Finkelstein MW, Vincent SD: Management of mucosal and related dermatological disorders. In: Principles of Oral and Maxillofacial Surgery, Peterson LJ, et al, (eds.), Philadelphia, JB Lippincott Co., 1991, pp. 881-900.

AUTHOR
Steven Vincent, DDS, MS

Glossopharyngeal Neuralgia

BASICS

DESCRIPTION
• A disorder of the somatosensory component of the 9th cranial nerve. Characterized by momentary episodes of paroxysmal, lancinating pain in the region of the larynx, tonsil, or ear. Less common than trigeminal neuralgia.
• Pain is most often unilateral and may be precipitated by yawning, swallowing, or contact of food with the tonsillar region.
• Presence of identifiable trigger zone is less common than in trigeminal neuralgia.
• Bradycardia, asystole, loss of consciousness, or seizure activity may occur during a paroxysm of pain.
• Predominant age: onset rare before age 20 years, slightly more common at age 50 years or older.

ETIOLOGY
• Unknown in most cases.
• Vascular compression of 9th and 10th cranial nerves has been postulated as a possible cause.
• Spillover of impulses from 9th cranial nerve to the motor nucleus of the vagus nerve via the tractus solitarius is likely cause of reflex bradycardia or asystole, and resulting seizures.

SYSTEMS AFFECTED
Nervous
  ◊ severe, lancinating paroxysmal pain in region of larynx, tonsil, or ear. Loss of consciousness or seizures occasionally seen.
Cardiovascular
  ◊ reflex bradycardia or asystole occasionally seen.
Digestive
  ◊ dysphagia.

DIAGNOSIS

SYMPTOMS AND SIGNS
• Severe, lancinating pain in larynx, tonsil, or ear.
• Pain elicited by yawning, swallowing, or contact of food with trigger area.
Neurosensory system
  ◊ no associated neurosensory deficit in affected dermatome; loss of consciousness, seizures.
Cardiovascular system
  ◊ bradycardia, asystole.
Respiratory/Digestive
  ◊ normal motility function of nasopharynx.

IMAGING/SPECIAL TESTS
Application of 10% solution of cocaine or other surface anesthetic to the tonsil and pharynx provides significant pain relief for 1 to 2 hours.

DIFFERENTIAL
• Geniculate neuralgia
• Eagle's syndrome
• Neoplasm
• Atypical facial pain

Glossopharyngeal Neuralgia

TREATMENT

General
◊ Pharmacologic management is initial/ preferred means of treatment for pain.

MEDICATIONS
• Drug(s) of choice
• Carbamazepine (200 to 1600 mg/day) and/or phenytoin (300 to 600 mg/day).
• Carbamazepine is used for initial therapy. Side-effects include drowsiness, ataxia, aplastic anemia, agranulocytosis, and thrombocytopenia. Serum carbamazepine levels and complete blood count with differential must be obtained at regular intervals during chronic carbamazepine therapy.

SURGERY
• Cardiac pacemaker placement is used for patients with associated bradycardia or asystole.
• If unresponsive to or unable to tolerate medications:
Intracranial sectioning of glossopharyngeal nerve and upper rootlets of the vagus nerve.
Sectioning of nervus intermedius of the 7th cranial nerve may be done in addition to intracranial sectioning when pain localizes to inner ear.

CONSULTATION SUGGESTIONS
Dentist with special training in facial pain disorders, Neurologist

REFERRAL SUGGESTIONS
Neurologist

COURSE/PROGNOSIS
Patients commonly experience periods of remission, ranging from several months to several years. Some patients report no periods of pain relief.

CODING

ICD-9-CM
784.0 Pain, facial

CPT
64716 Decompression/transposition, cranial nerve

MISCELLANEOUS

SYNONYMS
Vagoglossopharyngeal neuralgia
Vagal neuralgia

SEE ALSO
Trigeminal neuralgia
Styloid process hyperplasia

REFERENCES
Dalessio DJ: Diagnosis and treatment of cranial neuralgias. Med Clin N Am 75:605-615, 1991.

Rushton JG, Stevens JC, Miller RH: Glossopharyngeal (vagoglossopharyngeal) neuralgia, a study of 217 cases. Arch Neurol 38:201-205, 1981.

Saviolo R, Faisconaro G: Treatment of glossopharyngeal neuralgia by carbamazepine. Br Heart J 58:292-291, 1987.

AUTHOR
Warren P. Vallerand, DDS

Gout

BASICS

DESCRIPTION
Condition characterized by hyperuricemia in which uric acid is deposited within body fluids, particularly articular joints.

ETIOLOGY

• Hyperuricemia that is intermittent or sustained.
• Most commonly a result of under-excretion of urate (approximately 90% of gout afflicted patients). The primary mode of excretion is renal and a defect in renal handling of urate is the most common cause of primary hyperuricemia.
• Secondary hyperuricemia also occurs at the level of the kidney and may be caused by a variety of processes, including medications (diuretics, EtOH, pyrazinamide, ethambutol, salicylates at low doses), volume depletion states (nephrogenic diabetes insipidus, dehydration, diuretics) and states in which there is increased organic acid load (EtOH, diabetic ketoacidosis, lactic acidosis, starvation). Lead nephropathy may also be a cause of increased urate levels in serum.
About 10% of patients are overproducers of urate. Included are those with inborn errors of metabolism; complete (Lesch Nyhan syndrome) or partial deficiency of hypoxanthine
◊ guanine phosphoribosyl transferase or 5-phosphoribosyl-1-pyrophosphate synthetase overactivity. It may also be secondary to a variety of causes related to increased nucleic acid turnover; myeloproliferative disorders, hematologic malignancy, psoriasis, increased purine intake or uptake, and increased ATP degradation states such as glycogen storage disease, hypoxia, or various acidoses.
• Cancer chemotherapy with high tumor burden also results in increased urate levels.

SYSTEMS AFFECTED
• Predominantly affects the joints, typically in monoarticular fashion of lower extremities causing an extremely painful arthritis. With time, attacks may become polyarticular.
• Kidneys are affected by urate deposition in the interstitium and/or medullary compartments causing functional impairment. Nephrosclerosis due to concomitant hypertension is not uncommon and may be the more common cause of renal dysfunction and insufficiency.
• Obstructive uropathy is secondary to urate precipitants in the collecting tubules and ureters. This is most common in tumor lysis syndrome patients with high tumor burden.
• Nephrolithiasis may occur secondary to urate stones or calcium oxalate stones because gout patients are also more susceptible to calcium containing stones.

DIAGNOSIS

SYMPTOMS AND SIGNS
• Acute intermittent bouts of monoarticular arthritis with joint swelling, erythema, and warmth, particularly of lower extremities. The first metalarsophalangeal joint is affected in approximately 90% of patients.
• Urinary calculi, lithiasis.
• Articular deposition, gouty tophi.

LABORATORY
Increased serum urate > 7 mg/dL in men, 6 mg/dL in women.
Definitive diagnosis
◊ synovial fluid with negative birefringent crystals, particularly intracellular needle-shaped crystals. Increased WBC of 10,000 to 60,000 is not uncommon in synovial fluid of acute gouty joints.
24 hour urinary urate excretion > 1,000 mg/dL
• Increased ESR.

DIFFERENTIAL
• Crystal induced synovitis
• Septic arthritis
• Pseudogout (Calcium pyrophosphate dihydrate deposition disease).
• Primary versus Secondary
• Medication induced (eg, diuretics)
• Lead toxicity
• Endocrine
• Hypovolemia
• Metabolic

TREATMENT

Recurrent Acute Gout
General
◇ rest, immobilization of joint, weight reduction, avoidance of high purine loads, aspirin, diuretics, (especially hydrochlorothiazide and furosemide), and alcohol.
Chronic Gout
◇ Treated with synthesis inhibition (eg, allopurinol) or uricosurics, eg, sulfinpyrazone, probenicid.
Renal disease of gout
◇ Best treated by control of hypertension.
Urinary lithiasis: maintain high urine output, alkalinize urine.

MEDICATIONS
• Recurrent Acute Gout
• Oral or IV colchicine usually provides good clinical response when initiated early. Colchicine is less frequently used today due to gastrointestinal side effects.
• Indomethacin and other NSAIDs are effective in acute attacks.
• Intra-articular corticosteroids may be used for recalcitrant gout.
• Avoidance of serum urate level altering drugs eg, allopurinol, probenicid which can prolong acute attacks.

CONSULTATION SUGGESTIONS
Rheumatologist

REFERRAL SUGGESTIONS
Primary Physician

PATIENT INSTRUCTIONS
Decrease intake of fat, ethanol, sardines, anchovies, liver.

COURSE/PROGNOSIS
If treated, excellent prognosis. During first 6 to 24 months of uricosuric or allopurinol therapy, acute gout may occur.

CODING

ICD-9-CM
274.0 Gout

MISCELLANEOUS

SYNONYMS
Crystal-induced synovitis

REFERENCES
Fox IH: Textbook of Internal Medicine, 2nd ed. Kelly WN (ed.), Philadelphia, JB Lippincott, 1992.

Levinson DJ, Becker MA: Arthritis and allied conditions. A Textbook of Rheumatology. 12th ed. McCarty DJ, Koopman WJ, (eds.), Philadelphia, Lea & Febiger, 1993.

Wolfe F: Gout and hyperuricemia. Am Fam Phys 43:2141-2150, 1991.

Ralston S: Management of gout. Practitioner 235:263-167, 1991.

AUTHOR
André Montazem, DMD, MD

Hairy Tongue

BASICS

DESCRIPTION
An elongation of the filiform papillae on the tongue dorsum that can be seen in debilitated patients giving the tongue a hairy or coated appearance.

ETIOLOGY

• Isolated elongation of filiform papillae has no known etiology.
• In debilitated patients, limited tongue movements by illness or painful conditions decrease the natural friction between the tongue and the teeth and palate. This lack of friction can result in elongation of the filiform papillae.
• Elongated papillae may retain debris and pigments from food, tobacco smoke, and other local agents.
• Systemic antibiotics and topical oxidizing agents (ie, hydrogen peroxide, perborate, and chlorhexidine) may result in secondary changes in oral flora, increasing the likelihood of developing hairy tongue.
• Frequently seen in patients who have received extensive head and neck radiotherapy.

SYSTEMS AFFECTED
Tongue
◇ increased length of the filiform papillae may result in gagging and/or halitosis.

DIAGNOSIS

SYMPTOMS AND SIGNS
General
◇ gagging sensation with halitosis and foul taste in the mouth.
Tongue
◇ elongated filiform papillae on the mid-dorsum of the tongue. May appear white or have a variety of discolorations through staining.

LABORATORY
HIV testing if suspected

IMAGING/SPECIAL TESTS
Due to characteristic clinical features, biopsy usually unnecessary. Will reveal elongated filiform papillae with keratization into midportions of stratum spinosum, but little basal cell hyperplasia.

DIFFERENTIAL
• Hairy leukoplakia (AIDS associated lesion of the lateral margins of the tongue)

TREATMENT

General
◇ Thorough cleaning, brushing and scraping of the tongue.
Investigation of patient's general health.

MEDICATIONS
• Applications of topical keratolytic agents.
• Use of yogurt or other Lactobacillus acidophilus cultures.
• Modification of drug regimens (ie, use of antibiotics and oxidizing agents).

SURGERY
Shearing the elongated papillae with scissors.

CONSULTATION SUGGESTIONS
Oral Medicine, Oral-Maxillofacial Surgeon

REFERRAL SUGGESTIONS
Oral Medicine, Oral-Maxillofacial Surgeon

PATIENT INSTRUCTIONS
Brush tongue at times of toothbrushing.

COURSE/PROGNOSIS
Signs and symptoms are reversible unless underlying debilitation prevents long-term control of the problem. This entity itself does not cause pain or impaired function.

CODING

ICD-9-CM
529.3 Hairy black tongue

CPT
41100 Biopsy, tongue, anterior 2/3
41110 Excision, lesion of tongue without closure

MISCELLANEOUS

SYNONYMS
Hypertrophy of foliate papillae
Hypertrophy of tongue papillae
Coated tongue
White hairy tongue
Black hairy tongue
Lingua villosa nigra

SEE ALSO
HIV and AIDS

REFERENCES
Burket's Oral Medicine Diagnosis and Treatment, 9th ed. Lynch MA, Brightman VJ, Greenberg MS (eds). Philadelphia, JB Lippincott, Co., 1994, pp. 260-261.

Addy M, Al-Arryed F, Moran J: The use of an oxidizing mouthwash to reduce staining associated with chlorhexidine. Studies in vitro and in vivo. J Clin Periodontol 18:267-271, 1991.

Regezi JA, Sciubba J: Oral Pathology Clinical Pathologic Correlations, 2nd ed. Philadelphia, WB Saunders, 1993, pp. 112-113.

AUTHOR
Dale J. Misiek, DMD

Halitosis

BASICS

DESCRIPTION
• A general term applied to foul, offensive, or bad smelling breath arising from a person's oral and/or nasal cavities.
• Can be related to local/oral or metabolic/systemic causes. Also termed bad breath.

ETIOLOGY

• Can clearly be related to location of the source of the odor.
• Local oral conditions such as periodontal disease produce volatile sulfur-containing compounds and other cell-degradation byproducts that result in oral malodors. Other oral conditions include dental abscesses, oral cancer, xerostomia, and candidiasis.
• Systemic conditions such as diabetic ketoacidosis (ketone), liver failure (fetor hepatitis), and renal failure (uremia) can produce metabolic products that are detectable as halitosis. Diets involving skipping meals may result in halitosis due to gastric air returning to the oral cavity.
• Bacterial infections of the gastrointestinal tract such as Helicobacter pylori or local conditions such a esophageal reflux, hiatal hernia, pyloric stenosis, etc.
• Bacterial infections of the respiratory tract including sinusitis, localized abscesses, etc.
• Patient self-complaints of halitosis with no detectable oral malodor may indicate a psychiatric disorder.

SYSTEMS AFFECTED
• Oral cavity, including the mucosa and periodontal tissues.
• Upper respiratory passages, including nasal cavities and sinuses.
• Lower respiratory passages, including bronchi, alveoli, and other parts of the lungs.
• Gastrointestinal tract, including esophagus, stomach, intestines, and liver.

DIAGNOSIS

SYMPTOMS AND SIGNS
• Self-perception of bad breath, dysguesia, or parosmia.
• Presence of a foul odor emanating from the oral/nasal cavities.
• Evidence of infection in the oral soft tissues, including periodontal disease, ulcer, dental caries, and abscesses.

LABORATORY
• Specific laboratory blood and urine studies may be indicated if a systemic disorder is suspected.

IMAGING/SPECIAL TESTS
• Imaging of the nasal passages indicated when upper respiratory tract etiology is indicated.
• Chest radiographs indicated when looking for lower respiratory tract etiologies.
• Gastrointestinal disorders can be determined with appropriate radiographic or endoscopic examinations.
• Gas chromatographic techniques are available to identify and measure certain volatile agents associated with halitosis.

DIFFERENTIAL
Ozostomia
◊ oral malodor arising from the upper respiratory tract.
Stomatodysodia
◊ oral malodor arising from the lower respiratory tract.
Physiological halitosis
◊ temporary oral malodor related to volatile food-related substances released into the lungs.
Pathologic halitosis
◊ oral malodor caused by systemic disorders releasing metabolic byproducts into the blood that are then released through the lungs into the oral cavity.
Fetor oris/fetor ex ore
◊ oral malodors arising from local conditions in the oral cavity.

TREATMENT

General
◇ Identification and elimination of the underlying abnormalities should eliminate halitosis.
◇ Oral care, including improved oral hygiene, professional cleaning of the periodontal tissues, and elimination of the infection.
◇ Recommendations to change dietary habits to eliminate foods with offensive volatile components.
◇ Treatment of the underlying metabolic disorder or the local or systemic pathology in the respiratory or gastrointestinal tracts.

MEDICATIONS
• Mouthwashes do not treat halitosis but can mask the problem.
• Oils of spearmint, wintergreen, and peppermint can mask the halitosis.

CONSULTATION SUGGESTIONS
Oral Medicine, Otolaryngologist, Periodontist

REFERRAL SUGGESTIONS
Oral Medicine

PATIENT INSTRUCTIONS
If dental causes of halitosis ruled out, medical causes should be considered.

COURSE/PROGNOSIS
Without removal of the underlying etiology, the halitosis will continue unabated.

CODING

ICD-9-CM
112.0 Candidiasis of mouth
300.4 Anxiety
311.0 Depression
527.7 Xerostomia
710.2 Sjögren's
784.9 Halitosis
990.0 Radiotherapy, adverse effect

CPT
70220 Radiologic examination of sinuses, complete, minimum of three
70310 Radiologic exam of teeth, less than full mouth
70320 Radiologic exam of teeth, full mouth
87060 Culture of throat or nose
87070 Culture of any source

MISCELLANEOUS

SYNONYMS
Bad breath
Ozostomia
Stomatodysodia
Fetor Oris/fetor ex ore
Morning breath

SEE ALSO
Sinusitis
Renal insufficiency
Liver failure

REFERENCES
Durham TM, Malloy T, Hodges ED: Halitosis: Knowing when 'bad breath' signals systemic disease. Geriatrics 48:55-59, 1993.

Johnson B: Halitosis, or the meaning of bad breath. J Gen Internal Med 7:649-656, 1992.

Kleinberg I, Westbay G: Salivary and metabolic factors involved in oral malodor formation. J Periodontol 63:768-775, 1992.

McDowell JD, Kassebaum DK: Diagnosing and treating halitosis. JADA 124:55-64, 1993.

Preti G, Clark L, Cowart BJ, Feldman RS, Lowry LD, Weber E, Young JM: Non-oral etiologies of oral malodor and altered chemosensation. J Periodontol 63:790-796, 1992.

Rosenberg M, McCulloch CAG: Measurement of oral malodor: Current methods and future prospects. J Periodontol 63:776-782, 1992.

Tiomny E, Arber N, Moshkowitz M, Peled Y, Gilat T: Halitosis and Helicobacter pylori: A possible link? J Clin Gastroenterol 15:236-237.

Touyz LZ: Oral malodor: a review. J Can Dent Asso 59:507-610, 1993.

Yaegaki K, Sanada K: Biochemical and clinical factors influencing oral malodor in periodontal patients. J Periodontol 63:783-789, 1992.

AUTHOR
Frank A. Catalanotto, DMD

Headache, Migraine

BASICS

DESCRIPTION
• A recurrent vascular headache disorder usually associated with nausea, vomiting, and visual disturbances.
• Migraines are classified as:
• Classical-occurring in 15 to 20% of patients and associated with neurologic symptoms that precede the headache (scintillating scotoma, paresthesia of the hands, tongue, or face, or motor weakness).
• Common
  ◇ no prodromal neurologic symptoms.
• Complicated
  ◇ the neurologic prodrome outlasts the headache.
• Migraine is an apparently common problem in the U.S. with some reports showing 17% of women and 6% of men suffering from migraine. First presentation of the migraine occurs in childhood and rarely later than 30, and then the attacks can remit completely after the age of 50.

ETIOLOGY

A familial pattern is seen in the majority of cases. The etiology of migraine is still unknown. Traditionally, the pain has been thought to be a direct result of changes in cerebral blood flow, but these changes have been shown to be too slight to be responsible for ischemic changes or pain. Decreased blood flow often coexists with an aura but continues long after the aura has disappeared and the headache phase is well instituted. Serotonin concentrations have been shown to change during migraine attacks and are now thought to cause the vasomotor changes.

SYSTEMS AFFECTED
Central nervous system
  ◇ headache

Eyes
  ◇ visual disturbance
GI
  ◇ nausea, vomiting
Precipitating factors include specific food and ethanol, missed meals, oral contraceptives and menses, fatigue, stress.

DIAGNOSIS

Important features of migraines that distinguish them from other headaches include their unilateral nature, a family history of migraine, nausea and vomiting associated with the headache, and a positive response to ergot preparations.

SYMPTOMS AND SIGNS
The aura of a migraine can be any focal neurologic function; however, it is usually visual and follows a phasic pattern. The visual aura consists of an active leading edge (the scintillation), followed by visual loss (the scotoma), and then restoration of vision. Other nervous system signs can include paresthesias, aphasia, hemiparesis, taste or smell disorders. Migraine headaches occur as recurrent, usually severe headaches, often starting unilaterally. Patients will usually follow a pattern, and the attacks can be precipitated by identifiable factors such as emotional stress, menses, foods such as aged cheese, chocolate or nuts, and also red wine. These attacks can also occur on a regular, almost daily, basis or on a more infrequent basis. The headache is often accompanied by malaise, nausea, vomiting, and photophobia that cause the patient to lay down in a quiet, dark room. Increased amplitude of pulsation of the scalp arteries has been recorded, and the scalp arteries become more prominent. Scalp tenderness may be present.

LABORATORY
• Sedimentation rate if temporal arteritis suspected.
• CBC if meningitis suspected.

IMAGING/SPECIAL TESTS
Temporal artery biopsy if temporal arteritis suspected.

DIFFERENTIAL
• Cluster headache
• Tension headache
• Drug seeking
• Epilepsy

TREATMENT

General
◇ Prophylaxis. Nonpharmacologic prophylaxis includes dietary changes (avoidance of monosodium glutamate, nitrates, alcohol, and spreading caffeine intake evenly over the course of the day); eating meals on a regular schedule; maintaining regular sleep patterns; and exercising regularly. Stress management, biofeedback, and relaxation training are all to be recommended.

MEDICATIONS
• Treatment of an acute attack:
• Caffeine and aspirin are of use in treatment of mild attacks. Ergotamine 2 mg sublingual or ergotamine 1 mg with caffeine every 30 minutes to a maximum dose of 6 mg of ergotamine is frequently effective. Ergotamine carries with it the problem of physical tolerance and/or dependence that can lead to vasoconstrictive problems when used for more than 48 hours. Sumatriptan has been shown in several trials to abort migraines with 80% of cases reporting significant reduction to complete elimination of the headache. The parenteral form of the drug has been approved by the FDA and the oral form should be approved soon. Sumatriptan works by binding to the serotonin receptors found on small peripheral nerves in the intracranial vasculature.
• Pharmacologic prophylaxis include methysergide 4 mg b.i.d. (but requires periods off the drug every 3 to 4 months); propanolol, sustained release, 160 mg every morning that is effective in approximately 50% of patients; and verapamil, sustained release, 240 mg every morning. Tricyclic antidepressants (amitryptyline or nortriptyline 150 mg) at bedtime have been reported to be successful in some cases.
• Avoid administration of narcotics.
• Ketoralac (Toradol) 30 to 60 mg IM may be useful in emergency situations.

CONSULTATION SUGGESTIONS
Neurologist

REFERRAL SUGGESTIONS
Primary Care Physician, Neurologist

FIRST STEPS TO TAKE IN AN EMERGENCY
• Administer anti-emetics and non-narcotic analgesics.

PATIENT INSTRUCTIONS
Avoid known precipitating factors or substances.

COURSE/PROGNOSIS
As patient ages, frequency and severity of migraines tend to decrease.

CODING

ICD-9-CM
346.9 Migraine

MISCELLANEOUS

SYNONYMS
Hemicrania

SEE ALSO
Cluster headache
Tension headache
Giant cell arteritis

REFERENCES
Dalessio DJ: Wolff's Headache, 5th ed. New York., Oxford University Press, 1987.

Walling A: Migraine. In: Griffith's 5 Minute Clinical Consult. Dambro MR, Griffith J. (eds). Baltimore, Williams and Wilkins, 1995, pp. 668-669.

Raskin NH: Headache. In: Harrison's Principles of Internal Medicine. 13th ed. Isselbacher KJ, et al (eds). New York, McGraw-Hill, 1994, pp. 65-71.

AUTHOR
Janet Leigh, BDS, DMD

Headaches, Cluster

BASICS

DESCRIPTION
• Paroxysmal, unilateral headaches focusing around the eye and temporal areas occurring in clusters.
• They occur in 0.08% of the population and affect men much more so than women, usually presenting between the 3rd and 6th decade. The clusters often present in the spring or autumn and can last from 4 to 12 weeks at intervals of 6 months to 5 years, though in 10% of patients, the pain continues without remission.

ETIOLOGY

The pathogenesis is unknown, but cluster headaches are thought to be vascular in origin and related to migraine. May be related to disordered serotonin or histamine kinetics. Tend to be triggered by ethanol or specific foods.

SYSTEMS AFFECTED
Central nervous system

DIAGNOSIS

The pain originating from cluster headaches is too intense and unique to be mistaken for anything else.

SYMPTOMS AND SIGNS
Cluster headaches present as a sudden onset of unilateral, crescendo, severe, piercing pain in the nostril, zygoma, teeth or behind the eye, that then spreads to the forehead. The attack lasts from 30 minutes to 2 hours, and is accompanied by ipsilateral lacrimation, nasal congestion, and watering (rhinorrhea) and ptosis. May also see nausea, bradycardia, restlessness, and perspiration. The headache stops as suddenly as it starts and leaves no residual effects. Recurrence can occur 1 to 3 times daily, and will wake the patient from sleep. There are no such symptoms as nausea or vomiting when the headache ceases.

IMAGING/SPECIAL TESTS
MRI to investigate when presentation not typical.

DIFFERENTIAL
• Tension headache
• Migraine headache
• Giant cell arteritis
• CNS neoplasm

TREATMENT

General
◇ Prophylaxis during a cluster epoch is the preferable treatment modality as the pain is frequently too short-lived to be successfully treated during an attack.
◇ Some individuals find that the initiation of a vigorous physical activity at first symptom of attack may abort it.
◇ Ipsilateral compression of superficial temporal artery relieves pain in some patients, but may increase it in others.

MEDICATIONS
• The serotonin inhibitor, methysergide, has been shown to have a useful role in prevention of cluster headache as has verapamil 120 mg t.i.d. or prednisolone 40 mg per day.
• Sumatriptan, 6 mg sub Q useful for acute headache.
• Ergotamine or dihydroergotamine may also be helpful in treating acute attack.
• 100% oxygen and intranasal lidocaine have also been used.

CONSULTATION SUGGESTIONS
Neurologist

REFERRAL SUGGESTIONS
Primary Care Physician, Neurologist

PATIENT INSTRUCTIONS
Avoid ethanol, tobacco products, and other precipitating factors.

COURSE/PROGNOSIS
Although remissions may occur, recurrent attacks are likely without therapy.

CODING

ICD-9-CM
784.0 Cluster headache

MISCELLANEOUS

SYNONYMS
Histamine cephalgia
Migrainous neuralgia
Sphenopalatine neuralgia

SEE ALSO
Migraine headache
Tension headache

REFERENCES
Dalessio DJ: Wolff's Headache and other Head Pain. 5th ed. New York, Oxford University Press, 1987.

Walling A: Cluster headache. In: Griffith's 5 Minute Clinical Consult. Dambro MR, (ed), Baltimore, Williams and Wilkins, 1995 pp. 446-447.

AUTHOR
Janet Leigh, BDS, DMD

Headaches, Tension

BASICS

DESCRIPTION
• A steady, nonpulsatile, unilateral or bilateral aching pain originating in the occipital region, but also including the frontal and temporal regions. Tension headache variants include depressive headaches, post-traumatic headaches, temporomandibular joint dysfunction, and atypical facial pain.
• Tension headaches are more frequently seen in women and recur on a daily basis. Complaints of dull, aching pain feeling, like a constricting band around the head, are common in the early afternoon and evening.

ETIOLOGY

• Etiology is unknown but there are many symptoms of tension headache that overlap with migraine despite the different origins of the two disorders. Traditionally, tension headaches have been felt to be myogenic in origin and related to muscle tension and tenderness. These headaches are more commonly found in patients whose work or posture requires sustained contracture of the neck and shoulder muscles. Some 56% of patients with tension headaches have been shown to exhibit higher levels of hyperchondriosis, depression, and hysteria on the MMPI scales.
• Stress or anxiety is commonly seen in the lives of those regularly afflicted.
• May be seen associated with obstructive sleep apnea or excess caffeine consumption.

SYSTEMS AFFECTED
Nervous system

DIAGNOSIS

SYMPTOMS AND SIGNS
• The cervical, frontal, and temporal muscles exhibit tenderness on palpation, and the patient complains of pain in the occipital or frontal regions that is often described as vice-like or a constricting band around the head.
• Pain usually bilateral.
• Intensity varies through the day.
• Difficulty in concentrating.
• Nausea and vomiting are rarely seen in conjunction with these headaches, but tinnitus, dizziness, and blurring of vision can be frequent symptoms.

LABORATORY
ESR if giant cell arteritis suspected.

IMAGING/SPECIAL TESTS
MRI if brain lesion suspected.

DIFFERENTIAL
• Temporal arteritis
• Migraine
• Sinusitis
• TMJ problems
• Anemia
• Head injury
• Refractive error
• Depression

TREATMENT

General
◇ Tension headaches require a multidisciplinary approach if they are to be treated successfully. Identification of the triggering factors is essential before treatment can commence (ie, patient posture, stress levels, and habits have all been shown to play significant roles in the etiology of tension headaches). Elimination of these triggers will be necessary and should give the patient a strong sense of control in the management of their disease. Spray and stretch, physical therapy, and trigger point injections also have a useful role to play when myospasm is identified. Regular vigorous exercise may assist those in which daily stress is factor in etiology.

MEDICATIONS
• The use of analgesics alone to treat these headaches is not be encouraged without the elimination of tension in the affected muscles as it can lead to overuse of the analgesics and subsequent analgesic rebound headaches. Nonsteroidal analgesics have a role to play when myospasm with resultant muscle inflammation is present. If NSAIDs used, monitor for signs of gastric upset or bleeding.
• Antidepressants such as the tricyclics amitriptyline, desipramine, and imipramine may be of prophylactic value.
• Avoid use of narcotics.

CONSULTATION SUGGESTIONS
Primary Care Physician, Neurologist

REFERRAL SUGGESTIONS
Primary Care Physician, Neurologist

PATIENT INSTRUCTIONS
Contact National Headache Foundation for helpful literature, (800) 843-2256.

COURSE/PROGNOSIS
If provoking factors avoided, such as stress, prognosis good.

CODING

ICD-9-CM
307.81 Tension headache

MISCELLANEOUS

SYNONYMS
Muscle contraction headache
Cephalgia

SEE ALSO
Migraine headache
Cluster headache
Giant cell arteritis

REFERENCES
Dalessio DJ: Wolff's Headache. 5th ed. New York, Oxford University Press, 1987.

Bonica JJ: The Management of Pain. 2nd ed. Philadelphia, Lea and Febiger, 1990.

AUTHOR
Janet Leigh, BDS, DMD

Hemangioma (Oral/Facial)

 BASICS

DESCRIPTION
• A benign, enlarged vascular hamartoma or neoplasm most commonly presenting in the lips, tongue, and buccal mucosa. Usually the lesion appears weeks after birth.
• More common in females.

 ETIOLOGY

• Congenital hemangioma is a benign congenital neoplasm with increased endothelial turnover. Histologically, it can be subdivided into two types based on vessel diameter: capillary and cavernous.
• Lesion is the result of abnormal vessel proliferation.
• Differs from vascular malformations, which are the result of abnormal vessel morphogenesis.

SYSTEMS AFFECTED
• G.I.
• Respiratory
• Lesion may disfigure face

 DIAGNOSIS

SYMPTOMS AND SIGNS
• Swelling in area of lesion
• Possible loss of function
• Bleeding
• Ulceration
• Superficial lesions may be red, blue, or purple in color.
• Contour may vary
 ◊ flat, raised, bosselated, or nodular.
• Deep lesions will not alter the color of overlying mucosa.
• Hemangiomas will blanch when compressed.
• Size varies greatly.
• Rarely effects bone.
• No bruit or thrill.

LABORATORY
• Histologic exam reveals endothelium-lined vascular pattern without muscular support.

IMAGING/SPECIAL TESTS
• CT with contrast
• Magnetic resonance imaging (MRI)
• Angiography for larger lesions.

DIFFERENTIAL
• Vascular malformation
• Varicosity
• Rendu-Osler-Weber syndrome (hereditary hemorrhagic telangiectasia)
• Angio-osteohypertrophy syndrome
• Sturge-Kalischer-Weber syndrome (encephalocutaneous angiomatosis)
• CREST syndrome = calcinosis cutis, Raynaud's, esophageal dysfunction, sclerodactyly, and telangiectasia.

TREATMENT

General

Observation

◇ spontaneous resolution may occur due to internal bleeding and fibrosis; childhood hemangiomas commonly decrease in size with age.

◇ Large hemangiomas benefit from angiography followed by superselective embolization.

SURGERY

• Any lesion that may represent a hemangioma should be aspirated prior to incision.

• Small lesions amenable to injection of sclerosing agents, or can be removed with laser or surgical excision.

• Cryosurgery may be indicated and helpful for intraoral lesions.

CONSULTATION SUGGESTIONS

Interventional Radiologist (for embolization)

REFERRAL SUGGESTIONS

Oral-Maxillofacial Surgeon, Plastic Reconstructive Surgeon, Interventional Radiologist

FIRST STEPS TO TAKE IN AN EMERGENCY

• Bleeding from hemangioma should be temporarily controlled with direct pressure.

• Transport patient to emergency facility for more definitive treatment such as surgery with or without prior embolization.

PATIENT INSTRUCTIONS

Avoid trauma to areas of possible hemangiomas. Seek immediate care if bleeding occurs.

COURSE/PROGNOSIS

• May have a rapid growth phase followed several years later by an involution.

• If the lesion has been present from birth with no change in size or color and there is no functional or cosmetic impairment, no treatment is necessary.

CODING

ICD-9-CM

228.0   Hemangioma, any site

228.01 Hemangioma, skin and subcutaneous tissue

CPT

11440 Excision benign lesion face, nose, lips

11441 lesion 0.6 1 cm

11442 lesion 1.1 2 cm

11443 lesion 2.1 3 cm

17106 Destruction by laser benign facial vascular lesion

36469 Injection sclerosing solution, face

MISCELLANEOUS

SYNONYMS

Vascular nevus

Port-wine stain

Nevus flammeus

Strawberry nevus

SEE ALSO

Osler-Weber-Rendu Disease

REFERENCES

Baurmash H, DeChiara S: A conservative approach to the management of orofacial vascular lesions in infants and children. J Oral Maxillofac Surg 49:1222-1225, 1991.

Jackson IT, Carreno R, Potparic Z, Hussain K: Hemangiomas, vascular malformations, and lymphovenous malformations: classification and methods of treatment. Plast Reconstr Surg 91:1216-30, 1993.

Sexton J, O'Hare D: Simplified treatment of vascular lesions using the argon laser. J Oral Maxillofac Surg 51:12-16, 1993.

Hupp JR: Superselective angiography with digital subtraction and embolization of a maxillary hemangioma in a patient with Eisenmenger's syndrome. J Oral Maxillofac Surg 44:910-916, 1986.

AUTHOR

Paul A. Danielson, DMD

Hepatic Cirrhosis

BASICS

DESCRIPTION
Fibrosis of the liver parenchyma as a result of chronic, irreversible liver injury. Connective tissue replacement of parenchyma with formation of regenerative nodules resulting in progressive deterioration of hepatic function.

ETIOLOGY

• Most commonly a result of chronic alcohol ingestion or infectious hepatitis. Alcohol acts as a direct hepatotoxic agent, although malnutrition and undefined genetic determinants appear to play a role in the development and progression of alcoholic liver disease. It appears that the duration of consumption in years is more influencing than is the quantity of daily intake.
• Infectious hepatitis is the other major cause of liver cirrhosis. Chronic viral hepatitis B and C, which occur in approximately 10% and 50%, respectively, predispose to cirrhosis.
• Other causes of cirrhosis include toxins. Specific hepatocellular toxins include: acetaminophen, methotrexate, amiodarone, and halothane.
• Autoimmune chronic active hepatitis is an uncommon cause of liver failure and is seen predominantly in women.
• Primary biliary cirrhosis (PBC), also an autoimmune disease, and primary sclerosing cholangitis (PSC) are causes of liver cirrhosis related to chronic cholestatic conditions.
• Depositional diseases: Wilson's disease, glycogen storage diseases, and hemochromatosis are less common causes of cirrhosis.
• Postinfectious causes include schistosomiasis and toxoplasmosis.

SYSTEMS AFFECTED
CNS symptoms are usually secondary to gastrointestinal bleeding, increased nitrogen from dietary proteins, and increased ammonia production, as well as electrolyte disturbances. Hepatic encephalopathy results from shunting of blood and collateral circulation bypassing the liver. Failure to remove toxins, increased circulating levels of unbound drugs, increased ammonia levels, or azotemia cause mental status changes. Central hyperventilation is not uncommon.
Skin
  ◇ spider angiomata, palmar erythema.
General
  ◇ gynecomastia, Dupuytren's contractures, pruritus from bilirubin deposition in skin, testicular atrophy, and jaundice.
Pulmonary
  ◇ cyanosis, tachypnea, and central hyperventilation.
Glandular
  ◇ parotid and/or lacrimal gland enlargement.
Vascular
  ◇ telangiectasia, superficial abdominal collaterals, caput medusae, and formation of esophagogastric varices which are susceptible to hemorrhage.

Hematologic
  ◇ spur cell anemia, coagulopathy secondary to failure of coagulation factor synthesis, and thrombocytopenia with hypersplenism.
Abdominal
  ◇ portal hypertension with resultant ascites and hepatosplenomegaly. Only in end-stage cirrhosis does the liver become small.
Renal
  ◇ increased aldosterone and sodium retention due to reduced intravascular volume. Hepatorenal syndrome; progressive azotemia without an identifiable cause for renal failure.

DIAGNOSIS

SYMPTOMS AND SIGNS
• Fatigue, fever (if infectious), pruritus, distended abdomen.
• Jaundice, ascites, spider angiomata, collateral abdominal vessels, palmar erythema, enlarged salivary and lacrimal glands, gynecomastia, testicular atrophy, Dupuytren's contractures.

LABORATORY
Liver function tests
◇ AST (SGOT), ALT (SGPT), bilirubin, GGTP, alkaline phosphatase, increased serum IgM for PBC and PSC. Increased anti-mitochondrial antibody (AMA) is consistently elevated in PBC. PSC does not have increased AMA. Increased anti-nuclear antibody in autoimmune chronic active hepatitis with hypergammaglobulinemia. Hepatitis A, B, C, and D profiles for viral infection.
• Hyperglobulinemia with hypoalbuminemia.
Vitamin K dependent factors
◇ V, VII, IX, X reduced, causing coagulopathy and prolonged PT, PTT.

IMAGING/SPECIAL TESTS
• Copper and iron studies can be used to diagnose Wilson's disease or hemochromatosis.
• Definitive diagnosis is made only by biopsy. The approach may be via percutaneous needle or open liver biopsy, demonstrating a characteristic fibrotic pattern. Endoscopy and barium studies may be used to demonstrate esophagogastric varices.

DIFFERENTIAL
• Alcoholic liver disease
• Postinfectious
• Autoimmune
• Primary biliary cirrhosis, primary sclerosing cholangitis.
• Cryptogenic
• Hemochromatosis
• Wilson's disease

TREATMENT

General
◇ Presently there are no satisfactory treatments for liver cirrhosis and efforts are best made to prevent its occurrence. Early detection of etiologic factors and appropriate treatment are the most important form of therapy.
◇ Mainly supportive
◇ Abstinence from alcohol is imperative in halting the progression of cirrhosis.
◇ Avoidance of hepatotoxic drugs.

MEDICATIONS
• Colchicine has been shown to slow disease progression and increase survival in some recent studies.
• Multivitamins, adequate nutrition high in branched-chain amino acids, avoiding high protein loads.
• Control of ascites: sodium restriction, diuresis, spironolactone (cirrhotic have increased aldosterone production), and paracentesis.
• Spontaneous bacterial peritonitis, usually due to E.coli, is treated with antibiotic therapy.
• Hepatorenal syndrome
◇ there is no effective treatment and prognosis is extremely poor should this syndrome develop. Hepatic encephalopathy is treated with lactulose which lowers serum ammonia levels.
• Variceal bleeds are treated by local injection of vasoconstrictors (eg, vasopressin, epinephrine) or sclerotherapy.
• Treatment for PBC and PSC is unsatisfactory and liver transplantation may be required. However, biliary tract decompression may be used in chronic cholestatic disease as a palliative measure.
• Alpha interferon therapy has been proven to be effective in the early treatment of hepatitis B and C. Approximately 50% of patients demonstrate a complete response and another 25% show a partial relapse, but low-dose therapy has been effective in maintaining remission in hepatitis C. Maintenance therapy has not been proven effective in hepatitis B remission.
• Immunosuppression with corticosteroids and occasionally azathioprine has been successful in the treatment of autoimmune chronic active hepatitis. Therapy has been shown to greatly reduce the progression to cirrhosis and to prolong survival.

SURGERY
• Liver transplantation appears to be the treatment of choice for acceptable candidates. Transplant recipients have a good 5 year survival if able to withstand the perioperative period.

• Portal hypertension may be treated by shunting of blood past the portal system, eg, portocaval, splenorenal shunts. Persistent portal hypertension uniformly leads to esophageal varices and bleeding varices, which may be exsanguinating.
• Any patient with cirrhosis should have PT, PTT and platelet count prior to any surgical procedure.

CONSULTATION SUGGESTIONS
Primary Care Physician, Hepatologist, Transplant Surgeon

REFERRAL SUGGESTIONS
Primary Care Physician

FIRST STEPS TO TAKE IN AN EMERGENCY
• Transport to emergency care facility.

PATIENT INSTRUCTIONS
Alcoholics should contact local chapter of Alcoholics Anonymous.

COURSE/PROGNOSIS
Prognosis dependent upon etiology and severity.

CODING

ICD-9-CM
571.2 Alcoholic cirrhosis
571.5 Non-alcoholic cirrhosis
571.6 Biliary cirrhosis

MISCELLANEOUS

SYNONYMS
Cirrhosis of the liver

SEE ALSO
Hepatitis

REFERENCES
Ahord JL: Clinical management of cirrhosis. Comprehensive Ther 17:57-64. 1991.

Podolsky DK, Isselbacher KJ: In: Harrison's Principles of Internal Medicine. 13th ed. Isselbacher KJ, et al, (eds). New York, McGraw Hill, Co., 1994, pp. 1483-1495.

AUTHOR
André Montazem, DMD, MD

Hepatitis, Alcoholic

BASICS

DESCRIPTION
• Inflammatory condition of the liver caused by excessive ethanol intake.
• Alcoholic liver disease is a common problem in dentistry. In the U.S. approximately 10.6 million adults are alcoholics, and 7.3 million have drinking problems. Alcoholic hepatitis presents in three stages: 1) liver cells become infiltrated with fat; 2) diffuse hepatic inflammation resulting in cellular degradation; and 3) cirrhosis 10 to 15% (irreversible).
• Oral manifestations of alcoholic liver disease include: glossitis, candidiasis, angular and labial cheilosis, and erosion of papillae on the tongue that often results from poor nutrition: mucosal tissues may have ecchymosis, petechiae, or a yellowish hue reflecting hematologic disorders, with gingival bleeding being a common finding. The three major complications presenting in this population are hemorrhage, delayed healing, and impaired drug metabolism.

ETIOLOGY

Hepatic inflammation caused by long-term, excessive ethanol intake.

SYSTEMS AFFECTED
Liver
◇ changes occur in the parenchymal cells of the liver. This alteration results in hepatic infiltration by mononuclear cells with edema and variable amounts of degeneration, necrosis, and autolysis to occur. In early alcoholic liver disease, the hepatocytes become engorged with fatty lobules and distended with liver enlargement.
• Esophageal varices are often noted in alcoholic hepatitis.
Skin
◇ abnormal findings resulting from various forms of hepatitis include: hyperpigmentation, jaundice, purpura, vascular spiders, excoriations, lichenification, xanthelasma, and xanthoma.
Eyes
◇ jaundice.
Abdomen
◇ hepatomegaly, splenomegaly, ascites.
Extremities
◇ bone tenderness, digital clubbing, peripheral edema, palmar erythema.
Nervous system
◇ peripheral neuropathy, encephalopathy.
Oral cavity
◇ alcoholic hepatitis nutritional deficiencies may result in reduced papilla on the tongue, glossitis, and labial or angular cheilosis. Mucosal ecchymosis, petechiae, and reduced healing following trauma or surgery has been noted. Jaundiced mucosal tissue may also be present. Parotid gland enlargement, which is painless, may be seen in advanced liver disease.

DIAGNOSIS

SYMPTOMS AND SIGNS
• Fatigue, nausea, vomiting, diarrhea, joint and muscle pain, anorexia, jaundice, hepatomegaly, abdominal and gastric distention, clay-colored stools, dark urine, fever, bruising, rash and chills.
• Signs of alcoholic hepatitis include: parotid gland enlargement, palmar erythema, petechiae, bruising, spider angiomas of the skin, transverse white bands on the nails, ascites, and ankle edema.

LABORATORY
Universal tests: bilirubin, alkaline phosphatase, albumin, amylase, urate, prothrombin time, partial thromboplastin time, complete blood count with differential and platelets, AST (aspartate aminotransferase), ALT (alanine aminotransferase). GGT (gamma-glutamyl transferase) elevation specific for ethanol insult. Decreased levels of magnesium, calcium, phosphorus are suggestive of ethanol abuse.

IMAGING/SPECIAL TESTS
• CT scan diagnostic for cirrhosis.
• Percutaneous liver biopsy (punch-blind method).
• Laparoscopy with direct liver biopsy (greater degree of accuracy than punch).
• MRI (magnetic resonance imaging) may be used to evaluate cirrhosis.

DIFFERENTIAL
• In young adults:
Hepatitis B, C, D, E, F, G, HIV, and ethanol abuse.
• In middle-aged women:
Primary biliary cirrhosis, ethanol abuse.
• In middle-aged males:
Ethanol abuse, neoplasms, medications.

TREATMENT

General

◇ To assess hemostasis, a coagulation profile should be obtained PT, PTT, platelet count, and bleeding time to plan surgical procedures. Because chronic hepatitis can impair the synthesis of clotting factors, an increased PT and PTT may alert the practitioner to potential hemorrhagic tendencies. A depletion in platelet levels is also indicative of both chronic hepatitis and cirrhosis. If these tests are elevated beyond normal limits, recommendations for patients with bleeding tendencies may apply. If these tests are within normal limits, patients may receive dental care with minimal risk of postoperative bleeding.

◇ Liver enzymes, AST, ALT, and alkaline phosphatase are used to monitor the course of hepatitis. Two laboratory values that monitor disease severity are mean peak AST rise and bilirubin elevations. To assess the patient's healing capabilities, a complete blood cell count (CBC) with differential may be obtained. The differential may demonstrate neutropenia (decreased neutrophil count) or an increase in lymphocytes, which both occur in hepatic conditions. Because chronic hepatitis patients often manifest adverse reactions that result from the inability of the liver to metabolize drugs, all medications are administered with caution.

◇ While alterations in treatment planning for these patients may be minimal in early disease, practitioners should be aware that these patients have unpredictable metabolic processes throughout the entire spectrum of their disease. Patients having mild to moderate disease may have an enzyme induction (tolerance to anesthesia, tranquilizers, and hypnotic drugs) resulting in practitioners having to administer larger than normal doses of drugs such as anesthetics for optimum results. Whereas drug metabolism in advanced alcoholic liver disease may be reduced resulting in patients becoming toxic on medications routinely administered in dentistry such as acetaminophen, which (in a therapeutic dose) has resulted in severe hepatocellular degradation with a 20% mortality rate. For these reasons, a comprehensive medical consultation should be obtained from the patient's physician when they have signs/ symptoms/history indicating alcohol abuse.

◇ To evaluate if coagulation processes are intact, screening tests should be ordered. Screening tests should include: platelet count, bleeding time, prothrombin time (PT), and partial thromboplastin time (PTT).

◇ If these tests are not within normal limits, the following recommendations may be used as appropriate for surgical procedures.

1. Avoidance of all aspirin products.
2. A 10 mg dose of Vitamin K to be administered IM or IV prior to dental procedures. Recheck PTT.
3. Projected appointments with all invasive dental procedures (ie, surgeries and extractions) scheduled in small increments to avoid stress to the patient's coagulation mechanisms.
4. Gelfoam or topical thrombin in extraction sites and suturing of all overlying gingiva as needed to control hemorrhage after surgery.
5. Pressure dressings on operative sites as necessary.
6. Soft diet for 48 to 72 hours after surgical procedure.
7. Elevated head position.

SURGERY
Portal hypertension sometimes managed with portacaval shunting.

CONSULTATION SUGGESTIONS
Hepatologist, Gastroenterologist

REFERRAL SUGGESTIONS
Primary Care Physician

FIRST STEPS TO TAKE IN AN EMERGENCY
• If coma develops after oral surgery, consider swallowing of blood as source of nitrogen load to liver.

PATIENT INSTRUCTIONS
Stop all use of ethanol. Join local Alcoholic Anonymous group. If severe hepatic compromise, patient requires tight control of dietary protein.

COURSE/PROGNOSIS
Prognosis hinges on control of ethanol abuse.

CODING

ICD-9-CM
571.1 Alcoholic hepatitis
571.2 Cirrhosis with alcoholism
572.3 Portal hypertension

MISCELLANEOUS

SYNONYMS
Alcoholic cirrhosis
Laennec's cirrhosis

SEE ALSO
Hepatitis (general concepts)
Alcoholism

REFERENCES
Little WL, Falace DA: Dental Management of the Medically Compromised Patient. 4th ed. St. Louis, CV Mosby, 1993, pp. 258-275.

Podolsky DK, Isselbacher KJ: Alcohol-related liver disease and cirrhosis. In: Harrison's Principles of Internal Medicine, 13th ed. Isselbacher KJ, et al (eds), NY, McGraw-Hill, 1994, pp 1483-1495.

AUTHOR
Christine Wisnom, BS

Hepatitis (General Concepts)

BASICS

DESCRIPTION
Hepatitis is an inflammatory condition of the liver.

ETIOLOGY

- It may occur as a primary disease or secondary to another disease.
- Primary hepatitis may be caused by:
  Toxic medications (drugs)
  ◇ ethanol, prescription drugs, Fluothane (halothane), chloroform.
  Viral
  ◇ hepatitis A virus (HAV, infectious hepatitis), hepatitis B virus (HBV, serum hepatitis) hepatitis C virus (HCV, non-A non-B), hepatitis D virus (HDV, delta agent), hepatitis E virus (HEV), hepatitis F virus (HFV) and hepatitis G virus (HGV).
  Forms of Viral Hepatitis:
  Autoimmune
  Type I (lupoid hepatitis), Type II, Type III (variant form of autoimmune hepatitis).
- Secondary hepatitis may occur with:
  - Epstein Barr virus (infectious mononucleosis)
  - Tuberculosis (TB)
  - Secondary syphilis
  - Herpes simplex virus (HSV)
  - Cytomegalovirus (CMV)
  - Rubella virus (Measles)
  - Coxsackie B virus
  Parasitic infestation
  ◇ (amebic liver abscess, echinococcosis/tapeworm).
  - Other bacterial forms of hepatitis occur secondary to bacteremia, sepsis and pyogenic liver abscess.
- In immunocompromised patients:
  - Hepatitis may result secondary to hepatitic candidiasis, infection, and liver tumors. Neoplasms such as Kaposi's sarcoma and non-Hodgkin's and Hodgkin's lymphomas occur secondary to the human immunodeficiency virus (HIV).
  - Primary biliary cirrhosis (PBC) an uncommon but not rare form of hepatitis, has no identified cause to date.
  - Metabolic diseases such as Wilson's disease and alpha-1-antitrypsin deficiency cause hepatitis.
- In neonates (birth to 28 days of age)
  ◇ four types of hepatitis are noted
  1) Neonatal jaundice which is the most common abnormal finding in this patient population. It may occur as the result of an immature liver, hemolytic disorder, or limited functioning of the albumin binding sites. Other conditions such as RH and ABO incapability, sepsis, and in utero infections also contribute to this condition.
  2) Neonatal hepatitis (giant cell hepatitis) is a disease of unknown etiology.
  3) Hyperbilirubinemia (serum bilirubin levels in excess of normal limits) may occur from maternal diabetes, maternal infections, or ingestion by the mother of hepatic inflammatory medications such as salicylates, diazepam, oxytocin, or other irritating drugs. Viral hepatitis (hepatitis B virus) may also transfer from mother to neonate at birth.
  4) Kernicterus (is most often found with blood group incapability), where high bilirubin levels cause brain toxicity.

SYSTEMS AFFECTED
Liver
  ◇ regardless of the etiology all types of hepatitis cause changes to occur in the parenchymal cells of the liver. This alteration results in hepatic infiltration by mononuclear cells with edema and variable amounts of degeneration, necrosis, and autolysis to occur. In early alcoholic liver disease, the hepatocytes become engorged with fatty lobules and distended with liver enlargement.
Thorax
  ◇ the most common site of drainage from rupture of a liver abscess, resulting in empyema or hepatobronchial fistula.
Peritoneum
  ◇ second most common site of drainage from rupture of a liver abscess resulting in peritonitis.
Esophageal varicies are often noted in alcoholic hepatitis.
Skin
  ◇ abnormal findings resulting from various forms of hepatitis include: hyperpigmentation, jaundice, purpura, vascular spiders, excoriations, lichenification, xanthelasma, and xanthoma.
Eyes
  ◇ pigmented corneal rings, jaundice.
Abdomen
  ◇ hepatomegaly, splenomegaly, ascites.
Extremities
  ◇ bone tenderness, digital clubbing, peripheral edema, palmar erythema, white or banded nails.
Nervous system
  ◇ peripheral neuropathy, encephalopathy.
Oral region
  ◇ in many types of hepatitis, the odor of the breath is described as musty and sweet. Gingival bleeding may be noted. In alcoholic hepatitis, nutritional deficiencies may result in reduced papillary on the tongue, glossitis, and labial or angular cheilosis. Mucosal ecchymosis, petechiae, and reduced healing following trauma or surgery has been noted. Jaundiced mucosal tissue may also be present. Parotid gland enlargement, which is painless, may be seen in advanced liver disease.

DIAGNOSIS

SYMPTOMS AND SIGNS
• Physical abnormalities vary greatly dependent upon the etiologic source of infection, and physical assessment may be normal in early or asymptomatic disease.
• Fatigue, nausea, vomiting, diarrhea, joint and muscle pain, anorexia, jaundice, hepatomegaly, abdominal and gastric distention, clay-colored stools, dark urine, fever, bruising, rash, chills, distaste for cigarettes and food.
• Note: symptoms are not specific to the etiologic agent; therefore, type-specific diagnosis cannot be made on physical examination alone.

LABORATORY
Universal tests for liver problems
◇ bilirubin, alkaline phosphatase, albumin, prothrombin time, partial thromboplastin time, complete blood count with differential and platelets, AST (aspartate aminotransferase), ALT (alanine aminotransferase).
Primary biliary cirrhosis (PBS)
◇ antinuclear antibody (ANA), antimitrochondrial antibody (AMA).
Echinococcosis (tapeworm)
◇ hemoagglutination (ELISA)
Wilson's disease
◇ ceruloplasmin, serum and urinary copper.
Alpha-1
◇ antitrypsin deficiency
◇ serum alpha-1-antitrypsin positive phenotype.
Autoimmune hepatitis
◇ ANA, smooth muscle antibody (SMA), liver kidney microsomal antibody Type 1 (anti-LKM-1), antibody-soluble liver antigen (anti-SLA).
Candidiasis
◇ blood cultures for: Candida albicans, C. pseudotropicalis, C. stellatoidea.
Bacterial hepatitis (ie, sepsis, bacteremia)
◇ bilirubin, alkaline phosphatase, AST and ALT.
Hepatitis virus (HAV)
◇ antiviral antibodies.

IMAGING/SPECIAL TESTS
• Ultrasonogram to diagnose abscesses, tumors, hepatic vessels, and stenosis.
• CT scan diagnostic for cirrhosis.
• Endoscopic retrograde cholangiopancreatography (ERCP) for diagnosing cystic ruptures and biliary stones.
• Percutaneous liver biopsy (punch-blind method).
• Laparoscopy with direct liver biopsy (greater degree of accuracy than punch).
• Chest radiograph to diagnose M. tuberculosis and atypical mycobacterium dissemination from a pulmonary site.
• Cholangiogram to assess extrahepatic and intrahepatic biliary tracts (gall bladder ducts).
• MRI may evaluate cirrhosis when a nodular linea is noted.
• Peritoneoscopy for diagnosing cirrhosis with visual sampling.
• Hepatic iron and copper for diagnosis of Wilson's disease and hemochromatosis.

DIFFERENTIAL
• In Neonates:
  Kernicterus, hyperbilirubinemia, hepatitis B and C (neonatal transmission), congenital abnormalities.
• In children:
  Hepatitis A
• In young adults:
  Hepatitis B, C, D, E, F, G, HIV, and ethanol abuse.
• In middle-aged women:
  Primary biliary cirrhosis, ethanol abuse.
• In middle-aged males:
  Ethanol abuse, neoplasms, medications, (eg, treatment for hypercholesterolemia).
• In immunocompromised patients (25 to 45 years):
  1) Neoplasms
  ◇ Kaposi's sarcoma and lymphomas (non-Hodgkin's and Hodgkin's).
  2) Infections
  ◇ Mycobacterium, cytomegalovirus, toxoplasmosis, histoplasmosis, cryptococcoses, candidiasis, syphilis, leptospirosis.
  3) Parasitic disease
  ◇ amebic liver abscess and echinococcoses.
• In older patients (>45 years):
  Liver diseases are noted at greater frequency during bacteremia and sepsis. Cirrhosis and heptocellular carcinoma, hepatitis B and C (blood transfusion).

TREATMENT

General
◇ Avoidance of substances such as ethanol and some medications that may cause hepatic inflammation. This is of primary importance to dental practitioners due to dental medications prescribed routinely which are metabolized in the liver. These include analgesics, such as aspirin, acetaminophen, codeine and meperidine; anesthetics including lidocaine and mepivacaine; sedatives including the barbiturates, diazepam, and many antibiotics such as tetracycline and ampicillin. Maintaining adequate hydration and bed rest in early disease are also beneficial. In advanced cirrhotic liver disease and fulminant hepatic failure, liver transplantation may be necessary. These universal treatment modalities may be prescribed for numerous forms of hepatitis.
Autoimmune hepatitis
◇ (types I, II and III)
◇ treatment with corticosteroids. For dental treatment, consult with patient's physician regarding possible alteration in prescribed therapy.
Primary biliary cirrhosis
◇ treatment includes corticosteroids, methotrexate, ozathiprine, and D-penicillamine.
HIV disease
◇ (for the most common fungal, bacterial, and parasitic infections of the liver.) Treatment includes ketoconazole, fluconazole, rifampin, isoniazid, zidouvidine (AZT), pentamidine, acetaminophen, trimethoprim-sulfamethoxazole and amphotericin B.

MEDICATIONS
• See general treatment section

CONSULTATION SUGGESTIONS
Hepatologist, Gastroenterologist

REFERRAL SUGGESTIONS
Primary Care Physician

(continued)

Hepatitis (General Concepts) *continued*

FIRST STEPS TO TAKE IN AN EMERGENCY
• If bleeding a problem in liver disease patient, order a coagulation profile: PT, PTT, platelet count, and bleeding time.

PATIENT INSTRUCTIONS
Avoid ethanol and other substances known to be hepatotoxic or require hepatic metabolism.

COURSE/PROGNOSIS
Hepatitis
◇ may either have an acute course with resolution and no sequellae, run chronic, indolent course with or without signs and symptoms, or a fulminant course causing death in a few days or weeks.

CODING

ICD-9-CM
286.9	Coagulopathy
570.0	Acute hepatitis
571.1	Alcoholic hepatitis
571.4	Chronic hepatitis
571.41	Chronic, persistent hepatitis
573.8	Cholestatic hepatitis
573.3	Drug induced hepatitis

MISCELLANEOUS

• Patients with hepatitis may experience coagulation defects. To evaluate if these processes are intact, screening tests should be ordered, including a platelet count, bleeding time, prothrombin time (PT), and partial thromboplastin time (PTT). The PT and PTT result will indicate if a defect in the coagulation phase has occurred. The bleeding time will indicate if the platelet phase is normal. If both are normal, surgical procedures may be performed with minimal risk of postoperative bleeding.

• If these tests are not within normal limits, the following recommendations may be used as appropriate for surgical procedures.

1) Avoidance of all aspirin products to prevent prolonged bleeding that can result from ingestion of even 10 grams of aspirin up to 5 days before treatment.

2) A 10 mg dose of vitamin K to be administered intramuscularly or intravenously prior to dental procedures if deficiency of vitamin K dependent clotting factors suspected.

3) Projected appointments with all invasive dental procedures (ie, surgeries and extractions) scheduled in small increments to avoid stress to the patient's coagulation mechanisms.

4) Gelfoam or topical thrombin in extraction sites and suturing of all overlying gingiva as needed to control hemorrhage after surgery.

5) Pressure dressings on operative sites as necessary.

6) Soft diet for 48 to 72 hours after surgical procedure.

7) Elevated head position.

8) If platelet count <20,000, platelet transfusion may be necessary.

• Corticosteroid therapy is the treatment of choice for patients with primary biliary cirrhosis, autoimmune hepatitis, and cryptogenic hepatitis. To receive dental care, these patients may require alterations to their steroid therapy. For patients receiving routine dental care who are well controlled with daily corticosteroids, no additional supplementation is required. If these patients have recently discontinued their steroids (less than 2 weeks), they should receive their previously prescribed daily dose on the day of their dental appointment. For patients who have discontinued their steroids for greater than 2 weeks, normally no medications are required for routine dental care. If, however, the patient who is or was taking steroids requires extensive or stressful dental treatment, their daily dose may be doubled both on the day of treatment and the first postoperative day.

• Alpha interferon is a man-made antiviral that mimics the body's naturally occurring antiviral mechanisms. It is an accepted therapy for chronic viral hepatitis. Treatment typically consists of 3 million units of alpha interferon administered subcutaneously 3 times per week for 24 weeks. While a decrease in clinical symptoms and a partial or complete normalization of aminotransferase has been noted in 50% to 60% of patients treated, relapse is common. Patients may experience side effects that include fever, malaise, headaches, weight loss, alopecia, and depression. Neutropenia and thrombocytopenia have also been noted. For patients who are receiving this medication, practitioners may elect to defer dental care until the patient has completed therapy.

SEE ALSO
Viral hepatitis
Alcoholic hepatitis

REFERENCES
Dienstag JL, Isselbacher KJ: Acute and chronic hepatitis. In: Harrison's Principles of Internal Medicine, 13th ed. NY, McGraw-Hill, 1994, pp 1458-1483.

Wisnom C, Kelly M: Medical/dental management of a chronic hepatitis C patient. Oral Surg, Oral Med, Oral Path 75:786-790, 1993.

Porter S, Scully C, Lakshman S: Viral hepatitis. Oral Surg, Oral Med, Oral Path 78:682-695, 1994.

Wisnom C, DePaola L, Lee R: A five year study of occupational exposures in dental health care workers. Am J Pub Health Dent, 1995. In press.

Edmond JC, Aren PP, Whitington PF, et al: Liver transplantation in the management of fulminant hepatic failure. Gastroenterology 96:1583-1589, 1989.

AUTHOR
Christine Wisnom, BS

Hepatitis, Viral

BASICS

DESCRIPTION
Inflammatory conditions of the liver due to viral infection.

ETIOLOGY

- Caused by:
  - hepatitis A virus (HAV, infectious hepatitis), hepatitis B virus (HBV, serum hepatitis) hepatitis C virus (HCV, non-A non-B), hepatitis D virus (HDV, delta agent), hepatitis E virus (HEV), hepatitis F virus (HFV), and hepatitis G virus (HGV).
- Variant Forms of Viral Hepatitis:
  - <u>hepatitis B viruses</u>
  ◊ 2 (HBV-2) which has been found in the United States, Spain, West Africa, New Zealand, Taiwan, France, and the Middle East. In Italy, an additional variant form of hepatitis B has also been identified.
  - hepatitis C virus (HCV) exists as at least six distinct genotypes that occur in various geographic locations. In North America HCV-1 and HCV-H; in Japan HCV-J, HC-J14, HC-J6, and HC-J8; in Europe HCV-E and GM 1, 2 are found. Hepatitis C also has at least 16 variant forms.

SYSTEMS AFFECTED
<u>Liver</u>
◊ changes occur in the parenchymal cells of the liver. Results in hepatic infiltration by mononuclear cells with edema and variable amounts of degeneration, necrosis, and autolysis.
<u>Abdomen</u>
◊ hepatomegaly, splenomegaly, ascites.
<u>Extremities</u>
◊ bone tenderness, digital clubbing, peripheral edema, palmar erythema, white or banded nails.
<u>Nervous system</u>
◊ peripheral neuropathy, hepatitic encephalopathy.
<u>Oral cavity</u>
◊ hepatitis C virus has been implicated as the onset Sjögren's syndrome in three studies; however, this is not a consistent finding. In Southern Europeans with chronic hepatitis disease, lichen planus has also been noted.

DIAGNOSIS

SYMPTOMS AND SIGNS
- Fatigue, nausea, vomiting, diarrhea, joint and muscle pain, anorexia, jaundice, hepatomegaly, abdominal and gastric distention, clay-colored stools, dark urine, fever, bruising, rash, chills, distaste for cigarettes and food.
- In addition to assessing a patient's signs and symptoms, practitioners should also evaluate a patient's risk group.

LABORATORY
- Universal tests: bilirubin, alkaline phosphatase, albumin, prothrombin time, partial thromboplastin time, complete blood count with differential and platelets, AST (aspartate aminotransferase), ALT (alanine aminotransferase).
- <u>Hepatitis A Virus (HAV)</u>
  ◊ anti-HAV IgM, antibody hepatitis A virus IgG immunoglobulin (anti-HAV IgG).
- <u>Hepatitis B Virus (HBV)</u>
  ◊ hepatitis B surface antigen (HBsAg), hepatitis B surface antibody (HGsAb), hepatitis B core antibody (HBcAb), hepatitis B core antigen (HBcAg), hepatitis B e antigen (HBe Ab), antibody hepatitis B virus immunoglobulin IgM (anti-HBV IgM), anti-HBVIgS.
- <u>Hepatitis B Virus (HBV) variant</u>
  ◊ hepatitis B virus DNA molecule (HBV-DNA), hepatitis B virus DNA Dane particle (HBV-DNA-P).
- <u>Hepatitis C virus (HCV)</u>
  ◊ antibody hepatitis C virus recombinant immunoblot assay 2 (anti-HCV RIBA 2).
- <u>Hepatitis C virus (HCV) variant</u>
  ◊ hepatitis C virus ribonucleic acid (HCV RNA).
- <u>Hepatitis D virus (HDV)</u>
  ◊ HDV Ag, Anti-HDV IgG, IgM, HDV RNA.
- <u>Hepatitis E Virus (HEV)</u>
  ◊ HEV Western blot, HEV ELISA, HEV polymerase chain reaction.

DIFFERENTIAL
- In neonates:
  Kernicterus, hyperbilirubinemia, hepatitis B and C (neonatal transmission), congenital abnormalities
- In children:
  Hepatitis A
- In young adults:
  Hepatitis B, C, D, E, F, G, HIV and ethanol abuse.
- In middle-aged women:
  Primary biliary cirrhosis
- In middle-aged males:
  Ethanol abuse, neoplasms, medications.
- In immunocompromised patients (25 to 45 years)

1. Neoplasms
   ◊ Kaposi's sarcoma and lymphomas (non-Hodgkin's and Hodgkin's)
2. Infections
   Mycobacterium
   Cytomegalovirus, toxoplasmosis, histoplasmosis, cryptococcoses, candidiasis, syphilis, leptospirosis.

TREATMENT

General

◊ Liver enzymes

◊ ALT, AST, and alkaline phosphatase will enable practitioners to estimate the degree of inflammatory disease present. (ie, liver function tests 2 1/2 times the normal value demonstrate significant liver diseases). Bilirubin levels that are elevated are indicative that the liver is not properly conducting its metabolic process and that patients may potentially become toxic on prescribed dental medications. In most patients, dental medications may be administered normally. In severe liver disease, drugs metabolized in the liver may be required in a lower dose or avoided.

HAV

◊ An IgG-anti-HAV immunoglobulin may be used prophylactically to prevent infection before an anticipated exposure or within 2 weeks following an exposure. The prescribed dose is 0.02 mL/kg of body weight-post exposure and 0.06 mL/kg of body weight prophylactically prior to an exposure. A new vaccine of inactivated HAV is currently available and may be prescribed to replace immunoglobulin therapy. Following a medical consultation, only emergency dental care should be provided for patients with an active hepatitis A infection.

◊ Basic tests in conjunction with the hepatitis A panel will enable dental care to be administered as safely as possible to the patient with an active hepatitis A infection. An acute HAV infection is diagnosed by an IgM anti-HAV seropositive result. It is usually present for 3 to 6 months. It is followed by a seropositive anti-HAV total, indicating patients have resolved their infections and may resume elective dental treatment with no special precautions required.

HBV in neonates and children

◊ vaccines for infants can be either a three-dose series: birth, 1 month, and 6 months, or a four-dose series: birth, 1 to 2 months, and 12-18 months. No booster recommendations currently exist. Awareness of, and compliance with, the pediatric recommendations made by the Immunization Practice Advisor Committee of CDC is especially relevant for dentistry due to the high rate of HBV seropositivity noted within our population. This fact, coupled with documentation of lateral transmission of HBV, makes vaccination of children imperative.

HBV in adolescents and adults

◊ vaccines (yeast or recombinant) have an approximately 95% efficacy rate when administered as a three-dose series. An initial dose, a 1-month and a 6-month dose usually confers maximum efficacy. However, these vaccines are not effective against the two variant forms of HBV. Additionally, postvaccination testing is recommended for dental personnel between 1 and 6 months following the third dose. In healthy adults and children, studies indicate that immunologic memory in vaccinated individuals remains intact for 9 years, conferring protection against chronic HBV. Following an exposure to HBV, HGIg immunoglobulin (0.06 mL/kg of body weight) may be administered within 7 days. Compliance with these CDC recommendations are critical to the control of the HBV in the dental setting.

HBV treatment

◊ for chronic HBV infections, alpha interferon

◊ 2b therapy may be prescribed. The efficacy rate is poor (approximately 50%) and side effects are often noted. Advanced disease resulting in cirrhosis may be treated with liver transplantation. Elective dental care should not be provided for a patient with signs or symptoms of hepatitis, and only emergency dental care should be provided for patients with active disease. In conjunction with the coagulation profile, liver enzymes, and bilirubin tests, a hepatitis B panel should be obtained. An HBsAg, HBeAg, and IgM anti-HBc seropositive result indicates that the patient has an acute HBV infection. As patients progress through their disease, these tests will become seronegative and the HBsAb, HBeAb, and IgG anti-HBc will become seropositive. Elective dental treatment may safely resume without additional precautions when the patient's HBsAg is seronegative and the anti-HBs is seropositive, and the ALT and AST are within normal limits. These markers indicate that recovery is complete, the patient had adequately acquired an immunity, and he/she is considered no longer infectious. If these markers are reversed (HBsAg+, anti-HBs, with elevations of the AST and ALT) for longer than 6 months, the patient is considered to be a "carrier" or has a chronic HBV infection. Ninety to 95% of adults recover within 6 months, while only 5% to 10% develop chronic hepatitis. If the patient develops a chronic condition, a consultation with gastroenterology should be obtained to evaluate the patient's ability to tolerate dental treatment. The major complications of the chronic hepatitis (CH) patient resulting from dental treatment are hemorrhage, poor wound healing, an increased risk of infection, and the inappropriate metabolism of prescribed medications.

(continued)

Hepatitis, Viral *continued*

◇ Dental Treatment for the Chronic Hepatitis (CH) Patient:

◇ To assess homeostasis, a coagulation profile should be obtained using PT, PTT, platelet count, and bleeding time to plan for surgical procedures. Because CH can impair the synthesis of clotting factors, an increased PT, PTT may alert the practitioner to potential hemorrhagic tendencies. A depletion in platelets is also indicative of both CH and cirrhosis. If these tests are within normal limits, patients may receive dental care with minimal risk of postoperative bleeding. Liver enzymes AST, ALT, and alkaline phosphatase are used to monitor the course of hepatitis. Two laboratory values that monitor disease severity are mean peak AST rise and bilirubin elevations. To assess the patient's healing capabilities, a complete blood cell count (CBC) with differential may be obtained. The differential may demonstrate neutropenia or an increase in lymphocytes, which both occur in hepatic conditions. Because CH patients often manifest adverse reactions that result from the inability of the liver to break down and metabolize drugs, all medications are administered and monitored with caution.

HCV treatment

◇ no vaccine exists currently for prophylaxis. However, occupational acquisition of HCV appears to be very low in a dental setting. The majority of patients with CHC are anicteric and asymptomatic. Diagnosis is based primarily on an elevated aminotransferase and/or a positive anti-HCV. Patients with these positive findings who are symptomatic are assumed to have an acute infection and only emergency dental care should be provided at this time. If these tests remain positive for greater than 6 months, the patient is assumed to have a CHC infection. Chronicity develops in approximately 75% of those infected. For patients requiring dental care, see "Dental treatment for CH Patient."

For chronic HCV infections, alpha interferon

◇ 2b therapy may be prescribed. However, the efficacy rate is low (approximately 50%) and side effects are often noted. Ribovirin and acyclovir may also be administered to reduce the degree of hepatic complications. Chronic HCV resulting is cirrhosis is frequently treated by liver transplantation.

HDV treatment

◇ vaccination of infants, children, adolescents, and adults for HBV will prevent an HDV infection because it is a defective virus and infects only HBV-infected individuals. Alpha interferon -2b therapy inhibits HDV replication in 50% of those treated. Liver transplantation is often indicated for patients with advanced cirrhosis. Only emergency care should be provided to patients with signs or symptoms of hepatitis D when the patient has an acute infection. The HDAg (hepatitis D antigen) and IgM anti-HD (IgM antibody to hepatitis D) seropositive results are indicative of an acute infection. The IgM anti-HD is rapidly replaced by the IgG anti-HD which persists and when it correlates with an elevated aminotransferase indicates a CHD infection. Ten to fifteen percent of all hepatitis D infections progress to chronicity. If dental treatment is required, follow recommendations "Dental Treatment of the CH Patient."

HEV, HFV, and HGV

◇ no vaccines are currently available. Treatment is generally palliative and supportive (see general treatment).

MEDICATIONS
• See general treatment

CONSULTATION SUGGESTIONS
Hepatologist, Gastroenterologist

REFERRAL SUGGESTIONS
Primary Care Physician

FIRST STEPS TO TAKE IN AN EMERGENCY
• If severe hepatitic disease present and oral bleeding a problem, check coagulation profile and consider Vitamin K or platelet administration.

PATIENT INSTRUCTIONS
Follow physician's recommendations carefully.

COURSE/PROGNOSIS
Viral hepatitis can have completely subclinical course or lead a fulminant course to death.

CODING

ICD-9-CM
570.0   Acute hepatitis
571.4   Chronic hepatitis
571.41 Chronic, persistent hepatitis

Hepatitis, Viral *continued*

MISCELLANEOUS

Treatment Recommendations for Infection Control
Viral hepatitis transmission in dentistry

1. Hepatitis A is commonly transmitted in via the fecal-oral route. However, saliva does contain HAV particles. Limited data exist regarding infection of dental personnel following occupational exposures. However, percutaneous injury (needlestick) has transmitted HAV. Cross-transmission of HAV (health care worker to patient) has also occurred but appears to be a minimal risk.

2. Hepatitis B is transmitted via blood and body fluids (saliva and gingival crevicular fluids) and HBV has the highest rate of transmissibility in dentistry (6% to 30%). Following an occupational exposure, the Hepatitis Branch of the CDC estimates that between 500 to 600 health care workers are hospitalized annually. Death occurs in 200, 12 to 15 resulting from fulminating hepatitis, 170 to 200 from cirrhosis, and 40 to 50 from liver cancer. Cross-transmission (health care worker to patient) has been documented in numerous studies. Patient infection occurs primarily during surgical procedures from an HBS Ag positive practitioner with poor infection control practices.

3. Hepatitis C has been transmitted to dental personnel occupationally. But, transmission rates are low. A recent study evaluated 343 Oral-Maxillofacial Surgeons and 305 General Dentists for anti-HCV following occupational exposures. Results indicated that 2% of the Oral-Maxillofacial Surgeons were anti-HCV positive and 0.7% of the General Dentists were anti-HCV positive. HCV is present in blood and body fluids, and up to 50% of patients with chronic hepatitis have hepatitis C viral particles in their saliva. Infection of health care workers has also resulted from a human bite. Cross-transmission (health care worker to patient) is under investigation because HCV is capable of remaining intact at room temperature for a period of at least 7 days.

4. Hepatitis D is transmitted via blood and body fluids, and the presence of HDV viral particles in saliva is being investigated. The occupational acquisition of HDV has also been noted in dentistry. Cross-transmission (health care worker to patient) has been documented in at least four dentists, with one HDV seropositive Oral-Maxillofacial Surgeon who infected several patients.

5. Hepatitis E is primarily a water-borne virus. But food is also a mode of transmission. In the U.S., HEV appears primarily in people traveling to areas endemic to HEV such as Asia, Africa, and Latin America. Parenteral and lateral transmission is rare. Hepatitis C, like hepatitis A, has no carrier state.

6. Hepatitis F and G, the most recent additions to the viral hepatitis family, are blood-borne viruses that are transmitted parenterally. Their impact on dentistry at this time is not clear, and further investigation is required to formulate recommendations relating to clinic practice.

Treatment recommendations relating to infection control include:

1. Vaccination of health care workers
◊ vaccines are available to protect against hepatitis A, B, and D.

2. Universal precautions as recommended by the CDC, which recommends the consistent use of blood and body fluid precautions for all patients regardless of their infectious disease status.

3. Compliance with the Department of Labor's Occupational Safety and Health Administration's Bloodborne Pathogen Standards as well as the State Regulatory Boards, as applicable.

4. Compliance with the continuing education requirements of the individual relicensure boards relating to infection control topics.

S-Suspected L-Low
Note: Hepatitis F & G risks are suspected to be parenteral.

SEE ALSO
Hepatitis (general concepts)

REFERENCES
Wisnom C, Kelly M: Medical/dental management of a chronic hepatitis C patient. Oral Surg, Oral Med, Oral Path 75:786-790, 1993.

Porter S, Scully C, Lakshman S: Viral hepatitis. Oral Surg, Oral Med, Oral Path 78:682-695, 1994.

Kelly M, Wisnom C: Heptatitis B vaccine and exposure protocol: update. J Gen Dent. Nov/Dec., 531-534, 1993.

Wisnom C, Lee R: Increased seroprevalence of hepatitis B in dental personnel necessitates awareness of revised pediatric hepatitis B vaccine recommendations. J Pub Health Dent 53:231-234, 1993.

Wisnom C, DePaola L, Lee R: A five year study of occupational exposures in dental health care workers. Am J Pub Health Dent, 1995, In press.

Thomas D, Gruninger S, Siew C, et al: Occupational risk of hepatitis C infections among general dentists and oral surgeons in North America. Am J Medicine 1995, In press.

AUTHOR
Christine Wisnom, BS

- 247 -

Herpangina

BASICS

DESCRIPTION
• An acute systemic viral infection, common in infants and children, and tends to occur in epidemics.
• Predominant age 3 months to 16 years.
• Highest incidence from June to October.
• Incubation period 2 to 10 days.

ETIOLOGY

• Group A Coxsackievirus principally A2, 4 through 6, 8 and 10.
• Disease usually transmitted by saliva from infected individuals, fecal contamination, or by fomites.

SYSTEMS AFFECTED
Oral mucosa
◊ small papulovesicular lesion (1 to 2 mm) with grayish-white surface surrounded by erythema. Most often found on the tonsillar pillars, hard and soft palate, tonsils, and uvula. Periodontium and buccal mucosa rarely involved.
Oropharynx
◊ often hyperemic
Parotid glands
◊ rare complication is parotitis.

DIAGNOSIS

SYMPTOMS AND SIGNS
Systemic
◊ sore throat, fever, malaise, myalgia, anorexia (all mild to moderate). Twenty-five percent of infected individuals experience vomiting and abdominal pain. Diarrhea may also be present.
Mouth
◊ dysphagia, pain from small vesicular lesions, drooling.
Oral mucosal
◊ lesions start as punctate macules, then evolve into papules and vesicles usually involving the posterior one-third of the oral cavity. Within 24 to 48 hours, vesicles rupture forming small (1 to 2 mm) ulcers. The ulcers have a white necrotic center surrounded by an erythematous base. Lesions may be multiple or occur in isolated small groups.
Pharynx
◊ hyperemic.

LABORATORY
• A diagnosis is usually based on the symptoms and characteristic oral lesions. When in doubt, a definitive diagnosis can be confirmed by demonstrating a rise in specific IgM titer or isolating virus from oral ulcer. Because Coxsackie A are enteroviruses, feces should also be cultured.
• Leukocytosis also present.

DIFFERENTIAL
• Primary herpetic stomatitis
• Aphthous ulcers
• Streptococcal pharyngitis
• Hand-Food-Mouth disease
• Varicella
• Mumps (if parotitis present)

Herpangina

 TREATMENT

General
◊ Palliative and supportive, including bed rest, soft diet, proper hydration, isolation of individual to prevent the spread of the disease.

MEDICATIONS
• Antipyretics
• Analgesics
• Palliative mouth rinse (topical anesthetic), such as diphenhydramine (Benadryl) syrup mixed with .05% dyclonine.

SURGERY
Biopsy not indicated.

CONSULTATION SUGGESTIONS
Oral Medicine, Oral-Maxillofacial Surgeon

REFERRAL SUGGESTIONS
Oral Medicine, Oral-Maxillofacial Surgeon

PATIENT INSTRUCTIONS
Maintain hydration orally.

COURSE/PROGNOSIS
• Disease is self-limiting with acute symptoms lasting about 3 to 4 days.
• Oral lesions generally heal in 7 to 10 days.

 CODING

ICD-9-CM
074.0 Herpangina

 MISCELLANEOUS

SYNONYMS
Aphthous pharyngitis

SEE ALSO
Pharyngitis
Herpes simplex

REFERENCES
Huebner RJ, et al: Herpangina, etiologic studies of a specific disease. JAMA 145:628, 1951.

Howlet, et al: A new syndrome of parotitis with herpangina caused by the Coxsackie virus. Canadian Med Assoc J 77:5-7, 1957.

Hypia T, Stanway G: Biology of Coxsackie A viruses. Adv Virus Res 42:343-373, 1993.

AUTHOR
John Jandinski, DMD

Herpes Simplex

BASICS

DESCRIPTION
• A family of six viruses with DNA cores, capsids, and envelopes. Five of the six, including herpes simplex I and II, Epstein-Barr, varicella-zoster, and cytomegalovirus can affect the oral and maxillofacial structures. Herpes simplex I most often affects oral and perioral structures, and occasionally the genitals. Herpes simplex II most often affects genital structures, and occasionally oral and perioral structures.
• During the first or primary infection, few show significant signs or symptoms. Most have subclinical disease. The incubation period lasts from several days to 2 weeks. Primary HSV oral infections manifest as oral region pain, lymphadenopathy, low-grade fever, and malaise followed by rapidly developing vesicles involving virtually all areas of oral mucosa. The gingiva is characteristically swollen and easily bleeds (primary herpetic gingivostomatitis). The vesicles are transient, lasting only a matter of hours before rupturing, leaving a well circumscribed 1 to 3 mm ulceration. The ulcers may stand alone or coalesce, forming larger areas of denuded mucosa. Untreated, the disease usually runs its course in 14 to 21 days.
• The initial symptom of a recurrent infection is usually a prodromal burning, tingling, or painful sensation at the terminal ends of the involved nerve branch. The recurrent infection gives rise to a small cluster of vesicles identical to those found in primary herpetic gingivostomatitis but usually involving an area no larger than 1 to 2 cm in diameter. The vesicles rupture usually in a matter of hours, forming a crust. A recurrent disease episode usually lasts 10 days to 2 weeks. Immunosuppressed patients may have recurrent episodes that mimic primary herpetic gingivostomatitis.

ETIOLOGY

• Herpes simplex is spread via direct physical contact.
• Following resolution of the primary disease, the virus travels to the trigeminal ganglion where it becomes latent. Recurrent herpes simplex infections occur in some but not all seropositive patients. Reactivation may be "triggered" by a subsequent illness (fever blisters, cold sores), hormonal changes, or environmental agents such as sunlight, mechanical trauma, or stress. The virus travels down a trigeminal nerve branch and infects the basal and parabasal cells in a localized area of keratinized mucosa, usually the vermilion of the lip, gingiva, or palatal mucosa.

SYSTEMS AFFECTED
Primary herpetic gingivostomatitis
◊ affects keratinized and nonkeratinized oral mucosa, regional lymphadenopathy, fever, malaise. Recurrent oral herpes type I or II: keratinized oral mucosa, including most often the gingiva and palate, or the vermilion of the lips.
Herpetic whitlow
◊ infection of nailbed and surrounding tissues.
Herpetic keratoconjunctivitis
◊ conjunctivitis with regional adenopathy.
Eczema herpeticum
◊ pox-like eruption complicating atopic dermatitis.

DIAGNOSIS

SYMPTOMS AND SIGNS
• Primary oral infections usually feature the symptoms common to many viral infections, including regional lymphadenopathy, low-grade fever, and malaise. Oral mucosal ulcerations, bleeding, fetid breath, drooling, dysphagia, and sore throat.
• Recurrent activations usually feature a prodromal pain sensation lasting several hours at the eventual site of vesicle formation.
• Transient 1 to 2 mm diameter vesicles that rupture in hours to form ulceration which may coalesce to form larger, irregular ulcerations.
• Intraoral ulcers will have the characteristic white, fibrin surface with a peripheral margin of erythema. Vermilion and skin ulcers usually become covered by relatively dark scabs made from serous exudate, blood, and foreign debris. Intact skin or vermilion around the ulcerated areas is also erythematous.

LABORATORY
For the primary infection, clinical laboratory studies will usually show nonspecific features of a viral infection, including an elevated sedimentation rate, and a lymphocyte shift in the CBC and differential.

IMAGING/SPECIAL TESTS
• Viral cultures can be done, but usually take 2 to 4 days.
• Cytologic preparations in ethanol fixative can be stained, usually with Papanicolaou's method (PAP) and will reveal giant, multinucleated epithelial cells, characteristic, but not diagnostic, of herpes simplex. (Papanicolaou smear). Varicella infection will have similar findings.
• Cytologic preps fixed in acetone can be stained immunologically to show cells specifically infected with HSV I or II.

DIFFERENTIAL
• Aphthous stomatitis
◊ occurs on nonkeratinized oral mucosa.
Lichen planus
◊ presence of hyperkeratotic striations.
Pemphigoid
◊ Nikolsky's sign and involvement of keratinized and nonkeratinized oral mucosa.
• Erythema multiforme/drug reaction may be impossible to distinguish from primary herpes without cytologic preps. Usually has less gingival involvement, and no fever or lymphadenopathy. Can be recurrent, whereas primary herpes should occur only once in an immunocompetent host.
• Herpangina
• Impetigo

TREATMENT

General
◇ Wash hands often to prevent spread.

MEDICATIONS
• Primary herpes
◇ palliative treatment, NSAIDs to relieve pain, topical oral anesthetics such as viscous lidocaine. Acyclovir, 200 mg × 5 daily (1 gm), is sometimes effective in shortening the overall course of the disease episode if administered within the first 24 to 48 hours.
• Recurrent Herpes
◇ intraoral recurrences usually require no treatment but palliative treatment can be administered with a topical anesthetic. Vermilion recurrences can, in some patients, be shortened in duration by the early (during the prodrome) application of topical acyclovir, with repeat applications every 1 to 2 waking hours for the first 24 to 48 hours. Topical ointments to prevent drying and contracture of the scab, which can result in enlargement of the wound and prolonged healing should also be used.

CONSULTATION SUGGESTIONS
Oral Medicine

REFERRAL SUGGESTIONS
Oral Medicine, Primary Care Physician

PATIENT INSTRUCTIONS
Avoid contact with infants or pregnant woman while active lesions present.

COURSE/PROGNOSIS
• Primary herpes usually runs its course if untreated in 14 to 21 days.
• Recurrent herpes usually runs its course if untreated in 10 to 14 days.

CODING

ICD-9-CM
054.0 Eczema herpeticum
054.1 Genital herpes
054.2 Primary herpes gingivostomatitis
054.9 Recurrent herpes, herpes labialis
079.9 Viral infection
528.0 Stomatitis
529.1 Glossitis
695.1 Erythema multiforme

CPT
11900 Intralesional injection
40812 Incisional biopsy
87252 Culture isolation
88160 Cytologic preparation

MISCELLANEOUS

SYNONYMS
Fever blisters
Cold sores
Acute herpetic gingivostomatitis
Herpes labialis

SEE ALSO
Herpangina
Oral ulcers
Herpes zoster

REFERENCES
Vincent SD, Finkelstein MW: Differential Diagnosis of Oral Ulcers. In: Principles of Oral Diagnosis. Coleman GC, Nelson JF, (eds), St. Louis, Mosby-Year Book Co., 1993, pp. 327-351.

Regezi JA, Sciubba JJ: Vesiculo-Bullous Diseases. In: Oral Pathology, Clinical Pathologic Correlations. Philadelphia, WB Saunders Co., 1993, pp. 4-9.

AUTHOR
Steven D. Vincent, DDS, MS

Herpes Zoster

BASICS

DESCRIPTION
Herpes Zoster is a painful, vesiculo-ulcerative cutaneous and/or mucosal viral infection (reactivation) characteristically occurring along specific dermatome areas in geriatric or immunocompromised individuals.

ETIOLOGY

• Varicella-Zoster virus (VZV) is a moderately sized (110 nm), lipid enveloped, double-stranded DNA virus with an icosahedral nucleocapsid. VZV exhibits specificity for infecting human tissues of ectodermal origin (ie, epithelium, neural tissue). Initial infection generally occurs through the respiratory route, although direct contact between the virus and open skin or mucous membranes may also present a pathway for infection in non-immune individuals.
• VZV affects over 90% of the population by the age of 15 as the well-known clinical disease referred to as chicken pox. Following infection, VZV localizes in the dorsal root and cranial nerve ganglia. There, latency and genomic integration of viral DNA occurs in the neurons.
• Although the precise mechanisms that trigger reactivation and structural viral assembly remain unclear, the ultimate clinical result is a vesiculo-ulcerative dermatitis or mucositis, which follows the dermatome or neural pathway of the affected ganglion known as shingles or zoster.
• Zoster (viral reactivation) occurs in 10 to 20% of all adults, usually after the 6th decade, or in patients who are immunosuppressed by organic disease, trauma (physical or psychogenic) or are taking certain medications (ie, steroids, cytotoxins).

SYSTEMS AFFECTED
Skin
◇ generally affecting single dermatomes distributed over the abdomen, neck or face, usually unilateral in distribution.
Ocular
◇ occasionally, eye involved resulting in corneal destruction and loss of sight following single or successive recurrences.
Oral
◇ lesions most commonly appear as unilateral vesicular erosions distributed across the palate, buccal mucosa, or gingiva.
Ear/Auditory Canal
◇ lesions affecting the geniculate ganglion producing a collection of symptoms, including facial paralysis, vertigo, and loss of taste (Ramsay-Hunt syndrome).

DIAGNOSIS

SYMPTOMS AND SIGNS
Symptoms usually begin with a prodrome, including paresthesia or vague tenderness in the affected dermatome. Erythema quickly follows by 48 to 72 hours, progressing to a vesicular eruption with extreme pain. This phase may persist for days or weeks, eventually leading to rupture, crusting, and resolution. Postdromal pain (postherpetic neuralgia) or paresthesia can persist for months or, rarely, even years with one or more recurrences.

IMAGING/SPECIAL TESTS
• Cell culture of material/fluid collected from vesicles allowing for VZV isolation.
• Cytologic evidence of Tzank cells in vesicular fluid of lesions.
• Seroconversion as measured by ELISA, HA, or FAMA.
• Immunofluorescent staining of cellular materials obtained from the base of affected skin or mucosa.

DIFFERENTIAL
• Contact dermatitis
• Bacterial impetigo
• Herpes simplex
• Pain may simulate biliary obstruction, pleural pain or pain due to myocardial ischemia.

TREATMENT

General
◊ Topical care to lesions on skin includes cool compresses and lotions such as calamine or diphenhydramine containing creams.
◊ Silvadene cream can be used if lesions look secondarily infected.
◊ Analgesics usually helpful.

MEDICATIONS
• Acyclovir 800 mg, 5 times daily for 1 to 2 weeks is especially effective if given in the prodromal stages. Severe cases are treated with IV acyclovir or vidarabine. Famyclovir may also be useful.
• Varicella-Zoster immune globulin is thought to be effective in preventing initial infection of susceptible individuals who come into contact with lesions due to either chicken pox or zoster. Few studies have examined the value of VZV immune globulin for preventing zoster outbreaks.
• A Varicella vaccine has been produced and used for preventing the initial infection. It has been of questionable value for the prevention of zoster, because the vaccine is a live-attenuated preparation and reports of subsequent zoster outbreaks in vaccines have been due to the vaccine strain. However, some feel that such preparation may be beneficial in boosting immunity in those previously infected from natural infections.
• Several instances of acyclovir resistance have been reported but this is a much less common finding when compared to Herpes simplex.
• Surface disinfection is achieved with any agent that acts as organic solvent disrupting the viral envelope.

CONSULTATION SUGGESTIONS
Neurologist, Ophthalmologist

REFERRAL SUGGESTIONS
Primary Care Physician

FIRST STEPS TO TAKE IN AN EMERGENCY
• If eye signs or symptoms, seek immediate ophthalmologic consult.

PATIENT INSTRUCTIONS
Warn patient that discomfort in affected areas may last weeks to months.

COURSE/PROGNOSIS
• Zoster is generally a self-limiting illness in otherwise immunologically intact patients. Duration of lesions is 2 to 3 weeks. Potential for significant morbidity (ie, vision loss, postherpetic neuralgia or paresthesia). Incidence of postherpetic neuralgia at ages 30 to 50 4%; ages over 80 50%.

• The likelihood of recurrence is generally thought to be low, although some patients are prone to one or more recurrences. Chronic zoster occurs in some immunocompromised patients. Fatalities from zoster are rare, although cases of motor paralysis mimicking polio have been reported.

CODING

ICD-9-CM
053.0　Herpes zoster
053.12　Postherpetic trigeminal neuralgia
053.13　Postherpetic trigeminal polyneuropathy
053.9　Herpes zoster without mention of complication

CPT
87252　Tissue culture inoculation and observation
87253　Tissue culture, additional studies

MISCELLANEOUS

SYNONYMS
Shingles
VZV
Zoster ophthalmicus

SEE ALSO
Herpes simplex
Contact dermatitis (allergy)

REFERENCES
Whitley RJ, Varicella-Zoster Virus. In: Principles & Practice of Infectious Disease. 4th ed. Mandell GL, et al. (eds, NY., Churchill Livingstone, 1995, pp. 1345-1351.

Fields BN, Knipe DM: Fundamental Virology. New York, Raven Press, 1986, pp. 313-321.

Habif TP: Clinical Dermatology. 2nd ed. St. Louis, CV Mosby, 1990, pp. 291-300.

AUTHOR
Peter G. Fotos, DDS, MS, PhD

Hiccups

BASICS

DESCRIPTION
• A paroxysmal involuntary contraction of the diaphragm creating a sudden inspiration.
• This is coupled with closure of the glottic opening, thereby producing the characteristic sound.
• Hiccups are usually a sign or symptom of another disease process rather than a disease in itself.
• Male:Female = 4:1.

ETIOLOGY

• Usually caused by central or peripheral stimulation of the phrenic nerve which innervates the diaphragm.
• Hiccup center located in upper spinal cord.
• May be a result of direct diaphragmatic irritation as well.
• May result from gastric distention or irritation.
• Known causes include alcoholism, CNS lesions, foreign material irritating tympanic membrane, pharyngitis, mediastinal lesions, hepatic lesions, pancreatic lesions, abdominal disease, psychogenic, drugs such as steroids, benzodiazepines, alpha methyldopa.

SYSTEMS AFFECTED
• Respiratory
• Gastrointestinal
• Nervous

DIAGNOSIS

SYMPTOMS AND SIGNS
• Repetitive-gulping inspiration occurring from 4 to 50 times per minute.
• Attack may last only a few minutes or can last 48 hours or more.

IMAGING/SPECIAL TESTS
Fluoroscopy may be used to determine if one hemidiaphragm is dominant.

DIFFERENTIAL
• Eructation (burping)
• Aerophagia
• See Etiology section

Hiccups

TREATMENT

General
◇ No treatment is indicated.
◇ Home remedies have variable response but include sucking on sugar or hard candy, Valsalva maneuver, drinking from far side of glass, inducing fright, sipping ice water.
◇ Treat underlying disease process if known, including relieving gastric distention, counterirritation of vagus nerve (ocular pressure, carotid sinus massage).

MEDICATIONS
• Chlorpromazine
◇ 25 to 50 mg PO, IM 3 to 4 times/day
• Haloperidol 2 to 12 mg IM
• Phenytoin 200 mg IV then 100 mg q.i.d.
• Quinidine 200 mg PO q.i.d.
• Metoclopramide 5-10 mg q.i.d.

SURGERY
Hiccoughs may persist despite bilateral phrenic nerve transection.

CONSULTATION SUGGESTIONS
Primary Care Physician

REFERRAL SUGGESTIONS
Primary Care Physician

PATIENT INSTRUCTIONS
Attempt home remedies; if unsuccessful, seek medical attention.

COURSE/PROGNOSIS
Most hiccups will spontaneously resolve in several hours to a few days if they are caused by a nervous irritation. Psychogenic hiccuping can persist for weeks.

CODING

ICD-9-CM
306.1 Psychogenic hiccups
786.8 Hiccups

MISCELLANEOUS

SYNONYMS
Hiccoughs
Singultus

REFERENCES
Lewis JH: Hiccups. In: Griffith's 5 Minute Clinical Consult. Dambro MR (ed), Baltimore, Williams and Wilkins, 1995, pp. 480-481.

Isselbacher KJ, et al (eds): Harrison's Principles of Internal Medicine. 13th ed. New York, McGraw-Hill Inc., 1994, pp. 209, 1233.

Tierney LM, et al: Current Medical Diagnosis & Treatment. Norwalk, Appleton and Lange, 1994.

AUTHOR
Alan L. Felsenfeld, DDS

Histiocytosis X (Langerhans' cell)

BASICS

DESCRIPTION
A non-neoplastic, proliferative, non-lipid reticuloendothelial disturbance that represents a spectrum of diseases with the similar histologic picture of histiocytes, eosinophils, granulocytes, and lymphocytes occurring in bone, lymphatics, and major organs.

ETIOLOGY

The cell of origin of histiocytosis X is thought to the Langerhans' cell, though this is not yet a consensus opinion. It is unknown whether the disease is due to abnormal cells, an accumulation of abnormally located cells, or a neoplastic proliferation of a precursor cell or some other cell of origin.

SYSTEMS AFFECTED
<u>Eosinophilic granuloma (monostotic disease)</u>
◊ localized, solitary, discrete lytic bone lesions often seen in the jaws; found in older children and young adults with a 2:1 male to female ratio. Other common sites include skull, humerus, and ribs.
<u>Hand-Schüller-Christian disease (chronic polyostotic and soft tissue disease)</u>
◊ chronic disseminated disease seen early in life (first and second decade), more common in boys (2:1). The classic triad of symptoms includes bony lesions, exophthalmos, and diabetes insipidus.
<u>Letterer-Siwe (acute polyostotic and soft tissue disease)</u>
◊ an acute, fulminant variant of histiocytosis X similar to Hand-Schüller-Christian disease only with earlier onset (within 1 year) and with a more aggressive course.

DIAGNOSIS

SYMPTOMS AND SIGNS
<u>Eosinophilic granuloma</u>
◊ there may not be symptoms associated with these lesions. A general malaise and fever are occasionally seen along with local pain, swelling, and tenderness.
  <u>Teeth</u>
  ◊ loosening of the teeth and dental pain is often a hallmark appearance.
  <u>Bone</u>
  ◊ swelling and tenderness are often associated with localized pain.
<u>Hand-Schüller-Christian disease</u>
◊ patients have a general malaise and fever with a cachectic appearance. They will usually have a sore mouth with halitosis and foul taste.
  <u>Mouth</u>
  ◊ soreness with or without mucosal ulcerations with halitosis and foul taste.
  ◊ loose and sore teeth with precocious exfoliation.
  <u>Gingiva</u>
  ◊ suppurative gingival and periodontal disease.
  <u>Mucosa</u>
  ◊ petechial and papular eruptions.
  <u>Skin</u>
  ◊ "punched-out" lesions all over the skull with the presence of unilateral or bilateral exophthalmos.
  <u>Face</u>
  ◊ facial asymmetry due to localized bone destruction.
  <u>Ears</u>
  ◊ otitis media is also associated with chronic mastoiditis.
  <u>Endocrine</u>
  ◊ diabetes insipidus with or without symptoms of dyspituitarism (polyuria, dwarfism, infantilism).
  <u>Visceral organs</u>
  ◊ nodular or disseminated invasion.
  <u>Skin</u>
  ◊ papular or nodular lesions are common.
<u>Letterer-Siwe</u>
◊ persistent, low-grade, spiking fever with general malaise and irritability.
  Signs of disease in Letterer-Siwe similar to those in Hand-Schüller-Christian disease but in addition:
  <u>Skin</u>
  ◊ rash of trunk, scalp, and extremities is the usual initial manifestation. This rash can be erythematous, purpuric, ecchymotic, or ulcerative.
  <u>Visceral organs</u>
  ◊ hepatomegaly, splenomegaly, and diffuse lymphadenopathy. There is also a nodular or diffuse involvement of the lungs and gastrointestinal tract.

Histiocytosis X (Langerhans' cell)

LABORATORY
Eosinophilic granuloma
◊ none
Hand-Schüller-Christian disease
◊ CBC with differential, pancytopenia is often seen with disseminated bony involvement.
Letterer-Siwe
◊ CBC with differential to demonstrate leukopenia, thrombocytopenia, and progressive anemia.

IMAGING/SPECIAL TESTS
Eosinophilic granuloma
◊ Panorex reveals irregular radiolucencies at the alveolar bone level. In the basal bone of the jaw, there may be single or multiple well-circumscribed radiolucencies. Long bone series may also be beneficial to determine single or multiple well-circumscribed radiolucencies that occur in the extremities and other bones of the skeleton.
Hand-Schüller-Christian disease
◊ Panorex to reveal alveolar and basal bone lucencies; CT
◊ especially of the temporal bone and mastoid for demonstration of otitis media and mastoiditis. Long bone series is also effective in demonstrated skeletal involvement, and magnetic resonance of the total body can help determine both nodular and diffuse invasion of the visceral organs.
Letterer-Siwe disease
◊ as in Hand-Schüller-Christian disease, facial radiographs, CT, and MR will be equally effective in determining the extent of the disease process. Facial radiographs in particular will demonstrate diffuse destruction of the facial bones and mandible.

DIFFERENTIAL
• Large, cyst-like lesions of the jaws only:
  • post-extraction sockets
  • dentigerous cysts and granulomas
  • xanthoma
  • xanthogranuloma
  • benign fibrous histiocytoma
  • basal cell nevus syndrome
  • cherubism
• Multiple, smaller lesions of jaws and other bones:
  • marrow spaces
  • metastatic disease
  • multiple myeloma
• Periodontal disease
• Periodontosis

TREATMENT

General
◊ Depends on the dissemination of the lesions.
Eosinophilic granuloma
◊ curettage with or without radiation therapy.
Hand-Schüller-Christian disease.
   Radiation therapy; local debridement of oral bone lesions for palliative purposes.
   Selected extractions and oral prophylaxis to maintain adequate oral hygiene.
Letterer-Siwe disease
◊ Radiation therapy.

MEDICATIONS
• Eosinophilic granuloma
◊ antibiotics to handle secondary infection in and around the bony lesion, and analgesics for pain.
• Hand-Schüller-Christian disease
◊ in addition to the previously described regimen, chemotherapy is instituted. This should be done with a well-documented protocol that will first get the disease process under control, and, second, maintain the patient in remission.
• Letterer-Siwe disease
◊ chemotherapy with recognized protocols.

CONSULTATION SUGGESTIONS
Hematologist/Oncologist

REFERRAL SUGGESTIONS
Primary Care Physician

FIRST STEPS TO TAKE IN AN EMERGENCY
• Patients with Hand-Schüller-Christian or Letterer-Siwe forms of disease are seriously ill, requiring immediate hospitalization.

COURSE/PROGNOSIS
Eosinophilic granuloma
◊ symptoms usually subside within 2 weeks of treatment. Because treatment is usually curative, prognosis is excellent.
Hand-Schüller-Christian disease
◊ patients improve, but side-effects of radiation and chemotherapy are serious. Cure is usually not seen and treatment is primarily palliative.
Letterer-Siwe disease
◊ usually fatal with an extremely small chance of becoming chronic with chemotherapy and radiation therapy.

CODING

ICD-9-CM
   202.5 Acute histiocytosis X
   277.8 Chronic histiocytosis X

CPT
   20220 Bone biopsy, trocar or needle, superficial
   20225 Bone biopsy, trocar or needle, deep
   20240 Bone biopsy, excisional, superficial
   20245 Bone biopsy, excisional, deep
   38500 Biopsy, excision of lymph nodes, superficial
   38505 Biopsy, excisional lymph nodes by needle, superficial
   41825 Excision, lesion tumor, without repair
   41826 Excision, lesion tumor with simple repair
   70355 Panorex

MISCELLANEOUS

SYNONYMS
Eosinophilic granuloma
Langerhans' cell granulomatosis
Hand-Schüller-Christian disease
Letterer-Siwe disease
Chronic histiocytosis X
Differentiated, progressive histiocytosis
Progressive histiocytosis X
Infantile reticuloendotheliosis
Reticulosis of infancy

SEE ALSO
Multiple myeloma
Leukemia
Lymphoma

REFERENCES
Pringle GA, Daley TD, Veinof LA, Wysocki GP: Langerhans' cell histiocytosis in association with periapical granulomas and cysts. Oral Surg Oral Med Oral Path, /4:186-192, 1992.

Dagenais M, Pharoah MJ, Sikorski PA: The radiographic characteristics of histiocytosis X. A study of 29 cases that involved the jaws. Oral Surg Oral Med Oral Path, 74:230-236, 1992.

Alessi DM, Maceri D: Histiocytosis X of the head and neck in a pediatric population. Arch Otolaryngol Head Neck Surg, 118:945-948, 1992.

AUTHOR
Dale J. Misiek, DMD

Histoplasmosis

BASICS

DESCRIPTION
Histoplasmosis is a fungal infection due to the soil-dwelling saprophyte Histoplasma capsulatum and is the most common systemic fungal infection in the United States. It primarily effects the pulmonary system.

ETIOLOGY

Infection with Histoplasmosis capsulatum, a dimorphic fungus that is endemic to the Ohio River Valley, exists in other regions internationally. Infection of humans results when airborne spores are inhaled and pass into the terminal passages of the lung.

SYSTEMS AFFECTED
• Pulmonary system
• In disseminated disease, multiple organs are infected:
    spleen, adrenals, liver, lymphatics, GI system, central nervous system, kidney, and oral mucosa (tongue, palate, and buccal mucosa).

DIAGNOSIS

SYMPTOMS AND SIGNS
• Most patients asymptomatic or have only mild symptoms.
• Symptoms are flu-like and persist 1 to 2 weeks.
• Acute histoplasmosis can cause fever, headache, myalgia, nonproductive cough, anorexia.
• Chronic histoplasmosis may produce tuberculosis-like presentation: cough, weight loss, fever, dyspnea, chest pain, hemoptysis, weakness, and fatigue.
• Disseminated histoplasmosis may spread to nonpulmonary sites with signs and symptoms accordingly. Oral lesions appear as ulcerations.

LABORATORY
• Serologic tests
• Identification of organisms on tissue examination

IMAGING/SPECIAL TESTS
Radiographs
    Hilar lymph node calcification (acute histoplasmosis).
    Upper lobe infiltrates and cavitation (chronic histoplasmosis).

DIFFERENTIAL
• Tuberculosis and other chronic pulmonary diseases.
• Intraoral malignancy
• Pulmonary malignancy
• Sarcoidosis

TREATMENT

• Acute histoplasmosis is usually self-limiting and generally requires no treatment.
• Chronic and disseminated forms are treated with antibiotics.

MEDICATIONS
• Chronic histoplasmosis
• Amphotericin B or ketoconazole (immunocompetent patient).
• Disseminated histoplasmosis
• Amphotericin B
◊ test dose of 1 mg followed by 0.25 mg/kg/dose slowly, increased to 0.5 mg/kg/dose 4 times a day.
• In selected cases, can use ketoconazole 400 mg daily.

CONSULTATION SUGGESTIONS
Infectious Disease Specialist

REFERRAL SUGGESTIONS
Primary Care Physician

FIRST STEPS TO TAKE IN AN EMERGENCY
• Seizures in patients with histoplasmosis can indicate cerebral metastasis of the infection. Amphotericin B should be considered if this occurs.

PATIENT INSTRUCTIONS
Failure to resolve infection usually due to poor patient compliance with medications or an immunodeficiency.

COURSE/PROGNOSIS
• Acute histoplasmosis
20% mortality if untreated. If treated, in immunocompetent patient, prognosis is good.
• Disseminated histoplasmosis
90% mortality if untreated, 7 to 20% mortality if treated.

CODING

ICD-9-CM
115.9 Histoplasmosis

CPT
40490 Biopsy of lip
40808 Biopsy, vestibule of mouth
42100 Biopsy, palate
87205 Smear and routine stain for fungi
99000 Transport specimen to outside laboratory

MISCELLANEOUS

SEE ALSO
Candidiasis
Tuberculosis

REFERENCES
Dijkstra JWE: Histoplasmosis. Dermatol Clin 7:251, 1989.
Wheat LJ: Diagnosis and management of histoplasmosis. Eur J Clin Microbiol Infect Dis 8:480, 1989.
Schuster GS: Viral and Fungal Diseases with Oral Manifestations. In: Oral and Maxillofacial Infections, 3rd ed. Topazian R, Goldberg M, (eds), Philadelphia, W. B. Saunders, 1994, pp. 596-597.
Hupp JR, Layne J, Glickman R: Solitary palatal ulcer: CPC. J Oral Maxillofac Surg, 43:365-371, 1985.

AUTHOR
Peter E. Larsen, DDS

Hodgkin's Disease

BASICS

DESCRIPTION
Uncommon malignancy of lymphoid tissue; more common in males in developed versus undeveloped countries. It has a bimodal age distribution with peaks at 20 and 70. Classification is important and is dependent upon background cells and ratios.
- Lymphocyte predominant
- Nodular sclerosis most common
- Mixed cellularity second most common
- Lymphocyte depleted

ETIOLOGY

Generally unknown, but risk factors include autoimmune diseases as well as acquired and inherited immunodeficiency syndromes. No genetic patterns have been identified. The Epstein-Barr virus (EBV) has been implicated as a possible contributory agent.

SYSTEMS AFFECTED
The initial presentation is painless swelling of lymph nodes in the neck, axillae, and groin. Other organs of the hemic and lymphatic systems can also be involved, including spleen, bone marrow, and liver. Because of the intimate association, the immune system also becomes compromised. The disease usually commences in a single lymph node group and spreads in an orderly fashion from one contiguous nodal group to another. Most begin above the diaphragm. The spleen is frequently involved early, and the liver and bone marrow only in advanced disease. The GI tract is involved by direct tumor extension rather than primary disease.

DIAGNOSIS

SYMPTOMS AND SIGNS
- Systemic symptoms may include weight loss, unexplained fever, and night sweats.
- Enlarged painless lymph nodes, splenomegaly. Advanced disease can show extra-lymphatic extension into skin, lungs, GI tract, and other soft tissue surrounding nodal areas.

LABORATORY
CBC with differential, ESR, electrolytes, renal and liver profiles.

IMAGING/SPECIAL TESTS
- Chest radiograph, CT scans of chest, abdomen, pelvis; bipedal lymphangiogram and gallium scanning are useful. Technetium bone scanning is less informative.

Lymph node biopsy
- ◇ entire node
- ◇ fresh to pathologist (do not send in fixative).
- The pathognomonic Reed-Sternberg cell must be identified to confirm the diagnosis of Hodgkin's disease. Entire nodes should be submitted fresh to the pathologist for evaluation. Fine needle aspirates and Tru Cut biopsies can be suggestive, but not conclusive. Flow cytometry is critical in evaluation and cannot be done if specimen has been placed in formalin or alcohol.
- Staging laparotomy with splenectomy and liver biopsy.
- Bone marrow biopsy/aspiration

Staging
Subclass "A"
- ◇ asymptomatic
Subclass "B"
- ◇ symptomatic
Stage I
- ◇ single nodal group
Stage II
- ◇ two or more nodal groups on same side of diaphragm or localized involvement of extra nodal tissue.
Stage III
- ◇ nodal groups on both sides of the diaphragm or extranodal involvement.
Stage IV
- ◇ disseminated disease involving one or more extra-lymphatic organs.
Subclass "X"
- ◇ bulky disease
- ◇ node greater than 10 cm or widened mediastinum

DIFFERENTIAL
- Non-Hodgkin's lymphomas
- Cat-scratch disease
- Tuberculosis
- Other inflammatory disease
- Metastatic tumors
- Sarcoid
- AIDS
- Drug reaction
- Reactive adenopathy

Hodgkin's Disease

 TREATMENT

<u>General</u>
◇ Aimed for complete remission in all cases. Factors influencing success include extent of extranodal disease, anemia, age, elevated ESR, and bone marrow involvement.
<u>Stage I & II</u>
◇ typically radiation or chemotherapy alone, unless bulky disease is present, then combined treatment should be advocated.
<u>Stage IIIA</u>
◇ primarily radiation but combined treatment is becoming more popular.
<u>Stage IIIB & IV</u>
◇ chemotherapy (with or without radiation).
◇ High-dose chemotherapy with bone marrow transplant for treatment failures.
◇ Psychological
◇ Patient education for long-term effects of treatment as well as the risk of future malignancies, recurrent and secondary.

MEDICATIONS
• Combination chemotherapy regimen, the most common being MOPP (Nitrogen mustard, Oncovin, Procarbazine, and Prednisone) and ABVD (Adriamycin, Bleomycin, Velban, and Dacarbazine).

IRRADIATION
See general treatment.

CONSULTATION SUGGESTIONS
Hematologist, Oncologist

REFERRAL SUGGESTIONS
Primary Care Physician

PATIENT INSTRUCTIONS
<u>Patient information bulletin</u>
◇ National Cancer Institute NIH publication #90-1555, What You Need to Know About Hodgkin's Disease.

COURSE/PROGNOSIS
Overall success rates are about 75%. "A" groups do better than "B" groups. Patients with combined therapy have slightly improved complete remission compared to those with single therapy. Generally accepted survival by stage:
<u>Stage I & II</u>
◇ 90+% 5 year survival
<u>Stage III</u>
◇ 80% 5 year, 75% 10 year survival
<u>Stage IV</u>
◇ 75% 5 year, 66% 10 year survival

 CODING

ICD-9-CM
<u>201.4x Hodgkin's disease</u>
◇ lymphocyte predominance
<u>201.5x Hodgkin's disease</u>
◇ nodular sclerosis
<u>201.6x Hodgkin's disease</u>
◇ mixed cellularity
<u>201.7x Hodgkin's disease</u>
◇ lymphocyte depleted
<u>201.9x Hodgkin's disease</u>
◇ unspecified
5th Digit
0 Unspecified site
1 Head and neck, facial
4 Axillary and arm nodes
5 Inguinal and leg nodes
8 Multiple site nodes

CPT
38500 Superficial lymph node biopsy
38510 Deep jugular lymph node biopsy

M **MISCELLANEOUS**

SYNONYMS
Malignant lymphoma

SEE ALSO
Cervical adenopathy
Cat-scratch disease
Sarcoidosis
Non-Hodgkin's lymphoma

REFERENCES
Urba WJ, Longo DL: Hodgkin's disease. N Engl J Med, 326:678-687, 1992.

Freedman AS, Nadler LM: Malignant lymphomas. In: Harrison's Principles of Internal Medicine, 13th ed. Isselbacher KJ, et al (eds), NY, McGraw-Hill, 1994, pp. 1774-1788.

AUTHOR
James Vopal DDS, MD

Hordeolum (Stye)

BASICS

DESCRIPTION
A common purulent infection of the glands of the eyelid.

ETIOLOGY

• Hordeolum is an external or internal acute glandular infection most often caused by Staphylococcus aureus or Staphylococcus epidermitis. Such infections often occur secondary to seborrheic, viral, allergic, or bacterial blepharitis (inflammation of the eyelids).

• External hordeolum (infection of the glands of Zeis) usually begins with tenderness and erythema of the eyelid margin, which is followed by the development of a small yellow pustular area of enlargement and induration ("pointing"). Patients may experience photophobia, excessive lacrimation, or a foreign-body sensation. The abscess eventually ruptures and drains, which brings relief.

• Internal hordeolum generally involves one of the Meibomian glands of the eyelid, and is more severe. Spontaneous rupture of the abscess is rare and recurrence is common.

SYSTEMS AFFECTED
Eye involved. No other system involved unless the lesion does not drain spontaneously and spreads, or in cases in which the patient is immunocompromised.

DIAGNOSIS

SYMPTOMS AND SIGNS
Pain, edema, erythema, lacrimation, unilateral occurrence, 2 to 5 day duration.

LABORATORY
Culture of the purulent material generally demonstrates pathogenic staphylococci. Culture usually not necessary.

DIFFERENTIAL
• Angioneurotic edema of the eyelid.
• Blepharitis
• Chalazion
• Acute conjunctivitis (viral or bacterial)
• Dacrocystitis/adenitis
• Eyelid neoplasm

Hordeolum (Stye)

TREATMENT

MEDICATIONS
• Suppuration may be averted by the early use of systemic antibiotics, which are effective against Staphylococci (ie, dicloxacillin or erythromycin 250 mg q.i.d.). May also use erythromycin ophthalmic ointment.

SURGERY
Early rupture and drainage is encouraged by the application of hot compresses for 10 minutes q.i.d., followed by incision with sterile, fine-tipped blade.

CONSULTATION SUGGESTIONS
Ophthalmologist

REFERRAL SUGGESTIONS
Primary Care Physician

PATIENT INSTRUCTIONS
Avoid squeezing abscess. Wash hands before touching involved area.

COURSE/PROGNOSIS
• Although transmission of infection is not described, it is felt by some that the transfer of pathogenic Staphylococci between individuals has the potential to produce related ophthalmologic infections.
• This disorder generally remains localized, and most mature lesions will rupture and drain spontaneously even when left untreated.

CODING

ICD-9-CM
373.0 Blepharitis
373.1 Hordeolum
373.2 Chalazion

CPT
67700 Blepharotomy, drainage of abscess eyelid
67800 Excision of chalazion

MISCELLANEOUS

SYNONYMS
Stye
Zeision stye
Meibomian stye

SEE ALSO
Blepharitis

REFERENCES
Mandell GL, Douglas RG, Bennett JE: Principles and Practices of Infectious Disease. 3rd ed. New York, Churchill Livingstone, 1990, pp. 1819-1827.

The Eyelids. In: Ophthalmology, 7th ed. Newell FW (ed). St. Louis, CV Mosby, 1992, pp. 187-201.

Schachat AP: The Red Eye. In: Ambulatory Medicine, 4th ed. Barker LR, et al (eds). Baltimore, Williams & Wilkins, 1995, pp. 1428-1435.

AUTHOR
Peter G. Fotos, DDS, MS, PhD

Horner's Syndrome

BASICS

DESCRIPTION
This syndrome consists of miosis, ptosis, and decreased sweating on the ipsilateral face.

ETIOLOGY

• Syndrome is caused by an interruption of the sympathetic nervous system pathways in the brain stem. Specifically:

Miosis
◇ (constriction of the pupil of the eye) due to paresis of the dilator of the pupil.

Ptosis
◇ (drooping eyelid) due to the paresis of the smooth muscle elevator of the upper lid.

Anhidrosis
◇ interruption of sudomotor and vasomotor control.

• Horner's syndrome indicates the presence of an underlying primary disease. Lesions in the brain stem (infections or tumors) or in the cervical or high thoracic spinal cord will produce Horner's syndrome. Infection, trauma, tumor, or aneurysm in the anterior spinal roots of the sympathetic chain affecting preganglionic fibers in the lower cervical or high thoracic areas will produce Horner's syndrome. Involvement of the sympathetic plexus of the carotid by lesions in the Gasserian ganglion or an aneurysm of the internal carotid can cause Horner's syndrome along with facial pain.

SYSTEMS AFFECTED
• Eye
Constriction of the pupil
Drooping of the eyelid
• Skin
Loss of sweating ability
Increased or decreased sensation depending on extent of the lesion.

DIAGNOSIS

SYMPTOMS AND SIGNS
• Miosis
• Ptosis
• Anhidrosis
• Occasionally facial pain
• Occasionally sensory loss

IMAGING/SPECIAL TESTS
CT or MRI to rule out a space occupying lesion, aneurysm, dissecting infection, or trauma.

DIFFERENTIAL
• Atypical facial pain
• Cluster headache
• Raeder's syndrome (oculosympathetic paralysis) or paratrigeminal neuralgia (incomplete Horner's due to involvement of carotid sympathetic plexus).
• Any involvement of the basilar artery or its branches.

TREATMENT

General
◇ Identification of the underlying etiology and correction, if necessary.

CONSULTATION SUGGESTIONS
Neurologist

REFERRAL SUGGESTIONS
Primary Care Physician, Neurologist

PATIENT INSTRUCTIONS
Follow referral recommendations.

COURSE/PROGNOSIS
The course and prognosis directly depends on the underlying pathology.

CODING

ICD-9-CM
337.9 Unspecified disorder of autonomic nervous system (Horner's)
954.0 Traumatic injury to cervical sympathetic nerve

MISCELLANEOUS

SYNONYMS
Sympathetic ophthalmoplegia

SEE ALSO
Cluster headache
Atypical facial pain

REFERENCES
Burns RA, Dhopesh V: Neurologic Disease. In: Internal Medicine for Dentistry, 2nd ed. Rose FL, Kay D. (eds), St. Louis, CV Mosby, 1983, pp. 789-791, 833.

Fields CR, Barker FM: Review of Horner's syndrome and a case report. Optometry Vision Sci 69:481-485, 1992.

Harpe KG, Roth RN: Horner's syndrome in the emergency department. J Emerg Med 8:629-634, 1990.

AUTHOR
Thomas P. Sollecito, DMD

Human Immunodeficiency Virus Infection and AIDS

BASICS

DESCRIPTION
• Human Immunodeficiency Virus, is the cause of an incurable sexually transmitted disease with an almost uniformly fatal prognosis once the illness has progressed to AIDS. Although the virus can infect many cell types, the infection of selective T-helper lymphocytes, and CD4 lymphocytes, results in quantitative and qualitative defects in cell count and loss of protective immune functions.

• Within the context of dental practice, this section will focus on HIV-related oral diseases and special considerations for the dental treatment of HIV-infected individuals. The commonly encountered oral manifestations of HIV infection and AIDS include:

CONDITION	ETIOLOGY
• Oral candidiasis	Candida, compromised host
• White hairy leukoplakia	Epstein-Barr Virus
• Kaposi's sarcoma	Endothelial/spindle cell tumor
• Atypical/persistent ulcerations:	
• Herpes simplex (HSV)	HSV in compromised host
• Cytomegalovirus (CMV)	CMV in compromised host
• severe/major aphthous	Immunologic defect
• Atypical, rapidly progressive periodontitis	Normal flora, compromised host; altered immune response
• Acute, necrotizing gingivitis	Normal flora, compromised host
• Oral warts	Human papilloma virus
• Salivary gland disease	altered immunity, lymphoepithelial infiltrate, cysts
• Herpes zoster, neuropathy	HZ in compromised host

ETIOLOGY

Transmission is by three major routes: (1) sexual; (2) parenteral or mucosal contact with HIV infected blood or blood products (including transmission among intravenous drug users, contaminated needle stick injuries, and recipients of blood and clotting factor transfusions); and (3) perinatally. Sexual contact is by far the single largest transmission route.

SYSTEMS AFFECTED
• No area of the mouth is spared the effects of AIDS.
• <u>Mucosa</u>
  ◊ candidiasis, leukoplakia, Kaposi's sarcoma, lymphoma, viral and aphthoid ulceration.
• <u>Periodontium</u>
  ◊ NUP, LEG, Kaposi's sarcoma.
• <u>Salivary gland</u>
  ◊ lymphoepithelial cystic degeneration.
• <u>Teeth</u>
  ◊ caries due to drug and HIV-related xerostomia.
• Side-effects of zidovudine include:
• Anemia and granulocytopenia
• Headaches
• Nausea
• Muscle weakness and fatigue

DIAGNOSIS

• The normal CD4 count in adults is 560 to 1400 cells/μL median about 650/μL. The 1993 revised classification system for HIV infection establishes a diagnosis of AIDS based on CD4 count when the number of cells drops below 200/μL. CD4 counts tend to fall at a rate of 50 to 80 per year with more rapid decline once below 200. However, several clinical conditions exist that are diagnostic of AIDS irrespective of the CD4 count. Oral conditions that are diagnostic for AIDS in HIV+ patients include: oro-pharyngeal candidiasis, chronic HSV ulceration (>1 month), unusual opportunistic infections such as CMV, cryptococcus, histoplasmosis, and tuberculosis, Kaposi's sarcoma, and non-Hodgkin's lymphoma.

SYMPTOMS AND SIGNS
<u>Candidiasis</u>
  ◊ removable white-red patches on palate and mucosa, with or without symptoms.
<u>White hairy leukoplakia</u>
  ◊ asymptomatic, nonremovable white corrugations on lateral tongue.
<u>Kaposi's sarcoma</u>
  ◊ blue-purple-red macule or tumor, more common on heavily keratinized mucosa.
<u>HSV ulceration</u>
  ◊ shallow to moderately deep ulcer, raised white border, keratinized mucosa.
<u>Major aphthous ulcer</u>
  ◊ persistent deep ulceration, flat or raised border with marginal erythema.
<u>Necrotizing periodontitis</u>
  ◊ diffusely painful, rapid attachment loss, mobility, bleeding.
Atypical gingivitis -diffuse, linear gingival erythema.
<u>Oral wart-condyloma</u>
  ◊ sessile or pedunculated mucosal papilloma with corrugated surface.
<u>Salivary gland disease</u>
  ◊ xerostomia, enlargement of major salivary gland(s), development of solitary or multiple parotid cysts.
<u>Herpes zoster</u>
  ◊ dermatomal distribution of vesicles-ulcers.
<u>Lymphoma</u>
  ◊ enlarging submucosal mass without obvious cause, may or may not be symptomatic.

Human Immunodeficiency Virus Infection and AIDS

LABORATORY
• Most diagnostic tests require tissue examination (see below). Antibody titers for HSV or CMV are likely to be elevated and are of little value.
• HIV infection is diagnosed by an initially positive enzyme immunoassay (ELISA) to detect antibody to proteins expressed in HIV infected cells and a confirmatory Western blot test for HIV-specific proteins. Progression to AIDS is based on a combination of clinical (development of HIV-related illnesses such as opportunistic infections) and laboratory (CD4 count) criteria. The reader should consult the references below for details of these criteria.

IMAGING/SPECIAL TESTS
Exfoliative Cytology
◊ smear from lesion useful for candidiasis and to identify viral (HSV, CMV) cytopathic changes.
Biopsy
◊ for chronic ulceration (viral, fungal, versus immunologic/aphthoid), oral papilloma, hairy leukoplakia, Kaposi's sarcoma, lymphoma (potential bleeding problem with Kaposi's sarcoma).
ELISA
◊ a simple office ELISA test is available to detect HSV from a simple smear of an ulceration, results available in 15 minutes.
CT Scan
◊ for salivary gland cystic disease or evaluation of oral-maxillofacial masses; axial cuts with and without enhancement.
Microbial culture
◊ for suspected bacterial, viral, or fungal lesions. Care must be exercised to collect uncontaminated specimen (ie, microbes in saliva unrelated to lesion). A smear or biopsy usually yields greater specificity and faster results.

DIFFERENTIAL
• Any patient with a negative history of HIV infection who presents with an apparent HIV-related oral disease should be questioned further regarding risk factors for HIV infection. Because immunosuppression in general can result in similar conditions, a screening CBC with differential is indicted. If leukopenia (more specifically lymphopenia) is present, HIV infection should be considered and further evaluation in consultation with a physician is indicated.
• Many chronic oral ulcerations may be indistinguishable on clinical grounds alone and the differential may include traumatic, infectious, or neoplastic processes. Biopsy will lead to a definitive diagnosis.
• Any unexplained, enlarging oral mass should be considered neoplastic until proven otherwise. Therefore, biopsy is essential to arrive at a definitive diagnosis.
Removable white patch
◊ candidiasis, material alba.
Nonremovable white patch
◊ hairy leukoplakia, hyperplastic candidiasis, idiopathic hyperkeratosis, white sponge nevus.
Chronic ulcer
◊ HSV, CMV, major aphthous, deep fungal infection (cryptococcus, histoplasmosis), malignancy, trauma.
Submucosal mass
◊ when red-blue: Kaposi's sarcoma, lymphoma, hemangioma, lymphangioma, salivary gland tumor.
Necrotizing periodontitis or linear gingivitis
◊ immunosuppression, ANUG.
Salivary gland enlargement
◊ salivary gland tumor, obstruction, bacterial sialadenitis, Sjogren's sarcoidosis, lymphoma.

TREATMENT

The treatment recommendations below are for patients with HIV infection. The same condition in non-HIV patients may be treated differently or less aggressively. When unfamiliar with the recommended therapy, seek the assistance of a clinician experienced with these techniques.

MEDICATIONS
• Candidiasis
◊ 100 to 200 mg fluconazole/day × 14 days; consider maintenance with nystatin rinse or clotrimazole troche after initial clearance; long-term fluconazole may be necessary and drug resistance can develop.
• White hairy leukoplakia
◊ does not require treatment unless desirable for cosmetic reasons. Surgical removal of small lesions or laser vaporization for larger lesions. Alternatively, oral acyclovir, 2 to 3 gms/day in divided doses for 2 to 3 weeks will reduce lesions. In all cases, recurrence is common but can be controlled with daily acyclovir, 1.2 to 2 gms/day.
• Kaposi's sarcoma
◊ surgical excision for smaller lesions (< 2 cm) or intralesional chemotherapy (vinblastine, alpha interferon) or sclerotherapy (3% sodium tetradecyl sulfate) is effective. Larger or multiple lesions respond well to fractionated radiotherapy (150 to 180 cGy × 10 to 12 doses).
• HSV ulceration
◊ oral acyclovir 800 mg 3 to 4 times/day. Maintenance may be necessary at 1 to 2 gms/day in divided doses. Resistant HSV may require IV acyclovir, foscarnet, or desciclovir.
• CMV ulceration
◊ IV ganciclovir or foscarnet.
• Major aphthous
◊ when accessible (anterior mouth), potent topical corticosteroid (clobetesol 0.05% ointment) 4 times/day. When less accessible, dexamethasone rinse. Systemic corticosteroids are indicated with inaccessible or multiple lesions. However, these lesions must be biopsy proven and the benefit/risk of steroids discussed with the physician and patient. Co-treatment with fluconazole is indicated to prevent candida infection.
• Oral wart, papilloma
◊ surgical excision with extension well into connective tissue. Combined treatment with topical podophyllum is useful with fast recurrence. Avoid ingestion of podophyllum.

(continued)

- Necrotizing periodontitis
  ◊ institute topical (chlorhexidine rinse t.i.d.) and systemic (metronidazole 500 mg b.i.d.) antibiotics first, followed within 2 days by mechanical debridement (scaling, root planing) with adjuvant povidine-iodine irrigation.
- Atypical gingivitis
  ◊ same as for periodontitis, pretreatment with metronidazole may not be necessary.
- Salivary gland disease
  ◊ the lesion itself is not treated. However, xerostomia may improve with pilocarpine 5 to 10 mg t.i.d., and caries prevention must include daily topical 5000 ppm neutral sodium fluoride.
- Herpes zoster
  ◊ oral acyclovir 800 mg t.i.d. × 15 days. Systemic corticosteroids may be necessary to reduce neuritis in herpetic neuralgia. Systemic foscarnet is used for acyclovir resistant infections.
- Lymphoma
  ◊ radiation and combination chemotherapy.

CONSULTATION SUGGESTIONS
Infectious Disease Specialist

REFERRAL SUGGESTIONS
Primary Care Physician

PATIENT INSTRUCTIONS
- Maintain good nutrition and regular exercise.
- Call National AIDS Hotline (800)342-2437 for helpful literature.
- Can call NIH for information about clinical trials (800)847-2572.

COURSE/PROGNOSIS
Almost without exception, most of these conditions continue or recur following treatment. However, every attempt must be made to aggressively treat these disorders because the degree of continued disease or rate of recurrence is significantly influenced by the degree of initial control. Once AIDS occurs, life expectancy is 2 to 3 years.

CODING

ICD-9-CM
- 018.9   Tuberculosis
- 042.1   Infection, HIV complication
- 042.9   Periodontitis, HIV complication
- 053.19 Herpes Zoster
- 053.2   Post-herpetic neuralgia
- 054.2   Lesion, Herpes Simplex
- 078.1   Condyloma, papillomavirus
- 078.5   Cytomegalovirus
- 101.0   Acute necrotizing periodontitis
- 112.0   Candidiasis
- 117.5   Cryptococcus
- 171.0   Kaposi sarcoma, (042.2, HIV complication)
- 523.0   Acute gingivitis
- 523.3   Acute periodontitis
- 527.2   Sialadenitis
- 528.2   Aphthous, major
- 528.3   Abscess
- 528.6   Leukoplakia

CPT
- 11100   Biopsy, 1st lesion, mucosa
- 11101   Biopsy, 2nd
- 11900   Therapeutic injection, intralesional, less than or equal 7 inj.
- 11901   Therapeutic injection, intralesional, >7 inj.
- 17001   Chemotherapy, intralesional
- 40490   Biopsy, lip
- 40808   Biopsy, vestibule
- 41100   Biopsy, ant. 2/3 tongue
- 41105   Biopsy, post. 1/3
- 42100   Biopsy, palate/uvula
- 64450   Diagnostic Injection
- 70355   Panoramic x-ray
- 87205   Exfoliative cytology
- 99000   Specimen handling to outside laboratory

MISCELLANEOUS

Other consideration:
1. Bleeding
   ◊ many patients with HIV infection develop auto-antibodies to platelets and other hematopoietic cells. Chronic anemia is common and can result in serious complications if there is sudden blood loss following surgery. Therefore, assessment of hemostasis and blood oxygenation is essential prior to dental surgery, including a CBC, platelet count, PT and PTT time. Transfusion prior to oral surgery with platelets, packed red blood cells, and/or FFP is necessary when there is a significant thrombocytopenia or anemia.
2. Antibiotic prophylaxis
   ◊ Prior to dental treatment is not necessary based on CD4 count alone. Neutropenia is a better indicator of the need for prophylaxis, in addition to the recommendations by the American Heart Association for all patients at risk for infective endocarditis.
3. Every attempt should be made to achieve primary closure of oral surgical wounds, if necessary, at the expense of bone.

SYNONYMS
Acquired immune deficiency syndrome

SEE ALSO
Kaposi's sarcoma
Candidiasis
Lymphoma

REFERENCES
Revised classification system for HIV infection and expanded surveillance case definition for AIDS. Centers for Disease Control, MMWR 41:1-15, 1992.

Eversole LR: Viral infections of the head and neck among HIV seropositive patients. Oral Surg Oral Med Oral Path 73:153-163, 1992.

Scully C, Laskaris G, Pindborg J, et al: Oral manifestations of HIV infection and their management. I. More common lesions, II. Less common lesions. Oral Surg Oral Med Oral Path 71:158-174, 1991.

AUTHOR
David A. Sirois, DMD, PhD

Hyperparathyroidism

BASICS

DESCRIPTION
• Primary hyperparathyroidism is a disorder of mineral and bone metabolism caused by increased secretion of parathyroid hormone (PTH).
• Secondary hyperparathyroidism occurs in response to chronic hypocalcemia, due to calcium malabsorption, excessive loss of calcium from the kidneys, or vitamin D deficiency. This form of hyperparathyroidism is discussed in the renal failure contribution of this book.

ETIOLOGY
• Associated most commonly (85%) with hyperfunctioning adenoma of a single parathyroid gland. The cause of the adenoma is unknown.
• In 10 to 13% of cases, diffuse hyperplasia of all four glands is noted.
• In less than 5%, parathyroid carcinoma is the cause of primary hyperparathyroidism.
• Neck radiotherapy may be an etiologic factor in some cases.

SYSTEMS AFFECTED
Renal
◇ increased incidence of urinary tract calculus formation and, less commonly, diffuse parenchymal calcification (nephrocalcinosis) due to excessive excretion of calcium and phosphate. Polyuria and polydipsia occur due to reduced renal tubule concentrating ability.
Skeletal
◇ increased turnover of bone may cause a reduction of cortical bone density. High levels of PTH may cause detectable subperiosteal bone resorption, marrow fibrosis and reparative, cystic bone lesions (brown tumors). Pathologic fractures are rare.
Neuromuscular
◇ proximal lower extremity muscle weakness, chondrocalcinosis leading to pseudogout.
Mental state
◇ depression, psychoses, emotional liability, or loss of mental acuity.
Gastrointestinal
◇ nausea, vomiting, anorexia, constipation, or abdominal pains.
Ocular
◇ calcification (band) keratopathy may occur.

DIAGNOSIS

SYMPTOMS AND SIGNS
May be asymptomatic or with vague symptoms, including:
General
◇ weakness, fatigability, depression, muscle weakness, psychosis, personality changes, anemia, anorexia, headaches, pruritus, paresthesia, weight loss, dysrhythmias.
Skeletal
◇ bone pain, joint pain, pathologic fractures. Bone cysts (brown tumors), tenderness in areas of high bone turnover, progressive kyphosis.
Urinary tract
◇ recurrent lower back pain, passage of stones/gravel, hematuria, chronic urinary tract infections, polyuria.
GI
◇ abdominal pain, nausea, vomiting, constipation.

LABORATORY
• Serum and urine chemistry, CBC, alkaline phosphatase, arterial blood gas (decreased CO_2, pH), renal function tests, increased total urinary cyclic AMP. Hypercalcemia seen early in disease process (greater than 10.2 mg/dL).
• Low serum phosphate (less than 2.5 mg/dL).
• Elevated serum chloride.

IMAGING/SPECIAL TESTS
• Abdominal series, neck ultrasound, Panorex, hand radiographs, radioimmunoassay of PTH (elevated), hydrocortisone suppression test, MRI of parathyroid glands, PTH levels using venous catheterization to localize site of abnormal production, ECG, needle biopsy of glands or open surgical removal for biopsy.
• Band keratosis of the cornea seen on slit lamp examination.

DIFFERENTIAL
Familial hypocalciuric hypercalcemia, multiple myeloma, metastatic and nonmetastatic cancer, hyperthyroidism, sarcoidosis and other chronic granulomatous diseases, vitamin D intoxication, acute bone atrophy, milk-alkali syndrome, idiopathic hypercalcemia of infancy, hypophosphatasia, myxedema, Addison's disease, secondary hyperparathyroidism.

TREATMENT

General
◊ Treatment of hypercalcemia with administration of fluids orally and parentally and limit calcium intake.
◊ Possible oral phosphate supplements.

MEDICATIONS
• Propranolol may be useful to prevent adverse cardiac effects. The use of calcitonin may be effective.

SURGERY
• Surgery is the definitive treatment. Indications of parathyroidectomy vary, but include a history of renal stones, progressive bone disease, symptoms of hypercalcemia or serum calcium greater than 11.5 mg per deciliter, and patients below 40 years of age.
• In cases of hyperplasia of all four parathyroid glands, the surgical rule has been to remove three and a half. Complete removal of all four glands with autotransplantation of a small amount of parathyroid tissue into the forearm is also performed.
• Essential that the surgery be performed by an experienced surgeon.

CONSULTATION SUGGESTIONS
Endocrinologist

REFERRAL SUGGESTIONS
Primary Care Physician, General Surgeon

FIRST STEPS TO TAKE IN AN EMERGENCY
• If signs of severe hypercalcemia, hyporeflexia, hypertension, dysrhythmia, mental status changes, begin rapid IV saline hydration, furosemide (Lasix) and phosphates.

PATIENT INSTRUCTIONS
Limit calcium intake. Maintain good fluid intake.

COURSE/PROGNOSIS
Hyperparathyroidism is often a chronic disease. Commonly, mild symptomatic hypercalcemia persists for years with little progression. In general, patients with more severe bone disease show a more progressive course. Acute hypercalcemia episodes may occur (parathyroid crisis) that require immediate treatment. The long-term course of untreated hyperparathyroidism is unknown.

CODING

ICD-9-CM
252.0 Hyperparathyroidism, unspecified
259.3 Hyperparathyroidism, ectopic
588.8 Hyperparathyroidism, secondary or renal origin

CPT
21040 Excision of benign cyst or tumor of mandible; simple
70355 Panorex
99000 Transport of specimens to outside laboratory

MISCELLANEOUS

SEE ALSO
Renal failure

REFERENCES
Spiegel AM: The Parathyroid Glands, Hypercalcemia, and Hypocalcemia. In: Cecil's Textbook of Medicine, 19th ed. Wyngaarden JB, Smith LH, Bennett JC (eds), Philadelphia, WB Saunders, 1992, pp. 1416-1417.

Rasmussen H: Mineral Metabolism and Metabolic Bone Disease. In: Internal Medicine for Dentistry, 2nd ed. Rose LF, Kaye D. (eds) St. Louis, CV Mosby, 1990, pp. 1051-1054.

Drury PL: Endocrinology, in Clinical Medicine, 2nd ed. Kumar PJ, Clark ML (eds), London, Bailliere Tindall, 1990, pp. 825-827.

Habener JF, Arnold A, Patts, Jr, JT: Hyperparathyroidism. In: Endocrinology, 3rd ed. DeGrost LJ (ed), Philadelphia, WB Saunders, Co., 1995, pp. 1044-1060.

AUTHOR
Daniel S. Sarasin, DDS

Hypertension

BASICS

DESCRIPTION
• Elevation of blood pressure, either systolic and/or diastolic. No uniformly accepted point at which hypertension defined. Recent trend is to define hypertension based on later appearance of hypertension-related complications statistically.
• Systolic pressure below 140 mm Hg is normal, 140 to 159 is borderline, and greater than 160 is severe systolic hypertension. Systolic pressure above 200 is considered malignant hypertension.
• Diastolic pressure below 85 normal, 85 to 89 is considered high normal, 90 to 104 is mild diastolic hypertension, 105 to 114 is moderate and 115 or greater is severe diastolic hypertension. Diastolic pressure over 140 is considered malignant hypertension.
• The prevalence of hypertension in white U.S. population is 20%, and is even higher in non-whites.
• Primary sites of damage from chronic hypertension are the heart, eyes, kidneys, and central nervous system.

ETIOLOGY
• Ninety percent of all hypertension is of unknown etiology (essential hypertension).
• Isolated systolic hypertension may be due to decreased aortic compliance (atherosclerosis) or due to increased cardiac stroke volume (aortic valve insufficiency, thyroid disease, fever).
• Hypertension due to increased peripheral resistance can be due to renal disease, endocrine disorders (pheo., Cushing's, myxedema), neurogenic (increased intracranial pressure), psychogenic (fear), or increased intravascular volume.
• Essential hypertension shows a multifactorial inheritance pattern.
• Environmental factors associated with hypertension include obesity, occupation, sodium intake (60% of hypertensives are sodium sensitive), smoking, age, gender, and use of oral contraceptives.

SYSTEMS AFFECTED
Cardiac
◇ left ventricular hypertrophy, accelerated coronary artery disease.
Eyes
◇ retinopathy with narrowing of A-V ratio, hemorrhages, exudates, papilledema, arteriolar spasms, and A-V crossing defects.
Neurologic
◇ headaches, dizziness, vertigo, tinnitus, syncope, encephalopathy, stroke.
Renal
◇ arteriosclerotic changes in arterioles and glomerular capillary tufts.

DIAGNOSIS

SYMPTOMS AND SIGNS
• Essential hypertension is insidious disease with few symptoms until late effects produced. Blood pressure measurement most useful diagnostic modality.
• Symptoms and signs depend upon system(s) affected in particular individual.
Cardiac
◇ angina, left ventricular enlargement, S4, faint aortic regurgitant murmur, heart failure symptoms and signs.
Eyes
◇ scotomata, blurred vision, blindness, retinal changes.
Neurologic
◇ occipital headaches on morning awakening, dizziness, vertigo, tinnitus, syncope, disordered consciousness, seizures, focal neurologic defects due to stroke.
Renal
◇ hematuria, proteinuria, bruits over kidneys, enlarged kidneys, peripheral edema.
• Pheochromocytoma causes headaches, diaphoresis, palpitations, and postural dizziness.

LABORATORY
Basic studies
◇ renal (urine for protein, blood, glucose, serum for creatinine, potassium). Check for endocrine problems renin levels, 24-hour catecholamine metabolites, hypercalcemia, fasting glucose, 24-hour urine for cortisol.

IMAGING/SPECIAL TESTS
• Chest radiograph for cardiac size and appearance of lung fields.
• Intravenous pyelogram (IVP) for renovascular hypertension.
• Renal arteriogram for renal artery stenosis.
ECG
◇ for ischemic changes ventricular enlargement.

DIFFERENTIAL
See etiology section.

TREATMENT

General
◇ Except in the presence of malignant hypertension, the harm from hypertension on an acute basis is minimal. But long-standing hypertension makes the heart, kidneys, and brain susceptible to problems.

◇ Little reason to even temporarily defer most dental care in a hypertensive that is not in malignant ranges. But should be referred to primary care physician for evaluation. Malignant hypertension is urgent situation requiring immediate care by a physician.

◇ Nonpharmacologic therapy includes sodium restricted diet, weight control, cease smoking, regular exercise, and limit stress in life.

◇ Diastolic pressure that is persistently over 90 mm Hg, or any patient over age 65 with a systolic pressure over 160 mm Hg should be evaluated and treated.

MEDICATIONS
• Diuretics (thiazide, spironolactone).
• Adrenergic antagonists (metoprolol, atenolol, nadolol, propranolol, clonidine, guanethidine, prazosin).
• Vasodilators (hydralazine).
• Calcium channel blockers (diltiazem, nifedipine, verapamil).
• Angiotensin
◇ converting enzyme (ACE) inhibitors (captopril, enalapril).
• These drug classes are used individually or in various combinations for patients unable to control hypertension with diet and with other nonmedication therapies.

SURGERY
Renal artery stenosis and pheochromocytoma as causes of hypertension amenable to surgery.

CONSULTATION SUGGESTIONS
Primary Care Physician

REFERRAL SUGGESTIONS
Primary Care Physician

FIRST STEPS TO TAKE IN AN EMERGENCY
• Malignant hypertension is medical emergency. Transport to emergency care facility as rapidly as practical. Immediate control can be obtained with intravenous nitroprusside, nitroglycerine, or diazoxide. Control that is delayed in onset can be obtained with intravenous enalaprilate or labetalol, intravenous or intramuscular hydralazine, or sublingual nifedipine.

PATIENT INSTRUCTIONS
Despite lack of symptoms, hypertensive patients should be educated as to great harm that can result by not treating chronic hypertension. NIH publication 85-1244 gives guide to patients as to dangers of hypertension.

COURSE/PROGNOSIS
Uncontrolled hypertension leads to accelerated atherosclerosis, congestive heart failure, renal disease, visual disturbance and/or stroke.

CODING

ICD-9-CM
401.1 Essential hypertension

MISCELLANEOUS

SYNONYMS
Benign hypertension
High blood pressure
Chronic hypertension
Essential hypertension
Idiopathic hypertension

SEE ALSO
Congestive heart failure
Renal failure
Stroke
Cushing's disease

REFERENCES
Williams GH: Hypertensive vascular disease. In: Harrison's Principles in Internal Medicine, 4th ed. Isselbacher KJ, et al (eds). New York, McGraw-Hill, 1994, pp. 1116-1131.

Frohlich ED, et al: The heart in hypertension. N Engl J Med 327:998-1006, 1992.

Symposium on Hypertension: Part I Mayo Clin Proc 64:1403-1446, 1989.

Pickering TG, et al: How common is white coat hypertension? JAMA 259:225-228, 1988.

Gifford RW: Management of hypertensive crises. JAMA 266:829-835, 1991.

Fletcher AE, Bulpitt CJ: How far should blood pressure be lowered? N Engl J Med 326:251-254, 1992.

AUTHOR
James R. Hupp, DMD, MD, JD, FACS

Hyperthyroidism

BASICS

DESCRIPTION
The second most common endocrine disorder (second to diabetes mellitus) which results from excess production of thyroid hormone. It encompasses a group of diseases, all of which cause the hyperthyroid state.

ETIOLOGY

Graves' disease
◊ represents the most common cause. An autoimmune disease that produces an IgG type immunoglobulin known as thyroid stimulating immunoglobulins (TSIs). The TSIs bind to the receptors for thyroid stimulating hormone (TSH) in the thyroid gland and cause the release of triiodothyronine (T3) and thyroxine (T4).

Toxic adenoma (uninodular goiter)
◊ is usually a benign neoplasm with autonomous hyperfunction. The remaining gland is commonly hypofunctional.

Toxic multinodular goiter
◊ is usually a benign process that occurs late in life and is generally insidious in nature with a subclinical presentation.

Thyroiditis
◊ may transiently present as hyperthyroidism as a result of the destruction
◊ repair mechanism within the damaged gland. Eventually hypothyroidism develops and persists.

Factitious hyperthyroidism
◊ results from the surreptitious ingestion of synthetic T4 (levothyroxine). Most commonly seen in the mentally handicapped, the elderly, and individuals using thyroid hormone inappropriately as a device for weight control.

Other rare causes
◊ excess exogenous iodine ingestion (Jod-Basedow disease), trophoblastic tumor that secretes beta-hCG which at high serum concentration can cross react with the TSH receptor, TSH secreting pituitary tumors.

SYSTEMS AFFECTED
Behavioral
◊ patients typically complain of anxiety, irritability, insomnia, and fatigue. Depression is more commonly found in the elderly patient.

Endocrine
◊ thyroid enlargement or goiter is commonly found as a result of the hyperfunctioning thyroid gland. Irregular menses in women, impotence and gynecomastia in men, and decreased libido and infertility in both sexes have been noted.

Metabolic
◊ weight loss is common as well as heat intolerance. Bone turnover is often accelerated as evidenced by hypercalciuria and elevated serum alkaline phosphatase.

Cutaneous
◊ excess sweating, urticaria, thyroid acropachy (clubbing) or onycholysis (Plummer's nails), vitiligo, and alopecia are often associated with autoimmune hyperthyroidism.

Ocular
◊ exophthalmos, conjunctivitis, periorbital edema, and extraocular muscle dysfunction are features of Graves' disease and occur much less commonly with the other causes of hyperthyroidism.

Cardiovascular
◊ tachycardia, palpitations, and systolic hypertension are common. The elderly may present with worsening congestive heart failure or angina pectoris. Hyperthyroidism must be included in the differential diagnosis of atrial fibrillation at any age.

Gastrointestinal
◊ diarrhea may be present especially with coexisting celiac disease. Liver enlargement may also be found as a result of hepatosteatosis secondary to weight loss.

Neuromuscular
◊ tremors, proximal muscle weakness and atrophy may occur in severe and long-standing cases.

DIAGNOSIS

SYMPTOMS AND SIGNS
- Nervousness and agitation
- Excessive sweating
- Palpitation
- Fatigue
- Heat intolerance
- Weight loss
- Tremor
- Diarrhea
- Increased appetite
- Emotional lability
- Tachycardia
- Dyspnea
- Fever
- Exophthalmos
- Goiter
- Muscle weakness

LABORATORY
- Radioimmunoassay of serum T3, T4, and TSH
- Free thyroxine index
- Radioactive iodine uptake
- Thyroid binding globulin (TBG)

IMAGING/SPECIAL TESTS
Thyroid scan using radiolabeled iodine

DIFFERENTIAL
- Anxiety disorder
- Malignancy
- Pregnancy
- Menopause
- Diabetes
- Pheochromocytoma

TREATMENT

General
◇ Three treatment options: (1) radioiodine therapy, (2) thioamide (eg, propylthiouracil or methimazole) therapy, and (3) surgery. For children and pregnant women thioamide therapy is the treatment of choice. Surgery is usually reserved for the patient who is noncompliant or does not want to take radioiodine.
◇ Activity should be modified based upon the disease severity.
◇ Diet should include an adequate number of calories to maintain weight.
◇ Hospitalization required for life-threatening thyroid storm (thyrotoxicosis).
◇ Minimize or avoid exogenous administration of epinephrine.

MEDICATIONS
- Initial therapy with propylthiouracil 100 to 900 mg per day in three divided doses. Maintenance usually requires 50 to 600 mg per day in two divided doses.
- Initial therapy with methimazole 15 to 60 mg per day given once daily. Maintenance dose ranges from 5 to 30 mg per day once daily.
- Radioiodine (I-131) is administered by an experienced radiotherapist with a varying dosage.
- Propranolol 40 to 240 mg is used to treat tachycardia and hypertension associated with hyperthyroid state. It is also used as a first line drug in treating thyroid storm.

CONSULTATION SUGGESTIONS
Endocrinologist

REFERRAL SUGGESTIONS
Primary Care Physician

FIRST STEPS TO TAKE IN AN EMERGENCY
- Thyroid crisis is medical emergency requiring very aggressive therapy with intravenous iodine, beta blockers, and treatment of triggering condition.

COURSE/PROGNOSIS
- This disease carries a good prognosis when appropriately diagnosed and treated. Thyroid storm represents the major complication of the disease which poses serious morbidity and mortality if untreated.
- Patients with enlarged thyroids should not have thyroid palpation unless clinician capable of treating thyroid crisis.

CODING

ICD-9-CM
242.0 Hyperthyroidism with goiter, Grave's disease
242.9 Hyperthyroidism without goiter

M MISCELLANEOUS

SYNONYMS
Thyroid storm
Thyroid crisis
Thyrotoxicosis

SEE ALSO
Atrial tachycardia

REFERENCES
Becker KL: Principles and practice of endocrinology and metabolism. Philadelphia, JB Lippincott, 1990.

Schimke RN: Hyperthyroidism: the clinical spectrum. Post Grad Med 91:229-236, 1992.

Sawin CT: Thyroid dysfunction in older persons. Adv Intern Med 37:223-248, 1991.

AUTHOR
Joseph J. Sansevere, DMD

Hyphema

BASICS

DESCRIPTION
Blood in anterior chamber of the eye.

ETIOLOGY

• Blunt trauma to the globe with anterior chamber hemorrhage arising from a tear in the iris or ciliary body.
• Three to thirty percent re-bleed 3 to 5 days after initial bleed.

SYSTEMS AFFECTED
Secondary glaucoma can develop with elevation and intraocular pressure, corneal staining from blood products possible.

DIAGNOSIS

SYMPTOMS AND SIGNS
• Pain, blurred vision, history of trauma.
• Blood in anterior chamber of eye, clot, or suspended RBC's.
• Somnolence occurs in affected children.

IMAGING/SPECIAL TESTS
Complete ocular exam, including slit-lamp examination, measurement of intraocular pressure, CT scan to rule out orbital fractures, if suspected.

DIFFERENTIAL
• Leukemia
• Sickle cell disease
• Retinoblastoma
• Blood dyscrasias
• Ruptured globe

TREATMENT

General
◇ Bed rest
◇ Elevate head of bed 30 degrees
◇ Shield eye (no eye patch)

MEDICATIONS
• Atropine 1% drops 3 to 4 times per day
• Amicar 50 mg per kg po q4h
• Analgesics
• Antiemetics prochlorperazine (Compazine) 10 mg IM q8hr
• If intraocular pressure elevated, give topical beta-blockers.
• Topical steroids

CONSULTATION SUGGESTIONS
Ophthalmology

REFERRAL SUGGESTIONS
Ophthalmology

FIRST STEPS TO TAKE IN AN EMERGENCY
• Bed rest
• Cover eyes
• Ophthalmology consult

PATIENT INSTRUCTIONS
Avoid movement/use of affected eye because use may trigger further bleeding into anterior chamber.

COURSE/PROGNOSIS
• Good if diagnosis made early and treatment initiated.
• Prognosis worse if re-bleeding occurs. Corneal staining may occur with severe or persistent hyphema.

 CODING

ICD-9-CM
364.41 Non-traumatic hyphema
921.3   Traumatic hyphema

 MISCELLANEOUS

SEE ALSO
Glaucoma

REFERENCES
Vrabec MP, Reppucci VS, Skuta GL, Carter KD, Howard GR: Trauma. In: Ophthalmic Essentials. Vrabec M, Florakis G. (eds), Oxford, Blackwell Scientific, 1992, pp. 419-421.

Cullom R, Chang B: In: The Wills Eye Manual, Philadelphia, JB Lippincott Co., 1994, pp. 32-34.

Gupta LY, Levin PS: Ophthalmic consequences of orbital trauma. Oral Maxillofac Surg Clin N Am 5:443-455, 1993.

Duguid IM: Ophthalmic injuries. In: Maxillofacial Injuries. Williams JL (ed), Edinburgh, Churchill Livingstone, 1994, pp. 827-843.

AUTHOR
Michael J. Buckley, DMD, MS

Hypothyroidism

BASICS

DESCRIPTION
An endocrine disorder resulting from a deficiency of thyroid hormone production or resistance to thyroid hormone action.

ETIOLOGY

Most commonly acquired after treatment with radioiodine or thyroid surgery for a hyperthyroid state.

Primary hypothyroidism is frequently associated with circulating antithyroid antibodies and in some cases may result from the action of antibodies that block the thyroid stimulating hormone (TSH) receptor.

Goitrous hypothyroidism is most commonly associated with Hashimoto's disease. This autoimmune thyroiditis results from the impaired ability to synthesize adequate quantities of thyroid hormone and hypersecretion of TSH, which leads to goiter.

Drug-induced hypothyroidism has been noted with aminosalicylates, lithium, and phenylbutazone all of which may impair hormone biosynthesis.

Iodine deficiency is very rare in the U.S.

Suprathyroid hypothyroidism may result from inadequate production of TSH by the pituitary gland (pituitary tumors, postpartum necrosis) or thyroid releasing hormone (TRH) by the hypothalamus.

SYSTEMS AFFECTED
• Metabolism is affected and most patients experience fatigue, lethargy, cold intolerance, and weight gain.
• Gastrointestinal system is impaired secondary to decreased motility, resulting in constipation, adynamic ileus, megacolon, and intestinal obstruction.
• Skin and hair become dry and hair tends to fall out.
• Voice becomes deep and hoarse.
• Muscles may become stiff and cramp easily.
• Tongue may become enlarged.
• Cardiac function can be compromised in the advanced stages of the disease as a result of enlargement of the heart an pericardial effusion.
• Neurologic problems may include carpal tunnel syndrome, decreased memory, hearing impairment, paresthesias and, in advanced disease, prolongation of the deep tendon reflexes.

DIAGNOSIS

SYMPTOMS AND SIGNS
• Fatigue, lethargy
• Cold intolerance
• Muscle weakness and cramps
• Arthralgias
• Constipation
• Weight gain
• Hearing impairment
• Decrease in memory
• Paresthesias
• Carpel tunnel syndrome
• Depression
• Menorrhagia
• Hoarseness and deepening of the voice
• Dry skin and hair
• Sparse body hair
• Dull facial expression
• Periorbital edema
• Bradycardia
• Hypothermia
• Decrease pulse pressure
• Macroglossia
• Hyponatremia
• Anemia
• Cardiomegaly

LABORATORY
Thyroid functions: T3, T4, radioactive T3 resin; electrolytes, CBC.

IMAGING/SPECIAL TESTS
Chest radiograph, ECG, radioimmunoassay (TSH).

DIFFERENTIAL
• Nephrotic syndrome
• Chronic nephritis
• Depression
• Euthyroid sick syndrome
• Congestive heart failure

TREATMENT

General
◇ The main goal is to restore and maintain the euthyroid state.
◇ The diet is modified to avoid constipation mainly by including plenty of high fiber foods. Also, a low-fat diet may be required for the obese.
◇ Patient activities are as tolerated.
◇ Patient education is most important and should stress compliance with medications, adhering to dietary restrictions, and regular follow up examinations with the primary care physician.

MEDICATIONS
• Levothyroxine 50 to 100 μg/day increased by 25 μg/day every 4 to 6 weeks until the TSH is normal.
• Dosages of oral hypoglycemic and anticoagulants may require adjustment after levothyroxine therapy has been instituted.

CONSULTATION SUGGESTIONS
Endocrinologist

REFERRAL SUGGESTIONS
Primary Care Physician

FIRST STEPS TO TAKE IN AN EMERGENCY
• If congestive heart failure appears, admit to hospital and treat with diuretics and digoxin, while increasing levothyroxine administration.

COURSE/PROGNOSIS
Generally carries a good prognosis if treated early. A return to the normal state can usually be expected. However, if compliance is poor or treatment is interrupted, relapse will occur. If unattended, it may progress to myxedema and coma (severe hypothyroidism).

CODING

ICD-9-CM
244.0 Hypothyroidism due to surgery
244.1 Hypothyroidism due to radiation
244.9 Acquired hypothyroidism
246.1 Sporadic goiter

MISCELLANEOUS

SYNONYMS
Myxedema

SEE ALSO
Pituitary disorders

REFERENCES
Sawin CT: Thyroid dysfunction in older persons. Adv Intern Med 37:223-248, 1991.

Wolf PG, Meek JC: Practical approach to the treatment of hypothyroidism. Am Fam Phys 45:722-731, 1992.

Wartofsky L: Diseases of the Thyroid. In: Harrison's Principles of Internal Medicine. 13th ed. Isselbacher KJ, et al (eds), New York, McGraw-Hill Co., 1994, pp 1930-1941.

AUTHOR
Joseph J. Sansevere, DMD

Idiopathic Thrombocytopenic Purpura (ITP)

BASICS

DESCRIPTION
Idiopathic thrombocytopenic purpura (ITP) is a relatively common autoimmune bleeding disorder characterized by isolated thrombocytopenia in otherwise healthy individuals. Two clinical forms of the disease are recognized: 1) acute ITP is sudden in onset, seen in children following recovery from a viral infection and 2) chronic ITP can be sudden or gradual in onset, usually found in adults.

ETIOLOGY

• In acute (childhood) ITP, viral antigen is thought to trigger synthesis of antibodies that may react with virus antigen on the platelet surface or that may involve the platelet as an antigen-antibody immune complex.
• The pathophysiologic mechanism for chronic (adult) ITP is characterized by the development of antibodies to one's own platelets, which are destroyed by phagocytosis in the spleen and, to a lesser extent, in the liver.

SYSTEMS AFFECTED
Hematologic
 ◇ epistaxis, menorrhagia, gastrointestinal bleeding, hematuria, and prolonged bleeding following surgery. Major hemorrhage is rare in chronic ITP. Cerebral hemorrhage occurs in approximately 1% of cases.
Oral mucosa
 ◇ minimal to extensive gingival bleeding and petechiae may be present.
Skin
 ◇ easy bruising, petechiae, purpura.

DIAGNOSIS

SYMPTOMS AND SIGNS
Hematologic
 ◇ easy bruising, epistaxis, recurrent petechiae particularly in pressure areas, prolonged bleeding, menorrhagia, GI bleeding, hematuria.
Oral mucosa
 ◇ spontaneous or minor trauma-induced gingival bleeding, scant to numerous petechiae, hematomas.
Skin
 ◇ few to many areas of petechiae, ecchymoses, purpura, hematomas.
Spleen
 ◇ usually non-enlarged, although enlargement may occur in childhood ITP as a consequence of viral infection.

LABORATORY
CBC
 ◇ anemia
Platelet count
 ◇ 5000 to 75,000
PT, PTT
 ◇ normal
Bleeding time
 ◇ prolonged
ANA (antinuclear antibody) test

IMAGING/SPECIAL TESTS
• Bone marrow aspirate
• Isotopic platelet survival test
• Measure platelet associated antibodies

DIFFERENTIAL
• Impaired production
 Generalized bone-marrow failure
 • Leukemia
 • Anaplastic anemia
 • Megaloblastic anemia
 • Myeloma
 • Myelofibrosis
 • Marrow infiltration by solid tumors
• Selective reduction in megakaryocytes
 • Drugs, eg, alcohol, thiazide diuretics, chemotherapeutic agents
 • HIV
• Excessive destruction
 Immune
 • Secondary immune thrombocytopenia
 • Systemic lupus erythematosus
 • Chronic lymphocytic leukemia
 • Viral infections, eg, infectious mononucleosis, HIV, CMV
 • Drugs, eg, quinine, rifampin, gold salts
 • Alloimmune neonatal thrombocytopenia
 • Post-transfusion purpura
 Coagulation
 • Disseminated intravascular coagulation
 • Thrombotic thrombocytopenic purpura
 • Hemolytic uremic syndrome
 • Septic shock

• Sequestration
 • Hypersplenism
• Dilutional loss
 • Massive transfusion of stored blood

Idiopathic Thrombocytopenic Purpura (ITP)

TREATMENT

General
◊ Avoidance of trauma, contact sports, or elective surgery. All unnecessary medication and exposure to potential toxins should be discontinued.
◊ Childhood ITP is usually monitored and only severe cases are treated.
◊ Platelet Transfusion
◊ Limited usefulness because of short survival of platelets in ITP, but may be given in active or imminent, life-threatening bleeding.

MEDICATIONS
Corticosteroid
• Prednisone or similar corticosteroid at a dose of 1 to 2 mg/kg/day is used in adult ITP and severe childhood ITP until the platelet count is normal/stabilizes and symptoms resolve. The steroid is then tapered slowly with close monitoring of platelet count.
Immunosuppression
• Cyclophosphamide, azathioprine, vincristine, vinblastine or danazol is used in patients who are refractory to corticosteroid therapy and splenectomy to raise the platelet count.

SURGERY
• Splenectomy
• Indicated in patients with ITP greater than 1 year duration, patients with moderate/severe ITP who have relapsed 2 to 3 times after corticosteroid therapy, and for severe ITP patients who do not respond to corticosteroids.

CONSULTATION SUGGESTIONS
Primary Care Physician, Hematologist

REFERRAL SUGGESTIONS
Primary Care Physician, Hematologist

FIRST STEPS TO TAKE IN AN EMERGENCY
• If prolonged hemorrhage occurring, apply pressure to site of bleeding if possible and transport to emergency facility.

PATIENT INSTRUCTIONS
• Avoid exposure to injury-prone situation.
• If using steroids, notify doctors of potential need for supplementation prior to procedures and obtain medical alert identification.

COURSE/PROGNOSIS
• In 75% of childhood ITP and 25% of all adult ITP, there is spontaneous and permanent recovery.
• Splenectomy is curative in 50 to 60% of patients. Some patients with no apparent response to splenectomy become responsive to steroid therapy after splenectomy.
• A small percent of patients who do not respond to steroids or splenectomy require immunosuppressive agents.

CODING

ICD-9-CM
287.3 Idiopathic thrombopenia purpura

CPT
85103 Bone marrow biopsy, staining and interpretation

MISCELLANEOUS

SYNONYMS
Purpura hemorrhagica
Werlhof's disease

SEE ALSO
Coagulopathy
Platelet disorders

REFERENCES
Shuman M: Hemorrhagic Disorders: Abnormalities of platelets and vascular function. In: Cecil's Textbook of Medicine, 19th ed. Wyngaarden JB, Smith LH, Bennet JC (eds), Philadelphia, WB Saunders, 1992, pp. 992-993.

Malpas JS, Murphy M: Disease of blood. In: Clinical Medicine, 2nd ed. Kumar PJ, Clark ML (eds), London, Bailliere Tindall, 1990, pp. 339-340.

George JN, El-harake MA, Aster RH: Thrombocytopenia due to enhanced platelet destruction by immunologic mechanisms. In: Williams Hematology, 5th ed. Beutler E, et al (eds), New York, McGraw-Hill, 1995, pp. 1315-1355.

AUTHOR
Daniel S. Sarasin, DDS

Immunodeficiency Diseases (Other than AIDS)

BASICS

DESCRIPTION
• This broad category includes a long list of uncommon, primary (genetically determined) immunodeficiencies and an even longer, but more common, list of secondary immunodeficiencies. Discussion of these disorders individually is well beyond the scope of this book. Instead, this section will focus on the oral manifestations of immunodeficiency and make recommendations for evaluation and management when immunodeficiency is suspected. The most common causes for secondary immunodeficiency are AIDS, lymphoreticular malignancies, and cytotoxic drugs or therapeutic immunosuppression. Immunosuppression due to AIDS is omitted from this section and is reviewed separately under HIV infection and AIDS.
• Oral manifestations of immunosuppression result from impaired immune surveillance and a host-organism balance in favor of the organism. The most common problems are candidiasis, herpes simplex infection, and oral malignant neoplasms. Other opportunistic infections resulting from immunosuppression include cytomegalovirus, herpes zoster, Epstein-Barr virus, papillomavirus, histoplasmosis, cryptococcus, tuberculosis, atypical mycobacterioses, and coccidiomycosis.

ETIOLOGY

• Most primary or genetic immunodeficiencies are diagnosed during infancy or early childhood and, unfortunately, many individuals with these disorders die during childhood due to sepsis. The most likely primary immunodeficiency likely to be encountered in a dental office is a sub-class immunoglobulin deficiency. Among the secondary or acquired immunodeficiencies, the most likely to be encountered include immunosuppression due to:
Infections
◇ AIDS, hepatitis B, Epstein-Barr virus.
Drug-induced
◇ therapeutics for dermatologic, malignant, autoimmune disease.
Endocrine disorders
◇ diabetes, Cushing's syndrome.
Autoimmune disease
◇ lupus, rheumatoid arthritis, Sjögren's, chronic active hepatitis
• Neoplasm
◇ Hodgkin's disease, leukemia, multiple myeloma.

SYSTEMS AFFECTED
Mucosa
◇ all surfaces susceptible to opportunistic infection; petechiae with thrombocytopenia.
Periodontium
◇ periodontium may become source for bacteremia in severely immunosuppressed patient.
Teeth
◇ caries prone with autoimmune diseases with Sjögren's and xerostomia component.

DIAGNOSIS

• The two most common causes for immunosuppression likely to be encountered in a dental office are medicine-induced and diabetes-related. In general, the major oral manifestation of immunosuppression is infection, typically opportunistic infection by commensal organisms. Mucosal petechiae or frank oral bleeding may occur when immunosuppression is secondary to a blood dyscrasia or hematologic malignancy. Finally, mucosal ulceration and/or xerostomia can occur when an autoimmune disorder is the underlying disease.
• Systemic signs of immunosuppression include fatigue, malaise, weight loss, frequent infection, and delayed healing. Polyarthralgia, polymyalgia, and neurocognitive impairment are common symptoms associated with immunosuppressive autoimmune disorders such as lupus erythematosus, rheumatoid arthritis, and Sjögren's syndrome.

SYMPTOMS AND SIGNS
Candidiasis
◇ removable white-red patches on palate and mucosa, with or without symptoms.
Frequent or chronic HSV infection/ ulceration
◇ shallow-moderately deep ulcer, raise white border, keratinized mucosa.
Chronic ulcer(s)
◇ nonhealing ulcer may represent chronic infection, malignancy, or trauma.
Frequent aphthous ulceration
◇ frequent shallow ulceration, flat or raised border with marginal erythema.
Acute periodontitis
◇ sudden onset periodontal pain, erythema, edema, bleeding out of proportion to local factors.
Chronic salivary gland disease/ dysfunction
◇ xerostomia, enlargement of major salivary gland(s).
Frequent or persistent zoster
◇ dermatomal distribution of vesicles, ulcers.

Oral petechiae
◇ small, superficial red spots or larger purpura; spontaneous bleeding.

LABORATORY
When any of the oral conditions described above are present and there are systemic symptoms of immunosuppression, a screening hematologic and/or autoimmune examination is indicated, including a CBC with differential and blood chemistry (SMA 12). A basic autoimmune screening would include an ANA, rheumatoid factor, and erythrocyte sedimentation rate.

IMAGING/SPECIAL TESTS
• As a separate issue from identification of a potential associated medical disorder, the oral manifestation may require additional tests to arrive at a diagnosis. Some useful diagnostic tests include:
Exfoliative cytology
◇ smear from lesion useful for candidiasis and to identify viral cytopathic changes.
Biopsy
◇ for chronic ulcerations (viral, fungal, versus immunologic/aphthoid) or masses. When a blood dyscrasia is suspected, surgical procedures should be postponed until the CBC and platelet count is obtained. When an autoimmune exocrinopathy, such as Sjögren's syndrome, is suspected a minor salivary gland biopsy is indicated.
ELISA
◇ a simple office ELISA test is available to detect HSV from a simple smear of an ulceration, results available in 15 minutes.
Microbial culture
◇ for suspected bacterial, viral, or fungal lesions. Care must be exercised to collect uncontaminated specimen (ie, microbes in saliva unrelated to lesion).
• This is essential in known immunosuppressed patients with atypical infections to identify the pathogen and determine the organism's sensitivity to antimicrobial medications.

DIFFERENTIAL
See etiology section.

Immunodeficiency Diseases (Other than AIDS)

TREATMENT

• Three issues are important: (1) treatment of the oral condition; (2) modifications of or precautions for routine dental procedures; and (3) management of the underlying medical disorder. While management of the underlying disorder is the domain of the physician, the dentist must communicate with the physician to ensure an understanding of the patient's problems and treatment needs from both disciplines' perspective.

• The treatment regimens listed below are for non-HIV immunosuppressed patients and are different than treatment of the same conditions in non-immunosuppressed patients.

MEDICATIONS

• Candidiasis
◊ fluconazole 100 to 200 mg/day × 14 days; consider maintenance with nystatin rinse or clotrimazole troche after initial clearance; long-term fluconazole may be necessary and drug resistance can develop.

• HSV ulceration
◊ oral acyclovir 800 mg 3 to 4 times/day. Maintenance may be necessary at 1 to 2 gms/day in divided doses. Resistant HSV may require IV acyclovir, foscarnet, or desciclovir. Prophylactic acyclovir should be used before invasive procedures to prevent viral replication and lesions.

• Chronic ulcers
◊ treatment is based on specific diagnosis. Infections (bacterial, fungal, viral) are treated by antibiotics to which the organism is shown to be sensitive by culture and sensitivity. Malignancies are referred to a oncologic surgeon (head and neck) for further evaluation.

• Acute periodontitis
◊ institute topical (chlorhexidine rinse t.i.d.) and systemic (metronidazole 500 mg bid) antibiotics. If hematologic evaluation reveals a coagulopathy, take necessary measures (ie, transfusion) before conventional mechanical debridement (scaling, root planing) with adjuvant povidine-iodine irrigation. Active periodontal disease in an immunosuppressed patient is a potential constant source of bacteremia. Teeth in nonhealing areas and mobile teeth should be removed.

• Major aphthous
◊ associated nutritional or hematologic deficiency should be investigated further by an internist and the appropriate replacement therapy instituted. When the ulcerations are a manifestation of an autoimmune disease (lupus, Behcet's etc.), treatment is directed at both the local (oral) and systemic disease (in conjunction with the patient's physician). When accessible (anterior mouth), potent topical corticosteroid (clobetesol 0.05% ointment) 4 times/day. When less accessible, dexamethasone rinses are effective. Chlorhexidine or tetracycline rinses may also be of some benefit. Systemic corticosteroids are indicated with inaccessible or multiple lesions, in consultation with the patient's physician. For patients unable to take systemic prednisone, intralesional triamcinolone may be beneficial if the number of lesions is limited.

• Salivary gland disease
◊ Sjögren's-like salivary gland disease is not curable. However, symptoms of xerostomia may improve with pilocarpine 5 to 10 mg t.i.d. and caries prevention must include daily topical 5000 ppm neutral sodium fluoride. Mechanical gustatory stimulation with sugarless gum may also be beneficial.

• Herpes zoster
◊ oral acyclovir 800 mg t.i.d. × 15 days. Systemic corticosteroids may be necessary to reduce neuritis in herpetic neuralgia. Systemic foscarnet is used for acyclovir resistant infections.

• Bleeding
◊ patients whose immunosuppression is due to hematologic disorders often have thrombocytopenia. Additionally, several autoimmune disorders have qualitative platelet defects (ie, lupus anticoagulant). Appropriate actions should be taken based on the results of a CBC/diff, platelet count, PT/PTT. Consultation with hematologist is essential.

SURGERY
Consider prophylactic antibiotics prior to surgery.

CONSULTATION SUGGESTIONS
Primary Care Physician

REFERRAL SUGGESTIONS
Primary Care Physician

FIRST STEPS TO TAKE IN AN EMERGENCY
• If immunodeficient patient shows evidence of sepsis, immediate intensive care unit care necessary.

PATIENT INSTRUCTIONS
Seek medical attention at first hint of infection or other types of symptoms.

COURSE/PROGNOSIS
Related to type and degree of immunodeficiency.

CODING

ICD-9-CM
053.19 Herpes Zoster
053.2 Post-herpetic neuralgia
054.2 Lesion, Herpes Simplex
078.5 Cytomegalovirus
101.0 Acute necrotizing periodontitis
112.0 Candidiasis
117.5 Cryptococcus
136.1 Behcet's disease
523.0 Acute gingivitis
523.3 Acute periodontitis
527.2 Sialadenitis
528.2 Aphthous, major
528.3 Abscess
528.6 Leukoplakia
695.4 Lupus erythematosus
710.2 Sjögren's syndrome
909.3 Complication of chemotherapy

CPT
11100 Biopsy, 1st lesion, mucosa
11101 Biopsy, 2nd
11900 Therapeutic injection, intralesional, less than or equal to 7
11901 Therapeutic injection, intralesional, >7
17001 Chemotherapy, intralesional
40490 Biopsy, lip
40808 Biopsy, vestibule
41100 Biopsy, ant. 2/3 tongue
41105 Biopsy, post. 1/3
42100 Biopsy, palate/uvula
64450 Diagnostic injection
70355 Panoramic x-ray
87205 Exfoliative cytology
99000 Specimen handling

MISCELLANEOUS

SEE ALSO
Candidiasis
Human immunodeficiency virus (HIV)
Fungal diseases
Diabetes mellitus
Xerostomia
Herpes Zoster
Sjögren's

REFERENCES
Greenberg MS: Immunologic Diseases. In: Burket's Oral Medicine, 9th ed, Lynch MA (ed), Philadelphia, JB Lippincott, 1994.

Porter SR, Scully C, Greenspan D: Primary and Secondary Immunodeficiencies. In: Oral Manifestations of Systemic Disease. 2nd ed, Jones HJ, Mason DK (eds), London, Bailliere Tindall, 1990.

AUTHOR
David A. Sirois, DMD, PhD

Impetigo

BASICS

DESCRIPTION
Common, contagious epidermal bacterial infection initially characterized by either a vesicular or bullous stage, later followed by a crusting stage. The disease is self-limiting but appropriate therapy may have a protracted course.

ETIOLOGY

• Impetigo generally is caused by Gram positive bacterial genera including: Group A Streptococcus (Streptococcus pyogenes, beta-hemolytic streptococci; also Group B, C, and G in decreasing frequency), Staphylococcus aureus, Staphylococcus epidermitis, or a mixture of representatives from either genus.
• Both Strep. and Staph. genera are capable of producing a variety of exotoxins, and proteolytic enzymes (ie, hyaluronidases, collagenases, hemagglutinases) capable of producing aggressive skin lesions.
• Occurring most frequently in hot and humid climates, the spread of impetigo is facilitated by crowding and poor hygiene (ie, day-care centers, schools, and mass, urban dwelling situations).

SYSTEMS AFFECTED
Skin
◇ two distinct types of skin lesions are described based on the primary culturable etiologic genus from the infected skin: vesicular impetigo (streptococcal) and bullous impetigo (staphylococcal).
Renal
◇ depending on the strain involved, acute nephritis can complicate the disease course. Thought to occur when the infection is due to a nephritogenic streptococcal strain, it rarely causes severe problems in children older than 6 years of age.

DIAGNOSIS

SYMPTOMS AND SIGNS
• Vesicular impetigo can affect any age group and generally follows minor skin trauma or irritation, which allows for entry of the bacterium (ie, insect bite, shaving injury, burn). After several weeks of colonization, vesicular lesions appear with accompanying regional lymphadenopathy. The pustular lesion ruptures within several days and is followed by the formation of a honey-yellow to white-brown adherent crust that subsequently extends radially. The disease can last for many weeks and continue to extend onto previously unaffected skin regions.
• Bullous impetigo is most common in children and neonates. Initial colonization of the nasal and respiratory tract prior to affecting the skin. Although any skin surface can be involved, the face is a particularly common site. Lesions occur either as scattered or clustered vesicles, which rapidly expand and coalesce to form characteristic bullous lesions. Lesions collapse and produce 2 to 8 cm tender erythematous lesions of surrounded with a crusted halo. Lesions can persist for weeks to months, but surprisingly present with minimal associated lymphadenopathy. The potential for scaring is greater than that seen with vesicular impetigo.

LABORATORY
Gram stain smear of purulent fluid from vesicles demonstrates (+) cocci.

IMAGING/SPECIAL TESTS
• Anti-DNase B response is increased.
• Anti-hyaluronidase titer is elevated.

DIFFERENTIAL
• Varicella-zoster
• Herpes simplex
• Allergic dermatitis

TREATMENT

MEDICATIONS
• The standard for treating proven streptococcal infections has been Benzathine penicillin (300,000 to 600,000 units for children and 1,200,000 units for adults (IM) or penicillin V 500 mg q.i.d. for 10 days PO (since impetigo can be due to a mixed infection, one should consider cloxacillin, dicloxacillin, or cephalexin).
• In penicillin-allergic patients, erythromycin 250 to 500 mg q.i.d. for 10 days PO may be effective, although resistant strains are reported. When staphylococcus is isolated, penicillinase-resistant antibiotics such as oxacillin or nafcillin may also be considered in conjunction with culture sensitivity studies.
• Topical mupirocin (Bactroban) applied t.i.d. has been found to be effective even in the presence of methicillin resistant strains.
• Chlorhexidine gluconate 4% (Hibiclens) disinfectant washes of hands and affected sites has also been recommended to prevent spread to sites not involved in the initial infection.

CONSULTATION SUGGESTIONS
Primary Care Physician, Oral Medicine, Infectious Disease Specialist

REFERRAL SUGGESTIONS
Primary Care Physician, Oral Medicine, Infectious Disease Specialist

PATIENT INSTRUCTIONS
Follow medication recommendation and alert doctor if symptoms worsen or fail to improve.

COURSE/PROGNOSIS
• The disease is usually self-limiting, although when untreated, it can become chronic and widespread, and result in significant renal complications (nephritis).
• Splenectomized individuals are at extreme risk for Gram positive sepsis due to their inability to effectively opsonize these organisms.

CODING

ICD-9-CM
684 Impetigo
694.3 Impetigo herpetiformis
696.5 Pityriasis, unspecified
704.8 Folliculitis, Perifolliculitis

CPT
87070 Culture, bacterial, definitive, any source except nose, throat, blood
99000 Transport of specimen to outside laboratory

MISCELLANEOUS

SYNONYMS
Superficial cellulitis
Ecthyma
Scalded skin syndrome
Pyoderma
Carbuncles and furuncles

SEE ALSO
Erysipelas
Rheumatic fever

REFERENCES
Mandell GL, Douglas RG, Bennett JE: Principles and Practices of Infectious Diseases. 3rd ed. New York, Churchill Livingstone, 1990, pp. 1819-1827.

Habif TP: Clinical Dermatology. 2nd ed. St. Louis, C.V. Mosby, 1990, pp. 184-188.

AUTHOR
Peter G. Fotos, DDS, MS, PhD

Inappropriate Secretion of Antidiuretic Hormone (SIADH)

BASICS

DESCRIPTION
The syndrome of inappropriate secretion of antidiuretic hormone (SIADH) is caused by the continued secretion of antidiuretic hormone (vasopressin) inappropriate to the body's needs. This causes hyponatremia, overhydration, decreased serum osmolality, and concurrent, inappropriately elevated urine osmolality.

ETIOLOGY

- Drug or disease-induced release of vasopressin from the neurohypophysis:
  - CNS disorders; head trauma, sub-dural hematoma, sub-arachnoid hemorrhage, brain tumor, encephalitis.
  - Drugs that release or potentiate action of vasopressin: chlorpropamide, vincristine, vinblastine, cyclophosphamide, carbamazepine, general anesthetics, tricyclic anti-depressants.
- Ectopic AVP production and release:
  - From neoplastic tissue: small cell carcinoma of lung, pancreatic carcinoma, lymphosarcoma, Hodgkin's disease, thymoma, carcinoma of duodenum or bladder.
  - From inflammatory lung diseases: tuberculosis, lung abscess, pneumonia, emphysema.

SYSTEMS AFFECTED
- Endocrine
- Central nervous system

DIAGNOSIS

A positive diagnosis is made with a water-load test.

SYMPTOMS AND SIGNS
- Hyponatremia and hypercalemia lead to anorexia, nausea, irritability, drowsiness, lethargy, mental confusion, restlessness, headache, convulsions, and coma. Can be asymptomatic.
- The rate of fall of serum sodium concentration is more important in neurologic changes than is the absolute value of hyponatremia.

LABORATORY
- Low or normal BUN and Creatinine
- Urinary sodium > 20 mEq/L
- Low urate level

IMAGING/SPECIAL TESTS
- Elevated ADH
- Water-load test
- Serum sodium levels must be above 125 mEq/L.
  - the patient is challenged with a water load by mouth or IV in 10 to 20 minutes. The inability to maintain a concentrated serum or more dilute urine osmolality and ability to excrete 80% of the water volume in 5 hours suggests the diagnosis.

DIFFERENTIAL
- Postoperative stress
- Psychotic polydipsia
- Drug induced
- Mechanical ventilation induced
- Tumor induced (bronchogenic cancer)
- TB
- CNS irritation
- Factitious (elevated serum glucose, cholesterol or proteins)

Inappropriate Secretion of Antidiuretic Hormone (SIADH)

TREATMENT

• Restriction of fluid intake to 800 to 1000 mL/day.
  • necessary to monitor daily weight changes and serum sodium concentration.
• With severe CNS changes, patients may be acutely treated with 0.5% NaCl solution (200 to 300 ml given IV over 3 to 4 hr).
• The underlying cause of increased AVP should be identified and corrected.

MEDICATIONS
• Demeclocycline is a potent inhibitor of AVP action, and can be administered in doses of 900 to 1200 mg/day.

CONSULTATION SUGGESTIONS
Primary Care Physician, Endocrinologist

REFERRAL SUGGESTIONS
Primary Care Physician, Endocrinologist

FIRST STEPS TO TAKE IN AN EMERGENCY
• Treat serious changes in mental status with sodium chloride infusion.

PATIENT INSTRUCTIONS
Restrict fluid intake and increase sodium intake per physician's instructions.

COURSE/PROGNOSIS
Depends on cause of SIADH
  • Infections should be treated, causative drugs withheld or tumors secreting AVP treated with surgery, chemotherapy, or radiation therapy.

CODING

ICD-9-CM
253.6 Inappropriate secretion antidiuretic hormone

MISCELLANEOUS

SYNONYMS
SIADH

SEE ALSO
Sodium disorders

REFERENCES
Moses AM, Streeten DH: SIADH In: Harrison's Principles of Internal Medicine, 13th ed. New York, McGraw-Hill, 1994, pp. 1928-1930.

AUTHOR
Jerry L. Jones, DDS, MD

Influenza

BASICS

DESCRIPTION
• A viral disease of the respiratory tract.
• Associated with generalized or constitutional symptoms.
• Can be a significant disease for high risk patients.

ETIOLOGY

• Influenza virus types A, B, and C (orthomyxoviruses).
• Spreads via aerosols.
• Tends to have variation of causative strains.

SYSTEMS AFFECTED
• Respiratory
• Musculoskeletal
• Gastrointestinal

DIAGNOSIS

SYMPTOMS AND SIGNS
• Headache
• Chills
• Nausea and vomiting
• Fatigue
• Muscle weakness and pain
• Nonproductive cough
• Pharyngitis
• Rhinorrhea (clear nasal discharge)
• Sneezing
• Fever
• Nasal congestion
• Dry, warm skin
• Pharyngeal erythema
• Cervical lymphadenopathy

LABORATORY
• Generally not indicated
CBC
   ◇ May show leukopenia.
• Viral cultures in selected cases.
• Immune system assays.

IMAGING/SPECIAL TESTS
• Generally not indicated
• Chest radiograph

DIFFERENTIAL
• Common cold
• Bronchitis
• Mononucleosis
• Acute tonsillitis
• Pneumonia
• Streptococcal pharyngitis

TREATMENT

General
◊ Bedrest
◊ Hydration
◊ Symptomatic treatment
◊ Vaccination for virulent strains

MEDICATIONS
• Acetaminophen for discomfort and fever control.
• Avoid NSAIDs in children due to Reye's syndrome potential.
• Antitussives as indicated.
• Antibiotics for secondary bacterial infections.
• Amantadine for high risk patients with influenza A.

CONSULTATION SUGGESTIONS
Primary Care Physician

REFERRAL SUGGESTIONS
Primary Care Physician

PATIENT INSTRUCTIONS
Stay well hydrated by consuming as much fluid as possible.

COURSE/PROGNOSIS
• Acute symptoms may dissipate within 5 to 7 days.
• Lassitude can persist for 10 days to 2 weeks.

 CODING

ICD-9-CM
487   Influenza
487.0 with pneumonia
487.1 with laryngitis, pharyngitis

CPT
90724 Immunization, influenza
90737 Immunization, influenza B

 MISCELLANEOUS

SYNONYMS
Grippe
Flu

SEE ALSO
Common cold
Pharyngitis
Pneumonia
Bronchitis

REFERENCES
Zimmerman R: Griffith's 5 Minute Clinical Consult. Dambro MR (Ed), Baltimore, Williams and Wilkins, 1994, pp. 562-563.

Dolin R: Influenza. In: Harrison's Principles of Internal Medicine. 13th ed. Isselbacher K, et al, (eds). New York, McGraw-Hill Inc., 1994, pp. 814-819.

Tierney LM, et al (eds): Current Medical Diagnosis & Treatment. Norwalk, CT, Appleton and Lange, 1994.

AUTHOR
Alan L. Felsenfeld, DDS

Intermittent Claudication

BASICS

DESCRIPTION
A symptom characterized by pain, usually described as muscle cramping or burning, affecting predominantly the buttocks, thighs, and calves but can involve other muscles in body. Pain of claudication is exacerbated by exercise, and relieved by rest.

ETIOLOGY

• The most common cause is arteriocclusive disease of which tobacco use, diabetes mellitus, and hypertension are risk-increasing factors. The distal aorta, iliac, femoral, and popliteal arteries are most commonly affected. Diabetics tend to have distal popliteal and tibial artery disease. Atherosclerotic plaques form causing a progressive occlusion of blood supply resulting in claudication, the area of which denotes the level of occlusion.
• Rheumatologic conditions such as Takayasu's arteritis and giant cell arteritis will occasionally present as claudication.
• Buerger's disease (thromboangiitis obliterans) is a disease affecting small- and medium-sized vessels of the distal extremities, may have claudication, especially of the arch of the foot, as a presenting symptom.
• Infectious aortitis, vasospastic disease, arterial thromboembolic disease, and neurospinal disease may also rarely present as or similar to claudication.

SYSTEMS AFFECTED
• Atherosclerotic disease is a systemic condition that affects the entire vascular system. The heart, cerebrovascular circulation, and peripheral lower extremity vessels are most frequently affected.
• Coronary artery disease is common and is the primary cause of reduction in life expectancy.
• Cerebrovascular disease is also relatively common and may lead to stroke due to carotid artery occlusion.
• The lower extremities are most commonly affected by peripheral vascular disease. Atherosclerotic plaques progressively occlude arterial blood supply and may lead to claudication and rarely to rest pain, nonhealing ulcers, and tissue loss.

DIAGNOSIS

SYMPTOMS AND SIGNS
• Pain, cramping, usually of lower extremities brought on by exercise and relieved by rest. Rest pain is an ominous sign and signifies critical limb ischemia with severe vascular occlusion. Sexual impotence is not uncommon in males when there is iliac occlusive disease.
• Diminished or absent distal pulses.
• Progressive reduction in exercise capability.
• Loss of hair, thickened nails, thinning skin all signal reduction in arterial blood supply.

LABORATORY
Increase in ESR, presence of anemia in giant cell arteritis, Takayasu's arteritis.

IMAGING/SPECIAL TESTS
• Noninvasive arterial studies ie, segmental blood pressures of the extremities, pulse volume recording by Doppler exam, ankle-brachial indices comparing systolic blood pressures in the arm and foot.
• Invasive arterial studies ie, arteriography of the aorta and distal extremities.
• Biopsy for tissue diagnosis if giant cell arteritis is suspected.
• Spinal imaging to rule out neurospinal disease

DIFFERENTIAL
• Atherosclerotic occlusive disease
• Thromboembolic disease
• Giant cell arteritides (temporal arteritis, Takayasu's arteritis).
• Buerger's disease (thromboangiitis obliterans).
• Vasospastic disease (Raynaud's disease).
• Infectious aortitis
• Neurospinal disease

TREATMENT

<u>General</u>
◊ Cessation of smoking is the most important single factor in altering progression of disease.
◊ Exercise
◊ Diabetes control
◊ Control of hypertension
◊ Weight loss
◊ Cholesterol reduction

MEDICATIONS
• Vasodilators, antiplatelet agents, and hemorrheologic medications have been used but are of questionable therapeutic value; eg, aspirin (antiplatelet agent) and pentoxyfilline (blood viscosity reducer).

SURGERY
<u>Sympathectomy</u>
◊ allows vasodilation but the long-term effect does not appear to be significant.
• Angioplasty may be useful for localized solitary lesions.
• Bypass grafting if conservative therapy fails or if physical limitations are unacceptable to the patient. Definite surgical indications are for rest pain, tissue necrosis, or nonhealing ulcers despite optimal wound care. Graft patency at 5 years approaches 85% but is significantly lower if prosthetic graft material is used for reconstruction.

CONSULTATION SUGGESTIONS
Primary Care Physician, Vascular Surgeon

REFERRAL SUGGESTIONS
Primary Care Physician, Vascular Surgeon

FIRST STEPS TO TAKE IN AN EMERGENCY
• If pain does not disappear by ceasing use of painful limb, have patient go to emergency site for peripheral vascular evaluation.

PATIENT INSTRUCTIONS
Institute walking program and stop smoking.

COURSE/PROGNOSIS
Although sometimes improves, progression of problems to rest pain or tissue necrosis may occur.

CODING

ICD-9-CM
443.9 Claudication

MISCELLANEOUS

SYNONYMS
Claudication

SEE ALSO
Thromboangiitis obliterans
Diabetes mellitus

REFERENCES
Sabiston DC: In: Textbook of Surgery. The Biologic Basis of Modern Surgical Practice. 14th ed., Sabiston DC (ed), Philadelphia, WB Saunders Co., 1991.

Criade E, Ramadan F, Keagy BA, Johnson G: Intermittent claudication. Surg Gyn Obst 173:163-170, 1991.

Smith GD, Shipley MJ, Rose G: Intermittent claudication, heart disease risk factors, and mortality. The Whitehall Study. Circulation. 82:1925-1931, 1990.

Glover JL, Bunch T: In: Textbook of Internal Medicine 2nd ed. Kelly WN (ed), Philadelphia, JB Lippincott, 1992.

AUTHOR
André Montazem, DMD, MD

Jaw Cysts

BASICS

DESCRIPTION
• A cyst is an epithelial-lined pathologic cavity that may contain fluid or debris from degenerating cells. Cysts are common within the maxilla and mandible, and can be classified as odontogenic or non-odontogenic.

<u>Odontogenic Cysts</u>
• Radicular, or periapical cysts, are the most common cysts of the oral cavity. They develop within an existing periapical granuloma, with the inflammation invoking the proliferation of odontogenic rests within the periodontal ligament. A radicular cyst can be associated with any tooth, but most commonly occurs in the maxillary anterior region.
• Dentigerous cysts are associated with the crown of an unerupted or developing tooth, most commonly the mandibular third molar. They develop as the result of fluid accumulation between the follicle and enamel. Dentigerous cysts have the potential to attain a large size, and may expand and thin the cortical bone.
• The lateral periodontal cyst is a rare entity and most frequently occurs in the mandibular premolar or maxillary lateral incisor regions adjacent or lateral to the root of a tooth. The tooth is vital, unless caries has involved the pulp.
• The odontogenic keratocyst deserves special classification due to its potentially aggressive behavior and characteristic histology. May occur anywhere in the jaws, but has a predilection for the posterior mandible. Keratocysts can attain significant size and result in perforation of the mandible and extension into soft tissue.

<u>Non-Odontogenic Cysts</u>
• The globulomaxillary cyst was previously thought to be a fissural cyst occurring between the premaxilla and maxillary process. Currently believed not be a specific entity, but only a clinical term. Characteristic presentation is a radiolucency between the maxillary lateral incisor and canine, with possible displacement of these roots.
• Incisive Canal Cyst
• Develops within the canal containing the nasopalatine neurovascular structures. May result in swelling of the labial or palatal tissues, but most frequently the cyst has an asymptomatic presentation and is only discovered on radiographic exam.

ETIOLOGY

Radicular cysts form due to infection or degeneration of pulpal tissue, which extends into periapical region. Other odontogenic cysts are thought to arise due to activation of trapped epithelial cells that are then triggered by various stimuli to proliferate.

SYSTEMS AFFECTED
Mandible, maxilla.

DIAGNOSIS

SYMPTOMS AND SIGNS
Slow expansion of alveolar processes. Expansion may result in thinning of the cortical bone and palpation may produce crepitus. May develop facial swelling if the expansion reaches substantial size. Teeth can be displaced or may become loose when cysts become large.

LABORATORY
All removed tissue should be carefully examined, particularly in areas where mural ameloblastomas may be present.

IMAGING/SPECIAL TESTS
Plain films are usually sufficient for diagnosis and to determine the extent of the lesion. A CAT scan may be appropriate if cortical perforation and soft tissue extension are assumed to be present with an odontogenic keratocyst. Aspiration of the luminal contents may produce a fluid return; straw-colored fluid is associated with a dentigerous cyst, and thick, cream-colored fluid is often produced by a keratocyst. Vitality will be maintained by teeth associated with all cysts except periapical (radicular) cysts.

DIFFERENTIAL
• Ameloblastoma
• Central giant cell granuloma
• Arteriovenous malformation
• Periapical cemental dysplasia
• Odontogenic myxoma
• Adenomatoid odontogenic tumor
• Idiopathic bone cavity

TREATMENT

General
◊ Cysts are benign pathologic lesions, so the treatment is relatively conservative.

SURGERY
• The periapical, lateral periodontal, and incisive canal cyst are treated with enucleation and curettage. A similar treatment is appropriate for the dentigerous cyst, but should also include removal of the associated tooth. The odontogenic keratocyst has recurrence rates as high as 60% when treated with enucleation and curettage. Chemical curettage, with Carnoy's solution, or a peripheral ostectomy can significantly reduce the recurrence rate.
• Large cysts enveloping vital structures may be marsupilized to allow them to shrink, and then enucleated.

CONSULTATION SUGGESTIONS
Oral-Maxillofacial Surgeon

REFERRAL SUGGESTIONS
Oral-Maxillofacial Surgeon

PATIENT INSTRUCTIONS
Cyst should be enucleated to prevent continued enlargement. Keratocysts require removal of cyst and margin of macroscopically uninvolved bone to improve chances of complete cure.

COURSE/PROGNOSIS
A cure can usually be accomplished with enucleation and curettage. The bony defects will reossify, and any bony expansions will remodel to normal contours.

CODING

ICD-9-CM
522.8 Radicular/periapical cyst
526.0 Developmental odontogenic cysts
   dentigerous
   lateral periodontal
   odontogenic keratocyst
526.1 Fissural cyst of jaw
   globulomaxillary
   incisive canal

CPT
20230 Biopsy, bone; needle (aspiration); superficial
20240 Biopsy, bone; superficial
21030 Excision of cyst of facial bone other than mandible
21040 Excision of cyst of mandible; simple
21041 Excision of cyst of mandible; complex
41899 Extraction of tooth
70100 Radiologic exam, mandible; partial, less than four views
70300 Radiologic exam, teeth; single view
70355 Panorex
70486 Computerized axial tomography, maxillofacial area

MISCELLANEOUS

SEE ALSO
Basal cell nevus syndrome

REFERENCES
Regezi JA, Sciubba JJ: Cysts of the Oral Region. In: Oral Pathology Clinical Pathologic Correlations, 2nd ed. Philadelphia, WB Saunders, Co., 1993, pp. 322-361.

Eversole LR: Radiolucent Lesions of the Jaws. In: Clinical Outline of Oral Pathology, 3rd ed. Philadelphia, Lea & Febiger, 1992, pp. 226-289.

Coleman GC: Unilocular Radiolucencies of the Jaws. In: Principles of Oral Diagnosis. Coleman GC, Nelson JF (eds). St. Louis, CV Mosby, 1993, pp. 394-408.

AUTHOR
Robert Rudman, DDS

Kaposi's Sarcoma

BASICS

DESCRIPTION
• A malignant neoplasm of capillary origin generally presenting in three varying clinical patterns. The lesions are reddish-brown to blue in color and found in various locations.
• The first pattern is a rare, indolent skin tumor involving the lower extremities of older men of Mediterranean heritage.
• The second has been discovered in Africa and is now endemic there. It is seen in Blacks with preference for the extremities.
• The third can present with oral lesions and is found in patients suffering from immunodeficiency (ie, AIDS).

ETIOLOGY

• Endothelial cells and dermal and submucosal dendrocytes are considered to be the cells of origin of these lesions.
• Whereas the etiology is generally considered to be unknown, the following factors have been considered as to possibly playing a role in the genesis of these lesions: genetic predisposition, environmental factors, viral infections, and immune system breakdown.

SYSTEMS AFFECTED
Cutaneous
◇ primary system affected with the skin of the extremities the most common site. To a lesser extent, the face and other locations can be involved, depending upon the pattern of the disease.
Oral mucosa
◇ frequently the site of lesions when associated with acquired immunodeficiency syndrome (AIDS).
Lymph node and visceral
◇ involvement of these tissues may occur in advanced cases.

DIAGNOSIS

SYMPTOMS AND SIGNS
Skin
◇ lesions are usually painless but can be uncomfortable when ulceration or cellulitis occurs. Lesions typically are reddish-brown to blue patches, plaques, and nodules on the distal lower extremities. Initially unilateral or bilateral with gradual coalescence and proximal spread. Ulceration may also occur. Upper extremity and facial lesions may be seen in certain forms of the disease.
Oral mucosa
◇ lesions are usually asymptomatic but can be uncomfortable and disruptive, especially when exophytic in nature. Reddish-brown to blue, flat or exophytic lesions seen often in patients with AIDS. When ulceration occurs, these lesions can clinically resemble squamous cell carcinoma.
Lymph nodes
◇ nonpainful lymphadenopathy.
Visceral
◇ asymptomatic gastrointestinal lesions present in 50% of AIDS patients. Gastric outlet obstruction and occasional GI bleeding have been reported.
Pulmonary
◇ dyspnea and hemoptysis. Seen in advanced cases of AIDS.

LABORATORY
HIV testing
◇ to positively identify patients with acquired immunodeficiency syndrome (AIDS).
Stain and culture for oral candidiasis (often seen in AIDS patients).

IMAGING/SPECIAL TESTS
Chest radiograph reveals infiltrates, mediastinal enlargement, and pleural effusion.
Biopsy
◇ lesions are usually biopsied to render definitive diagnoses. Histology reveals bland-appearing spindle cells and multiple vascular channels. Advanced lesion may show atypical vascular channels with red blood cells, hemosiderin, and inflammatory cells in stroma.

DIFFERENTIAL
• Kaposi's sarcoma
• Hemangioma
• Pyogenic granuloma
• Melanoma
• Erythroplakia
• Squamous cell carcinoma

Kaposi's Sarcoma

TREATMENT

General
◊ Various forms of treatment have been attempted but none with uniform success.

MEDICATIONS
• Chemotherapy
◊ often employed in patients with disseminated disease that have not been helped by radiotherapy. Especially useful in patients with lymph node or visceral involvement.

SURGERY
Excision
◊ often used with success on small and localized lesions.
In AIDS patients, perform hematologic evaluation prior to elective surgery.

IRRADIATION
Low-dose application useful for larger, multifocal lesions. Helpful to reduce pain and improve appearance.

CONSULTATION SUGGESTIONS
Primary Care Physician, Oral-Maxillofacial Pathologist, Infectious Disease Specialist

REFERRAL SUGGESTIONS
Primary Care Physician

PATIENT INSTRUCTIONS
Diagnosis of Kaposi's mandates immediate investigation of patient's HIV status by primary care physician.

COURSE/PROGNOSIS
• This varies markedly depending upon the pattern of the disease (three forms).
• First pattern is seen predominantly in older men of Mediterranean origin. Here the lesions are usually multifocal and on the skin of the lower extremities. Oral lesions are rare. The clinical course is long with a fair to good prognosis.
• The second pattern is seen primarily on the extremities of African Blacks. Skin lesions are typical with oral lesions rare. The clinical course is long with a fair prognosis.
• The third pattern has been classically seen in patients with AIDS. Skin lesions can be found over the entire body and are often multifocal. Oral lesions are often seen and can be the initial site of involvement. Visceral and lymph node lesions can also be encountered. The clinical course can be rapid and aggressive, and the prognosis poor.

CODING

ICD-9-CM
176   Kaposi's sarcoma
176.0 Skin
176.1 Soft tissue
 • Includes: blood vessel, connective tissue, fascia, ligament, lymphatics, muscle.
 • Excludes: lymph glands and nodes (176.5).
176.2 Palate
176.3 Gastrointestinal sites
176.4 Lung
176.5 Lymph nodes
176.8 Other specified sites
 • Includes: oral cavity
176.9 Unspecified; viscera

CPT
11440 Excision face/lips/muc up to 5 cm
40490 Biopsy of lip
40808 Biopsy vestibule of mouth
41100 Biopsy anterior 2/3 of tongue
41105 Biopsy posterior 1/3 of tongue
41108 Biopsy floor of mouth
42100 Biopsy of palate
42104 Excise lesion plate, uvula

MISCELLANEOUS

SYNONYMS
Endothelial cell sarcoma

SEE ALSO
HIV
Melanoma

REFERENCES
Regezi JA, Sciubba J: Oral Pathology. 2nd ed. Philadelphia, WB Saunders Co., 1993, pp. 148-150.

Zurrida S, et al: Classic Kaposi's sarcoma: A review of 90 cases. Dermatology, 19:548-552, 1992.

Chor PJ, Santa Cruz DJ: Kaposi's sarcoma. A clinicopathologic review and differential diagnosis. J Cutan Pathol 19:6-20, 1992.

AUTHOR
Lawrence T. Herman, DMD

Keloids (and Hypertrophic Scars)

 BASICS

DESCRIPTION
• Proliferative healing response after integumentary wounding, more pronounced in certain ethnic groups.
• Ethnic group predilection: Afro-Americans > Mideast and Mediterranean peoples > Asians > Caucasians.

 ETIOLOGY

• Hypertrophic scars
◇ exuberant deposits of collagen in wound repair that remain within the wound margins.
• Keloids occur as an imbalance in wound repair due to:
  • Increased levels of hydroxyproline and hydroxylysine.
  • Pronounced collagen deposition.
  • Increased production of glycosaminoglycan and chondroitin-4-sulfate.
  • Ineffective or decreased collagen breakdown in wound maturation.

SYSTEMS AFFECTED
• Integument over tension areas, eg, shoulders, trunk, sternum, mandible, ears.
• Rarely occurs distal to knees and wrists.

 DIAGNOSIS

SYMPTOMS AND SIGNS
• Hypertrophic Scars
• Little progression beyond 6 months
• Remain within wound borders
• More cellular and vascular than normal scars.
• Keloids
• Progress beyond 6 months
• Accompanied by itching, increased pigmentation
• Extend beyond original wound margins
• Dense, thick bands of collagen with minimal cellular component.

IMAGING/SPECIAL TESTS
Histology of keloid reveals whorls of hyalinized collagen bundles with thinning of papillary dermis and minimal elastic tissue.

DIFFERENTIAL
• Hypertrophic scar
• Dermatofibroma
• Infiltrating basal cell carcinoma
• Keloid

Keloids (and Hypertrophic Scars)

TREATMENT

- Identify keloid-formers (previous keloids).
- Reduce inflammatory conditions early in wound repair.
- Pressure dressings after initial wounding.
- Surgery of scars

MEDICATIONS
- Small keloids may be treated with intralesional injection of triamcinolone (Kenalog) using 27 to 30 gauge needle and TB syringe. Inject into lesion every 4 weeks.
- Vitamin A (retinoids) reduce collagen production (contra-indicated in pregnancy).

SURGERY
- Surgery of scars
  - Intralesional triamcinolone acetamide injections (can mix local anesthetic with steroid for anesthesia at time of excision).
  - Administer preoperatively, intraoperative, postoperatively
  - Every 3 to 4 weeks over 3 to 4 month period
- Intralesional excision
- Consider W- or Z-plasty for hypertrophic scars to reduce tension.
- Minimal buried/deep sutures
- Pressure dressings for long period (6 to 12 months).
- Camouflage with dermabrasion or pigmentation techniques (tattoo) for mildly raised or depressed scars.

IRRADIATION
Not indicated.

CONSULTATION SUGGESTIONS
Oral-Maxillofacial Surgeon, Plastic Reconstructive Surgeon

REFERRAL SUGGESTIONS
Oral-Maxillofacial Surgeon, Plastic Reconstructive Surgeon

PATIENT INSTRUCTIONS
Always warn surgeons prior to surgery of abnormal scarring potential.

COURSE/PROGNOSIS
- Hypertrophic scars usually do not recur if treated correctly.
- Keloids recur often
  - conservative treatment indicated
  - patient compliance necessary for good result

CODING

ICD-9-CM
701.4 Keloid, or Hypertrophic scar

CPT
11440 Excision and layered closure scar tissue face 0.5 cm or less
11441 Excision and layered closure scar tissue face 0.6 to 1 cm
11442 Excision and layered closure scar tissue face 1.1 to 2.0 cm
11443 Excision and layered closure scar tissue face 2.1 to 3.0 cm
11444 Excision and layered closure scar tissue face 3.1 to 4.0 cm
11446 Excision and layered closure scar tissue face over 4 cm
  Add suffix modifier
◊ 22 for complex case.
11900 Intralesional injection, up to and including 7 lesions
11901 more than 7 lesions
15780 Dermabrasion, total face
15781 segmental face
40812 Incisional biopsy
99000 Transport of tissue specimen to outside laboratory

MISCELLANEOUS

SEE ALSO
Basal cell carcinoma

REFERENCES
Robson MC, Burns BF, Phillips LG: Wound repair: principles and applications. In: Plastic Surgery: A Core Curriculum. Ruberg RL, Smith DJ, (eds), St. Louis, CV Mosby Co., 1994, pp. 21-22.

Engrav LH: A comparison of inframarginal and extramarginal excision of hypertrophic scars. Plas Reconst Surg 81:40-48, 1988.

AUTHOR
Bruce Horswell, DDS, MD

Keratoacanthoma

BASICS

DESCRIPTION
A rapidly growing, locally infiltrating, self-limiting, benign neoplasm of keratinocytes. Occurs mainly on sun-exposed skin or lips.

ETIOLOGY

• Originates from squamous cells within the pilosebaceous apparatus.
• Most likely etiologic agent is sunlight.
• Other possible induction factors include trauma, viruses, chemical agents, and genetic factors.

SYSTEMS AFFECTED
A local lesion only; affects no other organ system.

DIAGNOSIS

SYMPTOMS AND SIGNS
• Asymptomatic
• Initially tends to appear as a small, red macule that rapidly grows into a papule over a period of 4 to 8 weeks. Multiple lesions can occur.
• The mature lesion appears as a firm, elevated, dome-shaped nodule with a central keratin plug.
• Laboratory
• Careful histologic examination is diagnostic.
• Histologically presents as a crater in which the keratin plug is surrounded by squamous epithelium. Marked pseudoepitheliomatous hyperplasia present with mixed inflammatory infiltrate. May be confused with a well-differentiated squamous cell carcinoma.

IMAGING/SPECIAL TESTS
Antigens such as involucrin may be histologic marker for this entity.

DIFFERENTIAL
• Squamous cell carcinoma
• Solar keratosis
• Verruca vulgaris

TREATMENT

MEDICATIONS
- Intralesional methotrexate.
- Oral retinoid therapy.

SURGERY
- Observation only with biopsy if lesion fails to regress.
- Excisional surgery or thorough curettage of base.

IRRADIATION
Not indicated

CONSULTATION SUGGESTIONS
Oral-Maxillofacial Pathologist

REFERRAL SUGGESTIONS
- Oral-Maxillofacial Surgeon
- Oral Medicine

PATIENT INSTRUCTIONS
Reassure lesion not malignant.

COURSE/PROGNOSIS
- With treatment no recurrence is expected.
- Lesions left untreated will usually spontaneously involute.
- Due to the lack of absolutely reliable clinical diagnosis, and the similarity both clinically and histologically to squamous cell carcinoma, all lesions should be followed closely.

CODING

ICD-9-CM
078.10 Viral warts, unspecified type
140.0   Malignant neoplasm of upper lip, vermilion border
140.1   Malignant neoplasm of lower lip, vermilion border
238.2   Keratoacanthoma

CPT
11440 Excision benign lesion, lips 0.5 cm or less
11441 Excision benign lesion, lips 0.6-1.0 cm
11442 Excision benign lesion, lips 1.1-2.0 cm
11443 Excision benign lesion, lips 2.1-3.0 cm
40490 Biopsy lip

MISCELLANEOUS

SEE ALSO
Squamous cell carcinoma
Solar Keratosis
Verruca vulgaris

REFERENCES
Hodak E, Jones RE, Ackerman AB: Solitary keratoacanthoma in a squamous-cell carcinoma: three examples with metastases. Am J Dermatopath 15:332-342, 1993.

Melto JL, et al: Treatment of keratoacanthomas with intralesional methotrexate. J Am Acad Derm 25:1017-1023, 1991.

Regezi JA, Sciubba JJ: Oral Pathology Clinical Pathologic Correlations. 2nd ed. Philadelphia, WB Saunders Co., 1993, pp. 184-187.

AUTHOR
Paul A. Danielson, DMD

Keratosis, Actinic

BASICS

DESCRIPTION
Lesion is a papular, scaly area that is usually of normal coloration, but can be slightly erythematous, pigmented, or fairly yellow. They are often best appreciated by touch rather than by appearance. Lesions are most often only a millimeter or two in size, but may be several centimeters as well. Lesion is common and premalignant, and often develops into squamous cell carcinoma if given enough time. Lesions are most common on the face and neck. Exposed areas of the arm and hand are also commonly affected. Recognition of lower lip lesions (actinic cheilitis) is extremely important due to its malignant potential.

ETIOLOGY

• Excessive sun exposure and fair skin are almost tantamount to guaranteeing a person has at least several actinic keratotic lesions.
• Increased recreational solar exposure has pushed the age of first appearance of lesions ever younger.
• Any source of UV radiation, even if artificially produced by tanning beds, may cause actinic keratosis.

SYSTEMS AFFECTED
Skin
◊ all surfaces at risk if chronically exposed to sunlight.
Oral mucosa
◊ vermilion of the lip is often affected. Loss of definition of the skin
◊ vermilion interface is common in chronic actinic damage. Atrophic changes are also more common on the vermilion of the lip than on the skin. The lower lip is more commonly involved than the upper lip due to increased exposure.
Conjunctival mucosa
◊ may also be affected.

DIAGNOSIS

SYMPTOMS AND SIGNS
• Generally asymptomatic, though there may be a vague sense of irritation.
• There are multiple clinical types in addition to the classic papular lesion. These include:
  • Lichenoid actinic keratosis
  • Actinic cheilitis
  • Hypertrophic actinic keratosis
  • Pigmented actinic keratosis
  • Actinic conjunctivitis
Loss of skin
◊ vermilion interface definition.
• Skin surface feels scaly.

LABORATORY
n/a

IMAGING/SPECIAL TESTS
• Lip, conjunctival, and burn scar lesions should be considered more ominous than the standard skin lesion. Biopsy of such lesions is recommended. It is imperative that node assessment is performed and recorded prior to biopsy of all lip lesions. This also applies to burn scars, conjunctival lesions and, to somewhat lesser extent, lesions involving the pinna of the ear.
• Actinic keratosis is considered a clinical diagnosis, so in most cases on the skin a biopsy is not performed unless there is increased suspicion or atypical features bring other lesion into the differential diagnosis.

DIFFERENTIAL
• Papular discoid lupus erythematosus
• Disseminated superficial actinic parakeratosis
• Squamous cell carcinoma
• Large cell acanthoma
• Coccidioidomycosis

TREATMENT

General
◇ Prevention is a key. Limit sun exposure and use sunscreens.

MEDICATIONS
• 5-fluorouracil (5-FU) is the most common therapeutic agent. It is used topically on affected areas. Systemic uses for other malignant disease may delineate unrecognized lesions.

SURGERY
• In actinic cheilitis, conservative excision is usually the treatment of choice. Severe extensive changes may warrant vermilionectomy with mucosal advancement.
• Cryotherapy is often employed on small focal lesions.
• Lasers have been used in actinic cheilitis.

IRRADIATION
Not indicated.

CONSULTATION SUGGESTIONS
Oral-Maxillofacial Surgeon, Oral Medicine Specialist

REFERRAL SUGGESTIONS
Oral-Maxillofacial Surgeon, Oral Medicine

PATIENT INSTRUCTIONS
Use sunscreens on face and lips.

COURSE/PROGNOSIS
• Premalignant if induration, ulceration, or erythema are present. The possibility of actual existing squamous cell carcinoma must be considered.
• Lower lip metastasis is generally localized to local lymph nodes. Central one-third of lip lesions most likely to metastasize to the submental triangle. Lateral one-third section lesions most likely to ipsilateral submandibular triangle.
• Excellent prognosis for standard skin lesions. Even though skin squamous cell carcinoma has a good prognosis, preventing progression will eliminate risk of disfigurement.

CODING

ICD-9-CM
370.20 Actinic conjunctivitis
370.24 Actinic keratosis
692.72 Actinic cheilitis
692.74 Solar elastosis
701.1 Hyperkeratosis

CPT
11100 Biopsy, skin
13131 Mouth, repair, complex
17340 Cryotherapy, skin
40400 Vermilionectomy with mucosal advancement.
40490 Biopsy, lip
41116 Mouth, excision, lesion
99000 Handling and transport of specimens

MISCELLANEOUS

SYNONYMS
Solar keratosis
Solar cheilitis

SEE ALSO
Basal cell carcinoma

REFERENCES
Regezi JA, Sciubba J: Oral Pathology, 2nd ed. Philadelphia, WB Saunders, 1993, pp. 102-140, 571-572.

Moschella SL, Hurley HJ: Dermatology, 3rd ed. Philadelphia, WB Saunders, 1991, pp. 1730-1731, 2087-2088.

AUTHOR
Joseph W. Hellstein, DDS

Lacrimal Disorders

BASICS

DESCRIPTION
Set of inflammatory conditions affecting the lacrimal gland (dacryoadenitis) or lacrimal sac (dacryocystitis) that results in changes in lacrimation and accompanied by infection.

ETIOLOGY

- Dacryoadenitis
- Autoimmune disorders affecting glandular structure, eg, rheumatoid arthritis, systemic lupus, Sjögren's disease.
- Granulomatous disease, eg, sarcoidosis, affects glands in 20 to 50% of patients, resulting in decreased tear production.
- Bacterial and viral infections.
- Age-related with glandular fibrosis and acinar destruction.
- Dacryocystitis
- Nasolacrimal duct obstruction
    - tumor
    - polyps
    - granulomatous disease
- Trauma to puncta and canaliculi.

SYSTEMS AFFECTED
Lacrimal

DIAGNOSIS

SYMPTOMS AND SIGNS
- Pain, swelling over lacrimal gland area or near lacrimal sac and puncta.
- Epiphora (tearing), discharge, fever.
- Erythema, enlargement or swollen gland and upper lid; swollen, tender inner aspect of eye when sac affected.
- Conjunctival infection
- Excessive tearing (nasolacrimal obstruction) or minimal tear secretion (lacrimal gland affected).
- Mucopurulent discharge expressed from puncta.
- Fever.

LABORATORY
CBC
◇ leukocytosis

IMAGING/SPECIAL TESTS
Lacrimal duct probing and/or cannulation

DIFFERENTIAL
- Acute sinusitis
- Orbital cellulitis
- Dacryocystitis secondary to orbital pseudotumors.
- Neoplasm of lacrimal gland or obstructing nasolacrimal system.
- Chalazion
- Viral infections (adenovirus)

TREATMENT

MEDICATIONS
- Bacterial
  - ◇ mild to moderate
  - ◇ amoxicillin/clavulanate.
    - • severe
  - ◇ ampicillin/sulbactam, ticarcillin/ clavulanate.
- Viral
  - ◇ cool compresses to affected area.
    - • Analgesics (no aspirin to children with viral illness because of risk of Reye's syndrome).
- Neoplasm
  - ◇ CT scan, biopsy, excision or resection if malignant.
- Dacryocystitis
- Antibiotics if acute infection
- Topical antibiotics
- Warm compresses
- Nasolacrimal system reconstruction (if due to obstruction) once acute infection resolves.
- Systemic treatment of autoimmune or granulomatous disease with immunosuppressant therapy.
- Artificial tears
- Massage of lids, lacrimal sac.

SURGERY
Incision and drainage if abscess present. Biopsy if neoplasm.

CONSULTATION SUGGESTIONS
Ophthalmologist

REFERRAL SUGGESTIONS
Ophthalmologist, Primary Care Physician

PATIENT INSTRUCTIONS
If eye dryness present, use ocular lubrication when sleeping. If swelling prevents eye closure while asleep, use ocular lubricants and tape eye closed while asleep.

COURSE/PROGNOSIS
- Most lacrimal gland disorders that are chronic (auto-immune, etc.) have a general, progressive downhill course and will require long-term therapy.
- Dacryocystitis and other acute infections respond to surgical and antibiotic therapy.

CODING

ICD-9-CM
- 375.01 Dacryoadenitis, acute
- 375.02 Dacryoadenitis, chronic
- 375.3 Dacrocystitis

CPT
- 68400 I & D, lacrimal gland
- 68420 I & D, lacrimal sac
- 68720 Dacryocystorhinostomy
- 68800 Dilation lacrimal punctum
- 68820 Probing of nasolacrimal duct
- 68830 Insertion of stent in nasolacrimal duct

MISCELLANEOUS

SEE ALSO
Sjögren's Disease
Xerostomia
Sinusitis

REFERENCES
Cullom RD, Chang B: Eyelid. In: The Wills Eye Manual. 2nd ed., Cullom RD, Chang B. (eds), Philadelphia, JB Lippincott Co., 1994, pp. 140-145.

Chowla HG: The Watering Eye. In: Ophthalmology. 2nd ed., Chowla HG (ed), London, Churchill Livingstone, 1993, pp. 127-131.

AUTHOR
Bruce Horswell, DDS, MD

Laryngeal Carcinoma

BASICS

DESCRIPTION
Cancer of the larynx is almost always squamous cell carcinoma. Lesions involving the free edge of the vocal cords are frequently detected early because of hoarseness or other vocal complaints. Lesions arising in areas adjacent to the larynx may remain silent until disease is advanced.

ETIOLOGY

Long-term tobacco abuse is the primary etiologic factor. Alcohol is probably not a significant cofactor, unlike oral or pharyngeal cancer.

SYSTEMS AFFECTED
Pulmonary
◇ laryngeal tumors may obstruct the airway and long-term smoking can produce concomitant chronic pulmonary disease that can complicate laryngeal cancer treatment.
Lymphatic
◇ laryngeal cancers metastasize first to cervical lymph nodes.

DIAGNOSIS

SYMPTOMS AND SIGNS
Throat
◇ persistent hoarseness
• recurrent sore throat
• hemoptysis
• difficult or painful swallowing
Neck
◇ slow onset of painless neck mass
General
◇ weight loss
Throat
◇ airway obstruction in advanced disease
Neck
◇ painless neck mass due to cervical metastasis

LABORATORY
No specific test or marker is available for laryngeal carcinoma

IMAGING/SPECIAL TESTS
• Direct laryngoscopy with biopsy
• Flexible fiberoptic laryngoscopy
• CT or MRI scan

DIFFERENTIAL
• Nonspecific laryngitis/pharyngitis
• Laryngeal tuberculosis
• Hoarseness due to vocal cord paralysis of benign etiology.

Laryngeal Carcinoma

TREATMENT

General
◊ Radiation therapy alone is used for small lesions (T1 and T2) without cervical metastases.
◊ Advanced lesions are often treated with initial chemotherapy and subsequent radiation and/or surgery.

MEDICATIONS
• Cis-platinum and 5-fluorouracil
• Analgesics
• Liquid nutritional supplements

SURGERY
Surgery may involve partial or complete removal of the larynx.

IRRADIATION
• Radiation fields for laryngeal carcinoma frequently include the oral region and communication with radiation oncologist is advisable prior to oral surgical, endodontic, or periodontal procedures.
• Construction of fluoride carrier trays may be requested by the radiation oncologist for those laryngeal carcinoma patients whose radiation fields significantly involve the oral region.

CONSULTATION SUGGESTIONS
Otolaryngologist, Speech Therapist, Dietitian

REFERRAL SUGGESTIONS
Otolaryngologist, General Surgeon specializing in head and neck surgery

PATIENT INSTRUCTIONS
Patients with new onset hoarseness or voice change that fails to resolve in a week should have careful evaluation of larynx.

COURSE/PROGNOSIS
• Varies with stage, patients with small lesions do well, larger lesions carry poorer prognosis.
• Presence of cervical metastases is unfavorable prognostic sign.
• Lesions that recur or persist following radiation therapy can often be successfully salvaged by laryngectomy.
• Laryngectomy patients breathe entirely through a tracheal stoma in the lower neck, ie, "neck breathers."
• Following laryngectomy, speech is possible by means of esophageal speech or through a battery powered sound producing device placed against the neck skin.

CODING

ICD-9-CM
161.9 Neoplasm, laryngeal

CPT
21085 Oral surgical splint
21089 Unlisted maxillofacial prosthetic procedure

MISCELLANEOUS

SYNONYMS
Glottic carcinoma
True/false vocal cord carcinoma
Carcinoma of supraglottis/glottis/subglottis

SEE ALSO
Laryngotracheobronchitis
Laryngitis
Epiglottitis

REFERENCES
Norris CM, Cady B: Head, neck and thyroid cancer. In: American Cancer Society Textbook of Clinical Oncology. Atlanta, GA, American Cancer Society, 1991.

Bailey BJ: Early glottic carcinoma. In: Head & Neck Surgery Otolaryngology. Bailey BJ (ed), Philadelphia, JB Lippincott Co., 1993, pp. 1313-1333.

Fried MP, Girdhar-Gopal HV: Advanced cancer of the larynx. In: Head & Neck Surgery Otolaryngology, Bailey BJ (ed), JB Lippincott Co., Philadelphia,, 1993, pp. 1437-1360.

Singer MI: Voice rehabilitation after laryngectomy. In: Head & Neck Surgery Otolaryngology, Bailey BJ (ed), Philadelphia, JB Lippincott Co., 1993, pp. 1361-1372.

AUTHOR
Eric J. Dierks, DMD, MD

Laryngitis

 BASICS

DESCRIPTION
• An infection of the larynx.
• May be an isolated infection or associated with the common cold.
• May be acute or chronic.

 ETIOLOGY

Viral-influenza virus, rhinovirus, others.
Bacterial
  ◊ usually streptococcal.

SYSTEMS AFFECTED
Upper respiratory

DIAGNOSIS

SYMPTOMS AND SIGNS
• Dysphagia
• Hoarseness
• Nonproductive cough
• Lymphadenopathy
• Erythematous vocal cords
• Laryngeal edema and erythema
• Fever

LABORATORY
CBC
  ◊ rarely indicated

IMAGING/SPECIAL TESTS
• Direct and/or indirect laryngoscopy.
• Culture and sensitivity

DIFFERENTIAL
• Tracheitis
• Bronchitis
• Diphtheria
• Foreign body or chemical substance irritation.
• Croup
• Neoplasm
• Supraglottitis/epiglottitis

TREATMENT

General
◇ Bed rest
◇ Voice rest
◇ Steam inhalation
◇ Warm gargles
◇ No smoking

MEDICATIONS
• Generally not indicated
• Antitussives
• Topical analgesics
• Antipyretics

CONSULTATION SUGGESTIONS
Primary Care Physician, Otolaryngologist

REFERRAL SUGGESTIONS
Primary Care Physician, Otolaryngologist

PATIENT INSTRUCTIONS
Process typically resolves in 2 to 4 days.

COURSE/PROGNOSIS
• Self-limiting in a 1 to 2 week period
• Persistent or chronic laryngitis should be referred for additional evaluation and treatment.

CODING

ICD-9-CM
034.0 Strep laryngitis
464.0 acute laryngitis
464.1 acute tracheitis
464.2 acute laryngotracheitis
476.0 Chronic laryngitis
476.1 Chronic laryngotracheitis
478.6 edema of larynx

CPT
87060 Throat/nose culture

MISCELLANEOUS

SYNONYMS
Hoarseness
Acute laryngitis
Chronic laryngitis

SEE ALSO
Bronchitis
Common cold
Laryngotracheobronchitis
Pharyngitis

REFERENCES
Mosser K: Laryngitis. In: Griffith's 5 Minute Clinical Consult. Dambro MR (ed), Baltimore, Williams & Wilkins, 1995, pp. 598-599.

Myerhoff WL, Rice DH: Otolaryngology Head and Neck Surgery. Philadelphia, WB Saunders, Co., 1992.

AUTHOR
Alan L. Felsenfeld, DDS

Laryngotracheobronchitis (Croup)

BASICS

DESCRIPTION
A childhood (age 1 to 3) viral infection of the larynx and lower respiratory tract that with rapid progression can lead to airway obstruction.

ETIOLOGY

Viral infection.

SYSTEMS AFFECTED
<u>Respiratory</u>
◊ infection involving larynx and lower respiratory tract.

DIAGNOSIS

SYMPTOMS AND SIGNS
<u>General</u>
◊ fever, malaise, clear rhinorrhea.
<u>Respiratory</u>
◊ abundant, thick airway secretions. Characteristic barky cough, inspiratory stridor.

LABORATORY
Leukocytosis

IMAGING/SPECIAL TESTS
None routinely. AP neck radiograph will show edematous narrowing of the subglottic airway.

DIFFERENTIAL
• Pharyngitis
• Epiglottitis
• Asthma

Laryngotracheobronchitis (Croup)

TREATMENT

General
◇ Humidification of inspired air Hospitalization if dehydrated or impending airway obstruction.

MEDICATIONS
• Racemic epinephrine breathing treatments.

SURGERY
Rarely, tracheotomy required for impending airway obstruction.

CONSULTATION SUGGESTIONS
Primary Care Physician

REFERRAL SUGGESTIONS
Primary Care Physician

FIRST STEPS TO TAKE IN AN EMERGENCY
• Transport to emergency care facility.

PATIENT INSTRUCTIONS
Humidify sleeping quarters.

COURSE/PROGNOSIS
Self-limiting viral infections usually not requiring hospitalization. Rarely impending airway closure may warrant tracheotomy.

CODING

ICD-9-CM
464.2   Acute laryngotracheobronchitis
464.21   with obstruction
476.1   Catarrhal, chronic

MISCELLANEOUS

SYNONYMS
Croup

SEE ALSO
Epiglottitis
Laryngitis

REFERENCES
Leonard G, Lafreniere DC: Infections of the Ear, Nose and Throat. In: Management of Infections of the Oral and Maxillofacial Regions. 3rd ed.

Topazian RG, Goldberg MH (eds), Philadelphia, WB Saunders Co., 1994, pp. 371-372.

Schuller DE, Schleuning AJ: Deweese and Saunders' Otolaryngology Head and Neck Surgery, 8th ed. St. Louis. CV Mosby Co., 1994, pp. 263-264.

AUTHOR
Samuel J. McKenna, DDS, MD

Leukemias

BASICS

DESCRIPTION
• Malignant neoplasms of the hematopoietic tissues. Leukemias are divided histologically into lymphoblastic and nonlymphoblastic forms. Leukemias are also classified into acute or chronic based upon cellular maturity.
• Acute leukemia may occur at any age, but acute lymphoblastic leukemia (ALL) is most commonly found in childhood.
• Chronic myelogenous leukemia (CML) occurs between ages 30 to 50. Chronic lymphocytic leukemia (CLL) is the only leukemia that has a male predilection and occurs in middle to old age.

ETIOLOGY

• The cause of human leukemias remains undefined. A viral association between human T-cell lymphotropic virus (HTLV-1) and human adult T cell lymphoma/ leukemia is widely accepted. However, a viral role in other leukemias has not been definitely established. Exposure to ionizing radiation and certain chemicals (benzene, chloramphenicol), as well as certain antineoplastics such as alkylating agents, has been found to be associated with leukemia.
• A role for genetic and hereditary factors is suggested by the predisposition of Down's syndrome and Fanconi's anemia patients to develop leukemia. In addition, there is an increased incidence of leukemia among identical twins when one is affected by the disease.

SYSTEMS AFFECTED
Oral mucosa
◇ predisposed to bleeding if thrombocytopenia is present.
General oral/dental
◇ increased susceptibility to infection such as pericoronitis.
• Reactivation of herpes simplex.
• Presence of candidiasis.
• Increased susceptibility to infection by aerobic Gram-negative enteric bacilli.
Teeth
◇ may become prone to caries because of xerostomia caused by chemotherapy.
Bones
◇ bone and joint pain may be a dominant complaint especially in children.
CNS
◇ paresthesia, anesthesia due to leukemic infiltrates.
  Mental state
◇ severely affected by symptoms, treatment and prognosis.

DIAGNOSIS

SYMPTOMS AND SIGNS
General
◇ ease fatigability, dyspnea, fever, anorexia, easy bruising, pallor, petechiae, purpura, cervical or peripheral lymphadenopathy, epistaxis, hepatomegaly, splenomegaly, recurrent infections of lungs, urinary tract, skin, rectum, and upper respiratory tract.
Bones and joints
◇ pain (especially in children).
Head and neck
◇ painful lymph-nodes, sore throat, flu-like symptoms.
Mouth
◇ petechiae, gingival bleeding, ecchymosis, gingival hyperplasia (due to leukemic infiltrates in acute myelomonoblastic leukemia or acute promyelocytic leukemia), generalized pallor of the oral mucosa due to increased red blood cells, soreness. Presence of candidiasis, recurrent infection, tonsillar enlargement.
Nervous system
◇ cranial nerve palsy, paresthesia, anesthesia, paralysis, headaches, vomiting, irritability.

LABORATORY
• Leukemic cells on peripheral blood smear.
• Serum immunoglobulin level (low in CLL).
• Presence of Philadelphia (Ph) chromosome for CGL t(9;22).

IMAGING/SPECIAL TESTS
• Periodic acid-Schiff (PAS) stain (positive for lymphoblasts).
• Sudan black and myeloperoxidase will be negative for lymphoblasts.
• Neutrophil alkaline phosphatase score (low or 0 in CML).

DIFFERENTIAL
• Mononucleosis
• Bleeding Disorder
• Rheumatic fever
• Aplastic anemia
• Lymphoma
• Megaloblastic anemia
• Leukemoid reaction
• Myelofibrosis with myeloid metaplasia
• Polycythemia vera
• Pertussis
• Tuberculosis
• Thyrotoxicosis
• Addison's disease

TREATMENT

General
◇ Sources of potential infection of irritation within the oral cavity should be eliminated.
◇ Orthodontic bands and brackets should be smoothed or replaced.
◇ Frequent re-evaluation during medical treatment phase for infection, bleeding, and oral ulcers.
◇ Scaling, root planing, oral hygiene instruction, and fluoride rinses.
Management of infections
◇ diagnosis of periodontal, pulpal, and pericoronal infections can be difficult in a neutropenic leukemia patient because normal inflammation may be absent.

MEDICATIONS
• Management of oral ulcers
◇ may be chemotherapy or Herpes Simplex (HSV)-related. Oral acyclovir should be used for treatment and prophylaxis of HSV-related ulcers
    treatment
◇ 200 mg q4h for 5 days;
    prevention
◇ 400 mg b.i.d. for up to 12 months.
• Chemotherapy induced ulcers
◇ should be gently debrided and treated with topical antibiotics such as povidone iodine solutions, bacitracin-neomycin ointments, or chlorhexidine rinses. Chlortetracycline compresses or pastes may be used.
• Use of topical anesthetics such as 4% viscous xylocaine, diphenhydramine oral rinses, or dyclonine 0.5% to 1% to relieve pain (15 to 30 ml swish, hold, spit).
• Both Gram-positive and Gram-negative organisms (Streptococcus viridans, Klebsiella, Proteus, Pseudomonas, Enterobacter and Eschericia coli); therefore, treat with broad spectrum antibiotic coverage (penicillin and an aminoglycoside).
• Management of candidiasis
◇ Nystatin oral suspension, Mycelex oral troches, oral ketoconazole, oral fluconazole, oral itraconazole, or IV amphotericin B for more severe cases (ketoconazole, fluconazole, and itraconazole may also be given IV). Clotrimazole (Mycelex) troches
◇ 10 mg dissolved slowly in mouth 5-6 times/day. Nystatin oral suspension 400,000 to 600,000 units 4 times daily, hold in mouth for several minutes prior to swallowing. Oral ketoconazole 200 to 400 mg/day
◇ single dose. Oral fluconazole 100 to 400 mg/day. Oral itraconazole 200 to 400 mg/day.

• Management of graft versus host disease in bone marrow transplantation-topical or systemic steroid therapy for lichenoid reactions (desquamative gingivitis, atrophy, and ulceration). Topical steroids include 0.05% clobetasol and 0.05% fluocinonide.
• Treatments for xerostomia associated with Sjögren's-like syndrome. (See Xerostomia).
• For ALL, weekly IV vincristine and prednisone are used most often for remission.
• Other agents such as 6-mercaptopurine and methotrexate with or without cyclosphamide are used long-term.
• For AML, arabinosyl cytosine and anthracycline antibiotics are given.
• Chronic leukemia
◇ goal of treatment is palliative.
• CLL treated with antineoplastics, corticosteroid therapy, local radiation therapy.

SURGERY
• Partially erupted third molars that present a problem as a source of pericoronitis should be extracted.
• Any teeth with a questionable prognosis should be removed, particularly while white counts are normal.
• Periodontally unsound teeth should be removed.
• Manage gingival bleeding with localized treatment such as absorbable gelatin sponge with topical thrombin or microfibrillar collagen. If unsuccessful, consider platelet transfusion.
• Young patients should undergo bone marrow transplantation. Children with AML may receive radiation to the cranium that may result in craniofacial deformities and dental anomalies.

CONSULTATION SUGGESTIONS
Hematologist, Oncologist, Oral-Maxillofacial Surgeon

REFERRAL SUGGESTIONS
Primary Care Physician, Hematologist

FIRST STEPS TO TAKE IN AN EMERGENCY
• Manage any suspected infection aggressively.

PATIENT INSTRUCTIONS
• Strict attention should be paid to cleaning removable appliances, which may be a source of infection.
• Education about maintaining proper hydration during chemotherapy.

COURSE/PROGNOSIS
• Half of properly treated children with ALL are cured.
• Adults with ALL have a 20% cure rate.
• 20 to 40% of adults with AML survive disease-free long term.
• Bone marrow transplantation of AML results in disease-free survival of 40-50%.

• Median survival is 3 to 4 years after clinical onset for patients with CML.
• CLL may be indolent or progress rapidly. Longevity may range from 18 months to over 12 years.
• Acute leukemia
◇ remission induction followed by consolidation of remission and then remission maintenance.

CODING

ICD-9-CM
204.0 ALL
204.1 CLL
205.0 AML, AGL
205.1 CML, CGL

CPT
40808 Biopsy, vestibule of mouth

MISCELLANEOUS

SEE ALSO
Lymphoma

REFERENCES
Greenberg MS, Garfunkel A: Hematologic disease. In: Burket's Oral Medicine, 2nd ed. Lynch MA, Brightman VJ, Greenberg MS, (eds). Philadelphia, JB Lippincott Co., 1994, pp. 510-543.

Omura GA: The leukemias. In: Internal Medicine for Dentistry 2nd Ed., Rose LF, Kaye D (eds). St. Louis, CV Mosby Co., 1990, pp. 317-324.

Principles and Practice of Oral Medicine, 2nd ed., Sonis ST, Fazio RC, Fang L, (eds). Philadelphia, WB Saunders, Co., 1995.

Ihde DC: Consensus Development Conference on Oral Complications of Cancer Therapies: Diagnosis, Prevention, and Treatment, N.C.I. Monographs, 1990, #9.

AUTHOR
John Jandinski, DMD

Leukoplakia, Oral

BASICS

DESCRIPTION
A white plaque or patch of oral mucosa that does not rub off, and cannot be diagnosed clinically as any other disease. Excluded are diseases that can be diagnosed, such as lichen planus and candidiasis. Leukoplakia is a clinical term that encompasses a group of diseases. Microscopic examination of leukoplakia will usually reveal hyperkeratosis, epithelial dysplasia, carcinoma-in-situ, or superficially invasive squamous cell carcinoma.

ETIOLOGY

• Many leukoplakias are idiopathic.
• Use of combustible or smokeless tobacco can produce leukoplakia, and the lesion may resolve if tobacco is discontinued.
• Candida albicans is associated with many leukoplakias, although its role as an etiologic agent is not proven.
• Mechanical trauma from dentures, restorations or habits.
• Ultraviolet radiation on vermilion border of lower lip.

SYSTEMS AFFECTED
Oral mucosa
◊ leukoplakia can occur on any oral mucosal surface.

DIAGNOSIS

SYMPTOMS AND SIGNS
Oral mucosa
◊ leukoplakia is a asymptomatic thickening of oral epithelium, not a soft tissue tumor. The surface is white, yellow or gray. Some lesions have interspersed red areas ("speckled leukoplakia").
• It may appear wrinkled, fissured, nodular or smooth, and is typically rough to palpation.
• Leukoplakia cannot be removed by rubbing or scraping.

LABORATORY
Biopsy with histopathologic examination is necessary for definitive diagnosis.

IMAGING/SPECIAL TESTS
Toluidine blue vital staining may be helpful in determining where an incisional biopsy would be most diagnostic, but it should never be used as a screening tool.

DIFFERENTIAL
Lichen planus
◊ multiple lesions bilaterally distributed; often has striations.
Candidiasis
◊ white plaques rub off leaving an erythematous base; usually symptomatic.
White sponge nevus (familial epithelial hyperplasia)
◊ familial history, present from childhood, multiple diffuse lesions.
Nicotinic stomatitis
◊ located on hard palate of smokers.
Discoid lupus erythematosus
◊ painful ulcers often associated with white areas; skin lesions common.
Verrucous carcinoma
◊ indurated, folded, attached to underlying structures.

Leukoplakia, Oral

TREATMENT

General
◇ Location of lesion is important in determining treatment. If the lesion is located on keratinized oral mucosa, including gingiva, attached alveolar mucosa, hard palate and dorsum of tongue, and appears to be the result of chronic mechanical irritation, the lesion probably represents a callus (hyperkeratosis). Lesion can be observed rather than performing immediate biopsy.

◇ If a leukoplakia appears to be associated with a tobacco habit, the patient may be given the option of discontinuing tobacco and then having the lesion reevaluated in several weeks. If the lesion is still present at follow-up, an incisional biopsy should be performed.

◇ If an incisional biopsy is performed on a leukoplakia, and the microscopic diagnosis is hyperkeratosis, no further surgery is necessary. If the diagnosis is dysplasia, carcinoma-in-situ or squamous cell carcinoma, complete surgical removal of the lesion is necessary.

SURGERY
• Leukoplakias located on nonkeratinized mucosa in high-risk area such as floor of the mouth, ventral-lateral tongue, soft palate and retromolar trigone, are more likely to represent epithelial dysplasia, carcinoma-in-situ or superficial squamous cell carcinoma. These lesions should be biopsied.

• Lesions that have speckled erythematous or nodular areas are especially serious and should be biopsied as soon as possible.

• Large areas of leukoplakia may require multiple biopsies to adequately examine the lesion.

IRRADIATION
Not indicated.

CONSULTATION SUGGESTIONS
Oral Pathologist, Oral Medicine, Oral-Maxillofacial Surgeon

REFERRAL SUGGESTIONS
Oral Medicine, Oral-Maxillofacial Surgeon

PATIENT INSTRUCTIONS
Smoking cessation necessary for resolution.

COURSE/PROGNOSIS
The clinical course and prognosis of leukoplakia depend upon the microscopic diagnosis and removal of etiology.

Hyperkeratosis
◇ the lesion is benign, at least in the short-term. Persistent hyperkeratosis, especially on nonkeratinized mucosal surfaces, can rarely progress to a more serious lesion.

Dysplasia
◇ some dysplastic lesions regress spontaneously, while others progress to invasive squamous cell carcinoma. They should be considered a premalignant lesion.

Carcinoma-in-situ
◇ surgical excision should be curative. If untreated, this lesion will progress to invasive squamous cell carcinoma.

Squamous cell carcinoma
◇ excision of superficial lesions should be curative. Prognosis of more deeply invasive lesions depends upon microscopic differentiation and clinical staging.

CODING

ICD-9-CM
528.6 Leukoplakia

CPT
11100 Biopsy of mucous membrane
11101 each additional lesion
11440 Excision, benign lesion 0.5 cm or less
11441 lesion 0.6 to 1 cm
11442 lesion 1.1 to 2 cm
11443 lesion 2.1 to 3 cm
40490 Biopsy of lip
40808 Biopsy, vestibule of mouth
40820 Destruction of lesion vestibule of mouth by physical method (laser, cryo)
41100 Biopsy of tongue
42100 Biopsy of palate
42104 Excision, lesion of palate without closure

MISCELLANEOUS

SYNONYMS
Hyperkeratosis

SEE ALSO
Lichen planus
Candidiasis
Nicotinic stomatitis
Squamous cell carcinoma

REFERENCES
Silverman S, Gorsky M, Lozada F: Oral leukoplakia and malignant transformation. A follow-up study of 257 patients. Cancer 53:563-568, 1984.

WHO Collaborating Centre for Oral Precancerous Lesions. Definition of leukoplakia and related lesions: An aid to studies on oral precancer. Cancer 46:518-539, 1978.

Coleman GC. Differential diagnosis of white mucosal lesions. In: Principles of Oral Diagnosis. Coleman GC, Nelson JF (eds), St. Louis, CV Mosby, 1993, pp. 278-299.

Brightman VJ: Red and white lesions of the oral mucosa. In: Burkett's Oral Medicine, 9th ed. Lynch MA (ed), Philadelphia, JB Lippincott, Co., 1994, pp. 51-120.

White lesions. In: Principles and Practice of Oral Medicine, 2nd ed. Sonis ST, Fazio RC, Fong L (eds), Philadelphia, WB Saunders, Co., 1995, pp. 360-369.

AUTHOR
Michael W. Finkelstein, DDS, MS

Lichen Planus

BASICS

DESCRIPTION
A chronic, recurrent, noninfectious, inflammatory disease affecting the mucosa and/or skin of about 0.5 to 2.0% of the population.

ETIOLOGY

The cause of lichen planus is unknown. CD4 and CD8 T-cells account for the inflammatory infiltrate noted microscopically and account for the basal cell liquefaction degeneration of the epithelium. This same reaction is noted in lichenoid drug and skin eruptions and in graft-versus-host disease. Lichen planus can be associated with systemic disease to include diabetes mellitus, rheumatic disease, and hypertension. Some investigators believe lichen planus is premalignant and report malignant transformation rates of 2 to 10%.

SYSTEMS AFFECTED
Oral mucosa
  ◊ hyperkeratotic striations (lacey pattern) and plaques, mucosal atrophy resulting in clinical erythema, and ulceration.
Skin
  ◊ erythematous macules with overlying keratotic crusts.

DIAGNOSIS

SYMPTOMS AND SIGNS
• Recurrent oral discomfort usually with exacerbations and partial or complete remissions.
• Sensitivity to hot, spicy, and citric foods and beverages.
• Pruritis in extensor surfaces of extremities, and on palms and soles.
• Hyperkeratotic striations, usually widespread orally, involving buccal, glossal, labial, palatal, and gingival mucosa, unilaterally or bilaterally. The pattern of mucosal involvement will change over the course of days or weeks.
• Mucosa associated with or underlying the striations will be relatively erythematous.
• During exacerbations, ulcerations will characteristically be found associated with the erythematous and hyperkeratotic mucosa.

LABORATORY
• No clinical laboratory tests are of value.
• An incisional biopsy may be indicated to establish the diagnosis. A biopsy should be considered for any area not responsive to therapy.

IMAGING/SPECIAL TESTS
Microscopic features include areas of surface epithelial hyperkeratosis, atrophy, and sometimes ulceration. Liquefaction degeneration of the basal cell layer replaced by a band of fibrin is noted. A band-like, superficial infiltrate of lymphocytes is found in the underlying connective tissue.

DIFFERENTIAL
• Lichenoid mucositis (drug induced)
• Graft-versus-host disease
• Lupus erythematosus
• Epithelial dysplasia

TREATMENT

General
◇ Avoid hot and spicy foods during exacerbations.
◇ Avoid exacerbation "triggers" if identified.

MEDICATIONS
• Topical steroid suspension: triamcinolone acetonide 0.1% aqueous suspension, Disp 200 mL, sig: 5 mL oral rinse and expectorate q.i.d., p.c., and h.s. n.o.p. 1 hr. (Directions to the Pharmacist: Injectible triamcinolone q.s. into water for irrigation, add 5 ml of ethanol to increase solubility). May alter suspension to include viscous lidocaine as a topical anesthetic.
• Prednisone burst therapy, 40 mg q.d. in the morning 30 minutes after arising for 5 days, then 20 mg q.o.d. also 30 minutes after arising for an additional 1 to 2 weeks.

SURGERY
Incisional biopsy

CONSULTATION SUGGESTIONS
Oral Medicine, Oral-Maxillofacial Pathologist, Oral-Maxillofacial Surgeon

REFERRAL SUGGESTIONS
Oral Medicine

PATIENT INSTRUCTIONS
• Patient education is important because therapy may promote healing of current ulcers and atrophic mucosa and, if used at subtherapeutic doses, can prevent recurrences, but cannot "cure" the patient of the disease.
• Lesions may have malignant potential so monitoring by professional important.

COURSE/PROGNOSIS
• Long-term management is aimed at finding the minimum amount of therapy that will keep the ulcers from recurring. This can usually be accomplished by using the topical triamcinolone t.i.d., b.i.d., o.d., q.o.d., or even p.r.n. Most patients in remission (asymptomatic) will continue to show hyperkeratotic striations.
• The most common complication/side effect of long-term topical triamcinolone use is oral candidiasis. In these cases, an antifungal such as nystatin can be used in the topical triamcinolone suspension (replacing the water).

CODING

ICD-9-CM
054.2	Primary herpes
054.9	Recurrent herpes
079.9	Viral infection
112.9	Candidiasis
136.9	Bacterial infection
141.2	Squamous cell carcinoma
141.3	Carcinoma in situ
400.0	Burn
528.0	Stomatitis
528.2	Aphthous
528.92	Ulcer
529.1	Glossitis
694.6	Cicatricial pemphigoid
694.4	Pemphigus
695.1	Erythema multiforme
695.4	Lupus
697.0	Lichen planus

CPT
11900	Intralesional injection
40812	Incisional biopsy, mouth with simple repair
87252	Culture isolation
88160	Cytologic preparation
99000	Transport specimen to outside laboratory

MISCELLANEOUS

SEE ALSO
Candidiasis
Aphthous stomatitis
Pemphigoid
Lupus erythematosus

REFERENCES
Vincent SD, Fotos PG, Baker KA, Williams TP: Oral lichen planus: the clinical, historical, and therapeutic features of 100 cases. Oral Surg Oral Med Oral Path 70:165-171, 1990.

Silverman S, Gorsky M, Lozada-Nur F: A prospective follow-up study of 570 patients with oral lichen planus-persistence, remission and malignant association. Oral Surg Oral Med Oral Path 60:30-34, 1985.

Regezi JA, Sciubba JJ: Ulcerative Conditions. In: Oral Pathology: Clinical-Pathologic Correlations. 2nd ed. Philadelphia, WB Saunders 1993, pp. 114-120.

Vincent SD, Finkelstein MW: Differential Diagnosis of Oral Ulcers. In: Principles of Oral Diagnosis. Coleman GC, Nelson JF. (eds), St. Louis, Mosby-Year Book Co., 1993. pp. 328-351.

AUTHOR
Steven D. Vincent, DDS, MS

Local Anesthetic Toxicity

BASICS

DESCRIPTION
Adverse local or systemic effects related to an imbalance between absorption and elimination of local anesthetic.

ETIOLOGY

Toxic reactions can be related to choice of drug (eg, bupivacaine > lidocaine), dose administered, too rapid a speed of injection, extra- versus intra-vascular injection, use of a vasoconstrictor, and pre-existing local or systemic pathology. Children, merely by virtue of smaller size, are at greater risk for toxic reactions.

SYSTEMS AFFECTED
While all excitable membranes can be affected, primary symptoms relate to the central nervous system with secondary involvement of the cardiovascular system. If the toxic reaction is due to the vasoconstrictor, symptoms will be primarily cardiovascular in nature.

DIAGNOSIS

SYMPTOMS AND SIGNS
• Toxic reactions to local anesthetic may be immediate (within 30 to 60 seconds) if accidental intravascular injection has occurred; symptoms from simple overdose will present from 5 to 20 minutes after injection, but could be delayed by more than 1 hour. Symptoms related to vasoconstrictor toxicity are invariably immediate.
• Local anesthetic toxicity
• Mild to moderate -
  circumoral or lingual anesthesia, visual disturbances, lightheadedness, dizziness, restlessness, tinnitus, mild drowsiness, nausea, slurred speech, excitability, hypertension, tachycardia, tachypnea, diaphoresis, shivering, muscle twitching or tremors, nystagmus.
• Moderate to severe -
  lethargy, disorientation, loss of consciousness, seizure activity, hypotension, bradycardia, apnea, cardiac arrest.
• Vasoconstrictor toxicity
• Nervousness, tremors, chest tightness, palpitations, apprehension, headache.
• Diaphoresis, tachycardia, hypertension, tachypnea, dysrhythmias.

LABORATORY
Continual monitoring of vital signs to assure adequate ventilation and perfusion, including electrocardiogram if possible.

DIFFERENTIAL
• Allergic reaction
• Idiosyncratic reaction
• Vasovagal reaction
• Reaction to the vasoconstrictor
• Cerebrovascular accident
• Myocardial infarction
• Epileptic seizure

TREATMENT

MEDICATIONS
• Sympathomimetics (eg, ephedrine, epinephrine) may be needed to support blood pressure.
• Benzodiazepines (diazepam, midazolam) for seizures.

CONSULTATION SUGGESTIONS
Cardiologist, Allergist, Anesthesiologist

REFERRAL SUGGESTIONS
Primary Care Physician

FIRST STEPS TO TAKE IN AN EMERGENCY
• "ABC's"
◊ ensure an open Airway, adequate Breathing and Circulation. If hypotension is present, place the patient in the Trendelenburg position, begin IV fluids, and administer pressor support as needed with ephedrine or epinephrine.

PATIENT INSTRUCTIONS
If adverse reaction to local anesthesia occurs, determine etiology before administering additional local anesthesia. Most untoward reactions due to anxiety and not the drug itself.

COURSE/PROGNOSIS
If the episode was mild and transient, the patient should be observed for a short period of time to assure stabilization and reassured. Consider postponing the procedure and reappointing. If the episode involved frank hypotension, loss of consciousness, airway compromise, or seizure activity, patient should be transferred to local Emergency Department for observation and treatment.

CODING

ICD-9-CM
289.7 Methemoglobinemia
780.2 Vasovagal syncope
780.3 Convulsive seizure
968.4 Overdose of anesthetic
995.2 Complication or reaction to anesthetic

CPT
90780 IV infusion for therapy
90784 Intravenous therapeutic injection

MISCELLANEOUS

A toxic reaction peculiar to the anesthetic prilocaine (Citanest, Astra) is methemoglobinemia. Excessive administration of prilocaine leads to a buildup of the metabolite ortho-toluidine, which converts hemoglobin to methemoglobin. Patients with congenital methemoglobinemia are at particular risk for this toxic reaction. Cyanosis, the primary symptom, may occur anywhere between 30 minutes to several hours after prilocaine administration. Healthy individuals are not usually compromised and may report only mild respiratory distress; patients with cardiopulmonary compromise may experience significant symptoms related to hypoxemia. Treatment includes administration of 1% methylene blue 1 to 2 mg/kg IV, repeated every 4 hours if cyanosis returns.

SEE ALSO
Circulatory shock
Seizures

REFERENCES
Denson D: Physiology, pharmacology, and toxicity of local anesthetics. In: Handbook of Regional Anesthesia. Raj PP (ed) New York, Churchill Livingstone, 1985.

Covino BC: Clinical pharmacology of local anesthetic agents. In: Neural Blockade, 2nd ed. Cousins NJ, Bridenbaugh PO (eds), Philadelphia, JB Lippincott, 1988.

Malamed SF: Handbook of Local Anesthesia, 3rd ed. St. Louis, CV Mosby, 1990.

AUTHOR
Jeffrey B. Dembo, DDS, MS

Ludwig's Angina

BASICS

DESCRIPTION
Acute toxic cellulitis with bilateral involvement of the submental, sublingual, and submandibular spaces. Phlegmon formation occurs.

ETIOLOGY

• Spread of odontogenic infection, usually from a mandibular second or third molar, into the submandibular space (most common cause).
• Oral trauma and penetrating injuries of the floor of the mouth.
• Infected malignancies of the perimandibular region.
• Sialoadenitis caused by aerobic or anaerobic organisms.

SYSTEMS AFFECTED
Respiratory
◊ breathing is labored and deliberate due to mechanical obstruction of the airway as the cellulitis progresses, forcing tongue up and back.
Gastrointestinal
◊ swallowing is difficult and painful.

DIAGNOSIS

SYMPTOMS AND SIGNS
• Moderate to severe pain that is aggravated by swallowing and speech.
• Difficulty eating and patient may be unable to ingest solids or liquids.
• Speech is impaired and patient is commonly unable to control saliva.
• Massive, bilateral submandibular space and neck swelling.
• Brawny edema with elevated tongue and floor of the mouth.
• Increased salivation, oral fetor, trismus, and drooling from sides of the mouth.
• Systemic signs including malaise, fever, and tachypnea.
• Respirations are deliberate and labored.

LABORATORY
• Leukocytosis on CBC.
• Stain and culture aspirate or drainage for infective bacteria, including anaerobic organisms.
• Monitor electrolytes if fluid intake has been compromised.

IMAGING/SPECIAL TESTS
• If poor fluid intake, monitor electrolytes.
• If available, cephalogram can be used to assess airway in emergency situation.
• CT, possibly MRI to monitor airway

DIFFERENTIAL
• Sublingual space infection
• Malignant tumor
• Hematoma

TREATMENT

General
◇ Rehydration and assisted nourishment (nasogastric feedings) if no oral intake.

MEDICATIONS
• High-dose, broad-spectrum, intravenous antibiotics.
• Empiric therapy may begin with penicillin G, 2 million units intravenously every 4 hours. This regimen can be augmented with metronidazole if an anaerobic infection is suspected.
• Patients allergic to penicillin should be given 200 to 400 mg of clindamycin intravenously in three to four divided doses each day.

SURGERY
• Surgical exploration and drainage of the involved fascial spaces with extraction of any offending teeth. Neck needs to be widely opened to decompress and allow multiple small pockets of pus to drain.
• Secure the airway with intubation or tracheotomy if patient is unable to maintain airway.

CONSULTATION SUGGESTIONS
Infectious Disease Specialist, Anesthesiologist

REFERRAL SUGGESTIONS
Oral-Maxillofacial Surgeon, Otolaryngologist

FIRST STEPS TO TAKE IN AN EMERGENCY
• Requires immediate hospitalization, blood cultures, empiric antibiotics, and probably surgery.

PATIENT INSTRUCTIONS
Immediate hospitalization for antibiotics and surgery mandatory.

COURSE/PROGNOSIS
• Rarely fatal if managed aggressively.
• Adequate surgical drainage and antibiotic therapy are usually successful in resolving the infection. However, incomplete therapy can lead to re-infection or spread to masticator and parapharyngeal spaces.

CODING

ICD-9-CM
528.3 Ludwig's angina

CPT
21501 I & D, soft tissues, neck
31500 Emergency endotracheal intubation
31600 Tracheostomy, planned
31603 Tracheostomy, emergency procedure
41015 Extraoral I & D, sublingual
41016 Extraoral I & D, submental
41017 Extraoral I & D, submandibular
41800 Drainage of abscess from dentoalveolar structure
70350 Cephalogram
70355 Panorex
70360 Radiologic exam, soft tissue neck
87040 Culture blood
87070 Culture any source other than nose, throat, blood
87205 Smear, 1° source with interpretation
99000 Transport specimen to outside laboratory

MISCELLANEOUS

SEE ALSO
Pharyngitis
Odontogenic infection

REFERENCES
Owens BM, Schuman NJ: Ludwig's angina. Gen Dent 42:84-87, 1994.

Fritsch DG, Klein DG: Ludwig's angina. Heart Lung 21:39-46, 1992.

Goldberg MH, Topazian R: Odontogenic infections and deep fascial space infections of dental origin. In: Topazian RG, Goldberg MH (eds). Oral and Maxillofacial Infections. 3rd ed. Philadelphia, WB Saunders, 1994, pp. 232-236.

AUTHOR
Vivek Shetty, DDS, DMD

Lung Abscess

BASICS

DESCRIPTION
Necrotic cavity in lung parenchyma containing purulent material usually caused by bacterial, fungal, mycobacterial, or parasitic infection. Can be secondary to bronchogenic or metastatic carcinoma, septic emboli, cysts, or conglomerate lesions (silicosis, coal miners lung).

ETIOLOGY

Necrotizing infections
◇ from aerobic, anaerobic, and microaerophilic bacteria, mycobacterial (TB), fungus and parasites (liver flukes).
Aspiration pneumonia
◇ usually from pyogenic bacteria.
Septic embolism
◇ usually from tricuspid valve endocarditis or septic thrombophlebitis.
Mechanical obstruction
◇ includes bronchial stenosis, obstructing tumors, mucous plugs.
Cavitary infarction
◇ due to pulmonary embolism or vasculitis.
Hematogenous spread
◇ bacteremia or septic emboli.
Risk Factors
1. Oropharyngeal and paranasal infections; tonsillitis, periodontal disease, dental abscesses, sinusitis.
2. Drug and alcohol abuse
3. Altered mental status
4. Diabetes mellitus
5. Steroid therapy
6. Immunodeficiency; acquired or inherited.
7. Pulmonary neoplasms
8. Pulmonary tuberculosis
9. Aspirated foreign body
10. Chronic aspiration; vocal cord paralysis, gastro-esophageal reflux, cardiovascular accident.

SYSTEMS AFFECTED
Pulmonary

DIAGNOSIS

SYMPTOMS AND SIGNS
• Dyspnea, chest pain, cough, sanguinous and/or purulent sputum, fever, chills, rigors, diaphoresis, night sweats, malaise, fatigue, anorexia, weight loss.
• Tachycardia, tachypnea, rales, rhonchi, shortness of breath, pleuritis, dull chest pain.
• Decreased breath sounds, bronchial breath sounds, dullness to percussion.

LABORATORY
• Neutrophilic leukocytosis with left shift (increased bands or immature forms).
• Anemia
• Hypoalbuminemia
• Sputum gram stain and culture should be done for aerobic, anaerobic bacteria, mycobacterium (acid fast), and fungus.
• Blood cultures are usually sterile with anaerobic abscesses but positive with septic emboli.
Predominant organisms
Aerobic
◇ S. aureus and enteric gram negative bacilli.
Anaerobic
◇ usually mixed with two or more including Peptococcus, Peptostreptococcus, fusobacterium and bacteroides.
Mycobacterium
◇ Mycobacterium tuberculosis, M. kansasaii, M. intracellularis.
Fungus
◇ histoplasma, Coccidioides, aspergillus.

IMAGING/SPECIAL TESTS
• Chest radiograph confirms the diagnosis but varies in presentation depending on etiology:
  multiple oval or wedge-shaped opacities from septic emboli.
  consolidation with radiolucency.
  cavitary lesion with air fluid levels in dependent segments.
  occasional pleural effusion, empyema or pneumothorax.
• CT scans are valuable in delineating extent of disease.
• Bronchoscopy for aspiration or lavage, specimen for cultures.
• Transtracheal or transthoracic aspiration.

DIFFERENTIAL
• Actinomycosis/Nocardiosis
• Bronchiectasis
• Bronchogenic carcinoma
• Empyema
• Infected pulmonary bulla
• Tuberculosis
• Wegener's granulomatosis
• Subphrenic abscess with perforation through diaphragm

TREATMENT

General
◇ Supportive measure including hydration, oxygen supplementation, control of fever, and nutritional support and treatment of underlying etiology.
Respiratory
◇ chest physiotherapy and nebullizers to loosen and mobilize secretions.

MEDICATIONS
• Sensitivities on culture will determine antibiotic of choice.
• Penicillin has traditionally been the antibiotic of choice. 10 to 12 million units daily intravenously followed by oral dosing 750 mg to 1 g four times daily for a total of 6 weeks.
• Clindamycin is recommended for anaerobic infections, 600 mg every 8 hours followed by 300 mg four times daily by mouth for duration of treatment.
• Multidosing therapy for mycobacterium and antifungals for fungal infections.
• Multiple new generation cephalosporins, and combination antibiotics, now available for resistant and nosocomial infections.

SURGERY
• Bronchoscopic aspiration and lavage for refractory cases.
• Tube thoracostomy for empyema or symptomatic pleural effusions.
• Surgery is rarely indicated.

CONSULTATION SUGGESTIONS
Pulmonologist, Thoracic Surgeon

REFERRAL SUGGESTIONS
Primary Care Physician

FIRST STEPS TO TAKE IN AN EMERGENCY
• Severely septic patient requires admission to medical intensive care unit.

PATIENT INSTRUCTIONS
Odontogenic source of abscess warrants complete dental evaluation and therapy to remove source from aspirated bacteria.

COURSE/PROGNOSIS
• Treatment needs to continue for at least 6 weeks because relapses are frequent.
• If etiology is not identified and corrected, recurrences occur.
• Sequelae are common especially with concomitant illnesses.

CODING

ICD-9-CM
513.0 Abscess; lung

MISCELLANEOUS

Related Illnesses
Pneumonia
Bronchogenic neoplasm
Dental caries
Peritonitis
Altered mental states secondary to alcoholism, seizures, or drug overdose.
Tuberculosis

SYNONYMS
Pulmonary abscess

SEE ALSO
Bronchiectasis
Pneumonia, aspiration
Lung malignancy

REFERENCES
Levison ME: Pneumonia, including necrotizing pulmonary infections. In: Isselbacher KJ, et al (eds). Harrison's Principles of Internal Medicine, 13th ed. New York, McGraw-Hill, 1994, pp. 1184-1191.

Cunningham J: Lung Abscess. In: Griffith's 5 Minute Clinical Consult. Dambro MR (eds). Baltimore, Williams & Wilkins, 1995, pp. 624-625.

AUTHOR
James Vopal, DDS, MD

Lung, Primary Malignancy

BASICS

DESCRIPTION
• Malignant neoplasm originating in lung tissue.
• Primary carcinoma of the lung is increasing annually. It has long been the leading cause of cancer related death in men, and recently has become one of the principal causes of cancer in women. At the time of diagnosis, more than 50% have distant metastasis and only 20% have only local disease. Most patients die within 1 year.
• The common malignancies of the lung can be divided into two major classifications:
  • Small-cell carcinoma (oat cell)
  • Non-small-cell carcinoma, which includes epidermoid (squamous cell) carcinoma (most common), adenocarcinoma, and large-cell carcinoma.
Other malignancies (sarcoma, lymphoma, carcinoid, melanoma, and mesotheliomas) are uncommon.
Peak incidence is between age 55 and 65. Males predominate with an incidence of 70/100,000.

ETIOLOGY

• Cigarette smoking; benzo(a)pyrene is a major carcinogen in tobacco smoke.
• Environmental pollutants
• Industrial pollutants
• Radioisotopes
• Asbestos exposure
• Inorganic arsenic

SYSTEMS AFFECTED
• Pulmonary
• Brain, bone, and liver are predominant sites of metastases with resultant seizures, neurologic deficits, pathologic fractures, liver dysfunction, and pain.

DIAGNOSIS

SYMPTOMS AND SIGNS
Asymptomatic
  ◇ five to fifteen percent diagnosed on routine chest radiograph.
General
  ◇ weakness, malaise, and shortness of breath, dyspnea on exertion, and clubbing (hypertrophic pulmonary osteoarthropathy), anorexia, cachexia/ weight loss.
Central or endobronchial lesion
  ◇ cough, dyspnea, hemoptysis, fever, productive sputum, wheezing.
Peripheral growth lesion
  ◇ cough, pleuritic pain, restrictive shortness of breath.
Regional spread
  ◇ hoarseness, cervical or axillary adenopathy, Horner's syndrome, superior vena cava syndrome, pleural effusion, cardiac dysrhythmia or tamponade. Shoulder, bone, or chest pain.

LABORATORY
CBC
  ◇ anemia secondary to chronic disease or bone marrow involvement.
Calcium
  ◇ increased secondary to bone metastases or ectopic parathormone production (epidermoid cancer).
Coagulation
  ◇ disseminated intravascular coagulation (DIC), migratory venous thrombophlebitis (Trousseau's syndrome).
Sodium
  ◇ decreased with syndrome of inappropriate secretion of antidiuretic hormone (SIADH) from small-cell cancer.
Liver profile
  ◇ increased bilirubin, transaminases, and alkaline phosphatase with metastases.

IMAGING/SPECIAL TESTS
Chest radiograph
  ◇ basic study to detect lung cancer.

CT scan of chest
  ◇ to evaluate extent of disease including hilar/mediastinal extension.
Bone scan
  ◇ to document metastases if symptomatic.
Other CT scans
  ◇ brain, abdomen to document metastases.
Ventilation/Perfusion lung scan
  ◇ evaluation of functional lung parenchyma.
Barium swallow
  ◇ for esophageal symptoms.
Special Diagnostic Procedures;
    Pulmonary function tests (PFTs)
    Fiberoptic bronchoscopy with brushings and biopsy
    Mediastinoscopy
    Fine needle biopsy
  ◇ accessible or CT guided
    Lymph node biopsy
  ◇ scalene, axillary or mediastinal

DIFFERENTIAL
• Metastatic carcinoma
• Granulomatous disease
• Fungal infection
• Hamartoma
• Lung abscess

TREATMENT

General
◊ Supportive care, including respiratory care, nutritional supplementation, and correction or treatment of laboratory abnormalities.
◊ Encourage patient to stop smoking.
◊ Avoid occupational and environmental toxins (ie, asbestos).
◊ Small cell carcinoma
Most have spread and are not resectable at time of diagnosis.
Combination chemotherapy and radiotherapy.
Radiotherapy alone.
◊ Non-small cell carcinoma
Pulmonary resection is the treatment of choice for operable tumors.
Radiotherapy for unresectable and node positive tumors.
Radiotherapy for inoperable tumors and to extra-thoracic sites.
Chemotherapy for inoperable tumors in patients with good performance status and extra-thoracic disease.

MEDICATIONS
• Analgesics
◊ pain control.
• Antibiotics
◊ pulmonary infection.
• Chemotherapy
◊ combination drug therapy.

SURGERY
See general treatment section.

IRRADIATION
See general treatment section.

CONSULTATION SUGGESTIONS
Primary Care Physician, Oncologist, Pulmonologist, Thoracic Surgeon

REFERRAL SUGGESTIONS
Primary Care Physician

COURSE/PROGNOSIS
Small-Cell Carcinoma
◊ cure rates of 15 to 25% for limited disease and 1 to 5% for extensive disease. Ninety to ninety-five percent will show objective tumor shrinkage.
Non-Small-Cell Carcinoma
◊ operable Stage I tumors resected for cure have 55%, 5-year survival with 15%, 10-year survival. Stage II and Stage III tumors vary between 35% and 10%, 5-year survival varying with cell type and extent of nodal involvement. The majority of patients thought to have had a curative resection die in 2 years indicating need for adjunctive therapy.

CODING

ICD-9-CM
162.9 Neoplasm, lung

CPT
38510 Biopsy deep cervical nodes
38520 Biopsy of deep cervical nodes with scalene fat pad

MISCELLANEOUS

SYNONYMS
Lung cancer
Mesothelioma
Bronchoalveolar carcinoma

SEE ALSO
Fungal disease
Pneumonia
SIADH
Lung abscess

REFERENCES
Minna JD: Neoplasms of the Lung. In: Harrison's Principles of Internal Medicine 13th ed. Isselbacher KJ, et al (eds). New York, McGraw-Hill 1994, pp. 1221-1228.

AUTHOR
James Vopal, DDS, MD

Lyme Disease

BASICS

DESCRIPTION
Originally called Lyme arthritis, Lyme disease is a multisystem illness caused by a tick-borne spirochete that produces a wide range of atypical arthritic, dermal, neurologic, cardiovascular, and ocular signs and symptoms usually occurring over a period of many months.

ETIOLOGY

• First recognized in 1975, Lyme disease (Lyme borreliosis) is caused by a spiral-shaped bacterium called the Borrelia burdorferi spirochete. It is carried and transmitted by several species of the tiny Ixodes (deer ticks), which are predominantly located in the northeastern, midwestern, and western United States, as well as other Asian and European countries.
• Transmission to humans most often occurs in June or July (May to November range) when the tick attaches to the host and regurgitates mid-gut contents into the wound site. Studies suggest that tick attachment of 24 hours or more are necessary for spirochetal transmission to the host.
• Following inoculation, the spirochete spreads laterally in the dermis eventually reaching regional lymphatics and disseminating in blood to the internal organs, distant skin, and musculoskeletal sites. The organism can be cultured from the blood within weeks of infection.
• An apparent immunosuppression occurs initially following infection with an increase in T-suppressor cell activity and poor mononuclear cell responsiveness to Borrelia antigens. This early hypo-responsiveness to these antigens is later supplanted by B-lymphocyte hyperactivity resulting in elevated serum IgM, cryoprecipitates, and circulating immune complexes. Over a period of months to years, a specific antibody response to the spirochete gradually develops. Although the organism is phagocytosed by PMNs and activated macrophages in vitro, it has been suggested that the organism may be capable of surviving intracellularly.

SYSTEMS AFFECTED
Skin
 ◊ characterized as erythema chronicum migrans (macular, intensely red migrating rings, hot to touch but nontender), which initially occur at the site of the tick bite.
Musculoskeletal
 ◊ within several weeks to 2 years after onset, most patients develop intermittent arthritis or chronic synovitis.
Neurologic
 ◊ early in the disease, patients develop severe headaches or neck pain and stiffness typically lasting for hours. Within months abnormalities such as meningitis, encephalitis, chorea, myelitis, and facial palsy (Bell's palsy) can develop. These abnormalities typically last for months, can recur, or become chronic.
Cardiac
 ◊ invasion of the heart muscle can result in myocarditis leading to varying degrees of heart block.

Ocular
 ◊ involvement of the deeper eye tissues can result in panophthalmitis and blindness with spirochetal invasion of the vitreous humor.

DIAGNOSIS

SYMPTOMS AND SIGNS
• Malaise, fatigue, lethargy, headaches, fever, arthralgias, nausea, photophobia, vertigo, cough, chest and abdominal pain, diarrhea, backache.
• Regional or generalized lymphadenopathy, conjunctivitis, and periorbital edema, neck pain on flexion, malar rash, chronic dermal erythema migrans or annular lesions, muscular tenderness, abdominal tenderness.

LABORATORY
Culture of Borrelia, detection of Borrelia specific serum IgM or IgG (ELISA), elevated serum AST, APT, LDH.

DIFFERENTIAL
• Rheumatic-collagen disorders
• Epstein-Barr virus
• Cytomegalovirus

TREATMENT

MEDICATIONS
• Tetracycline 250 to 500 mg p.o., q.i.d., (or) penicillin V 500 mg p.o., q.i.d., (or) doxycycline 100 mg p.o., b.i.d. for 2 to 4 weeks depending on stage of infection.
• Established Lyme disease may require repeated course of therapy given a frequent incidence of relapse.

CONSULTATION SUGGESTIONS
Infectious Disease Specialist

REFERRAL SUGGESTIONS
Primary Care Physician

FIRST STEPS TO TAKE IN AN EMERGENCY
• If acute arthritis appears, immediately confer with infectious disease specialist and/or rheumatologist.

PATIENT INSTRUCTIONS
Examine children for attached ticks and tell-tale characteristic rash if exposed to areas with deer.

COURSE/PROGNOSIS
• Fifty percent of all patients treated experience late complications of disease (ie, chronic headache, myalgia, arthralgia, lethargy) lasting hours to days.
• The development of complicating cardiac conduction blockage, meningitis, or peripheral or cranial neuropathies indicates a need for intravenous antimicrobial therapy.

CODING

ICD-9-CM
088.81 Lyme disease

CPT
86618 Borella burgdorferi immunologic identification

MISCELLANEOUS

SYNONYMS
Lyme Borreliosis
Lyme arthritis
Bannwarth's syndrome
Acrodermatitis chronica atrophicans

REFERENCES
Mandell GL, Douglas RG, Bennet JE: Principles and Practices of Infectious Disease. 3rd ed. New York, Churchill Livingstone, 1990, pp. 1819-1827.

A New Test for Lyme Disease. Johns Hopkins Med Letter, 6(6):3. 1994.

Steere AC: Proceedings of the First International Symposium on Lyme Disease. Yale J Biol Med 57, 1984.

AUTHOR
Peter G. Fotos, DDS, MS, PhD

Lymphoma (Non-Hodgkin's)

BASICS

DESCRIPTION
• A malignant disease of the lymphoreticular system that may present within lymph nodes or at extranodal sites. Lymphoma is broadly divided into Hodgkin's disease and non-Hodgkin's lymphoma.
• The treatment and prognosis vary widely according to the specific type of non-Hodgkin's lymphoma and the extent of disease present.
• Burkitt's lymphoma is endemic in Central Africa and New Guinea.

ETIOLOGY

• Viral etiology is purported for some non-Hodgkin's lymphomas such as high association between Epstein-Barr virus and Burkitt's lymphoma.
• The diagnosis of a non-Hodgkin's lymphoma is increasingly associated with the AIDS virus.

SYSTEMS AFFECTED
• Lymphoreticular: site of origin.
• Other organ systems may be involved via direct extension, invasion, or by extranodal sites of involvement. Burkitt's lymphoma commonly involves bone marrow and central nervous system.

DIAGNOSIS

SYMPTOMS AND SIGNS
• Specific symptoms vary widely with the site(s) of involvement and many patients are asymptomatic at the time of diagnosis.
• Only 12% of patients affected have general symptoms of weight loss, malaise, fever, chills, night sweats.
• Painless rubbery lymphadenopathy in a young adult that frequently appears as multiple nodes matted together.
• Oropharyngeal lymphoid involvement is more common with non-Hodgkin's lymphoma than with Hodgkin's disease.

IMAGING/SPECIAL TESTS
• Fine needle aspirate (FNA) biopsy often does not provide adequate diagnostic material and open biopsy of a lymph node is often required for specific histologic subtyping.
• Monotonous sea of cells with round to oval nuclei.
• Burkitt's type shows starry sky pattern.
• Jaw involvement shows radiolucent areas with bony expansion.
• CT scanning of chest and abdomen has supplanted staging laparotomy to identify potential hidden areas of involvement and to determine stage.

DIFFERENTIAL
• Extranodal lymphomas mimic neoplastic or inflammatory lesions at any site.
• Squamous cell carcinoma, primary or metastatic
• Reactive lymphadenopathy due to regional inflammatory process.

Lymphoma (Non-Hodgkin's)

TREATMENT

General
◊ Chemotherapy and radiation will alter immune system and vascularity, respectively. Confer with treating physician prior to dental therapy for information related to white cell counts and radiation fields.

MEDICATIONS
• Chemotherapy combination include:
• "CVP"
◊ Cyclophosphamide + vincristine + prednisone.
• "CHOP"
◊ Cyclophosphamide + doxorubicin + vincristine + prednisone.
• "M-BACOD"
◊ Methotrexate + leucovorin + bleomycin + doxorubicin + cyclophosphamide + vincristine + dexamethasone.

SURGERY
• Biopsy for diagnosis and staging.
• Avoid elective dental care when white blood cell counts are low due to chemotherapy. Consider removal of unrestorable teeth prior to neutropenic periods.

IRRADIATION
• Early, localized non-Hodgkin's lymphomas are often treated with local radiation therapy, whereas intermediate and high-grade lesions require chemotherapy with or without radiation.
• Radiation fields for lymphoma can include the oral region. Communication with a radiation oncologist is advisable prior to oral surgical, endodontic, or periodontal procedures.
• Construction of fluoride carrier trays may be requested by the radiation oncologist for patients with lymphoma involving the oral region.

CONSULTATION SUGGESTIONS
Oncologist, Oral-Maxillofacial Surgeon, Radiation Oncologist

REFERRAL SUGGESTIONS
Primary Care Physician

COURSE/PROGNOSIS
• Outcome varies significantly with specific histologic subtype, stage, and site.
• Lymphomas, in general, are among the most curable cancers.

SYNONYMS
• Lymphocytic lymphoma
• African lymphoma
• Monomorphic lymphoma

CODING

ICD-9-CM
200.2 Burkitt's lymphoma
202.0 Lymphoma, nodular or mixed
202.8 Lymphoma (malignant), non-Hodgkin's

CPT
21085 Oral surgical splint
21089 Unlisted maxillofacial prosthetic procedure

MISCELLANEOUS

SEE ALSO
Hodgkin's disease
AIDS
Immunodeficiency

REFERENCES
Eyre HJ, Farver ML: Hodgkin's disease and non-Hodgkin's lymphomas. In: American Cancer Society Textbook of Clinical Oncology, Atlanta, American Cancer Society, 1991.

Longo DL, DeVita VT, Jaffe ES, Mauch P, Urba, WJ: Lymphocytic lymphomas. In: Cancer, Principles & Practice of Oncology, 4th ed. Devita VT, Hellman S, Rosenberg SA (eds), Philadelphia, JB Lippincott Co., 1993, pp. 1859-1927.

Hupp JR, Collins F, Ross A, Myall R: A review of Burkitt's lymphoma: importance of radiographic diagnosis. J Maxillofac Surg 10: 240-245, 1982.

AUTHOR
Eric J. Dierks, DMD, MD

Malignant Hyperthermia

BASICS

DESCRIPTION
Identified as a distinct condition in the mid-1960s, malignant hyperthermia (MH) is a hypermetabolic state of skeletal muscle triggered by certain anesthetic agents in genetically susceptible individuals, resulting in a variety of systemic complications leading to a potentially fatal outcome.

ETIOLOGY

• An abnormality or hypersensitivity of calcium channels in the sarcoplasmic reticulum leading to decreased control of intracellular calcium. Upon exposure to certain anesthetic agents, there is excessive release of calcium causing increased muscle contraction and metabolism. The chromosomal deficit associate with MH has been tentatively localized to chromosome 19 at a locus associated with the ryanodine receptor.
• MH susceptibility is a genetic trait that is usually (but not always) autosomal dominant.
• Individuals to be considered at increased risk are:
  a) patients who survived a previous MH episode or had a positive muscle biopsy (see below),
  b) patients with a 1st degree relative having the above,
  c) a member of a family with suspected MH tendency and known muscle abnormality and increased resting creatine phosphokinase (CPK).
• There should be increased suspicion for MH susceptibility in patients who have Duchenne-type muscular dystrophy, increased muscle bulk, scoliosis, or strabismus.

SYSTEMS AFFECTED
Primarily skeletal muscle, subsequently affecting other organ systems (especially cardiovascular and renal).

DIAGNOSIS

SYMPTOMS AND SIGNS
• Awake individuals may undergo a MH episode, experiencing stress- or heat-induced muscle cramps, fever, or dark-colored urine. Most often, however, the MH episode occurs during a general anesthetic in which known triggering agents (eg, Halothane, succinylcholine) have been used.
• Hypercarbia
• Cyanosis
• Skin mottling
• Masseter and/or generalized muscle rigidity
• Unexpected tachycardia within the first 30 min of induction
• Hypertension
• Rapid temperature rise (>0.25° C in 10 min)
• Tachypnea
• Cardiac dysrhythmias
• Cardiac arrest

LABORATORY
During the crisis, arterial and venous blood gases should be drawn, as well as potassium, calcium, bicarbonate, myoglobin levels, and coagulation studies. Frequently found are acidosis, hyperkalemia, and myoglobinuria. An elevated creatinine kinase (CK) occurs within 24 to 48 hours.

IMAGING/SPECIAL TESTS
• To confirm the presence of MH susceptibility if an intraoperative event has occurred or if the preoperative history indicates a possible family history, a MH diagnostic muscle biopsy is performed. Fresh skeletal muscle taken from the thigh is exposed in vitro to halothane and caffeine. Contracture responses are compared to expected norms – muscle of MH-susceptible patients requires lower than average amounts of caffeine to stimulate contracture, and even less if Halothane is present.
• Of the medications frequently used in dental practice, the following are NOT considered to be triggering agents: nitrous oxide, benzodiazepines, lidocaine, propofol, barbiturates.

DIFFERENTIAL
Other causes for intraoperative fever include atelectasis, aspiration, sepsis, excessive body heat retention, thyroid storm, pheochromocytoma, cocaine toxicity, sepsis. Masseter muscle spasm (MMS) may occur without developing into a full-blown MH crisis, but it is unclear whether this is a separate pathologic entity or merely a subclinical MH event arrested in the early stages. Therefore, controversy exists regarding treatment of MMS absent other signs of MH. Neuroleptic malignant syndrome (NMS), also treated with dantrolene, is accompanied by many of the same symptoms as MH but usually occurs more slowly than MH and is associated with administration of certain neuroleptic agents, not known anesthetic triggering agents.

Malignant Hyperthermia

TREATMENT

General
◊ Cooling core of body by any means possible.
◊ Important using intubation and lavage with chilled saline and immersion in cool bath. IV chilled saline also administered.

MEDICATIONS
• Dantrolene sodium, a muscle relaxant, is the primary drug of choice. Approved in 1979, dantrolene blocks calcium release from the sarcoplasmic reticulum and reverses the hypermetabolic events; dantrolene is also an anti-pyretic and helps prevent true hyperthermia from developing.
• Furosemide (Lasix) to promote diuresis to limit myoglobin renal damage.

CONSULTATION SUGGESTIONS
Anesthesiologist

REFERRAL SUGGESTIONS
Anesthesiologist, Emergency Medicine Physician

FIRST STEPS TO TAKE IN AN EMERGENCY
1. Discontinue all triggering agents
2. Hyperventilate with 100% O_2
3. Reconstitute and administer dantrolene 2.5 mg/kg IV, repeat as needed every 5 to 10 minutes until heart rate and end-tidal CO_2 decrease.
4. If possible, insert central arterial and venous catheters and urinary catheter.
5. Cool the patient with a chilled IV infusion or by surface cooling.
6. Diurese with furosemide (Lasix) 1 mg/kg.
7. Draw blood samples for serum electrolytes, arterial blood gases, PT/PTT, platelet count, fibrinogen, myoglobin.
8. Treat hyperkalemia with glucose + insulin (10 units regular insulin mixed in 50 mL 50% dextrose in water, titrate to effect).
9. Treat metabolic acidosis with sodium bicarbonate, titrated in 1 to 2 mEq/kg increments.
10. Monitor ECG, temperature, urine output, arterial blood pressure, central venous pressure.
11. Treat dysrhythmias as needed, but avoid calcium channel blockers.
12. Call MH Hotline: (209)634-4917 (ask for Index Zero) for additional assistance.
13. Transfer patient to nearest postanesthetic care unit or intensive care unit for at least 24 hours observation.
14. Report the incident to the North American Malignant Hyperthermia Registry: (717)531-6936.

PATIENT INSTRUCTIONS
• Patient should be counseled regarding the need for diagnostic muscle biopsy and should be encouraged to consult the Malignant Hyperthermia Association of the United States (MHAUS) (203)655-3007.
• A Medic-Alert bracelet should be issued to the patient.

COURSE/PROGNOSIS
Mortality can be 40% or greater if dantrolene is not administered. With dantrolene and other appropriate treatment, mortality approaches 0%.

CODING

ICD-9-CM
995.89 Malignant hyperthermia

CPT
90780 IV infusion for therapy
90782 IM therapeutic infection
99186 Total body hypothermia

MISCELLANEOUS

SYNONYMS
Malignant hyperpyrexia

SEE ALSO
Fever of Unknown Origin

REFERENCES
Britt BA: Malignant hyperthermia. Boston, Martinus Nijhoff Pub., 1987.

Muldoon SM, Karan S: Hyperthermia and hypothermia. In: Principles and Practice of Anesthesiology. Rogers MC, Tinker JH, Covino BG, et al (eds), St. Louis, CV Mosby, 1993.

AUTHOR
Jeffrey B. Dembo, DDS, MS

Malignant Jaw Tumors

BASICS

DESCRIPTION
• Malignant Jaw Tumors may be classified as:
(1) Primary
  • Tumors of bony tissue,
    ◇ osteosarcoma, chondrosarcoma, Ewing's sarcoma.
  • Systemic neoplasms involving bone
    ◇ multiple myeloma, Burkitt's lymphoma.
  • Tumors in the jaw arising from soft tissue
    ◇ malignant ameloblastoma, primary intraosseous carcinoma, central salivary gland cancers, etc.
(2) Metastatic
  • Arising from lung, breast, prostate, kidney, thyroid, and colon.
• The commonest malignant tumors of jaw bones are secondary metastases. Multiple myeloma is the commonest primary bone cancer. (This section will not discuss tumors in the jaw bone arising from soft tissue.)

ETIOLOGY

• Radiation has been associated with inducing osteosarcoma both by strontium incorporation into the bone and radiation of benign lesions such as fibro-osseous lesions.
• Paget's disease is complicated by osteosarcoma in <1% of cases.
• Burkitt's lymphoma is associated with an 8 to 14 chromosome translocation. The African type has a very high incidence of Epstein-Barr virus; however, this is less common in the American type.

SYSTEMS AFFECTED
• Mandibular and maxillary bone, and associated structures, ie, teeth, nerves, mucosa, sinuses, nasal cavity involved, through local spread.
• Metastases may involve, lung, liver, and bones other than the mandible.
• Multiple myeloma may be associated with amyloid formation and renal failure.

DIAGNOSIS

SYMPTOMS AND SIGNS
• An enlarging mass in the jaws, commonly painful.
• Paresthesia or anesthesia of the inferior alveolar, intraorbital or spheno-palatine nerves.
• Loosening or extrusion of teeth.
• Localized bleeding.
• A mass in the jaws that may or may not be ulcerated, displacing and loosening the teeth.

LABORATORY
• Serum electrophoresis
• Urinalysis for Bence-Jones protein in myeloma.
• EBV titer in Burkitt's, plus chromosomal analysis.

IMAGING/SPECIAL TESTS
• Plain radiographs: May show radiopacity, moth-eaten radiolucency, or a mixed picture.
• Classical "sun ray" appearance of osteosarcoma rare in jaws. Widened periodontal membrane of involved teeth is a common early sign of osteosarcoma or chondrosarcoma. Onion skin appearance seen in Ewing's sarcoma. Punched out lesions in myeloma. CT scan better to show extent of lesion.
• Biopsy mandatory for diagnosis. If lymphoma suspected, touch preps and fresh specimen should be sent.
• If biopsy indicates the jaw lesion to be metastatic, thyroid scan, abdominal CT, chest radiograph, mammograph, barium enema will be indicated as dictated by the histology.

DIFFERENTIAL
• Osteomyelitis
• Infected jaw cyst
• Carcinoma invading the mandible
• Odontogenic tumor

Malignant Jaw Tumors

TREATMENT

• Osteosarcoma and chondrosarcoma are preferably managed by radical surgery.
• Ewing's sarcoma protocols include combination treatment with surgery, radiation, and chemotherapy.
• Burkitt's and myeloma are primarily treated by chemotherapy.
• Solitary metastasis will require, excision, radiation or chemotherapy as dictated by the primary tumor.

MEDICATIONS
• See treatment section above

SURGERY
• See treatment section above

IRRADIATION
• See treatment section above

CONSULTATION SUGGESTIONS
Oral-Maxillofacial Surgeon, Otolaryngologist, General Surgeon, Oncologist

REFERRAL SUGGESTIONS
Oral-Maxillofacial Surgeon, Otolaryngologist

COURSE/PROGNOSIS
The prognosis for these lesions will depend on site and type of neoplasm. Parosteal osteosarcomas have a better outlook than medullary osteosarcomas. In chondrosarcomas, the histologic grading is a major determinant of behavior and likelihood of metastasis. The prognosis for multiple myeloma remains poor, as is the case for metastatic lesions.

CODING

ICD-9-CM
170.0 Malignant tumor maxilla
170.1 Malignant tumor mandible
198.5 Secondary metastasis mandible/maxilla
200.2 Burkitt's lymphoma
203.0 Multiple myeloma

CPT
20134 Excision of malignant tumor facial bone other than mandible
20144 Excision malignant tumor mandible
20145 Radical resection
20220 Biopsy bone
31225 Maxillectomy without orbital enucleation

MISCELLANEOUS

SYNONYMS
Jaw Cancer

SEE ALSO
Lymphoma
Multiple myeloma
Osteoradionecrosis

REFERENCES
Dahlin D: Bone Tumors. General Aspects and Data on 6,221 cases, 3rd ed. Springfield, IL. Charles C. Thomas, 1978.

Gamington G, Schofield H, Coryn J, et al: Osteosarcoma of the jaws. Analysis of 56 cases. Cancer 20:377-391, 1967.

Arlen M, Tollefses H, Huvos A, et al: Chondrosarcoma of the head and neck. Am J Surg 120: 456-460, 1970.

Zarbo RJ: Malignant non-odontogenic neoplasms of the jaws. In: Oral Pathology: Clinical-Pathologic Correlations. 2nd ed. Regezi JA, Sciubba J (eds), Philadelphia, WB Saunders, Co. 1993, pp. 436-457.

AUTHOR
Robert A. Ord, MD, DDS, FRCS, FACS

Marfan's Syndrome

BASICS

DESCRIPTION
A chromosomal-based, connective tissue disorder that affects the musculo-skeletal system, the eyes, and the cardiovascular system.

ETIOLOGY

Passed as an autosomal dominant trait that may skip generations. Fifteen to 30% of the cases may be due to new mutations.

SYSTEMS AFFECTED
• Skeleton
  unusually tall
  unusually long limbs
  long lower body
  long slender fingers and toes
  chest deformities due to overgrowth
    of ribs
  scoliosis
  kyphosis
  hypermobility of joints
• Ocular changes
  subluxation of the lens (ectopia
    lentis), usually in an upward
    direction.
  axial length of the globe is greater
    than normal, predisposing the
    patient to myopia and retinal
    detachment.
• Cardiovascular
  mitral valve prolapse
  aortic dilation that is progressive
    and usually dissects and ruptures.
• Miscellaneous changes
  skin striae occur over the shoulders
    and buttocks
  spontaneous pneumothorax
  high arch palate
  high pedal arch

DIAGNOSIS

SYMPTOMS AND SIGNS
Cardiovascular
  ◇ heart murmurs related to mitral valve prolapse and/or aortic dilation.
Skeletal
  ◇ chest deformities
  ◇ pectus carintum, pectus excavatum. Scoliosis usually accompanied by kyphosis.
Long fingers
  ◇ arachnodactyly
Ocular
  ◇ myopia, subluxated lenses
  ◇ Visual changes

IMAGING/SPECIAL TESTS
• Echocardiogram to rule out aortic dilatation and mitral valve prolapse.
• Slit lamp examination; lens dislocation

DIFFERENTIAL
Typical marfanoid habitus, lens dislocation, and cardiovascular abnormalities can be inherited independently, so that the diagnosis is only made when a member of the family has characteristic changes in at least two of the three connective systems.

TREATMENT

General
◇ None well-established or predictably effective.
◇ Mechanical bracing of the back.
◇ Physical therapy for the muscles of the back.
◇ Frequent ophthalmologic exam for retinal detachment.
◇ Genetic counseling because at least 5% are familial.

MEDICATIONS
• Some advocate use of propranolol to delay aortic complications.

SURGERY
• Mitral valve, aortic valve, and aortic replacement have been advocated.
• Surgical correction of the back if the scoliosis is greater than 45°.
• Subluxated lens removal.
• Valvular replacement or surgery for aortic dilation may be necessary.
• Surgery used to correct scoliosis.
• If lens subluxation occurs, surgical correction possible.

CONSULTATION SUGGESTIONS
Primary Care Physician, Cardiologist, Orthopedic Surgeon

REFERRAL SUGGESTIONS
Primary Care Physician

PATIENT INSTRUCTIONS
• Patients should avoid highly aerobic sports.
• If heart murmur or prosthetic valve present, endocarditis prophylaxis necessary before invasive dental care.

COURSE/PROGNOSIS
• Women have greater cardiovascular risk if pregnant.
• Variable presentation of the syndrome is seen due to the heterogeneity of the disease.
• With appropriate treatment, most patients can live normal life span.

 ## CODING

ICD-9-CM
759.82 Marfan's syndrome

 ## MISCELLANEOUS

SEE ALSO
Mitral valve disorder
Aortic valve disorder
Endocarditis

REFERENCES
Prockop DJ, Kuivaniemi H, Tromp G: Heritable Disorders of Connective Tissue. In: Harrison's Principles of Internal Medicine 13th ed., Isselbacher KJ, et al (eds), New York, McGraw-Hill Co. 1994, pp. 2115-2117.

Woerner EM, Royalty R: Marfan's syndrome. What you need to know. Postgrad Med 87:229-236, 1990.

AUTHOR
Thomas P. Sollecito, DMD

Mastoiditis

 BASICS

DESCRIPTION
• An acute or chronic inflammatory process of the mastoid air cells usually occurring in children and young adults. The acute type is usually a suppurative process secondary to an acute otitis media, while the chronic type is often secondary to chronic ear disease or cholesteatoma.
• Extension from internal mastoid infection to mastoid tip may cause Bezold's abscess to form.

 ETIOLOGY

Acute otitis media
◊ represents the most common cause. In many instances it results from an inadequately treated severe suppurative otitis media with contiguous spread to the mastoid air cells.
Obstruction
◊ of the natural drainage of the mastoid air cells by a cholesteatoma or chronic ear infection.

SYSTEMS AFFECTED
Hearing
◊ is usually affected due to concurrent middle ear disease and may be conductive, mixed, or sensorineural hearing loss.
Neurologic
◊ involvement may include cranial nerve VII and VIII with ipsilateral paresis of the muscles of facial expression and vertigo. In addition, severe infections may extend intracranially causing meningitis or brain abscess.

 DIAGNOSIS

SYMPTOMS AND SIGNS
Ear
◊ otalgia, otorrhea, hearing loss, vertigo
• Fever
• Retroauricular pain, swelling, and erythema
• Bulging and erythematous tympanic membrane
• Protrusion of the pinna and concha of the ear

LABORATORY
CBC with differential; leukocytosis

IMAGING/SPECIAL TESTS
• Plain films of mastoid air cells
• CT scan in more complicated cases
• Audiogram if hearing loss suspected

DIFFERENTIAL
• Retroauricular lymphadenopathy
• Otitis externa
• Retroauricular cellulitis
• Fibrous dysplasia/benign neoplasm of the temporal bone

TREATMENT

General
◇ Manage otitis media with IV antibiotics, and surgical drainage via myringotomy and tube placement.
◇ Culture and sensitivity of drained material.
◇ Frequent otoscopic examinations to assess drainage and tube patency.
◇ Incision and drainage of subperiosteal abscess.
◇ Mastoidectomy usually necessary in cases refractory to above treatment or in cases with intracranial complications.

MEDICATIONS
• Antibiotic coverage for most common organisms, including group A beta hemolytic strep., Hemophilus influenza, Strep. pneumoniae, Staph. aureus.
• Ampicillin 250 mg with or without sulbactam IV every 6 hours, or
• Cefuroxime 750 mg IV every 8 hours, or
• Clindamycin 600 mg IV every 6 hours (doses must be adjusted by weight or body surface area in children).
• Cortisporin otic drops when cleaning the external auditory canal.

SURGERY
• Bezold's abscess requires drainage.
• Cholesteatoma requires removal.

CONSULTATION SUGGESTIONS
Otolaryngologist, Infectious Disease Specialist

REFERRAL SUGGESTIONS
Primary Care Physician, Otolaryngologist

FIRST STEPS TO TAKE IN AN EMERGENCY
• If patient becoming septic, immediately refer to otolaryngologist for surgery and IV antibiotics.

PATIENT INSTRUCTIONS
Carefully comply with antibiotic instructions.

COURSE/PROGNOSIS
Most signs and symptoms are reversible with early intervention. In severe cases, permanent hearing loss and neurologic dysfunction may persist after resolution of the acute disease.

CODING

ICD-9-CM
383.0 Acute mastoiditis
383.1 Chronic mastoiditis

MISCELLANEOUS

SEE ALSO
Otitis media

REFERENCES
Shanley DJ, Murphy TF: Intracranial and extracranial complications of acute mastoiditis: evaluation with computed tomography. J Am Osteopath Assoc 92:131-134, 1992.

Myer CM: The diagnosis and management of mastoiditis in children. Pediatr Ann 20:622-626, 1991.

English GM: Otolaryngology. New York, Harper & Row, 1989.

AUTHOR
Joseph J. Sansevere, DMD

Median Rhomboid Glossitis

BASICS

DESCRIPTION
• A well-demarcated, ovoid, diamond or rhomboid-shaped, nonulcerated, flat or slightly raised, pink or red area on the central, middle third of the tongue dorsum. It stands out from the rest of the tongue because it has no filiform papillae.
• Incidence is reported to be less than 1% with a 3 to 4:1, female to male predominance.

ETIOLOGY

• A developmental defect is hypothesized as a contributing factor for this anomaly. The lateral lingual swellings from the first branchial arch fail to completely fuse over a midline swelling, known as the tuberculum impar. This is discounted as the sole etiology because the lesion is rarely seen in children under the age of ten.
• Current evidence suggests a relationship with a localized, chronic Candida albicans infection. Fungal hyphae are seen in 85% of histologic sections associated with a significant decrease in the number and function of specialized macrophages (Langerhans' cells) in the epithelium of the lesion. It is particularly common in diabetics.

SYSTEMS AFFECTED
Tongue
◇ demarcated, pink or reddish area on the central portion of the tongue. If symptomatic, may affect speech, mastication, and/or deglutition.

DIAGNOSIS

SYMPTOMS AND SIGNS
Tongue
◇ lesion generally does not hurt and appears relatively innocuous. Occasional burning sensation or pain may be present if a Candida infection is diagnosed. Loss of papillae with a varying degree of hyperparakeratosis gives the area a distinct appearance from the rest of the tongue, which appears coated, or the papillae are heavy and matted.

LABORATORY
Serum chemistry
◇ if patient a diabetic, accumulation of ketone bodies, acetoacetate, betahydroxybutyrate, acetone, and hyperglycemia. Arterial blood gas
◇ depleted bicarbonate levels and lowered pH.
Urinalysis
◇ acetone and ketones in the urine. Stain and culture for candidiasis (PAS stain).

IMAGING/SPECIAL TESTS
Histology
◇ loss of papillae and hyperparakeratosis; proliferation of the spinous layer with elongation, branching, and anastomosis of rete ridges; increased vascularity, lymphocytic infiltrate in connective tissue; and degeneration and hyalinization within the underlying muscle.

DIFFERENTIAL
• Benign migratory glossitis
• Radiation mucositis
• Chemotherapy mucositis
• Chemical or thermal burn
• Pernicious anemia (vitamin B_{12} deficiency)

TREATMENT

General
◇ treatment is necessary only if the patient has symptoms.
◇ Control of systemic diabetes disease.
◇ Management of chronic Candida infections.

MEDICATIONS
• Modification of drug regimen to control diabetes (ie, insulin or oral hypoglycemic agents).
• Antifungal agents
◇ oral/topical clotrimazole, ketaconazole, nystatin.

SURGERY
Biopsy if necessary for diagnosis.

CONSULTATION SUGGESTIONS
Oral Medicine

REFERRAL SUGGESTIONS
Oral Medicine

PATIENT INSTRUCTIONS
Reassure lesion not premalignant.

COURSE/PROGNOSIS
• Sometimes lesions will regress spontaneously without treatment.
• Use of antifungal agents may cause lesions to regress.
• Control of underlying diabetic disturbance will occasionally result in regression.
• Because lesion is generally innocuous, elimination is usually not required.

CODING

ICD-9-CM
250.00 Type II, non-insulin dependent, adult onset, or unspecified, not stated as uncontrolled.
250.01 Type I, insulin dependent, juvenile type onset, not stated as uncontrolled.
250.02 Type II, non-insulin dependent, adult onset, or unspecified type, uncontrolled.
250.03 Type I, insulin dependent, juvenile type, uncontrolled.
592.2 Median rhomboid glossitis

CPT
41100 Biopsy, tongue, anterior 2/3
99000 Transport specimen to outside laboratory

MISCELLANEOUS

SYNONYMS
Central papillary atrophy of the tongue.

SEE ALSO
Glossitis
Diabetes mellitus
Candidiasis

REFERENCES
Farman AG, vanWyk CW, Staz J, Hugo M, Dreyer WP: Central papillary atrophy of the tongue. Oral Surg Oral Med Oral Path, 43:48-58, 1977.

Carter LC: MRG: A puzzling entity. Compend Contin Educ Dent, 11:446-451, 1990.

Walsh LJ, Cleveland DB, Cumming CG: Quantitative evaluation of Langerhans' cells in median rhomboid glossitis. J Oral Path Med, 21:28-33, 1992.

AUTHOR
Dale J. Misiek, DMD

Melanoma

DESCRIPTION
- Malignancy of melanocytes.
- There are five major forms:
  Superficial spreading melanoma (70%)
  Nodular melanoma (15%)
  Lentigo maligna melanoma (4 to 10%)
  Acral-lentiginous melanoma (2 to 8%)
  Mucosal melanoma

- Melanocytes are one type of dendritic cell found in the epidermis and in various mucosal epithelia. When malignant transformation of these cells occurs, tumor is called a melanoma. Melanocytic nevi are also composed of melanocytes and can undergo malignant transformation.
- Light complexion individuals have a higher predisposition to development of melanoma than darker complexion.
- Increased sun exposure plays a direct role, but history of even a single severe blistering sunburn may be as significant as chronic exposure.
- Dysplastic nevi especially in conjunction with familial history of melanoma display an increased relative risk.
- People having a total body count of greater than 20 melanocytic nevi (>2 mm) may begin to show an increased risk, and greater than 50 total nevi is considered to greatly increase the risk of melanoma.
- Familial history is important.
- Congenital nevi display an increased risk.
- Lentigo meligna lesions should be closely followed due to possible malignant transformation.
- Mucosal lesions do not follow race predilection of skin melanomas. Darker complexion individuals may have a slightly increased risk in mucosal, palmar and plantar lesions.

SYSTEMS AFFECTED
Skin
  ◊ all surfaces at risk with sun exposed > non-sun exposed.
Oral mucosa
  ◊ all mucosal surfaces may be affected. Gingiva and palate are the most common sites.
Eye
  ◊ conjunctiva, retina
- Nasal mucosa accounted for 55% of head and neck mucosal melanomas in one study. Oral mucosa accounted for 40%.
- In general, all upper aero-digestive tract mucosa can be involved.

DIAGNOSIS

SYMPTOMS AND SIGNS
- Lesions generally black, blue-black, or brown. Can be hypopigmented.
- Generally flat with or without visible spread beneath superficial epithelium. Can be raised.
- Nasal congestion
- Epistaxis/bleeding mucosa
- Remember ABCDE eponym
  A = asymmetry, lesion cannot be divided into mirror images
  B = border, edges display notches or other irregularities
  C = color, there is variation in color within the lesion
  D = diameter, should be able to cover the lesion with a pencil eraser
  E = evolution, if it is changing it needs to be biopsied.

LABORATORY
No specific laboratory tests are available.

IMAGING/SPECIAL TESTS
Biopsy lesion. Imperative that regional node assessment is performed and recorded prior to biopsy. All oral nevi should be excised. Periapical radiographs can be of help in confirming the diagnosis of amalgam tattoos if the metallic fragments are radiographically evident. Remember that deciduous teeth long since exfoliated may have had amalgam restorations.

DIFFERENTIAL
- Amalgam tattoo
- Melanocytic nevus
- Peutz-Jeghers syndrome
- Vascular/blood derived lesion
- Pigmented seborrheic keratosis
- Dysplastic nevus
- Pigmented actinic keratosis
- Lentigo maligna
- Sebaceous carcinoma

TREATMENT

MEDICATIONS
• Chemotherapy is generally aimed at palliation and quality of life. Various regimens have been used.
• Specific active immunotherapy continues to show promise for the future.

SURGERY
• Surgical excision is the therapy of choice with the general consensus being 1 cm margins, though 3 cm margins have also been recommended in areas where feasible. In lesions less than 1 mm in thickness it appears that simply clear margins does not improve prognosis versus larger margins.
• Excisions to limiting anatomic barrier, if applicable.
• Elective node dissections do not aid in survivability though it may be done when imaging studies display evidence of single chain involvement.
• Mohs surgery not indicated.

IRRADIATION
Not indicated

CONSULTATION SUGGESTIONS
Dermatologist, Oncologist, Head and Neck Surgeon

REFERRAL SUGGESTIONS
Primary Care Physician, Dermatologist, Oncologist, Head and Neck Surgeon

PATIENT INSTRUCTIONS
Visit physician frequently for careful examinations to detect recurrences or new lesions. Contact National Cancer Institute for helpful literature (301)496-5583.

COURSE/PROGNOSIS
• Most studies agree that oral lesions have a 10 to 25% 5-year survival. One M.D. Anderson study showed a 45% survival rate for head and neck mucosal melanomas.
• Overall skin survival at 10 years is 75% with histologic depth of invasion and histologic type being important prognostic factors.
• Presence of metastatic lesions is a dire predictor with most only surviving 6 months.

 CODING

ICD-9-CM
143.9 Malignant neoplasm, gingiva
145.0 Malignant neoplasm, buccal mucosa
145.2 Malignant neoplasm, hard palate
145.3 Malignant neoplasm, soft palate
145.9 Malignant neoplasm, mouth, unspecified
172.0 Melanoma, lip
172.3 Melanoma, unspecified parts of the face
172.4 Melanoma, neck and scalp

CPT
11100 Biopsy, skin
13131 Mouth, repair, complex
40808 Biopsy, mouth intraoral
41116 Mouth, excision, lesion

 MISCELLANEOUS

SYNONYMS
Malignant melanoma

SEE ALSO
Amalgam tattoo

REFERENCES
Regezi JA, Sciubba J: Oral Pathology. 2nd ed. Philadelphia, WB Saunders, 1992, pp. 167-171.

Moschella SL, Hurley HJ: Dermatology. 3rd ed. Philadelphia, WB Saunders, 1991, pp. 1745-1763.

Rhodes AR, Weinstock MA, Fitzpatrick TB, et al: Risk factors for cutaneous melanoma. A practical method of recognizing predisposed individuals. JAMA 258:3146-3154, 1987.

Breslow A: Thickness, cross-sectional areas and depth of invasion in the prognosis of cutaneous melanoma. Ann Surg 172:902, 1970.

Cochran AJ, et al: Malignant melanoma of the skin. In: Cancer treatment, 4th ed. Haskell CM (ed), Philadelphia, WB Saunders, Co., 1995, pp. 810-824.

Epithelial pathology. In: Oral and Maxillofacial Pathology. Neville BW, et al (eds), Philadelphia, WB Saunders, Co., 1995, pp. 312-321.

AUTHOR
Joseph W. Hellstein, DDS

Meniere's Disease

BASICS

DESCRIPTION
Meniere's disease (MD) is a complex, progressive disorder of the inner ear, characterized by recurrent vertigo, sensory hearing loss, tinnitus, and auricular fullness.

ETIOLOGY

• The exact cause and pathogenesis of MD is unknown.
• The most common explanation is a multifactorial genetic abnormality with disturbance of the endolymphatic duct or sac leading to endolymphatic dysfunctional absorption and then to hydrops.
• There may be contributing extrinsic causes, including:
  • Infection/Inflammation
  • Otosclerosis
  • Trauma
  • Syphilis
  • Allergy
  • Tumor
  • Leukemia
  • Autoimmunity

SYSTEMS AFFECTED
Cochlear
  ◊ progressive, fluctuating, unilateral or bilateral sensorineural hearing loss (usually low frequencies first), tinnitus, loudness intolerance, diplacusis (a perception of the same sound with different pitches in the ears), membrane rupture may be present. Bilateral hearing loss is reported in approximately 50% of patients followed long-term.
Vestibular
  ◊ episodic paroxysmal vertigo with possible nausea and vomiting.
Autonomic nervous system
  ◊ possible pathologic changes involving the brain and brain stem have been reported, including an abnormal pupillary reflex on the affected side during or close to the time of attacks of vertigo and nystagmus.

DIAGNOSIS

SYMPTOMS AND SIGNS
Vestibular
  ◊ severe, episodic vertigo associated with nausea, vomiting, and perspiration lasting from less than 1 hour to several days.
Cochlear
  ◊ progressive fluctuating unilateral or bilateral hearing loss, continuous tinnitus, intolerance to loud sounds, diplacusis.
Aural
  ◊ episodic pressure sensation described as a dull headache which can be diffuse or fullness in the affected ear.
• Fluctuating, low-tone sensorineural hearing loss, normal stance and gait between attacks without nystagmus, and usually a normal otoscopic exam.

LABORATORY
• Treponema antigen test, possible glucose metabolism test and thyroid function test.

IMAGING/SPECIAL TESTS
• Complete audiologic test
• Caloric vestibular test
• Electrocochleography
• Sinusoidal harmonic acceleration
• Electronystagmography
• Brain stem audiometry
• Routine mastoid radiographic series
• CT scan with enhancement
• MRI with enhancement
• Posturography

DIFFERENTIAL
Psychogenic vertigo, central nervous system causes of vertigo, idiopathic postural vertigo, benign paroxysmal positional vertigo and vertigo of childhood, vestibular neuronitis, labyrinthitis, labyrinthine fistula, herpes zoster, labyrinthine concussion or fracture of the temporal bone, otosclerosis, Paget's disease, latent congenital syphilis, ototoxicity, intermittent tubotympanitis, barotrauma with sudden hearing loss, intralabyrinthine hemorrhage, vertebral basilary ischemia, vascular disease, multiple sclerosis, tumor of the cerebellar pontine angle, hereditary ataxia, vestibular epilepsy, postural imbalance of the elderly.

TREATMENT

General
◇ Low salt diet may reduce major attacks.

MEDICATIONS
• Steroid therapy
◇ dexamethasone 4 mg a day for 2 weeks then tapered for 3 months.
• Hydrochlorothiazide 50 mg every other day.
• Meclizine (Antivert, Bonine) 25 to 100 mg p.o. hs may control vertigo.
• Transdermal scopolamine patches may be useful for nausea control.
• Atropine 0.2 to 0.4 mg IV diazepam, thought to cause vestibular sedation, may give acute vertigo relief.
• Aminoglycoside administration by various routes is used as a vestibular ablative agent although ototoxicity may occur.

SURGERY
• Used when MD becomes intractable or progressive for vestibular symptoms and deafness in spite of prolonged medical treatment.
• Conservative surgical procedure (endolymphatic enhancement), used commonly, has the potential to reverse the pathogenesis of MD.
• Destructive surgical procedure (labyrinthectomy or vestibular nerve section) is used for intractable vertigo.

CONSULTATION SUGGESTIONS
Otolaryngologist, Neurologist

REFERRAL SUGGESTIONS
Primary Care Physician

COURSE/PROGNOSIS
• MD is a chronic recurrent disease that persists for years.
• Remission or improvement of vertigo, tinnitus, and hearing loss after treatment may occur. Tinnitus and hearing loss may be permanent. The disease may progress to complete deafness.

CODING

ICD-9-CM
38600 Meniere's disease unspecified site
38601 Meniere's disease cochleovestibular
38602 Meniere's disease cochlear
38603 Meniere's disease vestibular

MISCELLANEOUS

SYNONYMS
Paroxysmal labyrinthine vertigo

SEE ALSO
Multiple sclerosis
Syphilis
Seizure disorders
Otitis

REFERENCES
Shea JJ: The classification and treatment of Meniere's disease. Acta Oto-Rhino-Laryngologica Belg 47:303-310, 1993.

Paparella MM: Methods of diagnosis and treatment of Meniere's disease. Acta Otolaryngol (Stockh) 485 (suppl):108-119, 1991.

Dickens JR, Graham SS: Meniere's disease: 1983-1989. Am J Otol 11:51-65 1990.

AUTHOR
Daniel S. Sarasin, DDS

Meningitis

BASICS

DESCRIPTION
An infectious process (usually viral or bacterial) involving the meninges and cerebrospinal fluid. The viral type is much more common and often much less virulent than the bacterial counterpart.

ETIOLOGY

• Viral type is most commonly caused by Coxsackie A or B, ECHO virus, cytomegalovirus, Herpes simplex or zoster, Epstein-Barr virus, and adenovirus.
• Bacterial type is most commonly caused by Hemophilus influenza, Strep. pneumoniae, Neisseria meningitidis, Listeria monocytogenism, and E. coli.
• Several factors predispose the patient to an increased risk of developing meningitis. The most common factor is an immunocompromised host. Previous neurosurgic procedures and open head injuries (eg, skull base fractures with involvement of the paranasal sinuses) are major factors with regard to the bacterial causes of meningitis.

SYSTEMS AFFECTED
Neurologic
◊ deficits are often found in both types of meningitis, including alteration in mentation, headache, photophobia, seizures, confusion, stupor, and coma.
Musculoskeletal
◊ problems are often characterized by stiff neck and back, polyarthralgia (especially viral syndromes) rigors, and muscle weakness.
Respiratory
◊ infections may in many cases precede or accompany both types of meningitis.
Gastrointestinal
◊ disturbances are usually limited to nausea and vomiting secondary to central nervous system pathology.
Integument and mucosa
◊ may have lesions which are commonly found during the acute phase of the viral infection (eg, blotchy skin rash found with Coxsackie A, multiple painful vesicles on the soft palate, and tonsillar pillars found with herpangina).

DIAGNOSIS

SYMPTOMS AND SIGNS
• Headache
• Nausea and vomiting
• Photophobia
• Fatigue
• Lethargy
• Fever
• Stiff neck (Kernig's and Brudzinski's signs)
• Seizures
• Muscle weakness
• Disorientation and confusion
• Focal neurologic deficits
• Upper or lower respiratory infection
• Rash

LABORATORY
• CBC with differential
• Cerebral spinal fluid (CSF) for WBCs, glucose, protein, CSF Gram stain and culture and sensitivity.
• Intracranial pressure measured during lumbar puncture (opening pressure).
• Blood cultures

IMAGING/SPECIAL TESTS
• CT scan or MRI of the brain
• Chest radiograph, if respiratory infection suspected.
• Sinus series, if sinus infection considered possible source.
• CSF for selected viral antibodies.
• CSF for selected bacterial antibodies.

DIFFERENTIAL
• Viral meningitis
• Bacterial meningitis
• Encephalitis
• Sepsis
• Brain abscess
• Viral syndrome
• Seizures
• Meningeal leukemia

Meningitis

TREATMENT

General
◇ Viral type
  ◇ bed rest, IV fluids, control fever, and manage nausea and vomiting.
Bacterial type
  ◇ usually more complicated, requires an ICU setting. IV antibiotics and fluids are instituted early, immediately after the lumbar puncture. Therapy is also directed at any coexisting disease.

MEDICATIONS
• Antibiotics are given empirically in suspected bacterial cases. The most commonly used regimens are ampicillin in combination with a third generation cephalosporin (eg, cefotaxime) or an aminoglycoside (eg, tobramycin).
• Acetaminophen to control fever.
• Narcotic analgesics often have to be used for pain control (eg, morphine 0.1 mg/kg q. 4 h).
• Antiemetics are used in cases of protracted nausea and vomiting (eg, phenergan 25 mg IM q. 4 h).
• There is usually no indication to administer any type of antiviral agent in cases of viral meningitis.

CONSULTATION SUGGESTIONS
Neurologist, Infectious Disease Specialist

REFERRAL SUGGESTIONS
Primary Care Physician

FIRST STEPS TO TAKE IN AN EMERGENCY
• Seizures or altered consciousness mandates admission to intensive care unit.

PATIENT INSTRUCTIONS
If bacterial meningitis diagnosed, notify recent contacts of infected individual and warn them of possible spread of disease to them.

COURSE/PROGNOSIS
• Viral meningitis runs a course of approximately 5 to 7 days and carries an excellent overall prognosis with complete recovery within 2 weeks.
• Bacterial meningitis carries an overall fatality rate of 10 to 20% depending on the causative bacteria. In severe cases, focal neurologic deficits may be permanent.

CODING

ICD-9-CM
047.9 Viral meningitis
320.9 Bacterial meningitis
322.9 Meningitis

MISCELLANEOUS

SYNONYMS
Viral meningitis
Aseptic meningitis
Abacterial meningitis

SEE ALSO
Seizure disorder
Headache

REFERENCES
Feigin RD, McCracken GH, Klein JO: Diagnosis and management of meningitis. Pediatr Infect Dis J 11:785-814, 1992.

Vetter R, Iverson GR, Kuzel MD: Adult meningitis: rapid identification for Scheld WM: Bacterial meningitis and brain abscess. In: Harrison's Principles of Internal Medicine, 13th ed. Isselbacher KJ, et al (eds), New York, McGraw-Hill, Inc. 1994, pp. 2296-2302.

AUTHOR
Joseph J. Sansevere, DMD

Mitral Valve Diseases

BASICS

DESCRIPTION
• The mitral valve lies between the left atrium and ventricle, and consists of five components: the mitral anulus, mitral leaflets, chordae tendineae, papillary muscles, and ventricular myocardium supporting these muscles. All five components must be effective for the valve to remain competent.

Mitral Stenosis:
• Mitral stenosis is generally caused by rheumatic fever and may rarely be congenital. The acute episode occurs in childhood, but may not become symptomatic until teenage years.
- the rheumatic process results in scarring and thickening of the leaflets, narrowing the valve orifice. Additionally, the chordae tendineae may shorten and contribute to associated mitral regurgitation.
- left atrial size may increase and thrombi may form as a result of stasis of blood in the left atrium.
- women predominate over men 3:1.

Mitral Regurgitation (Insufficiency):
• Mitral regurgitation results when any of the functional anatomic aspects of the valve fails
- if the anulus becomes calcified
- rheumatic fever may cause thickening and calcification of the leaflets. Commissures become adherent, the chordae shorten and retract the leaflets preventing proper opposition.
- myxomatous degeneration of the leaflets cause prolapse into the left atrium.
- papillary muscles may become ischemic or infarcted resulting in shortening during systole.
- left ventricular myocardial infarction or dilatation may cause malposition of the papillary muscles and cause regurgitation.
- women experience rheumatic mitral regurgitation three times more frequently than do men.
- patients over 40 years of age have higher incidence of coronary artery disease and secondary ischemia of papillary muscles or ventricular dilation.

Mitral Valve Prolapse
• Mitral valve prolapse (MVP) is characterized by redundant mitral leaflets that bulge into the left atrium during systole.
- most cases are idiopathic
- few cases of MVP are seen with Marfan's syndrome, atrial septal defect, congenital heart disease, or rheumatic valve disease.
- some patients may show echocardiographic evidence of myxomatous degeneration of the mitral leaflets.
- prolapse may occur secondary to bacterial endocarditis of the mitral valve.
- prevalence is unknown but estimates vary from 0.3% to 15%.
- most patients are under 40 years of age and women far outnumber men.

ETIOLOGY

Rheumatic fever is the most common cause of mitral valve disease.

SYSTEMS AFFECTED
Cardiac
◇ hypertrophy, atrial fibrillation, heart failure.
Pulmonary
◇ pulmonary edema due to congestive heart failure.
Central nervous system
◇ emboli from atrial thrombosis.
Musculo-skeletal
◇ weakness due to poor cardiac output.

DIAGNOSIS

SYMPTOMS AND SIGNS
Mitral Stenosis:
• As obstruction of flow into the left ventricle worsens, left atrial pressure increases and is transmitted to the pulmonary veins.
• The patient will complain of dyspnea and orthopnea.
• With increased dilation of the left atrium, atrial fibrillation may occur.
• Pulmonary hypertension may occur and can cause right ventricular failure with pedal edema, ascites, and hepatomegaly.
• The second heart sound is split with accentuation of P2 in pulmonary hypertension.
• An opening snap may be heard, followed by a low-frequency diastolic rumble.
• The diastolic rumble is best heard with the bell of the stethoscope at the apex of the heart in the left lateral decubitus position.
• When due to rheumatic fever, mitral stenosis has long, asymptomatic latency period, with symptoms developing 2 decades after insult, and disability not present until the fourth decade. Dyspnea and cough after exertion appear, with progressively less exercise producing symptoms. Atrial fibrillation occurs due to atrial enlargement with production of an irregularly, irregular pulse. Increased pulmonary vascular pressure can produce hemoptysis, chest pain, pulmonary infections, tricuspid regurgitation, and a right ventricular tap along left sternal border due to right ventricular enlargement. Heart sound changes include a loud S1, an opening snap followed by a low pitched, rumbling diastolic murmur and a soft systolic murmur. Atrial thrombus formation can lead to cerebral emboli, while damaged valve surfaces are predisposed to infective endocarditis, as well as respective associated symptoms and signs.
Mitral Regurgitation:
• Dyspnea secondary to an increase in left atrial pressure which is transmitted into the pulmonary veins with resultant pulmonary edema.
• Fatigue due to diminished cardiac output late in the course of the disease.
• Apex of heart displaced beyond mid-clavicular line secondary to ventricular dilatation.
• Holosystolic murmur radiating from apex to the base or to the axilla.
• With pulmonary hypertension, P2 (pulmonic valve closure) is increased and splitting of the second heart sound is accentuated.
• An S3 gallop can be heard representing early diastolic filling.

Mitral Valve Prolapse:
• Most important finding is a mid- or late systolic click before the first heart sound, followed by a late systolic crescendo-decrescendo murmur heard best at the apex.
• The click and murmur are accentuated by the Valsalva maneuver which decreases left ventricular volume, and is diminished by squatting and isometric exercise which increase left ventricular end-diastolic volume.
• Non-anginal chest pain is common.
• Atrial and ventricular premature beats and pre-excitation syndromes are frequent.
• Sudden death has been reported but is rare.
• Thoracic abnormalities are common such as pectus excavatum, straight back syndrome, and thoracic scoliosis.
• Click sound may vary in the same patients making diagnosis difficult.
• Most patients asymptomatic, but patient may experience palpitations, light-headedness, syncope, and fatigue. Dysrhythmias such as paroxysmal supraventricular and ventricular tachycardia, and frequent premature ventricular contractions may occur. On auscultation the heart will have a characteristic mid- or late systolic click followed by high pitched, late systolic crescendo-decrescendo murmur.

IMAGING/SPECIAL TESTS
• Mitral Stenosis:
• Chest radiograph
◇ reveals left atrial enlargement, shown by a double density beneath an elevated left main-stem bronchus.
    • pulmonary venous congestion may be evident.
    • a calcified mitral valve may be seen in the lateral chest film.
• ECG may show left atrial enlargement and right axis deviation.
• Echocardiogram
◇ can establish presence of mitral stenosis, but cannot quantify the severity.
• Angiocardiography
◇ can document the pressure gradient between the left atrium and ventricle in diastole.
• Mitral Regurgitation (MR):
• Chest radiograph reveals left ventricular enlargement and cardiomegaly.
    • the left atrium may enlarge and be seen as a "double density" under the left main-stem bronchus.
    • may see pulmonary congestion and signs of pulmonary edema.
• ECG
◇ may reveal left atrial enlargement with negative P waves in V1.
    • with increasing left atrial dilation, atrial fibrillation is common.
    • left ventricular hypertrophy causes increased QRS voltage and repolarization abnormalities in the ST segments and T waves.

• Echocardiography
◇ Doppler reveals dilated left ventricle and left atrium, and is best diagnostic study for MR.
    • may see reason for regurgitation such as structural abnormalities of the mitral valve.
• Cardiac catheterization
◇ can assess the hemodynamic burden and determine the presence of concomitant coronary artery disease.
• Mitral Valve Prolapse:
• ECG
◇ inverted T waves may occur in the inferior leads. Prolonged QT intervals are frequent and are associated with premature atrial or ventricular contractions.
• Echocardiogram
◇ shows late systolic displacement of one or both leaflets into the left atrium. Doppler studies may reveal associated MR.
• Angiocardiography will show mitral regurgitation and reveal the mitral leaflets protruding beyond their closure line into the left atrium.

DIFFERENTIAL
• Cardiomyopathy
• Myocardial infarction
• Infective endocarditis
• Congestive heart failure

(continued)

TREATMENT

Mitral Stenosis (MS):
Symptoms of pulmonary congestion and dyspnea respond to sodium restriction and diuretics.
• Atrial fibrillation should be treated with digoxin, but should have electrical cardioversion to decrease risk of emboli. MS patients with sinus rhythm get little benefit from digoxin.
• Patients with atrial fibrillation should be treated with anti-coagulation therapy to prevent systemic emboli.
• Patients who are symptomatic with minimal exertion should undergo surgical management with commissurotomy or valve replacement. Percutaneous balloon valvuloplasty is available that may be useful for young patients with MS.
• Diseased or valve replacement patients should be covered with antibiotic prophylaxis prior to surgical procedures.

Mitral Regurgitation:
While mild regurgitation is asymptomatic it requires only endocarditis prophylaxis during dental care.
• As symptoms of dyspnea, orthopnea, paroxysmal nocturnal dyspnea and fatigue appear, restriction of dietary sodium, diuretic therapy, exercise limitations, and digitoxin may be necessary.
• Atrial fibrillation should be converted to sinus rhythm, otherwise the rate of the ventricular response is controlled with digitalis.
• Patients may benefit from arterial vasodilators to reduce afterload and increase cardiac output.
• With increasing dyspnea, despite medical therapy, the mitral valve should be replaced.
    • these can be prosthetic disc or ball valve, or porcine heterograft. Prosthetic valves require lifelong anticoagulation. Both require antibiotic prophylaxis prior to invasive surgery.

Mitral Valve Prolapse:
Mitral valve prolapse patients are generally treated with antibiotic prophylaxis during dental/surgical procedures.
• The degree of mitral regurgitation determines the risk of sudden death as well as the prevalence of dysrhythmias. Use of beta-blocker such as propranolol may be helpful in treatment of atypical chest pain that accompanies MVP, but this is somewhat controversial.

MEDICATIONS
• See general treatment.

SURGERY
• See general treatment.

CONSULTATION SUGGESTIONS
Cardiologist, Thoracic Surgeon

REFERRAL SUGGESTIONS
Primary Care Physician, Cardiologist

FIRST STEPS TO TAKE IN AN EMERGENCY
• If severe dyspnea, consider pulmonary edema and treat accordingly.
• If severe chest discomfort, consider myocardial ischemia and treat accordingly.

PATIENT INSTRUCTIONS
• Inform all dental providers of need for endocarditis prophylaxis. (See Endocarditis p. 182).
• Can contact American Heart Association (214)373-6300 for useful patient information.

COURSE/PROGNOSIS
Mitral stenosis
    ◊ disability by 4th decade but good prognosis with commissurotomy and/or valve replacement.
Mitral valve prolapse
    ◊ runs typically benign course, particularly with proper care.

CODING

ICD-9-CM
  394.0 Mitral stenosis
  394.1 Mitral insufficiency
  394.2 Mitral stenosis with insufficiency
  394.9 Other and unspecified mitral valve diseases
  424.0 Mitral valve disorders

CPT
  90780 IV infusion for therapy
  90788 Intramuscular injection of antibiotic

MISCELLANEOUS

SYNONYMS
Mitral regurgitation
Mitral insufficiency
Mitral valve prolapse
Systolic murmur click syndrome
Mitral click murmur click syndrome

SEE ALSO
Aortic valve
Congestive heart failure
Rheumatic fever
Atrial fibrillation
Endocarditis
Pulmonary edema

REFERENCES
Internal Medicine for Dentistry 2nd ed.
Rose FL, Kaye D. (eds), St. Louis, CV
Mosby Co. 1990.

Braunwald E: Valvular Heart Disease. In:
Harrison's Principles of Internal Medicine
13th ed., Isselbacher KJ, et al (eds),
New York, McGraw-Hill, 1994, pp. 1052-
1059.

AUTHOR
Jerry L. Jones, DDS, MD

Mononucleosis, Infectious

BASICS

DESCRIPTION
Viral infection due to the Epstein-Barr virus (EBV) that generally involves persons in the range of ages 15 to 35 years old. It affects the lymphoreticular system and is earmarked by a classic triad of signs: fever, pharyngitis, and cervical lymphadenopathy. Infection is self-limited and leads to a carrier state which confers life-long immunity.

ETIOLOGY

EBV belongs to the DNA group of Herpesviruses. It was first identified in 1964 and etiologically linked to mononucleosis in 1973. The virus is shed in oropharyngeal secretions, which is also the main route of entry. It replicates in the oropharyngeal and nasopharyngeal epithelial tissues, salivary tissues, and in B lymphocytes. The peak incidence occurs between 15 and 19 years of age. The peak age for males occurs slightly later than for females, 18 to 23, and 15 to 16 years of age, respectively.

SYSTEMS AFFECTED
Oropharynx
◇ sore throat, edematous uvula, palatal petechiae. At risk for tonsillar enlargement resulting in airway obstruction.
Lymphatics
◇ generalized lymphadenopathy from the lymphocytosis, including marked cervical lymphadenopathy, enlarged tonsils.
Cardiac
◇ pericarditis, ECG changes.
Spleen
◇ splenomegaly; at risk for rupture either spontaneously or secondary to trauma.
Liver
◇ hepatitis, hepatomegaly, jaundice.
Renal
◇ nephrotic syndrome, glomerulonephritis.
Hematologic
◇ thrombocytopenia, lymphocytosis, hemolytic anemia (rare).
Skin
◇ nonspecific rash, urticaria.
Neurologic
◇ altered mentation, Guillain-Barre syndrome, Bell's palsy, encephalitis, optic neuritis, cerebellar ataxia, Reye's syndrome.
Ophthalmic
◇ periorbital edema, dry eyes, keratitis, uveitis, conjunctivitis, retinitis, ophthalmoplegia.

Pulmonary (rare)
◇ hilar and mediastinal lymphadenopathy, interstitial pneumonia

DIAGNOSIS

SYMPTOMS AND SIGNS
• Onset occurs within 4 to 7 weeks after exposure.
Prodrome
◇ lasts approximately 5 to 7 days with malaise, fatigue, headache, arthralgias, fevers/chills, dysphagia, and anorexia. In persons over the age of 40, the presentation is commonly atypical without many of the former symptoms. Instead, those older than 40 years of age present with fever, jaundice, and hepatomegaly, leading to diagnostic confusion.
Fever
◇ lasting for 3 or more weeks.
Pharyngitis
◇ results in sore throat, difficulty swallowing, possible dehydration.
Lymphadenopathy
◇ generalized and cervical in particular.
Splenomegaly
◇ tender and enlarged in the left upper quadrant of abdomen.
Hepatomegaly
◇ tender and enlarged in the right upper quadrant of abdomen.
Skin
◇ nonspecific rash, urticaria.
Ophthalmic
◇ periorbital edema, dry eyes, conjunctivitis, ophthalmoplegia.
Hematologic
◇ during active infection, there is an increase in IgG, IgM antibodies to viral capsid antigens (VCA) and transient antibodies to diffuse antigen, and no antibodies to EBV-nuclear antigen (EBNA). Because patients do not present early enough in the course of the disease prior to the VCA-IgG levels decreasing, the most accurate hallmark during the active phase is the VCA-IgM antibodies. When the disease progresses beyond the active phase, the antibody most sensitive as marker of recent infection is the VCA-IgG. The VCA-IgM and anti-EBNA are not present. In the carrier state, only moderate levels of VCA-IgG and anti-EBNA are found. If the patient is immunosuppressed, there is a different variation in the timing of the antibodies formed.

LABORATORY
CBC with differential
◇ lymphocytosis secondary to increased numbers of B and T cells.
Thrombocytopenia
◇ occurs in 50% of persons.

IMAGING/SPECIAL TESTS
Monospot test
◇ evaluates heterophil antibodies via latex agglutination. Is only about 80% sensitive in adults; has poorer sensitivity in children less than 4 years old; infants do not produce heterophil antibodies. In adults, has false-positive rate of approximately 15% secondary to other viruses like adenovirus, CMV, and toxoplasmosis.
ELISA, Western blot
◇ can also be performed.

DIFFERENTIAL
• Strep throat
• Diphtheria
• Hodgkin's
• Leukemias
• Lymphomas
• CMV
• Rubella
• HIV
• Hepatitis A/B
• Toxoplasmosis

TREATMENT

General
◇ Supportive, bed rest, no strenuous exercise for 3 to 4 weeks, particularly with splenomegaly.

MEDICATIONS
• Acetaminophen or ibuprofen for pain or discomfort. Avoid aspirin due to possibility of Reye's syndrome.
• May give gamma globulin for cases not responsive to corticosteroids in situations above.
• Acyclovir is not routinely recommended because it does not shorten the length of infection.
• No antibiotics indicated.
• In severe, life-threatening airway obstruction due to tonsillar hyperplasia may elect to give corticosteroids as adjunct treatment with intubation. Other indications for corticosteroids are neurologic changes, hemolytic anemia, thrombocytopenic purpura, myocarditis or pericarditis.

SURGERY
If splenic rupture occurs, this is a life-threatening emergency requiring splenectomy due to the internal hemorrhage. This the most common fatal complication.

CONSULTATION SUGGESTIONS
Primary Care Physician

REFERRAL SUGGESTIONS
Primary Care Physician

PATIENT INSTRUCTIONS
Rest during recuperation important for increased speed of recovery.

COURSE/PROGNOSIS
Generally, if patients recover without fatal or disabling organ system damage, the prognosis is excellent. Splenic rupture occurs in 0.1 to 0.5% of proven infectious mononucleosis.

CODING

ICD-9-CM
075 Infectious mononucleosis

MISCELLANEOUS

SYNONYMS
Mono

SEE ALSO
Herpes Simplex

REFERENCES
Schooley RT: Epstein-Barr virus infections. In: Harrison's Principles of Internal Medicine, 13th ed. Isselbacher KJ, et al (eds), New York, McGraw-Hill, 1994, pp. 790-793.

Tierney LM, McPhee SJ, Papadakis MA: Current Medical Diagnosis and Treatment. New York, Appleton and Lange, 1994, pp.1103-1104.

Axelrod P, Finestone AJ: Infectious Mononucleosis in older adults. Am Fam Phys 42:1599-1606, 1990.

Bailey RE: Diagnosis and treatment of infectious mononucleosis. Am Fam Phys 49:879-885, 1994.

AUTHOR
Roger S. Badwal, DMD, MD

Mucocele

BASICS

DESCRIPTION
• Mucocele is a generic clinical term referring to benign raised lesions consisting of collection of mucus in the oral soft tissues; because of distinctive etiology, pathogenesis, and microscopy, the terms mucus extravasation phenomenon, mucus retention cyst, and superficial mucocele are used to describe the lesions after microscopic evaluation.
• Mucus extravasation phenomenon is the most common "mucocele," usually found on the lower lip, with nearly half of these painless swellings being reported before the age of 21; a superficial lesion appears as a raised, circumscribed vesicle with a translucent or bluish hue; a deeper lesion presents as a swelling with a color similar to the adjacent mucosa; they range in size from a few millimeters to a few centimeters.
• Mucus retention cyst is a much less common "mucocele," usually appearing after 50 years of age; it may appear on the palate, buccal mucosa or floor of mouth, with only rare presentation on the lower lip. They present as mobile, nontender, painless swellings with a similar color to the adjacent mucosa; size ranges from 3 to 10 mm.
• Superficial mucocele is the most recently described "mucocele," usually presenting as 3 to 4 mm clear vesicles. They may be single or multiple, and appear on non-inflamed mucosa of the soft palate, retromolar area, or posterior buccal mucosa. They usually rupture within 24 hours and are more common in women than in men, with an age range of 20 to 70 years.

ETIOLOGY

Mucus extravasation phenomenon
◊ trauma to a minor salivary gland excretory duct, with collection of mucus in the adjacent connective tissue stroma.
Mucus retention cysts
◊ excretory duct obstruction of a minor salivary gland resulting in blockage of salivary flow.
Superficial mucocele
◊ there are no known etiologic or precipitating factors, although some appear related to various foods and beverages.

SYSTEMS AFFECTED
Oral cavity

DIAGNOSIS

SYMPTOMS AND SIGNS
Mucus retention phenomenon
◊ painless, movable swelling with a pink to bluish hue, sometimes with an inflammatory reaction.
Extremely large or ulcerated, secondarily infected mucus retention phenomenon may interfere with mastication or speech. Mucus-filled vesicles raised well above the adjacent mucosa with minimal inflammatory reaction.
Mucus retention cysts
◊ painless, movable swelling with a color resembling the adjacent mucosa. Mucus-filled cystic cavity lined with ductal epithelium.
Superficial mucocele
◊ clear, tense vesicles that may ulcerate leaving a pseudomembrane or ulcer making mastication difficult. Mucus-filled cystic cavity lined with ductal epithelium.

IMAGING/SPECIAL TESTS
Biopsy (incisional or excisional)

DIFFERENTIAL
• Pleomorphic adenoma
• Monomorphic adenoma
• Mucoepidermoid carcinoma
• Adenocystic carcinoma
• Adenocarcinoma
• Traumatic fibroma
• Ranula
• Vesiculobullous lesions (superficial mucocele of mucosa)

Mucocele

TREATMENT

SURGERY
Complete surgical excision of lesion and associated minor salivary glands with microscopic examination.

CONSULTATION SUGGESTIONS
Oral-Maxillofacial Surgeon, Oral Medicine

REFERRAL SUGGESTIONS
Oral-Maxillofacial Surgeon

PATIENT INSTRUCTIONS
Lesion have no malignant potential. Will tend to recur even if they spontaneously drain. Complete excision is curative.

COURSE/PROGNOSIS
Recurrence is rare except when incompletely excised; prognosis excellent as this is a benign condition.
Superficial mucocele
◊ may recur but prognosis excellent because of benign course.

CODING

ICD-9-CM
527.6 Mucocele

CPT
40810 Excision lesion of mucosa and submucosa, vestibule of mouth; without repair
40812 with simple repair
41116 Excision, lesion of floor of mouth
42100 Biopsy of palate, uvula
42104 Excision, lesion of palate; without closure
42106 with simple primary closure
99000 Transport of specimen to outside laboratory

MISCELLANEOUS

SYNONYMS
Mucus extravasation phenomenon
Mucus retention cyst
Superficial mucocele

SEE ALSO
Ranula

REFERENCES
Regezi JA, Sciubba J: Oral Pathology Clinical Pathologic Correlations, 2nd ed., Philadelphia, WB Saunders, 1993, pp. 239-246.

Eveson JW: Superficial mucocele: Pitfalls in clinical and microscopic diagnosis. Oral Surg Oral Med Oral Path 66:318-322, 1988.

Jensen JL: Recurrent intraoral vesicles. JADA 120:569-570, 1990.

Bouquot JE, Gundlach KK: Oral exophytic lesions in 23,616 white Americans over 35 years of age. Oral Surg Oral Med Oral Path 62:284-291, 1986.

Praetorius F, Hammarstrom L: A new concept of the pathogenesis of oral mucous cysts based on a study of 200 cases. J Dent Assoc S Afr 47:226-231, 1992.

Dilley DC, Siegel MA, Budnick S: Diagnosing and treating common oral pathologies. Pediatr Clin N Am 38:1227-1264, 1991.

Yamasoba T, Tayama N, Syoji M, Fukuta M: Clinicostatistical study of lower lip mucoceles. Head Neck 12:316-320, 1990.

Bodner L, Tal H: Salivary gland cysts of the oral cavity: clinical observation and surgical management. Compendium 12:150-156, 1992.

AUTHOR
Dennis L. Johnson, DDS, MS

Multiple Myeloma

 BASICS

DESCRIPTION
A malignant proliferation of plasma cells presenting as a prototype of monoclonal gammopathy. It is the most common primary malignancy of bone. The median age of incidence is 60, range 40 to 80, with peak incidence in the 70s. Males predominate, especially among Blacks.

 ETIOLOGY

Exposure to toxic chemicals (benzene) and radiation (atomic and radium-dial) has been implicated. Familial cases have been identified, indicating recessive heredity. In most cases cause is unknown.

SYSTEMS AFFECTED
Hemic
◇ anemia (normochromic, normocytic) is present in 60% of patients at diagnosis; thrombocytopenia also frequently seen.
Immunologic
◇ development of serious bacterial infections with Gram-positive and encapsulated organisms (eg, Streptococcus pneumoniae, Staphylococcus aureus, and Hemophilus influenzae).
Musculoskeletal
◇ bone pain and compression fractures of ribs and vertebrae. Accelerated bone dissolution from osseous lesions leads to hypercalcemia in 20% of patients.
Renal
◇ casts of Bence Jones protein in tubules, hypercalcemia, and dehydration all cause renal insufficiency. Twenty percent of patients present with renal impairment and an additional 20% develop this complication during the course of their disease.

 DIAGNOSIS

SYMPTOMS AND SIGNS
• Bone pain, weakness, fatigue, lethargy, weight loss, epistaxis, and recurrent infections.
• Pathologic fractures, dehydration, ecchymosis, purpura, gingival bleeding, seizures (from hypercalcemia).

LABORATORY
The presence of a monoclonal protein in serum or urine (eg, Bence Jones) found on:
    Serum protein electrophoresis
    Urine protein electrophoresis
CBC
◇ 70% present with anemia. Thrombocytopenia common.
Peripheral blood smear
◇ Rouleaux formation.
Chemistries
◇ Hypercalcemia
Renal functions
◇ increased BUN and creatinine (prerenal azotemia).
ESR
◇ elevated
LDH
◇ elevated

IMAGING/SPECIAL TESTS
Skeletal survey
◇ easiest and most cost efficient. 70% of patients have lytic lesions at diagnosis. Skull and jaw films may reveal solitary or multiple well-defined circular (punched out) radiolucencies.
MRI
◇ valuable in evaluating extent of disease in spine and other sites of marrow.
Technetium bone scan
◇ less diagnostic than in other malignant bone disease.
Bone marrow biopsy
◇ necessary to document bone marrow plasmacytosis.

DIFFERENTIAL
• Metastatic carcinoma to bone
• Primary bone malignancies (sarcomas)
• Solitary plasmacytoma
• Other monoclonal gammopathies
• Hyperparathyroidism and other metabolic bone disease
• Amyloidosis

TREATMENT

General
◇ Transfusion of packed red blood cells and platelets where indicated.
◇ Neupogen (leukocyte growth factor) for leukopenia.
◇ Hydration for dehydration and hypercalcemia.
◇ Encourage activity as immobility worsens condition.

MEDICATIONS
• Chemotherapy is the primary treatment for multiple myeloma. Melphalan and prednisone have provided the best regimen for control.
• IV fluids with normal saline and steroids usually provide a rapid response for treatment of hypercalcemia.
• VAD Therapy (Vincristine, Adriamycin, and Decadron).
• Allopurinol for hyperuricemia.
• Analgesics for bone pain (NSAIDs, narcotics).
• Antibiotics for bacterial infections, cephalosporins for the usual Gram-positive infections.

SURGERY
High-dose chemotherapy and bone marrow transplant for unresponsive cases.

IRRADIATION
Radiation therapy for control of painful bone lesions and pathologic fractures.

CONSULTATION SUGGESTIONS
Hematologist, Oncologist

REFERRAL SUGGESTIONS
Primary Care Physician

FIRST STEPS TO TAKE IN AN EMERGENCY
• Seizure due to hypercalcemia treated with hydration, mithramycin, and corticosteroids.

PATIENT INSTRUCTIONS
Contact American Cancer Society in local area for helpful literature.

COURSE/PROGNOSIS
• With melphalan and prednisone, 40% of patients respond, with complete remission in 5%.
• Median survival is 3 years.

CODING

ICD-9-CM
203.0 Multiple myeloma
238.6 Solitary myeloma

CPT
20134 Excision of malignant tumor or maxilla
20144 Excision of malignant tumor of mandible
70250 Radiologic exam of skull
70350 Cephalogram
70355 Panorex

MISCELLANEOUS

SYNONYMS
Myeloma
Plasmacytoma
Plasma cell dyscrasia monoclonal gammopathy

SEE ALSO
Hypercalcemia
Amyloidosis

REFERENCES
Longo DL: Plasma cell disorders. In: Harrison's Principles of Internal Medicine, 13th ed. Isselbacher KJ, et al (eds), NY, McGraw-Hill, 1994, pp 1618-1625.

Devita VT, Hellman S, Rosenberg SA: Principles and Practices of Oncology, Philadelphia, JB Lippincott, 1995.

Lesson M: Multiple myeloma. In: Griffith's 5 Minute Clinical Consult. Dambro MR (ed), Baltimore, Williams & Wilkins, 1995, pp. 684-685.

AUTHOR
James Vopal, DDS, MD

Multiple Sclerosis

BASICS

DESCRIPTION
Multiple sclerosis (MS) is a progressive degenerative neurologic disease characterized by demyelination of central nervous system axons. The average age at diagnosis is during the fourth decade. MS is a chronic disease with periods of remission and exacerbation; most patients live 25 years after the diagnosis. The earliest symptoms are visual disturbances, muscle weakness, and numbness. Facial numbness is the presenting symptom is 2 to 3% of cases. Trigeminal or glossopharyngeal neuralgia develops in 3 to 5% of MS patients.

ETIOLOGY

The etiology of MS is unknown, although mounting evidence supports the concept of an autoimmune disease with anti-myelin antibodies.

SYSTEMS AFFECTED
Ocular
   ◇ diplopia due to CN III, IV, and VI involvement.
Ophthalmologic
   ◇ loss of acuity, color blindness, total blindness.
Extremities
   ◇ weakness, paresthesia, hyper-reflexia, incoordination.
Maxillofacial
   ◇ mandibular tremor, weakness, dysarthria.
Sensation
   ◇ numbness, neuralgia
Other
   ◇ bladder dysfunction, euphoria

DIAGNOSIS

SYMPTOMS AND SIGNS
• The diagnosis is generally clinical based on the age, multi-focal neurologic symptoms not attributable to a single lesion, history of periods of remission and exacerbation, and slow progression. Ocular and ophthalmologic symptoms appear early. Flares of increased muscle weakness, numbness or paresthesia, and incoordination are suggestive of MS.
• In face, may see ocular paralysis, trigeminal neuralgia, hyperesthesia, sensory dysfunction, and blurred vision.

LABORATORY
There are no definitive laboratory tests for MS. Non-specific elevation of cerebrospinal fluid immunoglobulins is suggestive of MS, although specific serologic tests for MS are being pursued. Abnormal colloidal gold curve and IgG elevation seen in CSF.

IMAGING/SPECIAL TESTS
Magnetic resonance imaging accurately reveals MS-specific plaques in the central nervous system, but these may not be obvious from the onset. CT can also be used.
Visual evoked response
   ◇ abnormal in most MS cases.
Sensory evoked potentials
   ◇ abnormal in most MS cases.

DIFFERENTIAL
• Sarcoidosis
• Syphilis
• Trigeminal neuralgia, when presenting symptom is pain.
• A variety of connective tissue disorders and central nervous system neoplasms characterized by weakness, fatigue, and neurocognitive impairment.

Multiple Sclerosis

TREATMENT

General
◇ Dental treatment for MS patients may be difficult due to involuntary tremor and muscle weakness. Assisted opening and short appointments are simple measures to facilitate treatment. Oral hygiene is limited when there is significant motor incoordination, resulting in increased caries. When extensive dental treatment is required, treatment under general anesthesia is advisable.
◇ There is no cure for MS and treatment is symptomatic. Acute flares are managed with systemic corticosteroids.

MEDICATIONS
• Trigeminal neuralgia responds to conventional medications such as carbamazepine, baclofen, and phenytoin. Treat constipation with stool softeners and bulk producing products. Manage urinary problems with propantheline (Banthine) or oxybutynin (Ditropan).

SURGERY
When medications fail, radiofrequency neurolysis or surgical neurectomy may be considered.

CONSULTATION SUGGESTIONS
Neurologist

REFERRAL SUGGESTIONS
Primary Care Physician, Neurologist

PATIENT INSTRUCTIONS
Contact National Multiple Sclerosis Society for additional patient information (800) 624-8236.

COURSE/PROGNOSIS
MS is a non-curable, progressive degenerative disease. It has a highly variable course. Some patients have mild disease without much progression, others rapidly progress to total paralysis and blindness. Most patients live more than 25 years after diagnosis.

CODING

ICD-9-CM
340.0 Multiple sclerosis

MISCELLANEOUS

SYNONYMS
Disseminated sclerosis
Insular sclerosis

SEE ALSO
Behcet's disease
Sarcoidosis
Trigeminal neuralgia
Syphilis

REFERENCES
Olsson T: Immunology of multiple sclerosis. Curr Opin Neurol Neurosurg 5:195-203, 1992.

Mickey MR: Correlation of clinical and immunologic states in multiple sclerosis. Arch Neurol 44:371-383, 1987.

Friedlander AH, Zeff S: Atypical trigeminal neuralgia in a patient with multiple sclerosis. J Oral Surg 32:301-305, 1974.

Rushton JG, Olafson RA: Trigeminal neuralgia associated with multiple sclerosis. Arch Neurol 13:383-387, 1965.

Sadiq SA, Miller JR: Multiple sclerosis. In: Merritt's Textbook of Neurology, 9th ed. Rowland LP (ed), Baltimore, Williams & Wilkins, 1995, pp. 804-825.

AUTHOR
David A. Sirois, DMD, PhD

Muscular Dystrophy

BASICS

DESCRIPTION
Muscular dystrophy (MD) is an incurable inherited disease characterized by progressive muscle atrophy and weakness. The facial and masticatory muscles are affected to varying degrees and macroglossia, caused by fatty deposition, occurs. Several clinical variants are recognized, some which appear during early childhood and others during adulthood:

Duchenne's Muscular Dystrophy (DMD)
◇ Sex-linked, recessive inheritance with symptoms developing during the first 3 to 5 years of life. Difficulty walking, frequent falling, and muscle fatigability are the early signs. Affected individuals are bedridden by 10 years of age. Involvement of respiratory muscles requires positive-pressure breathing masks and most patients die due to respiratory failure by their second or third decade.

Facioscapulohumeral Dystrophy (FSH)
◇ Autosomal dominant inheritance with equal gender distributions with symptoms developing in the second decade of life. Muscle atrophy is not as severe as in Duchenne's and many patients will have a normal life span. The facial and upper extremity muscles are more severely affected and facial/masticatory weakness is common.

Becker's Myotonic Dystrophy (BMD)
◇ Autosomal recessive trait with adult onset of symptoms. Muscles of the head, neck, and distal extremities are most severely affected. These patients exhibit myotonia or sustained muscle contraction.

ETIOLOGY

The cause of MD is not yet fully known, although mounting evidence points to an enzyme defect at the muscle surface membrane.

SYSTEMS AFFECTED
Muscle is the primary organ affected by the disease. Involvement of the respiratory muscles or myocardium leads to death due to respiratory insufficiency and/or cardiac failure.

DIAGNOSIS

SYMPTOMS AND SIGNS
• Unexplained progressive muscle weakness is the cardinal diagnostic feature. May be seen as clumsiness, generalized or localized weakness particularly apparent in the face, or pseudohypertrophy of calf muscles. Kyphoscoliosis can cause respiratory compromise.
• Oral manifestations include masticatory weakness and macroglossia. Oral hygiene suffers due to limited physical dexterity, and caries is a significant problem.
• Temporomandibular joint dislocations and locking have been reported. Dental malocclusion, especially anterior open bite, is common due to poor masticatory muscle tone and macroglossia.

LABORATORY
Elevated serum creatine kinase, particularly high in DMD, moderate elevation in BMD and FSH, normal in congenital MD.

IMAGING/SPECIAL TESTS
• Electromyography; muscle biopsy immunohistochemistry.
• Biopsy in DMD reveals necrosis, fiber splitting, and attempts at regeneration with interspersed fibrosis.

DIFFERENTIAL
• Myasthenia gravis (in early stages).
• Polymyositis
• Viral myositis
• Congenital myopathies
• Periodic paralysis
• Encephalopathy

TREATMENT

General
◇ There is no cure for MD and treatment is largely symptomatic and limited. Physical therapy can prolong use of some muscle groups but with little effect on the inevitable outcome, paralysis.
◇ Involvement of the respiratory muscles leading to hypoventilation is often treated with positive pressure masks or nasal prongs.
◇ Unlike other patients with neuromuscular impairment (ie, multiple sclerosis), MD patients cannot receive general anesthesia to facilitate dental treatment. Post-anesthesia respiratory failure is not uncommon. Dental treatment is best performed with assisted opening and for short periods of time. Macroglossia can become a formidable barrier to dental treatment.

MEDICATIONS
• Prednisone 0.15 to 0.75 mg/kg/d improves strength in boys with DMD.

CONSULTATION SUGGESTIONS
Neurologist, Physical Therapist

REFERRAL SUGGESTIONS
Primary Care Physician, Neurologist

PATIENT INSTRUCTIONS
Contact Muscular Dystrophy Association for helpful patient information, (800)221-1142.

COURSE/PROGNOSIS
All forms of MD are incurable and progressive. Adolescent and adult onset MD is generally not as rapidly progressive as childhood MD (Duchenne's). Early death likely: DMD 16, BMD 42.

CODING

ICD-9-CM
359.0   Congenital muscular dystrophy
359.1   DMD, BMD, FSH
359.2   Myotonic dystrophy

M MISCELLANEOUS

SYNONYMS
Pseudohypertrophic muscular dystrophy
Steinert's disease
Fukuyama syndrome
Landouzy-Dejerine dystrophy

SEE ALSO
Myasthenia gravis

REFERENCES
Brooke MH: Clinician's View of Neuromuscular Diseases. 2nd ed. Baltimore, Williams and Wilkins, 1986.

Mendell JR, Griggs RC: Inherited, metabolic, and toxic myopathies. In: Harrison's Principles of Internal Medicine. 13th ed. Isselbacher KJ, et al (eds), New York, McGraw-Hill, 1994, pp. 2383-2387.

Rowland LP: Myopathies. In: Merritt's Textbook of Neurology, 9th ed. Rowland LP (ed), Baltimore, Williams & Wilkins, 1995, pp. 766-781.

AUTHOR
David S. Sirois, DMD, PhD

Myasthenia Gravis

BASICS

DESCRIPTION
Myasthenia gravis (MG) is an autoimmune disease characterized by easy fatigability of skeletal muscle. MG occurs more frequently in females during the fourth decade. Oro-facial symptoms are early and prominent, manifest as impaired eye blinking, mask-like facial expression, and masticatory weakness and fatigability.

ETIOLOGY

Autoantibodies directed against the acetylcholine receptor. The antibody prevents acetylcholine, the neurotransmitter at the neuromuscular junction, from binding and contraction is impaired. MG is seen as a secondary component in several other autoimmune disorders such as pemphigus, lupus erythematosus, and rheumatoid arthritis.

SYSTEMS AFFECTED
• Skeletal muscles throughout the body can be affected, but those supplied by the cranial nerves and cervical spinal nerves are usually more affected, leading to prominent facial and upper extremity weakness. Progression to respiratory insufficiency is uncommon.
• Difficulty chewing and swallowing food is common due to easy fatigability of the masticatory muscles. The muscle may become so tired that the jaw remains open after eating and the patient has to hold the jaw closed with his/her hand. Weakness of the tongue and palatal muscles is common.

DIAGNOSIS

SYMPTOMS AND SIGNS
• The earliest sign is typically "tired eyes" or impaired eye blinking. The patient will tire easily when asked to repeatedly blink the eyes.
• Other symptoms include fatigue on chewing, dysphagia, dysarthria (difficulty speaking properly), neck weakness, and generalized weakness.

LABORATORY
Thyroid function tests to rule out thyroid disorder.

IMAGING/SPECIAL TESTS
• Anti-acetylcholine receptor antibody.
• Specific clinical test is the administration of edrophonium chloride (Tensilon), resulting in dramatic improvement of the symptoms. Tensilon is a cholinesterase antagonist, thereby reducing the ability for cholinesterase to degrade acetylcholine, allowing the neurotransmitter to bind more neuromuscular receptors.
• Repetitive nerve stimulation.

DIFFERENTIAL
• Chronic fatigue syndrome
• Thyroid disorder
• Bell's palsy
• Polymyositis
• Multiple sclerosis

TREATMENT

MEDICATIONS
- Anticholinesterase antagonists such as neostigmine (Prostigmin) or pyridostigmine (Mestinon) are used in mild cases.
- In more severe cases, systemic corticosteroids, azathioprine, and/or cyclophosphamide are useful.
- Intravenous gamma globulin can be used.
- Finally, drugs that affect the neuromuscular junction should be avoided, including narcotics, tranquilizers, barbiturates, and certain antibiotics (clindamycin, tetracycline, sulfonamides).
- Dental considerations include assisted opening and short treatment visits. Respiratory crisis is a potential danger at any time due to the disease itself as well as over-medication. Treatment in a hospital setting where airway management can be provided is recommended.

SURGERY
Thymectomy may be useful.

CONSULTATION SUGGESTIONS
Neurologist

REFERRAL SUGGESTIONS
Primary Care Physician, Neurologist

PATIENT INSTRUCTIONS
Contact Myasthenia Gravis Foundation for useful patient information (800)221-1142.

COURSE/PROGNOSIS
Slow progression of symptoms is the rule. However, most patients respond to therapy and can lead a normal life. Mortality due to MG less than 10%.

CODING

ICD-9-CM
358.0 Myasthenia gravis

MISCELLANEOUS

SEE ALSO
Multiple sclerosis
Hypothyroidism

REFERENCES

Drachman DB: Biology of myasthenia gravis. Ann Rev Neurosci 4:195-201, 1981.

Farmbrough DM: Neuromuscular junction in myasthenia gravis. Science 182:293-295, 1973.

Mason DK: Oral aspects of myasthenia gravis. Dent Pract 15:23-27, 1964.

Penn AS, Rowland LP: Myasthenia gravis. In: Merritt's Textbook of Neurology, 9th ed. Rowland LP (ed), Baltimore, Williams & Wilkins, 1995, pp. 754-761.

AUTHOR
David A. Sirois, DMD, PhD

Myeloproliferative Disorders

BASICS

DESCRIPTION
• Neoplastic diseases of the multipotent hematopoietic stem cell. The four major diseases are chronic myelogenous leukemia (CML), polycythemia vera (PV), agnogenic myeloid metaplasia with myelofibrosis (AMM/MF), and essential thrombocytosis (ET). Incidence equal in males and females.
• These diseases arise as cloned expansions of single transformed stem cells. Nearly all the myeloid cells are derived from the neoplastic clone at the time of diagnosis.
CML
◇ Increased production of neutrophils and marked splenomegaly. Divided into chronic and blastic, or acute phase. The chronic phase is typified by hyperplasia of mature marrow elements. The blastic phase evolves into proliferation of immature marrow elements, ie, blasts and promyelocytes. Blast crisis can develop into acute myelogenous leukemia.
PV
◇ Increased production of all myeloid cells, but dominated by increased RBCs; with splenomegaly.
AMM/MF
◇ Neoplastic stem cells proliferate and lodge in multiple sites outside the bone marrow. Splenomegaly and fibrosis of marrow spaces occur.
ET
◇ Markedly elevated platelet count in the absence of a recognizable stimulus.

ETIOLOGY

Unknown for general population, although familial cases have been identified. Increased incidence of CML following atomic radiation and radiation therapy for cervical cancer and ankylosing spondylosis.

SYSTEMS AFFECTED
Hematopoietic
◇ proliferation of myeloid clone.
Lymphatic
◇ lymphadenopathy
Renal
◇ urate stones secondary to hyperuricemia due to increased cellular turnover; uric acid nephropathy.

DIAGNOSIS

SYMPTOMS AND SIGNS
General
◇ Most patients are asymptomatic at the time of diagnosis or have a vague complaint of malaise.
CML
◇ Symptomatic splenomegaly, anemia, weight loss, fever. Arthralgias may be severe.
PV
◇ Thrombotic or hemorrhagic event. Arterial or venous sufficiency, headache, tinnitus, syncope, vertigo, scotomas secondary to decreased cerebral perfusion; Splenomegaly develops late.
AMM/MF
◇ Symptomatic splenomegaly followed by hepatomegaly; petechiae and bleeding in 10 to 20%. Occasional ascites, jaundice, and lymphadenopathy.
ET
◇ Spontaneous bleeding and easy bruising; unusual bleeding after minor dental procedures; venous or arterial thrombosis, transient ischemic attacks or strokes may occur.

LABORATORY
General
Basophilia
Increased serum vitamin B_{12} and vitamin B_{12} binding capacity
Hyperuricemia
CML
　Marked granulocytosis
　Low or absent leukocyte alkaline phosphatase
　Near normal platelet morphology
PV
　Marked hemoglobin elevation
　Normochromic, normocytic RBC
　Leukocytosis in more than 60%
　Normal ESR
　Thrombocytosis in more than 50%
　Increased leukocyte alkaline phosphatase
AMM/MF
　Anemia
　Leukocytosis in 50%, leukopenia in 20%
　Thrombocytosis to thrombocytopenia as disease progresses
　Abnormal liver function tests (increased bilirubin and alkaline phosphatase)
ET
　Thrombocytosis which is polymorphic
　Abnormality in platelet aggregation

IMAGING/SPECIAL TESTS
Skeletal radiograph
◇ Identifies marrow sclerosis and increased bone density in axial skeleton and proximal long bones.
Bone marrow biopsy
◇ Essential to the diagnosis of AMM/MF

Philadelphia chromosome (Ph1)
◇ Present in 95% of CML
Red cell mass determination with 51Cr labeled autologous blood for PV.

DIFFERENTIAL
CML
　Leukemoid reaction secondary to infections, neoplasm or stress
　Blastic phase can resemble acute myelogenous leukemia
Paroxysmal nocturnal hemoglobinuria
AMM/MF
　Difficult to differentiate between other stages of CML, PV and ET
　Metastatic carcinoma
　Leukemia or lymphoma
　Tuberculosis
　Paget's disease
　Metabolic toxins exposure (benzene)
　Gaucher's disease
　Toxic exposure to radiographs
PV

　Secondary polycythemia
　Chronic cardiac or pulmonary disease
　Hypernephroma or other renal disease (Increased erythropoietin production)
　Decreased plasma volume (dehydration)
　Hemoglobinopathy
ET

　Secondary thrombocytosis

Myeloproliferative Disorders

TREATMENT

General
◇ Measures to maintain hydration, relieve arthralgias, prevent thrombotic episodes, and prevent infections. With massive splenomegaly, splenectomy will not prolong survival but can provide some symptomatic relief. However, hematologic/infectious complications from removal of the spleen can occur.

MEDICATIONS
• Chronic Myelogenous Leukemia
• Chronic phase treated with hydroxyurea (Hydrea) or busulfan (Myleran) (alkylating agent) does not alter inexorable progression to acute phase. Intense therapy only provides transient remission with no prolongation of survival.
• Bone Marrow Transplant (BMT)
• Syngeneic or allogeneic transplant provides increased disease free interval in 40 to 50% of patients; long-term survival in patients younger than 20 is 70%; older patients 40%. Hydroxyurea is the first line drug followed by other alkylating agents (busulfan, cyclophosphamide, melphalan).
• Alpha interferon provides better long-term results.
• Allopurinol for hyperuricemia and after chemotherapy.
• Polycythemia Vera
• Phlebotomy alone has extended survival 10 to 12 years. Reduce hemocrit to approximately 45%. Myelosuppressive therapy with radioactive 32P or chemotherapy with alkylating agents.
• Can also use hydroxyurea and allopurinol, and give cyproheptadine for pruritus.
• Agnogenic Myeloid Metaplasia with Myelofibrosis
• There is no definitive therapy. Transfusions or androgens with or without corticosteroids to improve anemia. Myelosuppressive therapy with alkylating agents rarely indicated except for splenomegaly or thrombocytosis. Splenectomy only for hemolysis, severe thrombocytopenia and intractable symptoms of splenomegaly. Androgens +/- glucocorticoids may be tried.
• Essential Thrombocytosis
• Indications for treatment are unsettled. With severe bleeding or thrombotic episodes, hydroxyurea is indicated. Alkylating agents or radioactive phosphorus can be used if hydroxyurea fails. Aspirin and dipyramidole may prevent symptoms. Platelet-pheresis can manage acute crisis. Non-steroidal anti-inflammatory drugs to prevent vaso-occlusive syndrome secondary to thrombocytosis.

CONSULTATION SUGGESTIONS
Hematologist, Oncologist

REFERRAL SUGGESTIONS
Primary Care Physician

FIRST STEPS TO TAKE IN AN EMERGENCY
• Infection in neutropenic patient requires hospitalization for intravenous antibiotics.

COURSE/PROGNOSIS
CML
    Dependent upon progression to blastic phase. 10% progress within the first two years after diagnosis, with 20% per year thereafter. BMT provides patients less than 20 with 70% long-term survival and those older, with 40% long-term survival.
    Median survival is 5 years after diagnosis, decreasing to 1 1/2 years after blastic stage and to 3 months after blast crisis. 85% die in blast crisis.

PV
    Median survival without treatment is only 1 year. "Phlebotomy alone" group had increased risk of death from hemorrhage or thrombosis in first four years.
    Similar survival rates for all treatment modalities until the 7th year.
    Alkylating agents predispose to acute leukemia later in course.
    Statistically significant incidence of second hematologic malignancy (Lymphoma or leukemia)
    Occasional asymptomatic survivor for more than 20 years.

AMM/MF
    Generally a prolonged course with median survival of 5 years from diagnosis; 25% live up to 15 years.
    Transformation to acute leukemia occurs in 5 to 10%.
    Major causes of death include congestive heart failure, renal failure, hemorrhage, portal hypertension and infection.

ET
    Median survival in not well defined; less than 10% transformation to acute leukemic phase.

CODING

ICD-9-CM
  205.1 Chronic myelogenous leukemia
  238.4 Polycythemia vera
  238.7 Essential thrombocytosis
  289.8 Agnogenic myeloid metaplasia/myelofibrosis

MISCELLANEOUS

SEE ALSO
Leukemia
Polycythemia vera
Gout

REFERENCES
Lichtman MA: Classification and clinical manifestations of the hemopoietic stem cell disorders. In: Williams Hematology, 5th ed. Beutler E, et al (eds), New York, McGraw-Hill, 1995, pp. 229-238.

Adamson JW: Myeloproliferative diseases, In: Harrison's Principles of Internal Medicine, 13th ed; Isselbacher KJ, et al (eds), New York, McGraw-Hill, 1994 pp. 1757-1764.

Dolin R: Myeloproliferative disorders. In: Griffith's 5 Minute Clinical Consult, Dambro M. (ed), Baltimore, Williams & Wilkins, 1995, pp. 696-697.

AUTHOR
James Vopal, DDS, MD

Myocardial Infarction

BASICS

DESCRIPTION
Necrosis of myocardial tissue from inadequate oxygen supply compared to myocardial oxygen consumption.

ETIOLOGY

Atherosclerosis involving coronary arteries complicated by platelet thrombus formation and narrowing or total occlusion of involved artery(s). Can also be due to:
 coronary artery vasospasm,
 coronary artery embolism,
 dissecting aortic aneurysm with
  occlusion of coronary artery, or
 sudden increase in myocardial
  oxygen demand in absence of
  coronary occlusion (cocaine,
  hypertension, physical exertion).

SYSTEMS AFFECTED
Myocardium
 ◇ necrosis and ultimately fibrosis of involved myocardium. This may lead to pump dysfunction, ventricular septal rupture, ventricular aneurysm, cardiac rupture. Pump dysfunction causes systemic problems of hypoperfusion and congestion of lungs, liver and other venous beds.
Heart valves
 ◇ overuse of papillary muscle can lead to mitral valve dysfunction.
Myocardial conduction disorders
 ◇ damage to pacemakers and/or conduction pathways may cause bradycardia, sinus arrest, atrioventricular blocks, atrial and ventricular dysrhythmias.

DIAGNOSIS

SYMPTOMS AND SIGNS
Chest discomfort similar to angina (pressure, burning tightness) but more severe, unaffected by rest or nitroglycerin. Pain may radiate or localize to neck, jaw, shoulder, arms particularly on the left. Epigastric pain may mimic indigestion. Twenty-five percent may have no pain.
General
 ◇ patient usually acutely distressed. Skin is cool, moist, pale.
Vital Signs
 ◇ heart rate and blood pressure may be normal, increased or decreased.
Heart
 ◇ faint heart sounds, often with S4 (atrial gallop) sound. May see jugular cannon venous "A" waves and jugular venous distension.
Lung
 ◇ dyspnea, rales, wheezing.
Other
 ◇ sweating, nausea, vomiting common. In elderly
 ◇ sudden dyspnea, cough, acute confusion, fever, dizziness, syncope may occur without pain.

LABORATORY
Blood creatinine kinase
 ◇ MB isoenzyme increased in proportion to size of infarct.
Serum lactate dehydrogenase, fraction 1 increased.
Cholesterol
 ◇ elevation indicates higher risk for atherosclerosis.

IMAGING/SPECIAL TESTS
Electrocardiogram
 ◇ specific changes reflect myocardial injury or necrosis such as ST elevation, ST depression with inverted T waves, and eventual appearance of Q waves.
Echocardiogram
 ◇ demonstrates ventricular wall motion abnormality that occurs with acute MI.
Radionuclide imaging
 ◇ technetium 99m Stannous pyrophosphate taken up by damaged myocardium allows estimation of infarct size. Thallium scanning useful to quantify ejection fractions.
Coronary arteriogram
 ◇ will demonstrate coronary artery disease.
MRI
 ◇ synchronized to heart beat can show areas of myocardial infarction. Primarily investigative role, not used routinely.

DIFFERENTIAL
• Unstable angina
• Coronary vasospasm
• Cocaine abuse
• Coronary artery embolism
• Pulmonary embolism
• Hypertension
• Pericarditis
• Dissecting aortic aneurysm
• Esophageal spasm
• Pancreatitis
• Gastroesophageal reflux

TREATMENT

General
◇ Pain relief. Minimize infarct size by decreasing myocardial oxygen consumption and increasing myocardial oxygen supply.

MEDICATIONS
• Nitroglycerin 0.4 mg sublingual spray or 0.25 mg tablets sublingually, repeat twice at 5-minute intervals unless hypotension present.
• Morphine sulfate 2 to 4 mg IV every 10 minutes for pain and pulmonary edema.
• Beta-adrenergic blocker (cardioselective)
◇ decreases sympathetic tone and myocardial oxygen consumption.
• Thrombolytic therapy
◇ streptokinase, recombinant tissue plasminogen activator (tPA); anisoylated plasminogen streptokinase activator complex
◇ most useful if given within 3 hours of onset of MI, but can be given up to 12 to 24 hours following onset of chest pain.
• Lidocaine
◇ infusion used selectively in patients with ectopic ventricular beats. 1 to 2 mg/kg bolus then 1 to 4 mg/min (some now question the value of this therapy).
• Antithrombotic therapy
◇ heparin, aspirin started after thrombolysis to decrease risk of reocclusion.
• Oxazepam, orazepam or diazepam for anxiolysis.
• Nitrous oxide may also be helpful in anxious patient.
• Nasal oxygen to cause nitrogen washout.

SURGERY
Balloon angioplasty
◇ an alternative or follow-up to thrombolytic therapy. Unclear if any better than thrombolysis.
Coronary artery by-pass grafting.

CONSULTATION SUGGESTIONS
Cardiologist, Cardiac Surgeon

REFERRAL SUGGESTIONS
Primary Care Physician

FIRST STEPS TO TAKE IN AN EMERGENCY
• Call emergency response team.
• Administer nitroglycerin up to maximum of three doses, if no hypotension.
• Administer morphine, nasal oxygen, and start IV.

PATIENT INSTRUCTIONS
Try to relax patient during infarction episode. Nitrous oxide may be used.

Wait at least 6 months following MI prior to doing any elective dentistry.

COURSE/PROGNOSIS
• In the best situation, mortality in the early phase of an MI is 1.5 %. Age > 70, previous MI, female gender, tachycardia, anterior location of MI, atrial fibrillation, and cardiac failure are associated with an increased mortality. Patients discharged from the hospital following MI have a 6 to 10 % mortality in the first year, with most deaths occurring in the first 3 months. Late morality is related to the degree of left ventricular dysfunction and ischemia, potential for dysrhythmias and is much higher in elderly patients.
• Patients may be placed on chronic anticoagulation therapy so inquire prior to dental care.

CODING

ICD-9-CM
410.9 Myocardial infarction

MISCELLANEOUS

SYNONYMS
Coronary thrombosis
Heart attack
Coronary occlusion

SEE ALSO
Congestive Heart Failure
Angina pectoris

REFERENCES
Hancock WE: Ischemic Heart Disease: Acute Myocardial Infarction. In: Rubenstein E, Federman D: (eds) Scientific American Medicine, Section I, Subsection X. New York, Scientific American, Inc., 1993. pp. 1-21.

Roberts R, et al: Pathophysiology, recognition, and treatment of acute myocardial infarction and its complications. In: The Heart, 8th ed. Schlent RC, Alexander RW (eds), New York, McGraw-Hill, Inc., 1994, pp. 1107-1184.

Hupp JR: Myocardial infraction: current management strategies. J Oral Maxillofac Surg, 51: 565-569, 1989.

AUTHOR
Samuel J. McKenna, DDS, MD

Neck Masses

BASICS

DESCRIPTION
Masses in the neck may be divided into four sites. Masses in the midline, the submandibular triangle, the anterior triangle, and posterior triangle.

ETIOLOGY

Mid-line masses include:
dermoid and thyroglossal cysts that are developmental; thyroid swellings: cystic, neoplasm, autoimmune, goiter; submental nodes:
inflammatory, neoplastic.
Submandibular triangle masses include:
enlarged submandibular gland usually infective, obstructive, rarely neoplasm; submandibular nodes: inflammatory, neoplastic, cystic hygroma (hamartoma).
Anterior triangle masses include:
branchial cyst: developmental; lymph nodes: inflammatory, neoplastic; parotid tail masses: neoplastic, cyst; carotid body tumor: neoplastic.
Posterior triangle masses include:
lymph nodes: reactive, inflammatory, neoplastic.

SYSTEMS AFFECTED
• Depends on the diagnosis:
Thyroid disease can cause hyperthyroidism and increased metabolic rate, sweating, tachycardia, atrial fibrillation, tremors, weight loss, and exophthalmos.
Infected nodes
◇ fever, sweating generalized toxic state, related to the primary infection.
Lymphoma
◇ skin rashes, itching, weight loss
TB nodes
◇ fever, cough, weight loss
AIDS lymphadenopathy
◇ weight loss, fever, hairy leukoplakia, Kaposi's sarcoma.

DIAGNOSIS

SYMPTOMS AND SIGNS
Painless neck mass
◇ usually neoplasm, or cystic.
Painful mass
◇ usually infective.
Midline masses
◇ Dermoid cyst: submental region, doughy to palpation, frequently raises floor of mouth.
Thyroglossal cyst
◇ Submental to thyroid region, feels cystic, moves on swallowing or protrusion of tongue.
Thyroid swelling
◇ May be unilateral or involve the entire thyroid, soft or hard
◇ moves on swallowing.
Sub-Mandibular mass
◇ Submandibular gland
◇ Firm, discrete, bimanually palpable
◇ stone palpable in duct, inability to milk saliva or purulent saliva;
Submandibular node, not bimanually palpable, see characteristics under nodes (below).
Anterior Triangle:
Branchial cyst
◇ round, half anterior to sternomastoid half deep to sternomastoid, cystic.
Painful swelling following injury from cat or other domestic animal, Cat-scratch disease.
Carotid body tumor
◇ firm, in line of carotid, can be moved side to side but not up and down.
Lymph nodes
◇ Tender, shotty nodes usually inflammatory, examine area of drainage for odontogenic infection, tonsillitis, etc. Bilateral generalized tender nodes may indicate tonsillitis, glandular fever
◇ examine junction hard and soft palate for ecchymosis in glandular fever. Generalized nontender nodes may indicate autoimmune disease, AIDS. Firm rubbery nodes with no obvious primary site in young or old may by lymphoma. Hard nodes in older patients frequently neoplastic. If nodes in upper neck examine mouth, pharynx, naso-pharynx, and larynx for primary site. If hard nodes supra-clavicular suspect lung or stomach cancer.
Posterior Triangle:
◇ usually node masses (as above). Matted shotty nodes may be tuberculous.

LABORATORY
• CBC, viral titers, monospot, HIV testing, where infective etiology for lymphadenopathy suspected.
• Auto-antibody screen if lupus, or other rheumatologic cause suspected.
• Thyroid function tests if thyroid etiology suspected.

IMAGING/SPECIAL TESTS
• CT scan for lymphoma, metastatic nodes, thyroid mass, thyroglossal cyst, carotid body tumor.
• Ultra-sound for thyroglossal cyst, branchial cyst, thyroid mass.
• Thyroid nuclear scan for solitary nodule
Carotid angiography
◇ Carotid body tumor
• Sialogram for sub-mandibular gland, swelling
• Fine-needle aspiration biopsy (FNAB)-metastatic node, thyroid mass, lymphoma.
Pan-endoscopy
◇ rule out head and neck primary before biopsy when enlarged node present.
Node biopsy
◇ touch prep., culture, histology

DIFFERENTIAL
(As above)

TREATMENT

General
◊ Treatment will depend on the diagnosis.
◊ Developmental lesions, thyroid gland cyst, dermoid cyst, and branchial cyst require surgical excision.
◊ Infective lymphadenopathy is treated with antibiotics as indicated for bacterial infections.
◊ Thyroid disease may be treated surgically or medically.
◊ Auto-immune disease will require medical therapy (eg, steroids).
◊ Lymphomas treated with chemotherapy or radiation.
◊ Metastatic nodes will be treated with surgery or radiation depending on the primary site.

MEDICATIONS
• See general treatment section.

SURGERY
• See general treatment section.

CONSULTATION SUGGESTIONS
Oral-Maxillofacial Surgeon, Otolaryngologist, General Surgeon

REFERRAL SUGGESTIONS
Oral-Maxillofacial Surgeon, Otolaryngologist, General Surgeon

FIRST STEPS TO TAKE IN AN EMERGENCY
• If neck mass seems inflammatory in nature and rapidly enlarging, move patient to emergency care facility for protection against airway compromise.

PATIENT INSTRUCTIONS
Biopsy generally necessary to establish diagnosis.

COURSE/PROGNOSIS
Developmental lesions are curable with surgery.
Bacterial infections or TB treated with specific antibiotics and are usually curable.
Neoplastic disease prognosis depends on staging
   the presence of a metastatic node is an ominous prognostic sign for head and neck cancer and reduces expected survival by 50%.

CODING

ICD-9-CM
017.2 Tuberculous cervical gland
196.0 Metastatic cervical node
200.1 Hodgkin's granuloma
202.1 Lymphomas depending on classification
202.8 Lymphoma (malignant)
240.9 Thyromegaly
245.9 Thyroiditis
527.2 Sub-mandibular sialadenitis
528.4 Oral dermoid cyst
744.42 Branchial cyst
759.2 Thyroglossal cyst

CPT
38500 Biopsy of lymph nodes
38550 Excision of cystic hygroma
38700 Suprahyoid neck dissection
38720 Radical neck dissection
38724 Modified radical neck dissection
42440 Submandibular gland excision
42810 Excision branchial cyst
60200 Excision thyroid cyst or tumor
60280 Excision thyroglossal cyst
88170 Fine needle aspiration thyroid, lymph node, salivary gland

MISCELLANEOUS

SEE ALSO
Salivary Gland Tumors
Squamous Carcinoma, Tongue
Squamous Carcinoma, Floor of Mouth
Hyperthyroidism
Tuberculosis
Parotid Swellings
Cat Scratch
Brachial Cleft Cyst
Thyroglossal Cyst

REFERENCES
Lindberg R: Distribution of cervical lymph node metastases from squamous cell carcinoma of the upper-respiratory and digestive tracts. Cancer, 29: 1446, 1972.

Catlin D: Surgery for head and neck lymphomas. Surgery 60:1160-1166, 1966.

Watts A: Fine needle aspiration of the thyroid. Clin Otolaryng 7:205-214, 1982.

Young JEM: Current status of needle aspiration biopsy of the head and neck. Can J Surg 25:410, 1982.

AUTHOR
Robert A. Ord, MD, DDS, FACS, FRCS

Nephrotic Syndrome

 BASICS

DESCRIPTION
Renal disease characterized by heavy proteinuria (more than 3.5 g protein/ 1.73m² body surface area/day) and is usually associated with hypoalbuminemia, hyperlipidemia, and edema.
- More than 70% of nephrotic syndrome cases are related to primary glomerular disease. Other causes are diabetes, amyloidosis, multiple myeloma, and collagen-vascular diseases.

 ETIOLOGY

Pathology
- Increased glomerular basement membrane permeability caused by immunologic, inflammatory or metabolic abnormality that results in proteinuria.
- With loss of albumin and some globulins, plasma oncotic pressure falls and fluid shifts to the interstitial space.
- Decreased intravascular volume decreases renal blood flow and stimulates aldosterone and antidiuretic hormone production. This causes retention of sodium and water with increased edema formation.
- In addition, large losses of plasma proteins may affect thyroid function, calcium metabolism, cause anemia secondary to decreased transferrin, and IgG deficiency contributing to increased frequency of infections.

SYSTEMS AFFECTED
Renal
Generalized edema

 DIAGNOSIS

SYMPTOMS AND SIGNS
- Patients show edema in the lower extremities followed by anasarca.
- When protein loss is large, patients may show signs of malnutrition (such as white bands on nails secondary to hypoalbuminemia).
- Hypertension may develop with other vascular diseases such as myocardial infarction, renal vein thrombosis, and deep vein thrombosis being common.

LABORATORY
- BUN and creatinine values are elevated.
- Proteinuria, lipiduria, RBC, granular, hyaline and fatty casts, glycosuria, and aminoaciduria.

IMAGING/SPECIAL TESTS
- Biopsy of kidney-percutaneous
- Complement levels
- Serum protein and urine immune-electrophoresis.
- Hypoalbuminemia, hyperlipidemia, azotemia, hypercholesterolemia
- Renal venogram
- Renal ultrasound
- Renal CT or MRI

DIFFERENTIAL
- Carcinoma
- Diabetes mellitus
- HIV infection
- Hodgkin's lymphoma
- Nephrosis
- Lupus

TREATMENT

• Protein rich diet (2 to 3g protein/kg body weight/day) is recommended.
• Supplemental vitamins replace those lost with proteinuria.
• Sodium intake is restricted.
• Specific treatment is guided by diagnosis of underlying cause.

MEDICATIONS
• Marked edema is treated with thiazide or loop diuretics.
• Antibiotics should be promptly started with bacterial infections, and prophylactic Pneumovax vaccination is recommended.
• Prednisone for steroid responsive causes of nephrotic syndrome.
• Treat high cholesterol with low cholesterol diet and cholesterol lowering drugs.

SURGERY
Renal failure treated with dialysis or transplantation.

CONSULTATION SUGGESTIONS
Nephrologist

REFERRAL SUGGESTIONS
Primary Care Physician

PATIENT INSTRUCTIONS
Patient can contact National Kidney Foundation for information, (800)622-9010.
Diet
◊ 1 g/kg/day protein, low fat, low sodium extra potassium, vitamins.

COURSE/PROGNOSIS
Varies with etiology.

CODING

ICD-9-CM
581.9 Nephrotic syndrome with unspecified lesion in kidney.

MISCELLANEOUS

SEE ALSO
Renal failure
Systemic lupus

REFERENCES
Glassock RJ, Brenner BM: The Major Glomerulopathies. In: Harrison's Principles of Internal Medicine, 13th ed. Isselbacher KJ, et al (eds), New York, McGraw-Hill 1994, pp. 1295-1299.

Internal Medicine for Dentistry 2nd ed. Rose LF, Kaye D: St. Louis, CV Mosby Co., 1990.

Kraus ES: Proteinuria. In: Principles and Practice of Ambulatory Medicine, 4th ed. Barker LR, Burton JR, Zieve PD (eds), Baltimore, Williams & Wilkins, 1995, pp. 521-526.

AUTHOR
Jerry L. Jones, DDS, MD

Neuralgia, Postherpetic

BASICS

DESCRIPTION
• Severe pain persisting or re-emerging following the healing of the cutaneous rash seen with reactivation of varicella-zoster virus infection (herpes zoster, "shingles").
• Nine to 14% of patients with herpes zoster develop postherpetic neuralgia.
• Pain may be spontaneous or triggered by light touch; affected area is usually insensitive to pinprick and local heat or cold.
• Pain may be persistent or re-emergent, developing 1 to 6 months after healing of the rash.

ETIOLOGY

• Primary infection with varicella zoster virus causes chickenpox. After skin lesions heal, the virus can pass from cutaneous sensory nerves to the dorsal root ganglia and lie dormant until reactivated. This reactivation produces the clinical condition known as herpes zoster or "shingles."
• Herpes zoster results in cell degeneration, death, and scarring in the spinal cord, sensory ganglia, and peripheral nerves; these changes result in cells in the afferent sensory pathway becoming hyperexcitable and prone to spontaneous discharge.
• Incidence, severity, and duration of postherpetic neuralgia all increase with age.
• Risk factors include ophthalmic herpes zoster, diabetes mellitus, cancer, severity of herpes zoster, and immunocompromise.

SYSTEMS AFFECTED
Nervous
  ◇ intense pain in affected dermatome.
Skin
  ◇ patient may avoid cleaning affected area resulting in localized accumulation of dirt, sebum, or debris. This may lead to lichenification, inflammation, and ulceration.
Mental state
  ◇ impacted by severe, chronic pain.

DIAGNOSIS

SYMPTOMS AND SIGNS
Skin
  ◇ spontaneous pain described as burning, throbbing, stabbing, shooting, sharp or aching. May be continuous with fluctuating intensity, or paroxysmal. Intense pain may also be triggered by normally nonpainful stimuli such as the light touch of clothing. Symptoms may be worsened by cold weather or stress.
Skin
  ◇ unilateral, dermatomal hypopigmented band of skin, often with residual scarring.
Nervous
  ◇ affected area usually insensitive to pinprick and local heat or cold. Mild, normally nonpainful stimuli may trigger pain (allodynia).

DIFFERENTIAL
• Trigeminal neuralgia
• Atypical facial pain
• Ramsay-Hunt syndrome

TREATMENT

<u>General</u>
◇ Avoidance of stimulation of trigger areas.

MEDICATIONS
• Somatic or sympathetic nerve blockade during herpes zoster attack may reduce acute pain and decrease likelihood of postherpetic neuralgia.
• Acyclovir therapy during herpes zoster attack substantially reduces risk of developing postherpetic neuralgia.
• Tricyclic antidepressants relieve postherpetic neuralgia-amitriptyline 75 mg/day, side effects include constipation, sedation, and urinary retention.
• Topical capsaicin cream applied to affected area may help some individuals, side effects include burning sensation after application.
  5% lidocaine-prilocaine cream (EMLA) and 5% to 10% lidocaine gels applied topically have been shown to be effective.

CONSULTATION SUGGESTIONS
Neurologist, Oral Medicine, Dentist Specializing in Facial Pain Disorders

REFERRAL SUGGESTIONS
Neurologist, Oral Medicine, Primary Care Physician

FIRST STEPS TO TAKE IN AN EMERGENCY
• Potent analgesics for mitigation of severe pain.

PATIENT INSTRUCTIONS
Use analgesics prudently to lessen possibility of dependence.

COURSE/PROGNOSIS
Usually resolves spontaneously in several months. Some patients may suffer for years, or permanently. Incidence, severity, and duration all increase with age.

 CODING

ICD-9-CM
  053.12 Postherpetic trigeminal neuralgia
  053.13 Postherpetic polyneuropathy
  053.19 Herpes zoster with nervous system complications

CPT
  64400 Anesthetic agent injection, trigeminal nerve
  64450 Anesthetic agent injection, peripheral nerve branch NOS
  64510 Anesthetic agent injection, stellate ganglion

 MISCELLANEOUS

SYNONYMS
Postherpetic trigeminal neuralgia
Postherpetic neuropathy

SEE ALSO
Trigeminal neuralgia
Immunocompromise

REFERENCES
Loeser JD: Herpes zoster and postherpetic neuralgia. In: Bonica JJ (ed), The Management of Pain, 2nd ed. Philadelphia, Lea & Febiger, 1990, pp. 257-263.

Pasqualuci V, et al: The early treatment of herpes zoster with continuous neural blockade prevents postherpetic neuralgia. American Pain Society 13th annual meeting abstracts. Abstract #94657:A-50, 1994.

Watson CPN: Herpes zoster and postherpetic neuralgia. Pain Research and Clinical Management, New York, Elsevier, 1993.

Cousins MJ, et al: Neural Blockade in Clinical Anesthesia and Management of Pain, 2nd ed. Philadelphia, JB Lippincott, 1988, pp. 899-933.

AUTHOR
Warren P. Vallerand, DDS

Nicotine Stomatitis

BASICS

DESCRIPTION
Common tobacco smoking induced type of mucosal keratosis.

ETIOLOGY

• Patient is nearly always a pipe smoker. Occasionally cigar smoking is involved.
• Unknown whether this characteristic lesion is related to heat or some byproduct of tobacco smoke.
• Red centers represent dilated, inflamed minor salivary gland ducts.

SYSTEMS AFFECTED
Oral mucosa of the hard and soft palate.

DIAGNOSIS

SYMPTOMS AND SIGNS
• Typically asymptomatic.
• Multiple white keratotic papules or plaques with depressed red centers. The papules can coalesce but normal oral mucosa may be preserved between them. Located on the hard and soft palate.

LABORATORY
Histologic examination reveals epithelial thickening with hyperkeratosis and acanthosis. Minor salivary gland tissue shows moderate inflammation and ducts may show squamous metaplasia.

DIFFERENTIAL
This lesion of white papules or plaque with red centers located on the hard and soft palate of a pipe or cigar smoker leads to a clinical diagnosis of nicotine stomatitis.

TREATMENT

• Treatment consists of cessation of tobacco usage.
• Carefully examine other areas of the oral mucosa for signs of malignancy.

SURGERY
Biopsy if diagnosis uncertain.

CONSULTATION SUGGESTIONS
Oral-Maxillofacial Surgeon, Oral Medicine

PATIENT INSTRUCTIONS
Stop, or at least limit, tobacco use.

Course/Prognosis
There is no evidence to support a premalignant potential to this lesion, but because this lesion only occurs in persons with a significant tobacco usage, the entire oral mucosa should be examined thoroughly on a regular basis for leukoplakia or erythroplakia occurring elsewhere. Reverse smoking (lit end in mouth) increases malignant potential.

CODING

ICD-9-CM
528.7 Leukokeratosis nicotina palati

CPT
42100 Biopsy of palate

MISCELLANEOUS

SYNONYMS
• Stomatitis nicotina
• Pipe smokers palate
• Nicotinic stomatitis

REFERENCES
Eversole LR: Clinical Outline of Oral Pathology: Diagnosis and Treatment, 3rd ed. Philadelphia, Lea & Febiger. 1992, pp. 24, 155.

Regezi JA, Sciubba J: Oral Pathology: Clinical Pathologic Correlations. 2nd ed. Philadelphia, W.B. Saunders, Co., 1993, p. 102.

AUTHOR
Michael J. Dalton, DDS

Nocardiosis

BASICS

DESCRIPTION
Rare infection with Nocardia species that usually begins in the lungs. Most common species is N. asteroides, but may involve N. farcinica, N. brasiliensis or N. caviac. Normally found in soil as saprophyte.

ETIOLOGY

• Acute, subacute, or chronic infection with Nocardia species.
• Infection from source in nature, not from infected person.
• Portal of entrance is the lung with hematogenous spread.

SYSTEMS AFFECTED
Pulmonary
  ◇ portal of entrance.
• Hematogenous spread to brain, subcutaneous tissue, and rarely other organs.
• Rarely mandibular osteomyelitis

DIAGNOSIS

SYMPTOMS AND SIGNS
• Fever
• Elevated temperature
• Productive cough for days to months
• Altered mental status

LABORATORY
• Difficult to isolate from sputum.
• Hyphae seen on Gram stain.
• Organism is aerobic, weakly Gram positive, weakly acid fast, beaded, branching filaments.

IMAGING/SPECIAL TESTS
Cavitation with radiodense central area on chest radiograph.

DIFFERENTIAL
• Bacterial pneumonia
• Histoplasmosis
• Malignancy
• Tuberculosis

Nocardiosis

TREATMENT

• Discontinue immunosuppressant drugs if possible.
• Hydration

MEDICATIONS
• Sulfadiazine 100 mg/kg/day divided in four daily doses.
• Sodium bicarbonate 50 mg/kg/day divided in four daily doses (prevent crystalluria seen with sulfadiazine).

SURGERY
Drainage of purulent collections.

CONSULTATION SUGGESTIONS
Infectious Disease Specialist

REFERRAL SUGGESTIONS
Oral-Maxillofacial Surgeon (for mandibular osteomyelitis)

COURSE/PROGNOSIS
92% survival
◇ isolated pulmonary infection
50% survival
◇ brain abscess

CODING

ICD-9-CM
039.9 Nocardiosis
730.2 Osteomyelitis

CPT
40808 Biopsy vestibule of mouth
42100 Biopsy palate
87070 Culture, bacterial, any source
87205 Smear and interpretation for fungi
99000 Transport specimen to outside laboratory

MISCELLANEOUS

SEE ALSO
Histoplasmosis
Actinomycosis

REFERENCES
Topazian RG: Osteomyelitis of the jaws. In: Oral and Maxillofacial Infections, 3rd ed. Topazian RG, Goldberg M (eds.), Philadelphia, WB Saunders, 1994, pp. 278-279.

Bennett JE: Nocardiosis. In: Internal Medicine for Dentistry. Rose LF (ed), St. Louis, Mosby, 1983, p. 247.

AUTHOR
Peter E. Larsen, DDS
Seidal JF, Younce DC, Hupp JR, Kominski ZC. Cervicofacial nocardiosis. J Oral Maxillofac Surg 52: 188-191, 1994.

Nonspecific Oral Ulcers

BASICS

DESCRIPTION
Oral ulceration may be the result of local mechanical or chemical trauma, neoplastic or infectious disease, or a manifestation of a systemic disorder including autoimmune, idiopathic, metabolic, and hereditary disease.

ETIOLOGY

• Mechanical trauma, including denture sores.
• Chemical burns such as those resulting from topical use of aspirin.
• Neoplastic disease, usually rapidly growing malignancies that outgrow their blood supply resulting in avascular necrosis.
• Infections such as primary and recurrent Herpes simplex or candidiasis.
• Autoimmune diseases, including the variants of pemphigus and pemphigoid.
• Idiopathic diseases, including lichen planus and aphthous stomatitis.
• Hereditary diseases such as epidermolysis bullosa.

SYSTEMS AFFECTED
• An oral ulcer is defined as an area of lost mucosal (epithelial) integrity.
• The epithelial membrane barrier is therefore lost allowing penetration of infectious agents and other antigens into the underlying connective tissues. If the resulting inflammatory response is profound, or if a primary or secondary infection is involved, regional lymphadenopathy, pain and swelling may occur.

DIAGNOSIS

SYMPTOMS AND SIGNS
• Ulcer consisting of a white plaque (fibrin clot) usually surrounded by a zone of mucosal erythema. Chronic ulcers, of more than 2 to 3 weeks duration may show a rolled border due in many cases to a buildup of granulation tissue. However, chronic ulcers with or without rolled borders may be the result of a more serious disease to include malignancy.
• Pain, superficial stinging and burning, usually exacerbated by consumption of salty, spicy or citric foods and beverages.

LABORATORY
Clinical laboratory tests may be indicated for the diagnosis of autoimmune diseases such as systemic lupus erythematosus (SLE) or metabolic disorders.

IMAGING/SPECIAL TESTS
• Biopsies are usually indicated to confirm a diagnosis for an autoimmune, idiopathic, infectious, or hereditary disease. For most, the biopsy must include mucosa with clinically intact (nonulcerated) surface epithelium to be diagnostic.
• Any ulceration of indeterminate etiology that fails to resolve after 2 weeks merits biopsy.
• Mechanical, chemical, and aphthous ulcers show nonspecific features microscopically and therefore the diagnosis depends primarily on historical and clinical features.

DIFFERENTIAL
Mechanical trauma
◇ Factitial or iatrogenic injury
Chemical trauma
◇ Aspirin burns
Temperature trauma
◇ "Pizza burns"
Autoimmune disease
◇ Pemphigus, pemphigoid, SLE
Infectious disease
◇ Viral, bacterial, fungal, parasitic
Neoplastic disease
◇ All malignancies, primary or metastatic
Hereditary disease
◇ Epidermolysis bullosa
Idiopathic disease
◇ Lichen planus, aphthous stomatitis, drug reactions

TREATMENT

General
◇ Depends entirely on the identification of the cause, either local or systemic.

MEDICATIONS
• Treatment of the primary disease when identified.
• Chronic traumatic ulcers or long standing ulcers due to inflammatory diseases including autoimmune and idiopathic processes may heal following intralesional steroid injections.
• Ulcers due to inflammatory disease in the oral cavity may be resistant to healing if the patient has a primary or secondary xerostomia.

SURGERY
For nonspecific traumatic ulcers, or chronic ulcers due to inflammatory disease nonresponsive to conventional topical or systemic therapy, excision with primary closure may be necessary.

CONSULTATION SUGGESTIONS
Oral Medicine, Oral Pathologist, Oral-Maxillofacial Surgeon

REFERRAL SUGGESTIONS
Oral Medicine, Oral-Maxillofacial Surgeon

PATIENT INSTRUCTIONS
If ulcer fails to improve within 2 weeks return for biopsy.

COURSE/PROGNOSIS
Dependent on proper management of the cause of the ulceration. Most ulcers resulting from trauma or inflammatory disease will normally take 1 to 2 weeks to heal following control of the disease or removal of the offending mechanical or chemical agent.

CODING

ICD-9-CM
054.2 Primary herpes
054.9 Recurrent herpes
079.9 Viral infection
112.9 Candidiasis
136.9 Bacterial infection
141.2 Squamous cell carcinoma
400.0 Burn
528.0 Stomatitis
528.2 Aphthous
528.92 Ulcer
529.1 Glossitis
694.4 Lupus (SLE)
694.6 Cicatricial pemphigoid
695.1 Erythema multiforme
697.0 Lichen planus

CPT
11900 Intralesional injection
40812 Incisional biopsy
87070 Culture for bacteria
87205 Gram stain
87220 KOH smear for fungi
87252 Culture isolation
88160 Cytologic preparation
99000 Transport of specimen to outside laboratory

MISCELLANEOUS

SEE ALSO
Aphthous ulcers
Candidiasis
Erythema multiforme
Herpes simplex
Lichen planus
Lupus (systemic and discoid)
Pemphigoid (cicatricial and bullous)
Pemphigus
Squamous cell carcinoma

REFERENCES
Vincent SD, Lilly GE: Clinical, historic and therapeutic features of aphthous stomatitis. Oral Surg Oral Med Oral Path 74:79-86, 1992.

Regezi JA, Sciubba JJ: Ulcerative conditions. In: Oral Pathology: Clinical-pathologic Correlations. Philadelphia, WB Saunders, 1993, pp. 34-92.

Vincent SD, Finkelstein MW: Differential diagnosis of oral ulcers. In: Principles of Oral Diagnosis. Coleman GC, Nelson JF (eds), St. Louis, Mosby-Year Book Co., 1993, pp. 328-351.

Greenberg MS: Ulcerative, vesicular and bulbous lesions. In: Burkett's Oral Medicine, 9th ed. Lynch MA (ed), Philadelphia, JB Lippincott, 1994, pp. 11-50.

Oral ulcerative disease. In: Principles and Practice of Oral Medicine, 2nd ed. Sonis ST, Fazio RC, Fong L (eds), Philadelphia, WB Saunders, Co., 1995, pp. 345-359.

AUTHOR
Steven D. Vincent, DDS, MS

Obsessive Compulsive Disorder

 BASICS

DESCRIPTION
• Anxiety disorder characterized by recurrent obsessions or compulsions that cause marked distress by being time-consuming (ie >1 hour per day), significantly interfering with the person's normal routine, occupational functioning or usual social activities, or impairing relationships with others. Obsessions are persistent ideas, thoughts, impulses, or images that are experienced, at least initially, as an intrusion and are senseless. The person attempts to ignore such thoughts or impulses, or to neutralize them with some other thought or action, and recognizes that they are the product of his or her own mind and excessive. Onset is usually during adolescence or early adulthood.
• Associated conditions seen include: avoidant behavior, hypochondriacal concerns, guilt, major depression, anxiety disorders, eating disorders, Tourette's disorder {high incidence of obsessive compulsive disorder (OCD)}, and dermatologic problems associated with excessive washing.

 ETIOLOGY

Theorized to be due to poor regulation of neurotransmitter, serotonin.

SYSTEMS AFFECTED
Nervous

 DIAGNOSIS

Diagnostic procedures
◊ psychiatric/psychologic interview, patient history.

SYMPTOMS AND SIGNS
• Common obsessions include thoughts about contamination, repeated doubts (ie, wondering if doors are locked), need to have things in order, aggressive or horrific impulses. Common compulsions (repetitive behaviors) include hand washing or mental acts like praying or counting.
• Patient may brush teeth excessively hard or long with secondary abrasion of gingival trauma.
• Compulsions regarding tooth brushing or factitious behaviors may occur.
• Patients may obsess about infections of the mouth or the possible spread of disease.
• Obsessions regarding dental esthetics may manifest. If the individual has obsessive or perfectionistic ideation, treatment may be perceived as unsatisfactory.
• Obsessions about a particular part of the body (ie, shape of jaw) result in individuals frequently doctor shopping. Such patients are rarely satisfied with treatment.

LABORATORY
No good test

IMAGING/SPECIAL TESTS
PET scan
◊ abnormal metabolism in frontal cortex and caudate nuclei.
Yale Brown OCD checklist.

DIFFERENTIAL
• Anxiety disorder due to a general medical condition
• Substance-induced anxiety disorder
• Body dysmorphic disorder
• Specific or social phobia
• Generalized anxiety disorder
• Hypochondriasis
• Delusional disorder
• Psychosis
• Impulse control disorders

TREATMENT

General
Psychotherapy
◇ usually outpatient
◇ Hypnotherapy
◇ Cognitive and behavioral therapy
◇ Continued follow-up is often indicated
◇ Support groups

MEDICATIONS
• Antidepressants, especially tricyclics, are useful; clomipramine may be successful when depression is also present; benzodiazepines are suggested with concurrent anxiety.

CONSULTATION SUGGESTIONS
Consultation with a mental health professional to address issues regarding unrealistic expectations with treatment or distorted perceptions of facial appearance is recommended.

REFERRAL SUGGESTIONS
Mental Health Professional

PATIENT INSTRUCTIONS
Patient can contact OCD Foundation (203)772-0565 or Obsessive-Compulsive Anonymous (516)741-4901 for useful information.

COURSE/PROGNOSIS
Majority of cases have a chronic waxing and waning course, exacerbated by stress. About 15% have progressive deterioration; about 5% have an episodic course.

SYNONYMS
Obsessive compulsive neurosis

CODING

ICD-9-CM
300.3 Obsessive compulsive

MISCELLANEOUS

SEE ALSO
Anorexia
Depression

REFERENCES
Scully C, Cawson RA: Medical Problems In Dentistry. Oxford, Butterworth-Heinemann, 1993.

American Psychiatric Association. Diagnostic and statistical manual of mental disorders, DSM-IV, Washington, DC, 1994.

Dambro M: Griffith's 5 Minute Clinical Consult. Baltimore, Williams & Wilkins, 1995, pp. 716-717.

Jenike MA: Obsessive-Compulsive disorder, In: Comprehensive Textbook of Psychiatry, 6th ed. Kaplen HI, Sadock BJ (eds), Baltimore, Williams & Wilkins, 1995, pp. 1218-1227.

AUTHORS
Hillary Broder, PhD, MEd
Kani Nicolls, DDS

Osler-Weber-Rendu Disease

BASICS

DESCRIPTION
A familial disease of vascular dysplasia presenting with recurrent epistaxis as the most prominent finding.

ETIOLOGY

Autosomal dominant disorder occurring with the frequency of approximately 1 to 2 per 100,000 births. This fibrovascular dysplasia occurs in localized and discrete segments of vessels from capillaries to large arteries and veins. Telangiectasias rupture easily. Lack of elastic fibers in the vessels weaken them and result in decreased ability to vasoconstrict.

SYSTEMS AFFECTED
Mucosa
◊ most common presenting feature is recurrent epistaxis which may begin in childhood and worsen with age.
Pulmonary
◊ arterial-venous malformations are found in 15 to 20% of patients. These may lead to embolism or cardiac failure.
Cerebral
◊ arterial-venous malformations may occur and may be multiple in number.
Hepatic
◊ arterial malformations may occur and cirrhosis may result.

DIAGNOSIS

SYMPTOMS AND SIGNS
Mucosa
◊ In 90% of patients the presenting symptom is recurrent, severe nasal bleeding.
Skin
◊ macular telangiectasis occurs at a later age than does nasal bleeding.
Gastrointestinal
◊ recurrent gastrointestinal bleeding occurs in approximately 17% of cases.

LABORATORY
CBC to identify anemia due to acute or chronic blood loss.

IMAGING/SPECIAL TESTS
Head CT, chest CT

DIFFERENTIAL
• Varicosity
• Angiokeratomas
• Spider telangiectasias
• Liver disease
Crest syndrome
◊ calcinosis cutis, Raynaud's, esophageal dysfunction, sclerodactyly and telangiectasia.

Osler-Weber-Rendu Disease

TREATMENT

SURGERY
• Management of epistaxis ranges from cautery to septodermoplasty to laser therapy.
• Skin and mucosal lesions effectively managed with laser ablation.

Pulmonary arteriovenous malformation (AVM)
◇ balloon embolization

Cerebral AVM
◇ balloon embolization

GI bleeding
◇ transfusions, management of esophageal varices.

CONSULTATION SUGGESTIONS
Oral Medicine, Oral-Maxillofacial Surgeon, Interventional Radiologist

REFERRAL SUGGESTIONS
Oral-Maxillofacial Surgeon

FIRST STEPS TO TAKE IN AN EMERGENCY
• Nasal bleeding managed acutely with intranasal packing or pressure catheters.

PATIENT INSTRUCTIONS
Avoid traumatizing lesions. Humidify air in winter conditions to produce dry air. Teach patient local measures that could be used to give themselves first aid should bleeding occur.

COURSE/PROGNOSIS
Genetic counseling is important for prevention. Primary morbidity of this disease is cerebral secondary to embolic complications of the pulmonary AVMs. Lesions appear early in life and tend to persist through adulthood.

CODING

ICD-9-CM
448.0 Hereditary hemorrhagic telangiectasia

CPT
11900 Injection, intralesional
17106 Destruction of cutaneous vascular lesion less than 10 sq cm
17107 10 to 50 sq cm
17108 over 50 sq cm
30620 Septal or other intranasal dermatoplasty
30901 Control nasal hemorrhage, anterior, simple
30903 Control nasal hemorrhage, anterior, complex
40820 Destruction of lesion of vestibule of mouth by physical method (eg, laser, cryo, thermal, chemical)
42960 Control of oropharyngeal hemorrhage
42970 Control of nasopharyngeal hemorrhage

MISCELLANEOUS

SYNONYMS
Hereditary hemorrhagic telangiectasia
Rendu-Osler-Weber syndrome

SEE ALSO
Epistaxis
Hemangioma

REFERENCES
Aasar OS, Friedman CM, White RI: The natural history of epistaxis in hereditary hemorrhagic telangiectasia. Laryngoscope 101:977-980, 1991.

Aesch B, Lioret E, deToffol B, Jan M: Multiple cerebral angiomas and Rendu-Osler-Weber disease: Case report. Neurosurg 29:599-602, 1991.

Guillen B, Guizar J, De LaCruz J, Salamanca F: Hereditary hemorrhagic telangiectasia: report of 15 affected cases in a Mexican family. Clin Genetics 39:214-218, 1991.

Porteous MEM, Burn J, Proctor SJ: Hereditary hemorrhagic telangiectasia: a clinical analysis. J Med Genet 29:527-530, 1992.

Rhodus NL, Kuba R: Hereditary hemorrhagic telangiectasis with florid osseous dysplasia. Report of a case with differential diagnostic consideration. Oral Surg Oral Med Oral Path 75:48-53, 1993.

Siegel MB, Keane WM, Atkins JP, Posen MR: Control of epistaxis in patients with hereditary hemorrhagic telangiectasia. Otolaryn 105:675-679, 1991.

AUTHOR
Deborah L. Zeitler, DDS, MS

- 381 -

Osteomalacia (Rickets)

BASICS

DESCRIPTION
Inadequate or delayed mineralization of both cortical and cancellous bone. Rickets affects patients prior to skeletal maturation and osteomalacia involves mature bone. Affects females slightly more often than males, and osteomalacia most common in 50- to 80- year-old group.

ETIOLOGY

• More than 50 disease processes of different etiologies manifest with either rickets or osteomalacia. Some etiologies can be categorized in groups:
  abnormalities of vitamin D metabolism [drug induced (Dilantin), renal failure], or deficiency of vitamin D, poor nutrition, malabsorption, inadequate exposure to sunlight.
  derangements of phosphorous or calcium metabolism.
  diseases without vitamin D or abnormalities of mineral metabolism.
• In the growing child, the zone of cartilage maturation is disorganized and increased in cellularity, resulting in delay of vascular ingrowth and calcification.
• In mature bone, abnormal amounts of osteoid coat the surfaces of bone.

SYSTEMS AFFECTED
Bone
  ◊ disorganized increase in cellular growth with decreased mineralization, osteopenia, pseudofractures, developmental deformities, and skeletal growth delay.

DIAGNOSIS

SYMPTOMS AND SIGNS
• Skeletal (bone) pain dull, poorly localized
• Weakness
• Muscle wasting
• Weight loss
• Tetany
• Restlessness
• Anorexia
• Skeletal deformities
• Fracture of long bones
• Pseudofractures
• Cranial softening in infants
• Rachitic rosary in children
• Bowing of the tibia and fibula in children

LABORATORY
• Calcium and phosphorus
  ◊ calcium low or normal, phosphorus low.
• Acidosis
• Alkaline phosphatase elevated
• Parathyroid hormone
• Aminoaciduria, glucosuria

IMAGING/SPECIAL TESTS
• Radiographs
  ◊ defective calcification of the ends of long bones, thinning of cortices, stress fractures, looser lines.
• Technetium-99 bone scans
• Bone biopsy

DIFFERENTIAL
• Hyperparathyroidism
• Dwarfism
• Osteoporosis
• Scoliosis
• Paget's disease
• Fibrous dysplasia
• Primary bone malignancies (myeloma, lymphoma)

TREATMENT

General
◊ Treatment should be based on the underlying disorder and is difficult to generalize.
◊ Calcium supplements or high dietary sources of calcium are necessary.
◊ Vitamin D intake in adequate amounts should be insured.

MEDICATIONS
• Vitamin D (ergocalciferol) 2000 to 4800 IV q.d. for 1 month, then gradually reduce amount.

CONSULTATION SUGGESTIONS
Primary Care Physician, Dietitian

REFERRAL SUGGESTIONS
Primary Care Physician

FIRST STEPS TO TAKE IN AN EMERGENCY
IV calcium salt if tetany occurs.

PATIENT INSTRUCTIONS
Get adequate sources of Vitamin D and calcium in diet, primarily with dairy products. Increase exposure to sunlight.

COURSE/PROGNOSIS
Varies with the nature of the underlying disorder.

CODING

ICD-9-CM
268.0 Rickets, active
268.1 Rickets, later effect
268.2 Osteomalacia
268.9 Unspecified vitamin D deficiency

CPT
20220 Biopsy, bone, trocar or needle, superficial
21450
21470 Mandible fracture treatments
70310 Dental periapicals, less than full mouth
70355 Panorex

MISCELLANEOUS

SEE ALSO
Multiple myeloma
Renal failure
Hyperparathyroidism

REFERENCES
Hutchison FN, Bell NH: Osteomalacia and rickets. Sem Nephro 12:127-145, 1992.

Mankin HJ: Rickets, Osteomalacia, and renal osteodystrophy: An update. Orthopedic Clin N Am 21:81-96, 1990.

Pitt MJ: Rickets and osteomalacia are still round. Radiol Clin N Am 29:97-118, 1991.

AUTHOR
Deborah L. Zeitler, DDS, MS

Osteomyelitis of the Jaws

BASICS

DESCRIPTION
An acute or chronic inflammation of bone and bone marrow that occurs in the jaws as a result of bacterial infection of odontogenic origin and other exogenous bacterial sources.

ETIOLOGY

• Osteomyelitis of the jaws differs from osteomyelitis of other bones in the body because it is a polymicrobial disease rather than the classic iatrogenic S. aureus/S. epidermidis of other bones that results from contamination from surgery or trauma.
• Organisms found include Streptococcus, Bacteroidies, Peptostreptococcus, Actinomyces, Eikenella, Arachnia, Veillonella, and other opportunistic organisms.
• Seen in noncompliant patients, patients who have limited access to health care, and patients with systemic, metabolic or immunologic compromise.
• Anatomic types
  Medullary
  ◊ hematogenous involving only cancellous bone.
  Localized
  ◊ less than 2 cm of bony involvement limited to one cortex.
  Diffuse
  ◊ greater than 2 cm of bony involvement with or without pathologic fracture.
Systemic factors affecting metabolism, vascularity or immunocompetence
  ◊ malnutrition, renal/hepatic failure, diabetes, chronic hypoxia, malignancy, immunosuppression, autoimmune disease, tobacco/alcohol abuse, age extremes.
Local factors affecting metabolism, vascularity or immunocompetence
  ◊ chronic lymphedema, venous stasis, major/small vessel disease, arteritis, scarring, radiation fibrosis, local neurologic deficits.
• Associated with acute apical infections secondary to caries, chronic or acute periodontal disease and trauma.

SYSTEMS AFFECTED
Bone
  ◊ local destruction of bone by bacteriologic and host immunologic mechanisms
  ◊ mechanical weakening of bone structure predisposes to fractures.
Teeth
  ◊ promotion and extension of periodontal disease.

Nerves
  ◊ extension of inflammation to inferior alveolar nerve can cause necrosis with subsequent pain, paresthesia and/or anesthesia.
Mucosa
  ◊ intraoral fistulas develop with exposure of sequestered necrotic bone.
Skin
  ◊ development of fistulas which drain extraorally as long as infected bone is present.
General
  ◊ fever, malaise, malnutrition secondary to reduced oral intake, and local or hematogenous extension of infectious process.

DIAGNOSIS

SYMPTOMS AND SIGNS
General
  ◊ fever, malaise, lymphadenopathy, weight loss, malnutrition signs.
Mouth
  ◊ acutely, severe pain, V3 paresthesia/anesthesia and halitosis. Chronically, mild/moderate pain with halitosis. Trismus may be seen.
Oral mucosa
  ◊ draining fistulae, ulceration with exposed bone, erythema, swelling.
Teeth
  ◊ caries, mobility, evidence of periodontal disease (ie, pocketing, gingivitis, bleeding).
Mandible
  ◊ swelling, pain to palpation, evidence of trauma (ie, fracture of alveolus or body).
Neck
  ◊ draining fistulas with indurated erythematous borders. Drainage may be intermittent.

LABORATORY
CBC with differential, blood culture, gram stain, culture and sensitivity testing (bone specimens must be obtained).

IMAGING/SPECIAL TESTS
Panorex or other films
  ◊ findings often delayed except in cases of fracture.
CT
  ◊ Radioisotope
  ◊ 99mTc methylene diphosphonate may identify occult areas of involvement but has poor resolution and margins are poorly define.
Positron emission tomography
  ◊ shows promise in mapping out margins of metabolic activity.

DIFFERENTIAL
• Avascular necrosis
• Benign fibro-osseous disease
• Fibrous dysplasia
• Cementifying/ossifying fibroma
• Central giant cell granuloma
• Metastatic disease
• Foreign body reaction
• Osteoradionecrosis

TREATMENT

General
◇ Debridement of foreign bodies, necrotic tissue, sequestra or teeth.
◇ Culture and identify specific organisms.
◇ Biopsy bone and associated soft tissue.
◇ Irrigation and drainage.
◇ Empiric antibiotic therapy based upon Gram-stain.
◇ Stabilization of bone to reduce fractures or prevent pathologic fractures by interjaw fixation, external pin fixation, or internal plate fixation.
Adjunctive treatment to enhance vascularity
◇ decortication, vascularized muscle flaps and/or hyperbaric oxygen therapy.
◇ Secondary reconstruction as necessary following resolution of infection.

MEDICATIONS
• Analgesics as indicated NSAIDs versus narcotics.
• Empiric antibiotic therapy is still penicillin.
• Local disease; oral therapy 500 mg q6h
• Diffuse disease; IV therapy 2 to 4 million units q4h
• Penicillin allergies
◇ cephalexin, clindamycin, cefazolin
• Definitive antibiotic therapy based on cultures. May include metronidazole, amoxicillin/clavulanate, sulbactam, ticarcillin, second and third generation cephalosporins, carbapenems, vancomycin, and fluoroquinolones.

SURGERY
Removal of sequestrum and devitalized bone. Send separate sample of removed bone for both histology and microbiology.

CONSULTATION SUGGESTIONS
Infectious Disease Specialist, Oral-Maxillofacial Surgeon

REFERRAL SUGGESTIONS
Oral-Maxillofacial Surgeon

PATIENT INSTRUCTIONS
Closely follow medications instructions.

COURSE/PROGNOSIS
• Local disease; generally good as long as nidus of infection is removed. Some may lapse into chronic cases which are slow to resolve and require long-term antibiotic therapy.
• Diffuse disease; also good but continuity defects left from eradication of involved bone may require later reconstruction.

• Complications can include neoplastic conversion to squamous cell carcinoma (.2 to 1.5% incidence) and progressive, diffuse sclerosis of the maxillofacial skeleton.

CODING

ICD-9-CM
522.5 Periapical abscess
523.3 Acute periodontitis
526.4 Inflammation (osteomyelitis) of jaw
528.3 Cellulitis of abscess mouth
682.0 Cellulitis of face
682.1 Cellulitis of neck
683 Acute lymphadenitis
906.0 Late effect open wound head/trunk
908.9 Late effect injury
909.2 Late effect of radiation
909.3 Late effect of surg/med complication
998.5 Postoperative infection

CPT
10060 I & D abscess, simple
10061 I & D abscess, complicated
10160 Puncture aspiration abscess
20000 Incisions of soft tissue abscess superficial
20005 Incisions of soft tissue abscess deep or complicated
20240 Bone biopsy, excisional superficial
20245 Bone biopsy, excisional, deep
21205 Excision of bone, mandible
21206 Excision of bone, facial bones
38300 Drainage lymph node abscess, simple
38305 Drainage lymph node abscess, extensive
40800 I & D abscess, vestibule of mouth simple
40801 I & D abscess complicated
41000 Intraoral I & D lingual
41005 Intraoral I & D sublingual, superficial
41006 Intraoral I & D deep
41007 Intraoral I & D submental space
41008 Intraoral I & D submandibular
41009 Intraoral I & D masticator space
41015 Extraoral I & D, sublingual
41016 Extraoral I & D, submental
41017 Extraoral I & D, submandibular
41017 Extraoral I & D, masticator space
41800 Intraoral I & D abscess, dentoalveolar
41830 Alveolectomy, sequestrectomy with curettage
42000 Drainage abscess of palate, uvula
42310 I & D abscess, submaxillary/sublingual, intraoral
42320 I & D abscess, submaxillary, external
42700 I & D abscess, peritonsillar
42720 I & D retro/parapharyngeal, intraoral
42725 I & D abscess, retro/parapharyngeal, external
70300 Radiologic exam, teeth, single view
70355 Panorex
99000 Transport specimen to outside laboratory.

MISCELLANEOUS

SEE ALSO
Cellulitis
Fibrous dysplasia

REFERENCES
Hudson JW: Osteomyelitis of the jaws: A 50 year perspective. J Oral Maxillofac Surg 51:1294-1301, 1993.

Adekeye EO, Cornak J: Osteomyelitis of the jaws: A review of 141 cases. Br J Oral Maxillofac Surg 23:24-35, 1985.

Koorbusch GF, Fotos P, Goll KT: Retrospective assessment of osteomyelitis. Etiology, demographics, risk factors, and management in 35 cases. Oral Surg, Oral Med, Oral Path 74:149-154, 1992.

AUTHOR
Dale J. Misiek, DMD

Osteoradionecrosis

BASICS

DESCRIPTION
Osteoradionecrosis (ORN) is a progressive, refractory necrosis of bone secondary to radiation-induced vascular changes.

ETIOLOGY

ORN is directly related to the radiation administered to treat head and neck cancer. More specifically, it is related to the vascular changes that occur 6 weeks after head and neck radiation therapy. Vascular changes include tissue fibrosis in the bone marrow, endarteritis, and periosteal degeneration.

SYSTEMS AFFECTED
Bone
◊ ORN usually involves the mandible rather than the maxilla. Presumably this is due to the increased vascularity in the maxilla.
Oral Mucosal
◊ many times the oral mucosa will be chronically infected allowing sequestration of necrotized bone.

DIAGNOSIS

SYMPTOMS AND SIGNS
• In the early stages patients may complain of toothache rather than jaw pain. Pain can be hypersensitivity to cold, percussion sensitivity or a dull throbbing toothache.
• Patients without teeth complain of a dull ache in the jaws without any clinical or radiographic signs to warrant the pain.
• Pain may be spontaneous and severe.
• Soft tissue breakdown is common, either intra- and/or extraorally.
• Bony sequestration results from the necrotizing of bone.

LABORATORY
• Many areas of ORN are infected such that appropriate culture and sensitivity testing is required.
• Soft tissue and osseous specimens should be sent for culture and sensitivity testing in addition to swab specimens of discharge or drainage.

IMAGING/SPECIAL TESTS
Serial radiographs can follow progression of disease.
Bone scan
◊ diseased area show as hot spots.

DIFFERENTIAL
• Osteomyelitis
• Malignant disease (primary or metastatic)

Osteoradionecrosis

TREATMENT

General
◊ Prevention of ORN is the best treatment.
◊ Fabrication of preradiation splints shielding the areas not being treated.
◊ Preradiation dental evaluation, including aggressively extracting hopeless or unhealthy teeth, fluoride treatments for remaining teeth.
◊ Hyperbaric oxygen treatment is used to stimulate neovascularization.

MEDICATIONS
• Antibiotics may help reduce secondary infection in the area of ORN
• Chlorhexidine rinses

SURGERY
Removal of necrotic bone ranging from limited sequestrectomy to partial mandibular resection is done in combination with hyperbaric oxygen therapy pre- and/or postsurgically. Resultant continuity defect may be corrected with bone graft reconstruction provided adequate, well-vascularized soft tissue bulk is present to provide graft coverage. Increase in soft tissue vascularity can be obtained with hyperbaric oxygen therapy. Increase in soft tissue bulk can be achieved with vascularized myocutaneous flaps such as the pectoralis major flap.

CONSULTATION SUGGESTIONS
Radiation Oncologist (who gave therapy), Oral-Maxillofacial Surgeon, Hyperbaric Oxygen Unit Director

REFERRAL SUGGESTIONS
Oral-Maxillofacial Surgeon

PATIENT INSTRUCTIONS
Inform all dentists of history of radiation prior to receiving any dental care.

COURSE/PROGNOSIS
• If extractions/surgery are required, then prophylactic antibiotic therapy, good surgical technique and a course of pre- and postextraction hyperbaric oxygen therapy is recommended.
• Overall prognosis is guarded once radiation necrosis begins.

CODING

ICD-9-CM
526.40 Osteomyelitis

CPT
14040 Adjacent tissue transfer
15732 Muscle flap, head and neck
21025 Excision of bone, mandible
21085 Oral splint (fluoride application)
21215 Graft mandible
21247 Reconstruct mandibular condyle
41830 Alveolectomy, incl. sequestrectomy
70355 Panorex
87040 Culture and sensitivity
99000 Transport specimen to outside laboratory
99183 Physician supervision of hyperbaric oxygen therapy

MISCELLANEOUS

SYNONYMS
Osteonecrosis
Radiation necrosis

SEE ALSO
Malignant jaw tumors
Squamous cell carcinoma
Osteomyelitis

REFERENCES
Friedman RB: Osteoradionecrosis: Causes and Prevention. NCI Monographs 9:145-149. 1990.

McKenzie MR, Wong FL, Epstein JB, Lepansky M: Hyperbaric oxygen and postradiation osteonecrosis of the mandible. Oral Oncol-Europ J Cancer: Part B 29B(3):201-207, 1993.

Galler C, Epstein JB, Guze KA, Bockles D, Stevenson-Moore P: The development of ORN from sites of periodontal disease activity: Report of 3 cases. J Perio 63:310-316, 1992.

AUTHOR
Thomas P. Sollecito, DMD

Otitis (Externa and Media)

BASICS

DESCRIPTION
• Otitis is an inflammation of the outer or middle ear. There are various types of otitis including:
• Externa
  Acute diffuse
  ◊ common, usually bacterial
  Acute circumscribed
  ◊ associated with furuncle
  Chronic
  ◊ long-standing
  Eczematous
  ◊ accompanying eczema
  Necrotizing (malignant)
  ◊ infection extends deep into adjacent tissues
• Media
  Acute
  ◊ bacterial infection
  Recurrent
  ◊ 3 or more episodes in 6 months
  With effusion
  ◊ middle ear fluid present but asymptomatic

ETIOLOGY

Acute otitis media
  ◊ Viral upper respiratory tract infection (URI) predisposes the ear to bacterial infection. Strep. pneumoniae (35%), Haemophilus influenzae (20%). Others include B. catarrhalis, Group A streptococcus and Staph. aureus. Mixed anaerobic bacteria occasionally cause otitis media.
Serous otitis media
  ◊ associated with URI and the bacteria listed above. Leaves fluid in ear even after symptoms abate.
Chronic otitis media
  ◊ commonly associated with Pseudomonas aeruginosa or Staph. aureus. Also implicated are E. coli and Proteus.
External otitis
  Trauma or foreign body
  Psoriasis
  Overgrowth of bacteria, mostly Staph., Strep. or Pseudomonas
  Can be mycotic or viral in origin
  Ramsey-Hunt syndrome
  ◊ Herpes zoster in the external auditory canal associated with the loss of sensory and motor functions of the VII nerve.
Necrotizing (Malignant) otitis externa
  Caused by P. aeruginosa and may result in osteomyelitis of the temporal bone.
  Most commonly seen in insulin dependent diabetics.

SYSTEMS AFFECTED
Auditory
  Ear Pain
  Loss of hearing
  Discharge from ear
  Loss of balance/vertigo
  Tinnitus (ringing in ear)

DIAGNOSIS

SYMPTOMS AND SIGNS
• Externa
  Itching
  Pain in ear
  Local adenopathy
  Erythema/purulence in canal
  Eczema
  Hearing loss
• Media
  Ear pain
  Hearing loss
  Tinnitus
  Vertigo
  Sense of fullness
• Fever
• Purulent otorrhea (discharge)
• Otoscopic exam reveals erythematous, dull, bulging tympanic membrane (TM). Mobility of TM decreased.
• Leukocytosis
• Serous otitis media will show a retracted TM.

LABORATORY
• Leukocytosis (may or may not be present)
• Culture for appropriate bacteria viral or fungal agent if otitis externa, and via tympanocentesis in otitis medica.

IMAGING/SPECIAL TESTS
• CT scan may be used to show thickening of mucosa in the middle ear space as well as extension into the mastoid cavity in chronic otitis media.
• CT scan is also helpful in diagnosis of necrotizing (malignant) otitis externa or especially if physical examination reveals granulation tissue in the posterior ear canal wall that is eroding into the temporal bone.
• Tympanometry, acoustic reflex measurement
Auditory testing
  ◊ if permanent loss suspected in serous otitis
• Standard audiometry and tympanometry can reveal conductive hearing loss.

DIFFERENTIAL
• TMJ pain
• Mastoiditis
• Trigeminal neuralgia
• Odontologic pain
• Pharyngeal pain
• Hearing loss due to inner ear disease
• Vertigo due to metabolic or central nervous system disease

Otitis (Externa and Media)

TREATMENT

General
◇ Control of predisposing factors (URI, allergy, etc.)

MEDICATIONS
• Externa
◇ topical therapy with 2% acetic acid, antibiotic drops and steroid drops.
• Necrotizing (malignant) otitis externa requires control of the patient's diabetes, IV antibiotics, local debridement.
• Media
◇ appropriate antibiotics
• Most often amoxicillin
◇ clavulanic acid, trimethoprim with sulfamethoxazole, or cefaclor.
• Antihistamines/decongestants not proven to be helpful.
• Glucocorticoids are useful in serous otitis media
• Recurrent acute otitis media give amoxicillin 20 mg/kg daily for 3 to 6 months or until summer arrives.

SURGERY
• Myringotomy with the insertion of a ventilation tube.
• Insufflation of the Eustachian tube.

CONSULTATION SUGGESTIONS
Otolaryngologist

REFERRAL SUGGESTIONS
Primary Care Physician, Otolaryngologist

PATIENT INSTRUCTIONS
Follow medication instructions closely. Take antibiotics 1 hour before meals to improve absorption.

COURSE/PROGNOSIS
• Good prognosis if appropriately managed as above.
• Recurrence of acute otitis media is common in younger children due to the limited size of the eustachian tubes.

CODING

ICD-9-CM
380.1 Infective otitis externa
380.14 Malignant otitis
380.16 Chronic otitis media
381.0 Otitis media with effusion
382.0 Acute otitis media

MISCELLANEOUS

SYNONYMS
Secretory otitis media
Swimmer's ear

SEE ALSO
Pharyngitis
Cleft deformities

REFERENCES
Lebovic R, Baker AS: Infectious diseases of the upper respiratory tract. In: Harrison's Principles of Internal Medicine, 13th ed. Isselbacher KJ, et al (eds), New York, McGraw Hill, 1994, pp. 515-520.

Klein, JO: Current issues in upper respiratory tract infections in infants and children. Ped Infections Dis J 13(Suppl 1):55-59, 1994.

AUTHOR
Thomas P. Sollecito, DMD

Pancreatitis

BASICS

DESCRIPTION
A state of acute or chronic inflammation of the pancreas resulting in secretion of active pancreatic enzymes. Auto-digestion may occur through secretion of proteases into pancreatic tissue. Enzyme secretion decreases as chronicity and pancreatic tissue destruction progress.

ETIOLOGY

- Gallstones
  - passage of stone through or near ampulla
  - 40% of acute pancreatitis
- Alcohol
  - 40% of acute pancreatitis
  - Ductal hypertension, edema
  - Often leads to chronic pancreatitis
- Hypertriglyceridemia (Type IV)
- Hypercalcemia (hyperparathyroidism)
- Postoperative pancreatitis
  - Stasis or hypotension
  - Abdominal trauma
  - Gastric or duodenal surgery

Familial pancreatitis
Pancreas divisum
Viral infection (Coxsackie; mumps)
Duodenal ulcer penetrating posteriorly

SYSTEMS AFFECTED
- Pancreas
  - Autodigestion
  - Pseudocyst and phlegmon
  - Associated ascites
  - Hemorrhagic
- Gastrointestinal
  - Portal vein thrombosis
  - Bowel inflammation and necrosis
  - Gastritis
- Cardiopulmonary
  - Hypotension
  - Pericardial effusion
  - Pleural effusion
  - Atelectasis
  - Adult respiratory distress syndrome (ARDS)
- Hematologic
  - Hemorrhage; may occur acutely, quickly
  - Disseminated intravascular coagulation
- Metabolic
  - Hypocalcemia
  - Hyperglycemia
- Acute Renal Insufficiency

DIAGNOSIS

SYMPTOMS AND SIGNS
- Abdominal pain (epigastric, severe) radiating to back
- Attack occurs after heavy meal or alcohol
- Nausea, vomiting, retching
- Hematemesis
- Cloudy sensorium if in shock
- Abdominal distension
- Epigastric tenderness
- Ileus
- Fever
- Hypotension, tachycardia
- Jaundiced, if obstructive (20 to 30%)
- Flank ecchymosis (Grey-Turner's sign) in hemorrhagic pancreatitis
- Umbilical discoloration (Cullen's sign)
- Pleural effusion
- Carpopedal spasm, if hypocalcemic
- Palpable mass (pseudocyst; chronic pancreatitis)

LABORATORY
- Elevated serum amylase and lipase
- Hypocalcemia, 2° hypoalbuminemia; Ca^{++} soaps from fat necrosis
- Elevated WBC (10,000 to 25,000)
- Elevated alanine aminotransferase and/ or aspartate aminotransferase
- Hyperglycemia 2° pancreatic endocrine insufficiency
- Hyperbilirubinemia

IMAGING/SPECIAL TESTS
- "Sentinel loop" (dilated bowel) seen on abdominal film
CT scan
  ◇ edematous pancreas; pseudocyst
HIDA scan
  ◇ biliary obstruction
Chest radiograph
  ◇ pleural effusion
- Ultrasound for pseudocysts
- Secretin stimulation test
- Endoscopic retrograde cholangiopancreatography (ERCP)

DIFFERENTIAL
- Cholecystitis
- Small bowel obstruction
- Duodenal or gastric ulcer (perforated)
- Acute bowel infarction
- Renal colic
- "Acute abdomen" due to a number of causes
- Macroamylasemia (salivary)
- Mesenteric vascular insufficiency

TREATMENT

- Acute pancreatitis
- Nothing by mouth (NPO),
- Keep pancreas at rest
- Nasogastric suctioning to keep stomach empty
- Monitor and replace fluids and electrolytes
    May require huge fluid replacement due to abdominal sequestration
- Management of complication
    Pericardial effusion; hypotension
    ◊ monitor central venous pressure
    Pleural effusion; atelectasis; ARDS
    ◊ may require ventilatory support.
    Disseminated intravascular coagulation
    ◊ factor replacement; fresh frozen plasma.
    - Bowel necrosis
    - Metabolic derangements
    - Renal insufficiency
- Chronic pancreatitis
- Nutritional supplementation
- Abstinence from ethanol

MEDICATIONS
- Endocrine deficiencies, eg, insulin administration
- Pancreatic enzymes for steatorrhea
- Antibiotics only in sepsis or abscess formation
- Pain control
    ◊ pentazocine, meperidine, or oxycodone
- H2 blockers to decrease gastric acidity

SURGERY
- ERCP to remove stones or to open duct.
- Ductal dilation procedures for stricture
- Pseudocyst drainage (usually internally) if > 6 weeks duration
- Cholecystectomy for biliary pancreatitis

CONSULTATION SUGGESTIONS
Gastroenterologist, General Surgeon

REFERRAL SUGGESTIONS
Primary Care Physician, Gastroenterologist

PATIENT INSTRUCTIONS
- Stop all ethanol use.
- High carbohydrate, low fat, low protein diet when able to eat.

COURSE/PROGNOSIS
Ranson's Criteria for Prognosis:
    On admission: Age >55; WBC >16,000; glucose >200 mg/dL; LDH >350 IU; ALT or SGOT >250 u.
    After 48 hrs: Hematocrit fall >10%; BUN rise >5%; Ca^{++} <8 mg/dL; PaO_2 <60 mm Hg; Base deficit >4 mg/L; Fluid sequestration >6L.
- If 3 or more of the above, increased number of complications and poor prognosis.
- Most common complication is pseudocyst formation
- Mortality 10 to 15% in acute pancreatitis
- 10% chronic pancreatitis develop adenocarcinoma

CODING

ICD-9-CM
577.0 Acute pancreatitis
577.1 Chronic pancreatitis

MISCELLANEOUS

SEE ALSO
Diabetes mellitus
Peptic Ulcer Disease
Cholecystitis

REFERENCES
Silen W, Steer ML: Pancreas. In: Principles of Surgery. 5th ed. Schwartz SI, Shires GT, Spencer FC, (eds), New York, McGraw-Hill Co. 1989, pp .1413-1440.

Reber HA, Way LW: Pancreas. In: Current Surgical Diagnosis and Treatment. 9th ed. Way LW, (ed), Norwalk, Appleton and Lange. 1991, pp. 558-579.

Steinberg W, et al: Acute pancreatitis. N Engl J Med 330:1198-1210, 1994.

AUTHOR
Bruce Horswell, DDS, MD

Panhypopituitarism

BASICS

DESCRIPTION
A congenital or acquired condition that results from the deficiency of all pituitary hormones, including:
adrenocorticotropic hormone (ACTH), follicle stimulating hormone (FSH), growth hormone (GH), luteinizing hormone (LH), prolactin, and thyroid stimulating hormone (TSH).

ETIOLOGY

Pituitary adenoma
◊ is the most common cause with or without infarction of the gland. The tumor suppresses normal gland function or enlarges, becoming ischemic, and subsequently necroses.
Pituitary surgery
◊ for pituitary tumors or tumors of the cranial base that result in significant destruction of the pituitary gland.
Irradiation
◊ for pituitary tumors.
Closed head trauma
◊ may lead to a disruption of the blood supply to the gland resulting in ischemia or necrosis.
Postpartum pituitary infarction (Sheehan's syndrome)
◊ occurs when the hypertrophied pituitary gland of pregnancy becomes vulnerable to ischemia. Postpartum hemorrhage followed by hypotension is the most common cause. Inability to lactate is usually the first indication.
Lymphocytic hypophysitis
◊ is an autoimmune process that results in pituitary destruction. It often occurs in conjunction with Hashimoto's thyroiditis and gastric atrophy.
Granulomatous diseases
◊ such as sarcoidosis, tuberculosis, etc, may result in destruction of the pituitary gland.

SYSTEMS AFFECTED
Endocrine/Metabolic
◊ Deficiency of ACTH and TSH may lead to potentially life-threatening crisis when the body is challenged with physiologic stresses beyond the norm. Both the pituitary/adrenal axis and pituitary/thyroid axis may be altered resulting in the signs and symptoms of hypofunction of the target organs.
Gonads
◊ are affected through the deficiency of LH and FSH.
Development and function of the male and female reproductive systems are affected and may result in infertility, impotence, amenorrhea, failure to develop secondary sexual characteristics, etc.
Breast
◊ lactation in the postpartum female may be affected and result in the inability to lactate.
Musculoskeletal
◊ growth and development is directly dependent on GH and the other GH-dependent hormones such as somatomedin C (insulin-like growth factor 1). A deficiency of GH in the growing individual leads to early closure of the epiphyseal areas of long bones and short stature.

Nervous system
◊ is affected by alterations in the pituitary/adrenal and thyroid axes—and the resultant deficiency of cortisol and thyroid hormones.
Gastrointestinal
◊ complications are due to derangements in the pituitary-adrenal/thyroid axes and result from a deficiency of cortisol and thyroid hormones.

DIAGNOSIS

SYMPTOMS AND SIGNS
- Impotence
- Infertility
- Decreased libido
- Fatigue
- Lethargy
- Cold intolerance
- Nausea
- Abdominal pain
- Amenorrhea
- Diabetic insipidus
- Fatigue
- Hypoglycemia
- Anorexia
- Inability to lactate (postpartum female)
- Growth failure
- Failure of secondary sexual characteristics to develop
- Psychosis/mental disturbances

LABORATORY
- CBC, electrolytes, thyroid function testing, ACTH stimulation test.
- Radioimmunoassay of all pituitary hormones.

IMAGING/SPECIAL TESTS
- Olfaction testing
- Visual field testing
Radiographs
  ◇ lateral skull, chest, hand/wrist
- CT scan and/or MRI of head

DIFFERENTIAL
- Addison's disease
- Primary hypothyroidism
- Primary growth hormone deficiency (pituitary dwarfism)
- Anorexia nervosa
- Primary psychosis

TREATMENT

General
  ◇ Surgery and/or irradiation for pituitary tumor.
  ◇ Hormone replacement therapy.
  ◇ Active physical exercise and strengthening program.
  ◇ High protein and high calorie diet.
  ◇ Patient education including the need for supplemental glucocorticoids during periods of major physical stress.

MEDICATIONS
Hormone replacement including:
- Cortisol (prednisone 5.0 to 7.5 mg every day as a single dose) during periods of stress (eg, surgery) the daily dose can be doubled the day before, the day of, and the day after surgery.
- Levothyroxine (Synthroid)
- Testosterone
- Estrogen and/or progesterone
- Growth hormone
Dosages and intervals are variable according to age, sex, and severity of disease.

CONSULTATION SUGGESTIONS
Endocrinologist

REFERRAL SUGGESTIONS
Primary Care Physician, Endocrinologist

PATIENT INSTRUCTIONS
Wear medic alert jewelry to warn doctors of need for steroid and thyroid hormone supplementation.

COURSE/PROGNOSIS
Careful monitoring and replacement of the appropriate hormones carry a favorable prognosis. Partial or complete recovery may occur after postpartum necrosis.

CODING

ICD-9-CM
  253.2 Panhypopituitarism

MISCELLANEOUS

SYNONYMS
Hypopituitarism syndrome
Simmond's disease
Sheehan's syndrome (postpartum pituitary infarction)

SEE ALSO
Hypothyroidism

REFERENCES
Blondell RD: Hypopituitarism. Am Fam Physician 43:2029-2036, 1991.

Crowne EC, Shalet SM: Adult panhypopituitarism presenting as idiopathic growth hormone deficiency in childhood. Acta Paediatr Scand 80:255-258, 1991.

Daniels GH, Martin JB: Neuroendocrine regulation and diseases of the anterior pituitary and hypothalamus. Harrison's Principles of Internal Medicine. 13th ed. Isselbacher KJ, et al (eds), New York, McGraw-Hill, Inc., 1994, pp. 1911-1913.

Abboud CF: Laboratory diagnosis of hypopituitarism. Mayo Clin Proc 61:35-48, 1986.

AUTHOR
Joseph J. Sansevere, DMD

Parkinson's Disease

BASICS

DESCRIPTION
Progressive debilitating movement disorder characterized by tremor, bradykinesia, rigidity, postural changes, and often mental changes. Affliction is a slowly progressive neurologic degenerative disorder of the basal ganglia associated with a localized deficiency of the neurotransmitter dopamine. More commonly seen in males. Predominately seen in the elderly, with onset between 50 and 65 years.

ETIOLOGY

• Loss of dopaminergic neurons in the substantia nigra, ventricular enlargement, and cortical atrophy.
• Environmental agents have been implicated in increased risk of Parkinson's disease (PD), (pesticides, wood pulp, paraquat, high blood mercury levels).
• May be idiopathic or caused by cerebrovascular disease of head injury. Drugs may cause parkinsonism such as phenothiazines and butyrophenones.

SYSTEMS AFFECTED
Musculoskeletal
    Stooped position
    Ill-defined aches and pains
    "Masked" facies
Speech
    Soft, monotonous voice, stammering-like speech
Cardiovascular
    Orthostatic hypotension increased with medications
    Ankle swelling
GI
    Sialorrhea (drooling, second to decreased swallowing with flexed neck)
    Constipation
Mental
    Depression
    Apathy
    Dementia, in 20 to 60%
    Impaired perceptual motor or visuospatial functions, especially inability to perform sequential voluntary movements.

DIAGNOSIS

SYMPTOMS AND SIGNS
• Ankle swelling
• Akinesia
• Anxiety
• Ataxia
• Behavioral disturbances (ie, impulsivity, loud verbal outbursts)
• Bradykinesia (slowness with paucity of movements)
• Cogwheel rigidity
• Constipation
• Dementia (cognitive and motoric slowness-executive dysfunction and impairment in memory retrieval)
• Depression
• Diplopia
• Drooling
• Dysarthria
• Joint aches
• Leg stiffness
• Loss of arm swing
• Loss of blinking
• Mask-like facies
• Muscle aches
• Ocular abnormalities
• Pill rolling motion of fingers
• Resting tremor
• Seizure
• Shuffling gait
• Slowness of movement
• Somnolence
• Stooped posture
• Urinary and gastrointestinal disturbance

LABORATORY
• Homovanillic acid (HVA)
• Measure metabolites of dopamine and serotonin in cerebrospinal fluid

IMAGING/SPECIAL TESTS
• CT or MRI of head. Structural brain imaging may reveal ventricular enlargement and cortical atrophy.
• Loss of dopaminergic neurons in the substantia nigra.

DIFFERENTIAL
• Subdural hematoma
• Hysterical tremor
• Familial tremor
• Depression
• Encephalopathy sequelae
• Neuroleptic medications
• Exposure to toxins
• Alzheimer's disease

TREATMENT

General

◇ Treatment is not curative, attempt to slow the progressive nature of the disease. Medical management consists of pharmacologic palliation in an attempt to control tremor and rigidity. Done on outpatient basis except for management of complications.

◇ May need special furniture and eating utensils at home. Will need assistance getting dressed.

◇ Wide variation in disease process. Carefully evaluate patient's tolerance of dental procedures and ability to maintain home care. Blankness of expression should not be interpreted as apathy. Empathetic responses are important. Muscular rigidity and tremor may make certain dental procedures difficult in advanced disease. Xerostomia may result from anticholinergic agents used for treatment of parkinsonism. L-dopa and bromocriptine may cause tardive dyskinesia, purposeless chewing, and grinding. If taking carbamazepine (Tegretol), erythromycin is contraindicated as may induce carbamazepine toxicity.

◇ Treatment may be facilitated with use of benzodiazepines, nitrous oxide, or IV conscious sedation. Family cooperation is critical for history taking, follow-up for dental treatment, and home hygiene.

MEDICATIONS

• For tremor, rigidity and behavior management include:
• Anticholinergics such as orphenadrine, benzhexol, trihexyphenidyl (Artane), benztropine (Cogentin)
• Anticholinergics may cause confusion, constipation, urinary retention, glaucoma or xerostomia.
• Amantadine
• Bromocriptine
• Levodopa/Carbidopa
• Levodopa for idiopathic Parkinson's disease with inhibitor of the degradative enzyme such as carbidopa (Sinemet) or benserazide (Madopar).
• L-dopa may cause dyskinesias or psychiatric side effects.

SURGERY

Adrenal brain transplants and thalamotomy being studied as possible therapies.

CONSULTATION SUGGESTIONS

Neurologist

REFERRAL SUGGESTIONS

Primary Care Physician

FIRST STEPS TO TAKE IN AN EMERGENCY

• Give antihistamine if dyskinesia occurs.

PATIENT INSTRUCTIONS

Patient can contact Parkinson's Education Program (800) 344-7872, or United Parkinson Foundation (312) 664-2344, for helpful information.

COURSE/PROGNOSIS

Progressive degeneration with increased muscle tremor and rigidity and increased mental changes.

CODING

ICD-9-CM

332.0 Parkinson's

CPT

21085 Oral splint (fluoride application)

MISCELLANEOUS

SYNONYMS

Paralysis agitans
Shaking palsy

SEE ALSO

Alzheimer's
Depression

REFERENCES

Hazzard W, et al: Principles of Geriatric Medicine and Gerontology. 2nd ed. New York, McGraw Hill, 1990, pp. 934-1096.

Scully C, Cawson RA: Medical problems in dentistry. Oxford, Butterworth-Heinemann, 1993.

American Psychiatric Association. Diagnostic and statistical manual of mental disorders, DSM-IV, Washington, DC, 1994.

Minteer J: Parkinson's disease. In: Griffith's 5 Minute Clinical Consult. Baltimore, Williams & Wilkins, 1995, pp. 760-761.

AUTHORS

Hillary Broder, PhD, MEd
Kani Nicolls, DDS

Parotid Swelling

BASICS

DESCRIPTION
Parotid swelling may be classified as:
• Localized
tumor, cyst, parotid lymph node
  abscess
• Diffuse
Unilateral infection, sarcoid, lymphomas,
  hemangioma/lymphangioma.
  Bilateral Sjögren's, sialosis, AIDS

ETIOLOGY

Parotid tumors (See Salivary Tumors)
Cysts
  ◊ may be developmental, traumatic,
obstructive.
Parotid lymph nodes swelling
  ◊ infective, inflammatory, lymphoma,
metastatic.
Diffuse swelling may be infective cause
by mumps, Echo, Coxsackie, CMV, or
AIDS viruses. Also bacterial,
Streptococci, Staphylococci, and TB.
Bilateral frequently autoimmune
  ◊ eg, Sjögren's, sialosis, associated
with diabetes and endocrine problems,
excess alcohol intake occasionally
secondary to drugs.

SYSTEMS AFFECTED
• Bilateral swelling may be associated
with xerostomia, and thus caries and dry
friable mucosa.
• Sjögren's associated with dry eyes,
lacrimal and submandibular gland
swelling. Also a systemic auto-immune
disease, eg, SLE, rheumatoid arthritis.
• Sarcoidosis affects many systems,
including the lung and uveal tract of the
eye.
• Lymphomas may involve cervical
nodes and have systemic involvement.

DIAGNOSIS

SYMPTOMS AND SIGNS
• Painless lump in the parotid is most
common symptom for tumor, cyst,
lymph node.
• Pain associated with mumps and
bacterial abscess
• Xerostomia, xerophthalmia, feeling of
grittiness of the eye
• Bilateral facial swelling
• Swelling of the parotid gland,
discrete, diffuse, or bilateral
• Facial palsy in sarcoidosis and
malignant parotid tumors
• Dry mouth, dry eyes in autoimmune
illness
• Pus or "snow storm" saliva from
Stenson's duct in sialadenitis
• Cervical lymphadenopathy in
lymphoma or malignant parotid tumors
• Fluctuant masses in cysts, polycystic
disease in AIDS, also lymphangioma and
hemangioma in children may be soft and
feel fluctuant.

LABORATORY
• ESR, Auto-antibody screen, AIDS
serology for bilateral swelling.
• Thyroid function tests in sialosis
• Mumps, CMV, Echo viral titers where
indicated

IMAGING/SPECIAL TESTS
• Sialography useful in obstruction,
sialadenitis and Sjögren's.
• CT scan for tumor, lymphoma, lymph
nodes or abscess
• MRI useful for tumor
• Lip biopsy and Schirmer test for
autoimmune disease

DIFFERENTIAL
• Tumors of skin or sebaceous cysts
overlying the parotid region may mimic
discrete swellings.
• Swellings of the mandibular ramus
due to large cysts, ameloblastoma, etc.
• Tumors of the condyle,
osteochondromatosis of the TMJ
• Masseteric hypertrophy
• Obesity, fat deposition

TREATMENT

<u>General</u>

◇ Tumors and cysts usually require parotidectomy. Parotid lymph nodes may require surgical removal if a diagnosis for primary cause cannot be made.

◇ Bacterial sialadenitis is treated with antibiotics. Once infection under control, sialogram for stone or strictures. Stone removal or dilation of stricture as indicated by sialogram.

◇ Recurrent unilateral sialadenitis frequently responds to sialography or dilation of the duct and irrigation.

◇ Parotid abscess requires drainage.

◇ Lymphomas are treated with chemotherapy or radiation.

◇ Sialosis is managed by treatment of the underlying problem, eg, thyroid disease, diabetes, alcoholism.

◇ Sjögren's syndrome is treated symptomatically, any associated underlying systemic disease is treated appropriately.

◇ Occasionally, large bilateral parotid masses in Sjögren's syndrome or HIV infection are removed for cosmetic purposes.

◇ Rapid growth or pain in an underlying immune disease of the parotid may indicate lymphomatous change.

SURGERY
See general treatment.

IRRADIATION
See general treatment.

CONSULTATION SUGGESTIONS
Oral-Maxillofacial Surgeon, Oral Medicine

REFERRAL SUGGESTIONS
Oral-Maxillofacial Surgeon, Primary Care Physician

PATIENT INSTRUCTIONS
Maintain hydration if recurrent parotiditis is a problem.

COURSE/PROGNOSIS
Many diseases with bilateral parotid swelling have a prolonged chronic course. Chronic conditions may benefit by superficial or total parotidectomy.

 CODING

ICD-9-CM
042.0 AIDS
072.9 Mumps
135.0 Sarcoid
142.0 Malignant parotid neoplasm
210.2 Benign parotid neoplasm
527.1 Mikulicz's
527.2 Sialadenitis
527.5 Sialolithiasis
527.6 Parotid cyst
527.8 Sialosis
710.2 Sjögren's

CPT
42400 Needle biopsy salivary gland
42405 Incisional biopsy salivary gland
42410 Parotidectomy (superficial) without nerve dissection
42415 Parotidectomy (superficial)
42420 Parotidectomy (total)
42425 Parotidectomy (radical)
42507 Parotid duct diversion
42550 Injection for sialography
42650 Dilation salivary duct
42660 Dilation and catheterization of salivary duct
42665 Ligation salivary duct
70355 Panorex
70380 Radiographic exam for salivary gland calculus
70390 Sialography

 MISCELLANEOUS

SEE ALSO
Xerostomia
Salivary Gland Tumors
Sjögren's
Sarcoid
Lymphoma

REFERENCES
Diamant H, Enfors A: Treatment of chronic recurrent parotitis. Laryngoscope 75:153, 1965.

Nesson VJ, Jacovay JR: Biopsy of minor salivary glands in the diagnostics of sarcoidosis. N Engl J Med 301:922, 1979.

Moatsopoulos HM, Chrised TM, Mann DL, et al: Sjögren's syndrome (sicca syndrome) & current issues. Ann Int Med 92:212, 1980.

AUTHOR
Robert A. Ord, MD, DDS, FACS, FRCS

Pemphigoid (Cicatricial)

 BASICS

DESCRIPTION
A chronic autoimmune disease causing vesicles (blisters) and ulcers that can involve oral mucosa, conjunctiva, and skin. The lesions sometimes heal with scarring. Onset in middle age and after.

 ETIOLOGY

• Autoantibodies react with constituents in the basal lamina.
• Separation occurs between epithelium and connective tissue, resulting in vesicle formation.

SYSTEMS AFFECTED
Oral Mucosa
◇ vesicles and ulcers. Gingiva commonly involved.
Skin
◇ involved less commonly than oral mucosa.
Conjunctiva
◇ ulceration, adhesion, and scarring can lead to blindness.
Other mucosal surfaces
◇ may involve nose, pharynx, and vagina.

 DIAGNOSIS

SYMPTOMS AND SIGNS
Oral mucosa
◇ multiple painful ulcers make eating difficult.
Conjunctiva
◇ soreness, pain, erythema, adhesions, and scarring.
Initial lesion is a fluid or blood-filled vesicle of variable size.
Vesicles are fragile and quickly rupture forming ulcers which heal slowly.
Individual ulcers may coalesce.
Gingiva
◇ vesicles, ulcers, erythema.
"Desquamative gingivitis" refers to sloughing of gingiva.
Nikolsky's sign-rubbing or blowing air on normal-appearing mucosa or skin causes formation of a vesicle.

LABORATORY
• Incisional biopsy needed for histopathologic and immunopathologic diagnosis.
• Subbasal clefting disorder with clean separation at basement membrane.
• Lamina propria variably infiltrated with lymphocytes.
• Dilated vascular channels in superficial lamina propria.

IMAGING/SPECIAL TESTS
Direct immunofluorescence shows linear pattern of homogeneous IgG fluorescence.

DIFFERENTIAL
Other chronic diseases causing oral vesicles and ulcers:
Bullous pemphigoid
◇ predominantly involves skin with limited oral involvement.
Pemphigus
◇ may have extensive skin lesions.
Erosive lichen planus
◇ usually white striae are evident.
"Desquamative gingivitis" may be present with pemphigus, erosive lichen planus, and cicatricial pemphigoid.

Pemphigoid (Cicatricial)

TREATMENT

General
◊ If conjunctival irritation is present, refer patient to ophthalmologist immediately.

◊ Educate patient that there is no cure for cicatricial pemphigoid. Goal of treatment is to control lesions using anti-inflammatory medications.

MEDICATIONS
• Systemic: Prednisone 40 to 60 mg, 1 hour after arising for 5 days followed by 10 to 20 mg every other day. Systemic corticosteroids are contraindicated for patients with peptic ulcers, active infections, and other conditions. Confer with the patient's physician before initiating treatment.

• Topical corticosteroids may be used as initial treatment, as an adjunct to systemic corticosteroids, or to maintain remissions. Triamcinolone acetonide 0.1% aqueous suspension, rinse with 5 mL and expectorate, four times a day, nothing by mouth for 1 hour. (Directions to pharmacist: Dilute injectable triamcinolone 40 into 200 mL of water for irrigation, add 5 mL of 95% ethanol).

• Candidiasis is a common side effect of steroid therapy.

CONSULTATION SUGGESTIONS
Oral Medicine

REFERRAL SUGGESTIONS
Oral Medicine, Ophthalmologist

PATIENT INSTRUCTIONS
Carefully follow medication instructions.

COURSE/PROGNOSIS
• Progressive disease with unpredictable exacerbations and remissions.

• Topical or systemic corticosteroids effectively control lesions in most patients.

• Major morbidity is conjunctival scarring and blindness.

CODING

ICD-9-CM
694.6 Benign mucous membrane pemphigoid, cicatricial pemphigoid

CPT
40490 Biopsy of lip
40808 Biopsy vestibule of mouth
42100 Biopsy palate, uvula
42800 Biopsy, oropharynx

MISCELLANEOUS

SYNONYMS
Benign mucous membrane pemphigoid

SEE ALSO
Pemphigus
Ulcers, oral

REFERENCES
Vincent SD, Lilly GE, Baker KA: Clinical, historic, and therapeutic features of cicatricial pemphigoid. A literature review and open therapeutic trial with corticosteroids. Oral Surg Oral Med Oral Path 76:453-459, 1993.

Lamey PJ, Rees TD, Binnie WH, Rankin KV: Mucous membrane pemphigoid. Treatment experiences at two institutions. Oral Surg Oral Med Oral Path 74:50-53, 1992.

Habif TP: Clinical Dermatology. A Color Guide to Diagnosis and Therapy, 2nd ed. St. Louis, CV Mosby Co., 1990, p. 418.

AUTHOR
Michael W. Finkelstein, DDS, MS

- 399 -

Pemphigus Vulgaris

BASICS

DESCRIPTION
A chronic autoimmune disease causing vesicles (blisters) and ulcers that can involve skin and mucosa. Onset is gradual and usually in mid-adult life, although children and elderly are sometimes affected. Other forms of pemphigus have been described, but pemphigus vulgaris is the most common type to involve oral mucosa.

ETIOLOGY

• Circulating autoantibodies develop against desmosomes of stratified squamous epithelium resulting in loss of cohesion of epithelial cells and vesicle formation.
• The cause of antibody formation is not known.

SYSTEMS AFFECTED
Oral mucosa
◇ lesions are almost always present some time during the course of the disease and often precede skin lesions.
Skin
◇ large areas of skin are typically involved, causing problems with infection.

DIAGNOSIS

SYMPTOMS AND SIGNS
• Multiple painful ulcers of oral mucosa and skin. Eating is difficult.
• Extensive areas of skin and mucosa can be involved.
• Initial lesion is a fluid-filled vesicle (blister) of variable size.
• Vesicles are fragile and quickly rupture forming ulcers which heal slowly. Individual ulcers may coalesce.
Nikolsky's sign may be present
◇ rubbing or blowing air on normal-appearing mucosa or skin causes formation of a vesicle.

LABORATORY
Incisional biopsy and direct immunofluorescence staining are usually diagnostic of pemphigus vulgaris.

IMAGING/SPECIAL TESTS
Indirect immunofluorescence
◇ autoantibodies against squamous epithelium are detected in blood. Level of autoantibodies correlates with activity of disease.
Cytologic smear (Tzanck preparation) of vesicle is of limited diagnostic value and not recommended.

DIFFERENTIAL
Other chronic diseases causing oral vesicles and ulcers include:
Cicatricial pemphigoid
◇ may involve conjunctiva
Bullous pemphigoid
◇ predominantly involves skin with limited oral involvement.
Erosive lichen planus
◇ usually white striae are evident
Herpetic stomatitis

TREATMENT

General
◇ If extensive skin lesions are present, consult with patient's physician.
◇ Patient should be informed that there is no cure for pemphigus. The goal of treatment is to use antiinflammatory medications, such as corticosteroids, to control the lesions.

MEDICATIONS
• Large doses of systemic corticosteroids are usually necessary to control the lesions of pemphigus. Systemic corticosteroids are contraindicated for patients with peptic ulcers, active infections, and other conditions. Confer with the patient's physician before initiating treatment. Burst therapy: prednisone 40 to 60 mg, 1 hour after arising, for 5 days followed by 10 to 20 mg every other day.
• Topical corticosteroids may be used as an adjunct to systemic corticosteroids or to maintain remissions. Triamcinolone acetonide 0.1% aqueous suspension, rinse with 5 mL and expectorate, four times a day, nothing by mouth for 1 hour. (Directions to pharmacist: Dilute injectable triamcinolone 40 into 200 mL of water for irrigation, add 5 mL of 95% ethanol).

SURGERY
Biopsy only

IRRADIATION
Not indicated.

CONSULTATION SUGGESTIONS
Oral Medicine

REFERRAL SUGGESTIONS
Oral Medicine, Oral-Maxillofacial Surgeon, Primary Care Physician

PATIENT INSTRUCTIONS
Follow steroid instructions carefully. Warn treating doctors of history of steroid use. Consider wearing medical alert jewelry referring to steroid use.

COURSE/PROGNOSIS
• Pemphigus is a chronic progress disease. Lesions exhibit unpredictable exacerbations and remission.
• Pemphigus is a serious disease that can be fatal due to extensive lesions or complications of corticosteroid therapy.

CODING

ICD-9-CM
694.4 Pemphigus vulgaris

CPT
40490 Biopsy of lip
40808 Biopsy, vestibule of mouth
42100 Biopsy of palate
99000 Transport specimen to outside laboratory

MISCELLANEOUS

SEE ALSO
Lichen planus
Herpes simplex
Pemphigoid
Oral ulcers

REFERENCES
Lamey PJ, Rees TD, Binnie WH, et al: Oral presentation of pemphigus vulgaris and its response to systemic steroid therapy. Oral Surg Oral Med Oral Path 74:54-57, 1992.

Habif TP: Clinical Dermatology. A Color Guide to Diagnosis and Therapy, 2nd ed. St. Louis, CV Mosby Co., 1990, pp. 412-415.

AUTHOR
Michael W. Finkelstein, DDS, MS

Peptic Ulcer Disease

 BASICS

DESCRIPTION

• A common chronic and occasionally acute disorder of the upper gastrointestinal mucosal tract that undergoes remission and recurrence. In this condition, there is an abnormal breakdown of the mucosal barrier secondary to hydrochloric acid and pepsin. The ulcers can form anywhere from the esophagus to the small intestine but occur most commonly in the stomach or duodenum. Current evidence points to the relative gastric hypersecretion as the cause of duodenal ulcers, and a deranged mucosal defense in gastric ulcers.

• Approximately 10% of the U.S. population suffers from this disease. The prevalence is approximately equally weighted among men and women. Duodenal ulcers usually occur before age 40, and gastric ulcers after 40. Only 1/3 of duodenal ulcer patients have increased acid secretions; the majority are normal. Gastric ulcer patients usually have normal or decreased acid secretions.

• Basal acid secretions follow a diurnal pattern in which they are highest at night and are lowest in the morning. Acid output is increased in response to the sight or thought of food, and is mediated by the hormone gastrin and indirectly by histamine. This effect can be inhibited by somatostatin and secretin. The integrity of the mucosa is dependent upon the endogenous prostaglandins these promote bicarbonate secretion, maintain mucosal blood flow, and are released during epithelial repair.

 ETIOLOGY

Risk Factors
  <u>Non-steroidal antiinflammatory drugs,</u>
  ◊ eg, aspirin, ibuprofen
  <u>Smoking (over 10 cigarettes/day)</u>
  ◊ not by increasing acid secretion, but possibly by inhibiting pancreatic bicarbonate secretion; also decreases response to therapy.
  <u>Family history</u>
  ◊ first degree relatives of duodenal ulcer patients have threefold incidence of duodenal ulcers.
  <u>Blood type O</u>
  <u>Stress,</u> eg, prolonged stress after major surgical procedures
  <u>Hypersecretory states</u>
  ◊ eg, Zollinger-Ellison syndrome (gastrinoma)
  <u>Chronic diseases</u> (chronic renal failure, alcoholic cirrhosis, chronic obstructive disease).
  <u>Helicobacter pylori:</u> colonization occurs in 95% of duodenal ulcer patients. In gastric ulcer patients there is 70% colonization. This bacteria does not invade tissue, instead it resides within the mucus of the epithelial cells. Its eradication leads to healing of ulcers. However, it is unclear how it interferes with the function of the epithelium.

SYSTEMS AFFECTED

• Esophagus; stomach; duodenum; proximal jejunum.
• Causes pain, "heart burn;" difficulty enjoying food, unable to tolerate certain medications, eg, NSAIDs; can have bleeding, resulting in life threatening hemorrhage; can perforate, resulting in spillage of digested foodstuffs into peritoneum.

 DIAGNOSIS

SYMPTOMS AND SIGNS

Symptoms of uncomplicated:
  <u>Duodenal ulcer</u>
  ◊ "heartburn;" episodic, bloating, belching, stomach pain, occasionally radiating to back; weight gain secondary to eating to relieve pain; vomiting, nausea.
  <u>Gastric ulcer</u>
  ◊ epigastric pain; pain may occur on eating; weight loss. It is difficult to reliably distinguish between duodenal or gastric ulcers by symptoms alone. In prospective studies it has been shown that approximately 50% of duodenal ulcer patients are symptom free.
<u>Midepigastric pain upon palpation</u>
  ◊ not specific
If a perforation occurs, it can lead to abdominal rigidity and generalized signs of peritonitis.
Hematemesis, melena, anemia.

LABORATORY

• CBC
• Gastrin levels
• Serum Ca^{++}
• Hemoglobin/hematocrit (reticulocyte count if anemic)
• Iron binding capacity and transferrin levels if iron deficiency anemia suspected
<u>Stool guaiac</u>
  ◊ test for occult GI bleeding
<u>Nasogastric tube aspirate</u>
  ◊ acutely for bleeding.

IMAGING/SPECIAL TESTS

• Barium swallow: Upper GI series with barium with double contrast radiography, 80 to 90% sensitivity
• Pentagastrin stimulation
• Endoscopy; with biopsy for H. pylorus

DIFFERENTIAL

• Nonulcer dyspepsia
• Reflex esophagitis
• Gastritis/duodenitis
• Pancreatitis
• Neoplasms e.g. Zollinger-Ellison syndrome (gastrinoma); Multiple Endocrine Neoplasia I
• Crohn's disease
<u>Infection</u>
  ◊ Giardiasis, Strongyloidosis, Tuberculosis
• Menetrier's disease
• Sarcoid

Peptic Ulcer Disease

TREATMENT

General
◇ Generally the initial course of uncomplicated duodenal or gastric ulcer is to relieve the pain, promote ulcer healing, and prevent recurrences. The use of the medications is usually carried out for 6 to 8 weeks, which results in a high cure rate. Gastric ulcers have a lower rate of healing than do duodenal ulcers, and usually require 3 months of medical therapy. Subsequent maintenance therapy is carried out for 1 year.
   1. Avoid risk factors if possible which promote, eg, smoking, caffeine products.
   2. Avoid alcohol consumption.

MEDICATIONS
• Antacids to neutralize acids (after meals)
• H2 blockers
   ◇ Cimetidine, ranitidine, famotidine, nizatidine
• Proton pump blockers
   ◇ Omeprazole
• Anticholinergic agents
   ◇ Atropine, pirenzepine
• Coating agents
   ◇ Sucralfate, colloidal bismuth
• Prostaglandins
   ◇ Misoprostol
• Antibiotics
   ◇ Tetracycline and metronidazole for treatment of H. pylori colonization/ infection.

SURGERY
Complicated peptic ulcers that do not respond to vigorous medical therapy, bleed, or perforate, require surgery. Approximately 15% of duodenal ulcer patients bleed, and approximately 6% perforate. Gastric ulcer perforation carries threefold morbidity associated with duodenal ulcer perforation.

CONSULTATION SUGGESTIONS
Gastroenterologist

REFERRAL SUGGESTIONS
Primary Care Physician

COURSE/PROGNOSIS
• The healing of peptic ulcers using medical therapy listed above results in the following success rates:

	H2-blocker	Sucralfate	Antacids
Weeks	4	6	8
Success	70%	80%	90%

• Complicated ulcers requiring surgery have a recurrence rate of about 8% at 5 years.

CODING

ICD-9-CM
531.9 Gastric ulcer
532.9 Duodenal ulcer

MISCELLANEOUS

SYNONYMS
Gastric ulcer
Duodenal ulcer

SEE ALSO
Gastroenteritis
Gastroesophageal reflux

REFERENCES
McGuigan JE: Peptic Ulcer and Gastritis. In: Harrison's Principles of Internal Medicine, 13th ed. Isselbacher KJ, et al (eds), New York, McGraw-Hill, 1994, pp. 1363-1373.

Rex DK: An etiologic approach to management of duodenal and gastric ulcers. J Fam Pract 38:60-67, 1994.

AUTHOR
Roger S. Badwal, DMD, MD

Pericarditis

 BASICS

DESCRIPTION
An inflammatory disease of the pericardium, with or without an associated pericardial effusion (fluid in the pericardial sac), resulting from a variety of causes. Acute pericarditis has rapidly progressive signs and symptoms. Constrictive pericarditis is a chronic disease with fibrosis and scarring of the pericardium that prevents adequate venous return to, and filling of, the heart.

 ETIOLOGY

Infectious:
Viral (Coxsackie B, echovirus), bacterial (Streptococcus pneumoniae, Streptococcus pyogenes, Staphylococcus aureus, Neisseria meningitidis, Haemophilus influenzae), granulomatous (Mycobacterium tuberculosis, Histoplasma capsulatum), other: syphilis, parasitic diseases.
Collagen vascular diseases:
(systemic lupus erythematosus, rheumatoid arthritis, scleroderma).
• Uremia (chronic renal failure)
• Hemodialysis
• Malignancy (lung cancer, breast cancer, melanoma, lymphoma).
• Hypothyroidism
• Trauma to the chest wall
• Radiation to the chest wall
• Drug-induced (procainamide, hydralazine, isoniazid)
• Myocardial infarction (Dressler's syndrome = pericarditis associated with myocardial infarction)
• Postcardiac surgery
• Idiopathic

SYSTEMS AFFECTED
Cardiovascular
◇ may lead to pericardial effusion and cardiac tamponade, with other systemic signs and symptoms of right heart failure.
Pulmonary
◇ may result in shortness of breath and pleural effusion.

 DIAGNOSIS

SYMPTOMS AND SIGNS
Constitutional symptoms
◇ fever, chills, sweats, cough.
Cardiovascular
◇ pleuritic chest pain, similar to an acute myocardial infarction; the pain is made worse with inspiration, and mildly relieved by sitting up, leaning forward, and exhaling; palpitations are common.
Pulmonary
◇ shortness of breath uncommon, unless cardiac tamponade or pleural effusion is present.
Cardiovascular
◇ pericardial friction rub, with three components heard in atrial systole, ventricular systole, and diastole (pathognomonic); rapid, irregular, thready pulse; distant heart sounds and pulsus paradoxus with cardiac tamponade (an inspiratory decrease in systolic blood pressure of at least 10 mm Hg); jugular venous distension.
Pulmonary
◇ shallow respirations due to pain and splinting, possible dyspnea and rales.

LABORATORY
CBC with differential
◇ leukocytosis with a left shift.
Erythrocyte sedimentation rate (ESR) elevated.
Viral swabs of pharynx and rectum for viral antibodies.
Purified protein derivative (PPD) skin test for TB.

IMAGING/SPECIAL TESTS
Electrocardiogram (ECG)
◇ typical, serial changes are initial ST elevation with PR depression in all leads, followed by T wave inversion, then normalization.
Pericardial biopsy (may be both diagnostic and therapeutic)
◇ submit tissue for diagnosis, and create pericardial window for drainage.
Pericardiocentesis (if pericardial effusion present)
◇ fluid analysis for cytology and culture.
Chest radiograph
◇ cardiomegaly (enlarged heart) with pericardial effusion.
Echocardiogram
◇ to detect associated pericardial effusion.

DIFFERENTIAL
• Acute myocardial infarction
• Aortic dissection
• Pulmonary embolism
• Pleurisy
• Pneumonia
• Costochondral or chest wall pain
• Peptic ulcer disease or hiatal hernia
• Cervical disc disease, including osteoarthritis
• Intercostal neuritis (herpes zoster)

Pericarditis

TREATMENT

General
◊ Therapy is directed toward treating the specific cause of the pericarditis.
◊ Determine if there is any hemodynamic compromise, especially if a pericardial effusion is present (this may necessitate sodium and fluid restriction, pericardiocentesis, or a surgical pericardial window).
◊ The development of chronic constrictive pericarditis may necessitate pericardial stripping, which has significant perioperative morbidity and mortality.
◊ Supportive care and analgesia may be necessary.
◊ Endocarditis antibiotic prophylaxis should be used in patients with myeloid metaplasia (myelofibrosis) during dental care.

MEDICATIONS
• Nonsteroidal anti-inflammatory agents medications of choice for decreasing inflammation and relieving chest pain: indomethacin 25 to 75 mg p.o., t.i.d.-q.i.d., aspirin 650 mg p.o., q.i.d., or ibuprofen 400 mg p.o., q.i.d.
• Steroids may be used for patients who do not respond to NSAIDs, if symptoms persist longer than 2 weeks, or if a congestive cardiomyopathy develops: prednisone 40 to 80 mg p.o., q.d. in divided doses, tapered over 2 to 4 weeks (rule out infective pericarditis prior to instituting steroid therapy).
• Colchicine 1 mg p.o., q.d. may be used (anti-gout medication).
• Antibiotics may be needed for an infective or purulent pericarditis.
• Tuberculous pericarditis should be treated with antituberculous multidrug therapy isoniazid (INH) 300 mg p.o., q.d. plus rifampin 600 mg p.o., q.d.; ethambutol 15 mg/kg p.o., q.d. may be used for INH resistance.
• Anticoagulation may further aggravate a pericardial effusion and contribute to the development of a cardiac tamponade.

SURGERY
Pericardial window

CONSULTATION SUGGESTIONS
Primary Care Physician, Cardiologist

REFERRAL SUGGESTIONS
Primary Care Physician

PATIENT INSTRUCTIONS
Frequent recurrences warrant educating patients of early signs and symptoms.

COURSE/PROGNOSIS
• Acute viral or idiopathic pericarditis is usually a self-limited disease that may resolve over days to weeks, but the course of the disease depends largely upon the underlying cause.
• May be recurrent.
• May result in pericardial effusion with hemodynamic compromise.
• Acute pericarditis may become chronic and lead to constrictive pericarditis, which may adversely affect cardiac output and lead to congestive heart failure.

CODING

ICD-9-CM
420.90 Acute pericarditis
423.2   Constrictive pericarditis
423.8   Chronic pericarditis

MISCELLANEOUS

SYNONYMS
Pericardial inflammation

SEE ALSO
Congestive Heart Failure

REFERENCES
Shabetai R: Acute pericarditis. Cardiology Clinics 8:639-644, 1990.

Ashman SG, Kahn S, Williams AC: Pericarditis secondary to tooth extraction in a patient with myeloid metaplasia: Report of a case. J Oral Surg 31: 881, 1973.

Braunwald E: Pericardial disease. In: Harrison's Principles of Internal Medicine, 13th ed. Isselbacher KJ, et al, (eds), New York, McGraw-Hill, 1994, pp. 1094-1101.

Spodick DH: Pericarditis in systemic diseases. Cardiology Clinics 8: 709-716, 1990.

Tuna IC, Danielson GK: Surgical management of pericardial disease. Cardiology Clinics 8: 693-696, 1990.

AUTHOR
Michael Miloro DMD, MD

Peutz-Jeghers Syndrome

BASICS

DESCRIPTION
A syndrome characterized by multiple hamartomatous polyps throughout the gastrointestinal tract and mucocutaneous pigmentation.

ETIOLOGY

• Peutz-Jeghers syndrome is a congenital disease transmitted as an autosomal dominant, by a single pleiotropic gene with a high degree of penetrance.
• Only about 50 percent of the reported patients have a familial history: the remainder are isolated cases resulting from sporadic mutation.

SYSTEMS AFFECTED
Oral mucosa and skin
◇ mucocutaneous pigmentation, which occurs as hairless melanotic spots found on the lips, buccal mucosa, gingiva, face, perianal area, and extremities.
Gastrointestinal tract
◇ have multiple hamartomatous polyps from the stomach to the rectum. Rarely, malignancies have been found with a preponderance in the gastric, colonic, or rectal areas. These patients may have hemorrhage, intestinal obstruction, and intestinal infarction resulting from torsion or intussusception.
Respiratory system
◇ polyps may be present in the nose and bronchioles.
Genitourinary system
◇ benign ovarian sex-cord stromal tumors and polyps of the bladder and ureter may occur.

DIAGNOSIS

SYMPTOMS AND SIGNS
Gastrointestinal
◇ recurrent, colicky abdominal pain, and GI bleeding may appear in childhood.
Oral mucosa and skin
◇ multiple brown to black macules 1 to 5 mm in diameter found on the lips, especially the lower lip, which appears at birth. In the oral cavity, the buccal mucosa is most frequently involved, followed by the gingiva, hard palate, and tongue. On the face, the macules appear to be grouped around the lips, eyes, and nostrils. Melanotic spots also occur on the forearms, hand, digits, soles, and perianal areas.
Gastrointestinal
◇ multiple hamartomatous polyps are noted from the stomach to the rectum, predominately in the small intestine. GI bleeding, intestinal obstruction, and intestinal infarction may be present.
Respiratory system
◇ polyps may be present in the nose as well as the bronchioles.
Genitourinary system
◇ benign ovarian sex cord stromal tumors and polyps of the bladder and ureter may occur.
Musculoskeletal
◇ clubbing of the fingers and occasional exostoses may be present.

IMAGING/SPECIAL TESTS
• Upper/lower GI series, fiberoptic enteroscopy, gastroscopy, and sigmoidoscopy
• Polyp biopsy

DIFFERENTIAL
• Addison's disease
• Heavy metal ingestion
• Hereditary pigmentation
• Medications eg, antimalarial drugs, birth control pills
• Hemochromatosis

Peutz-Jeghers Syndrome

TREATMENT

General
◇ Preventive surgery is not indicated. The only treatment is aimed at management of complications.
◇ Prevention of this disorder is through genetic counseling.

CONSULTATION SUGGESTIONS
Geneticist, Gastroenterologist, Dermatologist, Oral-Maxillofacial Surgeon

REFERRAL SUGGESTIONS
Primary Care Physician, Oral-Maxillofacial Surgeon

COURSE/PROGNOSIS
• Gastrointestinal carcinoma occurs in 2 to 3 % of patients, which is higher than the general population.
• Facial pigmentation often fades later in life, but the mucosal pigmentation persists.

CODING

ICD-9-CM
759.6 Other hamartomas not specified

CPT
30100 Biopsy, intranasal
30110 Excision, nasal polyp, simple
99000 Transport specimen to outside laboratory

MISCELLANEOUS

SYNONYMS
Hereditary Intestinal Polyposis Syndrome

SEE ALSO
Addison's disease
Melanoma

REFERENCES
Levin B: Neoplasms of the Large and Small Intestine. In: Cecil's Textbook of Medicine, 19th ed. Wyndgaarden JB, Smith LH, Bennett JC (eds), Philadelphia, WB Saunders, 1992, p. 716.

Regezi JA, Sciubba J: Pigmentations of oral and perioral tissues. In: Oral Pathology, 2nd ed. Philadelphia, WB Saunders, 1993, pp. 161-165.

AUTHOR
Daniel S. Sarasin, DDS

Pharyngitis

BASICS

DESCRIPTION
• An inflammation of the pharynx that is usually caused by an acute viral or bacterial infection.
• Group A streptococcus is a focus of diagnosis due to its potential for preventable rheumatic sequelae, particularly in individuals with a positive family history of rheumatic fever.
• Although pharyngitis is seen in all age groups, streptococcal infection is mostly seen in children and teenagers.

ETIOLOGY

Acute
◇ Bacterial causes of acute pharyngitis include group A β-hemolytic streptococci, Haemophilus influenzae, N. gonorrhoeae, and Corynebacterium diphtheriae. Viral causes of acute pharyngitis include the herpes simplex virus, Epstein-Barr virus, rhinoviruses, adenoviruses, and coxsackieviruses.
Chronic
◇ Most cases of chronic pharyngitis are non-infectious in origin. The inflammation may be caused by chronic irritation (smoking, alcohol), irritation from postnasal discharge of chronic allergic rhinitis, neoplasms, vasculitides, immunosuppression, and diabetes mellitus.

SYSTEMS AFFECTED
Respiratory

DIAGNOSIS

SYMPTOMS AND SIGNS
• Sore throat, especially on swallowing
• Headache
• Malaise
• Fever
• Anorexia
• Chills
• Absence of cough, hoarseness or lower respiratory symptoms.
• Enlarged tonsils
• Pharyngeal erythema
• Tonsillar exudates
• Enlargement and tenderness of cervical lymph nodes.
• Fever (>102.5°F frequently suggests streptococcal infection).
• Scarlatiniform rash with punctate erythematous macules appearing on neck and trunk, reddened flexor creases, palatal petechiae, white strawberry tongue that eventually turns beefy red (streptococcal pharyngitis).
• Gray pseudomembrane band that sloughs with considerable loss of tissue (diphtheria).
• Small clear vesicles with a characteristic erythematous base (herpetic pharyngitis).

LABORATORY
• Differential blood count and ESR.
• Leukocytosis (if pharyngitis is bacterial in origin).
• Throat culture inoculated on a sheep blood agar plate to evaluate hemolytic patterns. Bacitracin disc sensitivity of hemolytic colonies suggests group A streptococci.
• Rapid screening for streptococci can be done directly from throat swabs with commercial antigen agglutination kits. Negative direct antigen tests may need to be confirmed with blood agar culture.

IMAGING/SPECIAL TESTS
• Special tests performed only on the basis of suggestive history.
• Streptococcal isolates can be immunologically typed.
• Screening for gonococcal infection using warm Thayer-Martin plate.
• Viruses can be cultured in special media.
• Monospot test for Epstein-Barr virus.

DIFFERENTIAL
• Acute tonsillitis
• Viral or bacterial pharyngitis
• Blood dyscrasias
• Chronic pharyngo-esophagitis (Plummer-Vinson syndrome)
• Retropharyngeal abscess
• Tertiary syphilis
• Pharyngeal tumors

TREATMENT

General
◇ Rest
◇ Fluids
◇ Salt water gargles

MEDICATIONS
• Analgesics
• Benzocaine lozenges
• For streptococcal pharyngitis, systemic antibiotics are necessary for at least 10 days regardless of symptom response. Penicillin is the drug of choice and is administered as Penicillin V, 500 mg q.i.d. (25 to 50 mg/kg/day).
• For patients allergic to penicillin, give erythromycin ethyl succinate 300 to 400 mg t.i.d. (30 mg/kg/day) or cephalexin 500 mg q.i.d. (30 mg/kg/day).

CONSULTATION SUGGESTIONS
Primary Care Physician

REFERRAL SUGGESTIONS
Primary Care Physician

COURSE/PROGNOSIS
• The course of streptococcal pharyngitis is brief with the fever peaking at 2 to 3 days and abating by day 6. Constitutional symptoms and sore throat disappear shortly thereafter.
• Symptoms will resolve spontaneously without treatment but rheumatic complications are still possible.
• Suppurative complications include acute otitis media, sinusitis, and peritonsillar abscess — may require surgical intervention.
• Nonsuppurative sequelae of streptococcal pharyngitis with delayed onset include acute rheumatic fever and acute glomerulonephritis.

CODING

ICD-9-CM
034.0 Streptococcal
462 Acute pharyngitis

CPT
87060 Culture, bacterial, throat
90788 Intramuscular injection of antibiotic
99000 Transport specimen to outside laboratory

MISCELLANEOUS

SYNONYMS
Sore throat
Strep throat

SEE ALSO
Tonsillitis
Laryngitis
Epiglottitis

REFERENCES
Wyngaarden JB, Smith LH (eds): Cecil Textbook of Medicine. 19th ed. Philadelphia, WB Saunders Co., 1992.

Gray FR, Hawthorne M: Synopsis of Otolaryngology. 5th ed. Oxford, Butterworth-Heinemann Ltd., 1992.

Tierney LM, McPhee SJ, Papadakis MA, Schroeder SA (eds): Current Medical Diagnosis & Treatment. East Norwalk, CT, Appleton & Lange, 1993.

Wessels MR: Streptococcal infection. In: Harrison's Principles of Internal Medicine. 13th ed. Isselbacher KJ, et al (eds), New York, McGraw-Hill, Inc., 1991, pp. 617-619.

AUTHOR
Vivek Shetty, DDS, DMD

Pheochromocytoma

BASICS

DESCRIPTION
Pheochromocytoma is a benign or malignant tumor of chromaffin cells, located in the adrenal medulla (over 90%) or sympathetic ganglia ("extra-adrenal pheochromocytomas"), that produces catecholamines, namely epinephrine and norepinephrine. The clinical features of this disease, most commonly hypertension, are due to the release of catecholamines. Pheochromocytomas are a rare (incidence of <1%) and treatable cause of hypertension if properly recognized and treated, but can be fatal if not diagnosed and managed appropriately.

ETIOLOGY

Altered response of vascular smooth muscle to catecholamines
Idiopathic
Familial
   ◊ 5 to 10% are inherited as autosomal dominant occurring alone or in association with one of the following syndromes:
- Multiple Endocrine Neoplasia (MEN) Type IIA (Sipple's syndrome) (multiple pheochromocytomas, medullary thyroid carcinoma, and hyperparathyroidism)
- MEN IIB or III (mucosal neuroma syndrome)
- von Recklinghausen's neurofibromatosis
- von Hippel-Lindau's retinal cerebellar hemangioblastomatosis

SYSTEMS AFFECTED
Cardiovascular
   ◊ hypertensive crises, chest pain
Endocrine
   ◊ impaired glucose tolerance, hypercalcemia
Hematologic
   ◊ elevated hematocrit due to contracted blood volume, or production of erythropoietin by the tumor
Gastrointestinal
   ◊ cholelithiasis (gallstones) occurring in 20% of patients.

DIAGNOSIS

SYMPTOMS AND SIGNS
Symptoms can be paroxysmal or sustained in nature
   ◊ precipitated by exercise, urination, swallowing, induction of anesthesia, or palpation of the abdomen.
Apprehension, anxiety, a sense of impending doom, panic attacks
Hypermetabolic state
Physical Findings
General
   ◊ fever, excessive sweating, pallor, weight loss (severe), severe headaches, low body weight, tremors, Raynaud's phenomenon, livedo reticularis, cold and clammy extremities, cyanotic nail beds, nausea with or without vomiting, dyspnea.
Ocular
   ◊ dilated pupils, hypertensive retinopathy
Cardiovascular
   ◊ severe hypertension, tachycardia or reflex bradycardia, orthostatic hypotension, chest pain, flushing, supraventricular dysrhythmias, PVCs with palpitations.
Head and Neck
   ◊ MEN IIB-large, thick nodular lips, thick, everted upper eyelids, mucosal neuromas of the anterior dorsum of the tongue, lips, buccal mucosa, palate, mandible, and conjunctiva, possible thyromegaly or neck mass.
Abdomen
   ◊ possible palpable mass, abdominal pain.

LABORATORY
Electrolytes
   ◊ hyperglycemia, hypokalemia, hypercalcemia
Complete blood count
   ◊ increased WBC, decreased blood volume, increased hematocrit
Lactic acidosis

IMAGING/SPECIAL TESTS
Urinary catecholamines and their metabolites
   ◊ elevated norepinephrine and epinephrine (urinary free catecholamines)
   ◊ Elevated metanephrines (metanephrine and normetanephrine) and vanillylmandelic acid (VMA).
   24 hour urinary metanephrine excretion rate
Serum catecholamines
Clonidine suppression test (a specific test-clonidine normally reduces plasma norepinephrine by 50%, but not in patients with pheochromocytoma)
Glucagon stimulation test (a provocative test to reveal a paroxysmally-secreting pheochromocytoma)
ECG
   ◊ dysrhythmias, myocardial ischemia

Abdominal flat plate-may reveal a mass, or displacement of adjacent structures.
CT scan-usually, the initial imaging technique; will identify 95% of lesions: will show an adrenal lesion if greater than 1 cm, and an extra-adrenal lesion if greater than 2 cm.
MRI
   ◊ Considered by some to be the most reliable imaging method for pheos.
Diagnostic ultrasonography
Intravenous pyelogram with nephrotomography
Adrenal scanning (^{131}I metaiodobenzylguanidine (MIBG)
   ◊ concentrates in 85% of pheochromocytomas)
Central blood sampling for catecholamines from various sites along the inferior vena cava for localization of the tumor.

DIFFERENTIAL
Essential hypertension
- Anxiety
- Headaches (migraine and cluster)
- Diabetes mellitus
- Autonomic hyperreflexia
- Carcinoid syndrome
- Acute abdominal process
- Toxemia of pregnancy (eclampsia)
- Pseudopheochromocytoma (drug-induced)
- Dissecting aneurysm
- Acute myocardial infarction
- Congestive heart failure
- Renal artery stenosis
- Renal parenchymal disease
- Coarctation of the aorta
- Hyperaldosteronism
- Cushing's syndrome
- Clonidine withdrawal
- Use of MAO inhibitors
- Hyperthyroidism
- Intracranial tumors of the posterior fossa
- Subarachnoid hemorrhage

Pheochromocytoma

TREATMENT

General
◇ Avoid vasoconstrictors in local anesthetics during dental care.

MEDICATIONS
• Alpha-adrenergic blocking agents-phenoxybenzamine (Dibenzyline) 10 to 20 mg PO b.i.d. in increasing doses until blood pressure is controlled; phentolamine (Regitine) intravenously for hypertensive crises; or prazosin (Minipress) 1 to 2 mg PO t.i.d.
• Beta-adrenergic blockade is used occasionally, but only in combination with alpha-blockers-propranolol 10 mg PO t.i.d.
• Labetalol, an alpha- and beta-blocker, 100 mg PO q.i.d. increased as necessary to control BP.
• Calcium channel blockers-nifedipine 40 to 60 mg qd
• Sodium nitroprusside (Nipride) IV infusion for hypertensive crises.
• Esmolol (Brevibloc) IV infusion for hypertensive crises
• Lidocaine (Xylocaine) IV/IM, if beta-blockers are contraindicated.
• Amiodarone (Cordarone) IV infusion.
• Metyrosine may be used since it inhibits tyrosine hydroxylase, and blocks the formation of norepinephrine and epinephrine.
• Combination chemotherapy (cyclophosphamide, vincristine, dacarbazine) may be helpful with malignant pheochromocytomas.

SURGERY
Surgical removal is the treatment of choice (with preoperative (2 to 4 weeks) alpha- and beta-adrenergic blockade to prevent hypertensive crises, and allow volume expansion).

IRRADIATION
Radiation with or without MIBG, has had limited success in treating bony metastases.

CONSULTATION SUGGESTIONS
Endocrinologist, General Surgeon

REFERRAL SUGGESTIONS
Primary Care Physician

FIRST STEPS TO TAKE IN AN EMERGENCY
• If hypertensive crisis occurs immediately transport to emergency facility.

COURSE/PROGNOSIS
• Surgical removal relieves hypertension in 75% of patients, while the other 25% require chronic antihypertensive medications.
• Five-year survival after surgery is over 95%, with a recurrence rate less than 10%.
• Malignant pheochromocytomas carry a 5 year survival rate of <50%, with frequent recurrences despite adequate therapy.
• Catecholamine levels should be followed routinely.

CODING

ICD-9-CM
194.0 Pheochromocytoma

MISCELLANEOUS

PEARLS
Rule of 10s
• 10% familial
• 10% bilateral (adrenal)
• 10% malignant
• 10% multiple
• 10% extra-adrenal
• 10% occur in children
The six Hs (signs and symptoms)
• Hypertension
• Headache
• Hyperhidrosis
• Heart consciousness (palpitations)
• Hypermetabolism
• Hyperglycemia

SYNONYMS
Chromaffin cell tumor
Multiple endocrine neoplasia (MEN)
Adrenal gland neoplasm

SEE ALSO
Hypertension
Tachycardia

REFERENCES
Bravo EL, Gifford RW: Pheochromocytoma. Endocrin Metab Clinics N Am 22:329-341, 1993.

Manger WM, Gifford RW: Pheochromocytoma: current diagnosis and management. Cleveland Clinic J Med 60:365-378, 1993.

Perusse R, Goulet J-P, Turcotte J-Y: Contraindications to vasoconstrictors in dentistry: Part II. Oral Surg Oral Med Oral Path 74:687-691, 1992.

Rose LF, Kaye D: Internal Medicine for Dentistry. St. Louis, CV Mosby Co., 1983, pp. 1164-1168, 1207.

Stein P, Black HR: A simplified diagnostic approach to pheochromocytoma. A review of the literature and report of one institution's experience. Medicine 70:46-66, 1991.

AUTHOR
Michael Miloro, DMD, MD

Phobias

BASICS

DESCRIPTION
Agoraphobia
◇ Fear of being in situations from which escape might be difficult or in which help might not be available in the event of suddenly developing a symptom that could be embarrassing or incapacitating (ie, dizziness, falling). As a result of this fear, the person restricts travel or endures agoraphobic situations with great anxiety. (ie, crowded store, bridge).
Social Phobia
◇ A persistent fear of one or more situations in which the person is in contact with others and fears that he will behave in an embarrassing way. The fear of having a panic attack, stuttering or eating abnormally is not related to another disorder (ie, panic disorder). The fear evokes extreme anxiety and avoidant behavior, interferes with social activities or occupational functioning. The patient is aware that the fear is irrational.
Specific Phobia
◇ Is a persistent fear of a circumscribed stimulus (object of situation). Fears can include objects (ie, needle, blood), situations (ie, dental appointment), animals or natural environments (ie, storms, heights). The stimulus always evokes extreme anxiety. Marked anticipatory anxiety is typical; therefore, the stimulus is often avoided because of feared harm from some aspect of the object or situation. The phobic stimulus is unrelated to the obsessions of obsessive compulsive disorder (OCD) or the trauma of post-traumatic stress disorder (PTSD). Adults and adolescents may realize their fear is excessive, but children often do not. Social phobias more common in males; simple phobias more common in females. Agoraphobia four times more common in females.

ETIOLOGY

Persistence or exaggeration of learned response. Social phobia may be learned maladaptive response to social situations.

SYSTEMS AFFECTED
• Mental
• Nervous

DIAGNOSIS

Diagnostic Procedures
Careful history and observations of patient; description of the behavior by the patient, family and/or friends.

SYMPTOMS AND SIGNS
• Extreme anxiety when exposed to phobic stimulus
• Insomnia
• Sweating
• Hyperventilation
• Xerostomia
• Difficulty swallowing
• Abdominal or chest tightness or pain
• Tachycardia
• Dizziness
• Trembling
• Fatigue
• Dyspnea
• Irritability and restlessness
• Nausea
• Cold clammy hands
• Diarrhea
• Difficulty concentrating
• Palpitations

IMAGING/SPECIAL TESTS
Psychological/psychiatric evaluation (interview and psychometric testing).

DIFFERENTIAL
• Panic disorder with or without agoraphobia.
• Paranoid and psychotic states
• Post-traumatic stress disorder
• Obsessive compulsive disorder (avoidance associated with obsessions such as fear of blood)
• Avoidant Personality disorder schizophrenia.

TREATMENT

General
◇ Typically outpatient
◇ General Measures
Behavioral treatment
Biofeedback
Systematic desensitization
Cognitive therapy, or phobia clinic or group therapy
◇ Diet: Consider restriction of caffeine, nicotine, chocolate, stimulants.
◇ Treatment: Psychotherapy, biofeedback, relaxation, hypnosis.
◇ Approximately 20% of the general population have reportedly high dental related feats. Can be associated with previous experiences of the patient or a family member or may be generalized anxiety. Assessment of patients type and level of fear should include Dental Fears Survey or the Dental Anxiety Scale and a thorough patient social and dental history.
◇ Systematic desensitization, relaxation therapy, and mental imagery are recommended. Use distraction techniques and give patient as much control as possible (ie, hand raising to discontinue treatment). Anxiolytics such as oral diazepam, supplemented with intravenous or inhalational sedation during dental treatment should be considered.

MEDICATIONS
• Typically used in treatment are benzodiazepines, MAO inhibitors, buspirone, beta-adrenergic blockers, and antihistamines.
• For simple phobias
◇ alprazolam; for acute conditions
◇ beta blockers (propranolol) 10 to 40 mg about 45 minutes before anticipated encounter; for Generalized/Social Phobia
◇ atenolol 50 to 100 mg/day; for chronic social phobias, phenelzine (MAO inhibitor), up to 90 mg/day.
• Avoid sympathomimetics, tricyclic antidepressants, fluoxetine, CNS depressants.

CONSULTATION SUGGESTIONS
Mental Health Professional

REFERRAL SUGGESTIONS
Mental Health Professional

PATIENT INSTRUCTIONS
Consider group therapy

COURSE/PROGNOSIS
Variable
◇ Typically chronic without treatment
◇ rarely incapacitating. Simple phobias
◇ impairment can be minimal; agoraphobia
◇ usually progressive and unremitting without treatment.

CODING

ICD-9-CM
300.22   Agoraphobia
300.235 Social phobia
300.29   Simple phobia

MISCELLANEOUS

SYNONYMS
Dental phobic

SEE ALSO
Obsessive Compulsive Disorder
Depression

REFERENCES
Redding S, Montgomery M: Dentistry in Systemic Disease. Portland, JBK, 1990, pp. 301-325.

Ydofsky S, Hales R: Textbook of Neuropsychiatry, 2nd ed. Washington, DC, American Psychiatric Press, Inc. 1992.

AUTHORS
Hillary Broder, PhD, MEd
Kani Nicolls, DDS

Platelet Disorders

BASICS

DESCRIPTION
• Platelets are a necessary component for effective blood coagulation. Disorders are typically either due to too few platelets (quantitative disorder) or due to poorly functioning platelets (qualitative disorder).
• Platelets are produced by the fragmentation of bone marrow derived megakaryocytes. One-third of platelets released from the marrow are sequestered in the spleen, while two-thirds circulate for 7 to 10 days. Platelets circulate until they become senescent and are then removed from the circulation by phagocytic cells, primarily in the spleen and liver. For poorly understood reasons, a decrease in platelet numbers causes an increase in platelet production. The normal platelet count ranges from 150,000 to 450,000 per mL. However, with properly functioning platelets, counts can fall to 20,000 to 50,000 without serious coagulation problems occurring.

ETIOLOGY
• Thrombocytopenia (decreased numbers of platelets) can occur due to three mechanisms:
   (1) depressed bone marrow production of megakaryocytes
   (2) increased splenic sequestration
   (3) accelerated destruction.
• Decreased production can be due to any disorder or substance that injures marrow stem cells (irradiation, cancer chemotherapy, ethanol, estrogen, thiazide diuretics).
• Increased splenic sequestration seen in portal hypertension due to liver cirrhosis or situations where spleen infiltrated with tumor cells.
• Accelerated destruction seen due to mechanical injury of platelets (heart valves), or immunologic disorders such as HIV, hemolytic uremia, idiopathic thrombocytopenic purpura (ITP), or with administration of certain drugs (carbamazepine, digoxin, methyldopa, aspirin, gold salts, sulfa drugs, and high doses of penicillins).
• Platelet membrane defects seen as autosomal recessive traits. Two rare types are Bernard-Soulier syndrome and Glanzmann's disease (thrombasthenia). Nonsteroidal anti-inflammatory drugs (NSAIDs) can induce qualitative platelet problems due to impairment of platelet production of thromboxane A2, an important mediator of platelet secretion and aggregation. Effect occurs shortly after NSAID enters circulation and lasts for 5 to 7 days after NSAID administration stops.
• Use of therapeutic heparin in amounts necessary to produce systemic anticoagulation can also cause thrombocytopenia.

SYSTEMS AFFECTED
Coagulation
   ◊ any site subject to injury of local blood vessels at risk for problems when platelet disorder present.

DIAGNOSIS

SYMPTOMS AND SIGNS
• Prolonged bleeding after even minor injury or during menstrual flow seen with mild platelet disorder.
• Severe platelet disorder may lead to spontaneous bleeding from sites such as nose (epistaxis), cerebrum (stroke), or GI tract.
• Patients may report easy bruising, large bruising even with minor trauma, symptoms related to anemia in women with excessive menstrual blood loss.
• Exam may reveal bruises, splenomegaly, signs of anemia.

LABORATORY
• Prolonged bleeding time in face of normal PT and PTT.
• Platelet count low and peripheral smear shows few or no platelets.
• Measure IgG level.

IMAGING/SPECIAL TESTS
Bone marrow biopsy (aspirate)
   ◊ hypocellular

DIFFERENTIAL
• Hemophilia
• von Willebrand's disease
• Idiopathic thrombocytopenic purpura
• NSAID use
• Drug-induced thrombocytopenia
• HIV infection
• Sarcoid
• Systemic lupus
• Bernard-Soulier syndrome
• Glanzmann's disease
• Chediak-Higashi syndrome
• Hypersplenism
• Lymphoma or leukemia
• Prosthesis destruction of platelets
• Vessel wall disorders (TTP, Henoch-Schönlein purpura, Rocky Mountain Spotted Fever, Marfan's, Ehlers-Danlos, Osler-Weber-Rendu, Kasabach-Merritt).

TREATMENT

General
◇ Therapy depends primarily upon reaching correct diagnosis.
◇ Quantitative defects can be mitigated by platelet transfusions (usually administer 8 to 10 units of platelets at a time). Because banked platelets lose some of their useful life, they will have a shorter life span than marrow derived platelets.

MEDICATIONS
• Immune-mediated platelet disorders may benefit from corticosteroid administration. Particularly true for ITP.
• Patients who fail to respond after steroids or splenectomy are often given azathioprine, cyclophosphamide, or vincristine. Danazol, an impeded androgen, is also sometimes helpful.

SURGERY
Splenic sequestration of platelets sometimes managed with splenectomy.

CONSULTATION SUGGESTIONS
Hematologist, Primary Care Physician

REFERRAL SUGGESTIONS
Oral-Maxillofacial Surgeon (for dentoalveolar surgery)

FIRST STEPS TO TAKE IN AN EMERGENCY
• If oral bleeding thought to be due to platelet disorder, put direct pressure on bleeding site and obtaining PT, PTT, bleeding time, and platelet count.

PATIENT INSTRUCTIONS
• Patients with known platelet disorder should consider medic alert jewelry.
• Also should alert any treating doctors of bleeding potential.

COURSE/PROGNOSIS
Once diagnosis of platelet disorder made, treatment and prognosis varies. If disorder requires repeated platelet transfusions, patient may develop antibodies to platelets compounding problem.

CODING

ICD-9-CM
287.1 Bernard-Soulier, Glanzmann's
287.3 Thrombocytopenia purpura
287.4 Thrombocytopenia due to drug
287.5 Thrombocytopenia

MISCELLANEOUS

SYNONYMS
Thrombocytopenia
Idiopathic thrombocytopenic purpura

SEE ALSO
Coagulopathy

REFERENCES
Stuart MJ, Kelton JG: The platelet. In: Hematology of Infancy and Childhood. 4th ed. Nathan DG, Oskia FA (eds), Philadelphia, WB Saunders, 1992, pp. 1343-1479.

Williams WJ, et al (eds): Hematology. 4th ed. New York, McGraw-Hill Co., 1990.

Handin RI: Disorders of the platelet and vessel wall. In: Harrison's Principles of Internal Medicine, 13th ed. Isselbacher KJ, et al (eds), New York, McGraw-Hill, 1994, pp. 1798-1802.

George JN, Shattil SJ: The clinical importance of acquired abnormalities of platelet function. N Engl J Med 324:27-36, 1991.

AUTHOR
James R. Hupp, DMD, MD, JD, FACS

Pleural Effusion

BASICS

DESCRIPTION
An abnormal excess accumulation of fluid within the pleural space.

ETIOLOGY

Transudative pleural effusion
◊ due to elevated systemic or pulmonary venous pressure, or decreased plasma oncotic pressure. The primary mechanism is systemic, and does not directly involve the lung surface.
• Congestive heart failure
• Cirrhosis
• Nephrotic syndrome
• Pulmonary embolism
• Pericardial disease
• Starvation
• Ascites
• Peritoneal dialysis

Exudative pleural effusion
◊ due directly to pleural disease, inflammation, or lymphatic obstruction to fluid outflow. Local factors are responsible for an alteration in formation and/or absorption of pleural fluid.
• Neoplastic disease-bronchogenic carcinoma, metastatic disease, mesothelioma, lymphoma.
• Infectious disease-bacterial (parapneumonic effusion) pneumonia (gram +, gram −, Actinomyces), tuberculosis, fungal (Nocardia, Coccidioides), viral (Coxsackie), parasitic (Amoeba, Echinococcus), Pneumocystis carinii (six reported cases).
• Pulmonary embolism

Gastrointestinal disease
◊ esophageal perforation, pancreatic disease, intra-abdominal abscess, diaphragmatic hernia, Meig's syndrome.

Collagen-vascular disease
◊ rheumatoid arthritis, systemic lupus erythematosus, drug-induced lupus, Sjögren's syndrome, Wegener's granulomatosis, Churg-Strauss syndrome.
• Post-cardiac injury syndrome (Dressler's syndrome)
• Asbestosis
• Sarcoidosis
• Uremia
• Iatrogenic injury
• Trauma-hemothorax, chylothorax
• Lymphedema
• Drug-induced pleural disease
• Radiation therapy
• Myxedema

SYSTEMS AFFECTED
• Cardiovascular
• Pulmonary

DIAGNOSIS

SYMPTOMS AND SIGNS
• Pulmonary-pleuritic chest pain, exacerbated with full inspiration, dyspnea.
Auscultation over involved lung region may reveal:
• Pleural friction rub
• Absent or decreased vocal fremitus
• Dull-to-flat percussion
• Reduced-to-absent breath sounds
• Reduced chest wall movement
• Auscultation over adjacent compressed lung may reveal an area of bronchial breath sounds and/or egophony.

LABORATORY
CBC
◊ leukocytosis, anemia
• Thoracentesis
Note gross appearance (red due to red blood cells)
Total protein content
◊ greater than 3 g/dL in exudate
Lactate dehydrogenase (LDH) level
◊ greater than 200 IV
Differential cell count
Bacteriologic examination
◊ gram stain, culture
Cytologic examination
◊ look for tumor cells
Carcinoembryonic antigen (CEA) level (for malignant pleural effusions)
Glucose level
◊ usually less than 60 mg/dL
Amylase level
◊ elevated in effusion due to pancreatitis.
Triglyceride level
pH less than 7.2 in empyema
• Criteria for exudative pleural effusion (Light's criteria):
• Pleural fluid protein/serum protein >0.5
• Pleural fluid LDH/serum LDH >0.6
• Pleural fluid LDH more than 2/3 normal upper limit for serum
• Pleural fluid LDH > 200 IU/liter
• Pleural fluid protein > 3 g/dL
• The diagnosis of a transudative pleural effusion usually warrants no further investigation and requires treatment of the underlying disorder. Because the differential diagnosis of an exudative pleural effusion is extensive, further diagnostic testing is necessary.

IMAGING/SPECIAL TESTS
Chest radiograph (CXR-PA, lateral, and lateral decubitus)
◊ blunting of the costophrenic angle; will show an effusion with greater than 175 mL of fluid.
• Closed pleural biopsy (needle biopsy) is indicated if thoracentesis is nondiagnostic.

• Open pleural biopsy (thoracotomy) and/or biopsy of other sites is indicated if a malignancy is suspected, or if all other investigation has not been diagnostic.
• Fiberoptic thoracoscopy and pleuroscopy allow direct visualization of the pleural surface under video guidance.

CT scan
◊ shows excellent pleural anatomy; can differentiate between pleural and parenchymal disease, and can distinguish benign versus malignant pleural involvement.

MRI
◊ value limited by motion artifact of cardiac and respiratory activity

Ultrasonography
◊ may show a loculated effusion, or help in guiding a needle thoracentesis
• Pulmonary angiogram, or V/Q lung scan, to rule out pulmonary embolism
• Purified protein derivative (PPD) to rule out tuberculosis.
• Shift of heart and mediastinum away from side of effusion on chest radiograph, and possible tracheal deviation.

DIFFERENTIAL
• Transudative pleural effusions:
• Congestive heart failure
• Pericardial disease
• Cirrhosis
• Nephrotic syndrome
• Peritoneal dialysis
• Superior vena cava obstruction
• Pulmonary embolism
• Exudative pleural effusions:
• Neoplastic diseases
• Infectious diseases
• Pulmonary embolism
• Gastrointestinal diseases
• Collagen-vascular diseases
• Sarcoidosis
• Drug-induced pleural disease
• Radiation therapy
• Iatrogenic injury

TREATMENT

General
◊ The specific etiology of the pleural effusion must be established, and treatment is directed toward the underlying disorder.
◊ Symptomatic pleural effusions may require thoracentesis with removal of a large amount of fluid, with possible chest tube drainage.
◊ Depending upon the underlying disease process and the degree of physiological impairment, various treatment modalities include repeated thoracentesis, chest tube thoracostomy, chemical pleurodesis [using a sclerosing agent (eg, tetracycline) to obliterate the pleural space], thoracotomy with decortication (pleurectomy), or mediastinal radiation therapy.

MEDICATIONS
• Used to treat the underlying disorder.
• Antibiotic therapy for parapneumonic pleural effusions.
• Chemotherapeutic agents for malignant pleural effusions.
• Antituberculous therapy for tuberculous pleuritis.

SURGERY
See general treatments.

IRRADIATION
See general treatments.

CONSULTATION SUGGESTIONS
Thoracic Surgeon, General Surgeon

REFERRAL SUGGESTIONS
Primary Care Physician, General Surgeon

COURSE/PROGNOSIS
• Depends upon the identification and treatment of the underlying disorder.
• Repeated thoracentesis for symptomatic relief should be performed with caution, because there is significant protein loss with reaccumulation of fluid over the next few days.
• Rapid removal of large amounts of fluid can predispose to acute pulmonary edema.

CODING

ICD-9-CM
197.2 Secondary malignant neoplasm in pleura
511.1 Pleurisy with effusion
511.9 Unspecified pleural effusion

MISCELLANEOUS

SEE ALSO
Lung malignancy

REFERENCES
Sahn SA: The pathophysiology of pleural effusions. Ann Rev Med 41:7-13, 1990.

Berkman N, Kramer MR: Diagnostic tests in pleural effusion an update. Postgrad Med J 69: 12-18, 1993.

Strange C, Sahn SA: Management of parapneumonic pleural effusions and empyema. Infect Dis Clin N Am 5: 539-559, 1991.

Horowitz ML, Schiff M, Samuels J, Russo R, Schnader J: Pneumocystis carinii pleural effusion: Pathogenesis and pleural fluid analysis. Am Rev Resp Dis 148:232-234, 1993.

Stogner SW, Campbell GD: Pleural effusion: What you can learn from the results of a "tap?" Postgrad Med 91:439-454, 1992.

AUTHOR
Michael Miloro, DMD, MD

Plummer-Vinson Syndrome

BASICS

DESCRIPTION
A rare pathologic condition characterized by iron deficiency anemia, esophageal webbing with resultant progressive dysphagia, and glossitis.

ETIOLOGY

The cause of Plummer-Vinson syndrome (PVS) has been attributed to a number of factors, including esophageal innervation disturbances, nutritional deficiencies (ie, iron deficient anemia), autoimmune reactions, and infection.

SYSTEMS AFFECTED
Hematologic
◇ microcytic, hypochromic anemia is present.
Mucosal tissue
◇ degenerative changes occur in the oral cavity, pharynx, and esophagus, which cause decreased cellular regeneration. As a result, ulcers or cracking secondary to trauma occur. There is an increased incidence of carcinoma involving the oral cavity, hypopharynx, and esophagus.
Upper gastrointestinal tract
◇ progressive dysphagia with webbing of the esophagus. Low swallowing pressure in the hypopharyngeal area may occur.
Ocular
◇ numerous complications, including conjunctivitis, keratitis, blepharitis, and visual disturbances are reported.
Gynecologic
◇ increased incidence of inflammation and infection, as well as menorrhagia may occur secondary to chronic iron deficiency.
Skin and nails
◇ nail deformities, hyperkeratosis, and seborrheic dermatitis.

DIAGNOSIS

SYMPTOMS
General
◇ fatigability, decreased exercise tolerance, mild dyspnea on exertion, dizziness, soft finger nails which may show spooning or longitudinal splitting, brittle hair, possible splenomegaly.
Eyes
◇ visual changes, conjunctiva are pale, conjunctivitis.
Oral cavity
◇ soreness of the tongue with erythematous tongue devoid of papillae and glossitis, and at the angles of the mouth (angular cheilitis), dry, pallid mucous membrane.
GI
◇ progressive dysphagia with increased frequency of choking, and regurgitation.

LABORATORY
CBC, iron binding capacity, transferrin levels.

IMAGING/SPECIAL TESTS
Cine
◇ Esophagram
Esophagoscopy
◇ endoscopy

DIFFERENTIAL
• Esophageal tumors
• Achalasia
• Barrett's esophagitis
• Peptic esophagitis
• Benign stricture of the esophagus
• Lower esophageal ring
• Raynaud's phenomenon
• Scleroderma
• Systemic lupus erythematosus
• Esophageal diverticula
• Esophageal cysts

TREATMENT

Long-term follow-up is important in PVS patients, because this disease is felt to be a premalignant disorder by many investigators..

MEDICATIONS
• Supplemental iron therapy is required due to chronic iron deficiency anemia. Ferrous sulfate, 325 mg t.i.d., until iron stores replenished.

SURGERY
Esophageal endoscopy with biopsy, as well as lysis of esophageal webbing, and/or esophageal dilation is indicated. Dysphagia improves following surgery.

CONSULTATION SUGGESTIONS
Gastroenterologist, Oral Medicine

REFERRAL SUGGESTIONS
Primary Care Physician, Oral-Maxillofacial Surgeon

PATIENT INSTRUCTIONS
Malignant potential makes it important that the patient receive careful monitoring by Oral-Maxillofacial Surgeon or Otolaryngologist.

COURSE/PROGNOSIS
• Following iron supplementation and surgical treatment of the esophageal webs, dysphagia, glossitis, and iron deficient anemia improve.
• There is an increased incidence of carcinoma involving the oral mucosa, hypopharynx, and esophagus. Regular long-term follow-up is indicated. Any symptoms of esophageal disease warrants aggressive diagnostic investigation.

CODING

ICD-9-CM
280.8 Plummer-Vinson syndrome
280.9 Iron deficiency anemia
529.0 Glossitis
750.3 Esophageal web

CPT
40808 Biopsy vestibule of mouth
41100 Biopsy of tongue
43200 Esophagoscopy; diagnostic
43202 Esophagoscopy; for biopsy
43220 Esophagoscopy; for dilation, direct
99000 Transport specimen to outside laboratory

MISCELLANEOUS

SYNONYMS
Patterson-Kelly Syndrome
Waldenstrom and Kyellberg dysphagia
Sideropenia dysphagia

SEE ALSO
Dysphagia
Esophageal tumors
Glossitis

REFERENCES
Seitz ML, Sabatino D: Plummer-Vinson syndrome in an adolescent. J Adoles Health 12:279-281, 1991.

Geerlings SE, Statius van Eps LW; Pathogenesis and consequences of Plummer-Vinson syndrome. Clin Investig 70:629-630, 1992.

Bredenkamp JK, Castro DJ, Mickel RA: Importance of iron repletion in the management of Plummer-Vinson syndrome. Ann Otol Rhinol Laryngol 99:51-54, 1990.

AUTHOR
Daniel S. Sarasin, DDS

Pentumonia - Bacterial

BASICS

DESCRIPTION
Acute bacterial infection of the lung parenchyma. Most commonly seen in adults due to nosocomial or community acquired bacteria. Pneumonia in children usually viral in origin.

ETIOLOGY

Epidemiology:
 • Very common cause for hospitalization, ranking as the fourth leading cause for men and fifth for women. Most common organisms are Streptococcus pneumoniae and Haemophilus influenzae. Bacterial resistance to antibiotics is a concern as different strains of these primary organisms mutate. Other common organisms are S. aureous, Legionella pneumophilia, Moraxella catarrhalis, Mycoplasm, Klebsiella, and Pseudomonas.
Causes:
 • Aspiration of oropharyngeal fluids or inhalation of organisms that have colonized the nose or mouth. The lung has continuous contact with foreign substances in the air and many may enter during inhalation. Disturbances of the normal defense mechanisms (smoking, tracheal intubation, emphysema, malnutrition, immunologic compromise, malignancy, cystic fibrosis, upper respiratory infection, sepsis) predispose to pneumonia. Common terminal event in patients debilitated due to other serious disorders such as congestive heart failure or stroke.

SYSTEMS AFFECTED
Pulmonary

DIAGNOSIS

SYMPTOMS AND SIGNS
 • Fever, chills, malaise, and other general constitutional symptoms. Cough (productive or nonproductive); chest pain (particularly with pleuritis). In the elderly or immunocompromised, systemic symptoms, eg, fever, may not be pronounced.
 • Physical Examination and Findings:
 • Fever, sputum production, bronchial breath sounds, hemoptysis, dyspnea, diminished or absent breath sounds indicating consolidation, dullness to percussion particularly when pleural fluid is present, egophony, pleural friction rub, cyanosis.

LABORATORY
 • Complete blood count with white cell differential; serial CBC to help assess response. If not responsive to treatment, invasive studies may be necessary such as lung biopsy (transtracheal or open) or bronchoalveolar lavage.
 • Blood cultures

IMAGING/SPECIAL TESTS
Diagnostic Testing:
Sputum examination by Gram stain and culture and sensitivity; nasotracheal or bronchoscopic suction will obtain a more accurate specimen.
Blood cultures
 ◇ may be appropriate if suspect bacteremia, particularly with S. pneumoniae.
Thoracentesis
 ◇ to tap pleural effusion may be source of culture specimen. Fine needle aspiration of parenchyma may also be useful if neoplasm suspected.
Chest radiograph
 ◇ mandatory; serial studies allow assessment of response to therapy. Look for air bronchograms, lobar, or segmental consolidation and pleural effusion.
Serum or urine test for pneumococcal antigen.
Arterial blood bases
 ◇ hypoxia, altered CO_2, acidosis.
Cold agglutinins for Mycoplasma.

DIFFERENTIAL
Nonbacterial pneumonia
 ◇ viral, fungal, rickettsial, parasitic.
 • Pulmonary contusion
 • Tuberculosis
 • Aspiration pneumonitis
 • Hypersensitivity pneumonitis
 • Acute sarcoid lung

TREATMENT

General
◇ Hydration with IV fluids, bed rest, pulmonary therapy (oxygen, humidification, incentive spirometry, chest percussion, tracheal suction). In severe cases, particularly if patient becomes exhausted due to the effort of breathing, should intubate and mechanically ventilate; also allows direct access for tracheal suction and lavage.

MEDICATIONS
• Antimicrobial therapy is the mainstay of therapy, initially being guided by Gram stain findings of sputum specimens and by clinical setting (eg, nosocomial infection in immunocompromised individual versus community-acquired pneumonia in a healthy person). For the community-acquired infection in an otherwise healthy individual, initial therapy is usually IV penicillin or IV vancomycin if penicillin-allergic (p.o. erythromycin in less ill patients) because S. pneumoniae is common. H. influenzae pneumonia treated with ampicillin. In alcoholics, consider Legionella and Klebsiella. In immunocompromised individuals in general, consider Gram-negative organisms such as Pseudomonas or Gram-positive organisms such as Staphylococcus aureus. Human immunodeficiency virus infection predisposes to Pneumocystis carinii pneumonia. Nosocomial infections are often Gram-negative. Ultimately, usually within 24 to 48 hours, treatment is modified as needed based on culture results.
• Antipyretics for fever such as acetaminophen or NSAIDs.
• Polyvalent pneumococcal vaccine available (pneumovax) for older children (>2 years) and adults at increased risk.

CONSULTATION SUGGESTIONS
Primary Care Physician, Infectious Disease Specialist, Pulmonologist

REFERRAL SUGGESTIONS
Primary Care Physician

FIRST STEPS TO TAKE IN AN EMERGENCY
• Transport to emergency facility if respiratory failure suspected.

PATIENT INSTRUCTIONS
• Avoid unnecessary hospitalizations to minimize contact with unusual organisms.
• Can call American Lung Association for printed patient information (212)315-8700.
• Avoid debilitation

COURSE/PROGNOSIS
In younger, otherwise healthy patients full recovery expected following proper therapy. Older, debilitated patients often succumb to disease even if aggressively managed.

CODING

ICD-9-CM
136.3 Pneumocystis carinii
481 Pneumococcal pneumonia
482.1 Pseudomonas pneumonia
482.2 Haemophilis pneumonia
482.9 Bacterial pneumonia
483 Mycoplasma pneumonia

MISCELLANEOUS

SYNONYMS
Lobar pneumonia

SEE ALSO
Respiratory distress syndrome
COPD
Aspiration pneumonia
Viral pneumonia

REFERENCES
Sarosi GA: Bacterial pneumonia. S. Pneumoniae and H. influenzae are the villains. Postgrad Med 93:43-52, 1993.

Griffith DE: Pneumonia in chronic obstructive lung disease. Infect Dis Clin N Am 5:467-484, 1991.

AUTHOR
Robert Chuong, MD, DMD

Pneumonia - Viral

BASICS

DESCRIPTION
• Infection of the lung parenchyma by viral organisms. Commonly referred to in the medical literature as "atypical pneumonia," in contrast to bacterial pneumonia.
• Pneumonias caused by mycoplasma or chlamydia, nonviral organisms, are also in the atypical category and are extremely difficult to culture and therefore may be misdiagnosed as viral in origin. Viral causes of pneumonia have been found in approximately 17% of pediatric outpatient pneumonias and a similar percentage in adults in the community and in nursing homes. Improved culture techniques have enhanced diagnosis.

ETIOLOGY

Causative Organisms:
Respiratory syncytial virus (RSV)
  ◇ most common in children, but also seen in immunocompromised adults. Adenoviruses and parainfluenza viruses are common in children. Common in adults are cytomegalovirus (CMV). Influenza A and B viruses common in both children and adults. Varicella zoster may cause pneumonia in children and immunocompromised.
Bacterial superinfection may complicate diagnosis and treatment.

SYSTEMS AFFECTED
Pulmonary

DIAGNOSIS

Proper index of suspicion because bacterial cultures are negative unless there is bacterial superinfection.

SYMPTOMS AND SIGNS
• Onset tends to be subtle with mild symptoms initially including low-grade fever and absence of toxic appearance. Usually nonproductive cough, no pleuritic pain, sometimes preceded by upper respiratory symptoms. Physical findings may be minimal including absence of major changes on pulmonary auscultation, although wheezing is common in infants.
• Chills, dyspnea, rales and rhonchi, and friction rub may be present.

LABORATORY
White count may be elevated, but is usually less than 15,000.

IMAGING/SPECIAL TESTS
• Chest radiograph may be nonspecific, sometimes showing patchy infiltrates, usually without pleural effusion.
• Viral culture may be diagnostic particularly in conjunction with a four-fold or greater increase in antibody titers against a given virus.

DIFFERENTIAL
• Bacterial, mycoplasma pneumonia
• Pulmonary embolism
• Hypersensitivity pneumonitis
• Aspiration pneumonitis
• Cystic fibrosis

TREATMENT

General
◇ Hydration with oral or IV fluids, bed rest or limited activity, chest physiotherapy, oxygen supplementation, possible ventilatory support. Try to maintain good calorie intake.

MEDICATIONS
• Antipyretics
• Antiviral agents may be effective such as acyclovir for herpes simplex or Varicella zoster, ribavirin for RSV, ganciclovir for CMV, amantadine or rimantadine for influenza A (not B).

CONSULTATION SUGGESTIONS
Primary Care Physician, Infectious Disease Specialist

REFERRAL SUGGESTIONS
Primary Care Physician

PATIENT INSTRUCTIONS
Can contact American Lung Association for helpful patient literature (212)315-8700.

COURSE/PROGNOSIS
• Usually see full recovery except in debilitated patients in whom death may occur.
• May be complicated by bacterial pneumonia.

CODING

ICD-9-CM
480.9 Viral pneumonia

MISCELLANEOUS

SYNONYMS
Walking pneumonia

SEE ALSO
Bacterial pneumonia
Aspiration pneumonia

REFERENCES
Ruben FL: Viral pneumonias. The increasing importance of high index of suspicion. Postgrad Med 93:57-64, 1993.

Kauffman RS: Viral pneumonia. In: Respiratory Infections: Diagnosis and Management. Pennington JE, (ed), New York, Raven Press, 1983, pp 317-328.

AUTHOR
Robert Chuong, MD, DMD

Pneumonitis, Aspiration

BASICS

DESCRIPTION
• A potentially fatal process related to pulmonary aspiration of material from the pharynx, most commonly gastric contents after an emesis.
• Also known as "Mendelson's syndrome," after a classic description in the obstetric anesthesia literature.

ETIOLOGY

• The aspirate causes a direct chemical injury to the respiratory mucosa and alveoli; severity of this injury is related to volume and pH of aspirate, and the nature of the aspirate (particulate versus liquid). The resultant inflammatory response causes profound changes in the alveoli and interstitium that interfere with gas exchange. Aspiration can occur in any patient with an altered state of consciousness, although it most frequently occurs during general anesthesia.
• Predisposing risk factors include obesity, upper gastrointestinal disease (eg, hiatal hernia, peptic ulcer disease, etc.), pregnancy, noncompliance with NPO recommendations, patients requiring emergency surgery, and extremes of patient age.

SYSTEMS AFFECTED
Tracheobronchial tree, alveoli, and pulmonary interstitium

DIAGNOSIS

SYMPTOMS AND SIGNS
Coughing, wheezing, dyspnea, rales and/or rhonchi, tachycardia, cyanosis, increased inspiratory efforts and sternal retraction, rise in inspiratory pressures when mechanical ventilation is used, hypotension.

LABORATORY
• Diagnosis is usually made based on clinical findings and exclusion of other potential causes.
• Arterial blood bases, capnography, and pulse oximetry reveal varying degrees of hypoxia, hypercapnia, mixed metabolic/ respiratory acidosis. Arterial blood gases can help confirm the presence of compromised gas exchange and can be used to assess resolution over time.

IMAGING/SPECIAL TESTS
Chest radiographs, while helpful, may not show changes until hours to days after the event. When visible, fluffy infiltrates progressing to complete "white out."

DIFFERENTIAL
• Upper airway obstruction
• Bronchospasm
• Anaphylaxis
• Pneumothorax

TREATMENT

General
◇ Hydration with crystalloid solutions IV. No attempt should be made to neutralize acid with bicarbonate instillation into lungs. Lavage with sterile saline advisable.

MEDICATIONS
• Bronchodilators such as IV theophylline used to combat bronchospasm.
• Although some advocate steroids or antibiotics, clinical outcome analysis fails to reveal a benefit from either. And antibiotic administration may select for resistant organisms.

CONSULTATION SUGGESTIONS
Pulmonologist

REFERRAL SUGGESTIONS
Primary Care Physician, Pulmonologist

FIRST STEPS TO TAKE IN AN EMERGENCY
• The severity of the event dictates the treatment focus. In the conscious patient, adequate coughing should allow for clearance of most material. Supplemental oxygen should be administered. In the unconscious patient, the patient should be placed in a 15° head down position on the right side with aggressive suctioning. In either case, if large particulate matter cannot be cleared there may be partial or complete airway obstruction. (See Airway Obstruction contribution in this book.)
• If the episode was self-limiting and the patient is breathing without assistance and has a clear airway, supplemental oxygen should be continued and the patient referred to the local Emergency Department for observation. If respiratory distress continues, then emergency intubation needs to be accomplished; this will allow for delivery of positive pressure oxygen and direct suctioning of the trachea. Administration of a bronchodilator through the endotracheal tube or systemically may help to decrease airway resistance.

COURSE/PROGNOSIS
Fortunately, mortality from aspiration is low. However, because of the severity of the delayed sequelae that may result from aspiration, medical observation over the 24 to 48 hour period after the event is a critical component of proper treatment.

CODING

ICD-9-CM
507.0 Aspiration pneumonia

CPT
31500 Emergency endotracheal intubation
31511 Laryngoscopy with removal of foreign body

MISCELLANEOUS

Within the last decade, treatment of aspiration has become more conservative owing to lack of evidence to support earlier practices. Routine saline lavage of the airway, once performed routinely, is now reserved only to assist clearance of thick or particulate vomitus. Administration of corticosteroids and antibiotics empirically is no longer indicated.

SYNONYMS
Mendelson's syndrome
Aspiration pneumonitis

SEE ALSO
Bacterial pneumonia
Airway obstruction
Shock

REFERENCES
Ochs MW: Pulmonary complications and their management. Oral Maxillofac Surg Clin N Am 4:769, 1992.

Office Anesthesia Evaluation Manual (4th ed), Chicago, American Association of Oral and Maxillofacial Surgeons, 1991.

Hupp JR, Peterson LJ: Aspiration pneumonitis: etiology, therapy and prevention. J Oral Surg 39:430-435, 1981.

AUTHOR
Jeffrey B. Dembo, DDS, MS

Polyarteritis Nodosa

BASICS

DESCRIPTION
• A connective tissue disorder characterized by necrotizing inflammation of small- to medium-sized arteries that can involve and compromise the function of any organ in the body. The vascular effect results in secondary ischemia of tissues supplied by the involved arteries.
• Male:Female (2.5:1), and mean age 45.

ETIOLOGY

• The true etiology of polyarteritis nodosa is unknown, but an altered immunologic response appears to be the source of the pathogenicity. Frequently are positive for hepatitis B antigens.
• Onset of the disease has been associated with drugs, vaccines, bacterial infections, and viral infections.

SYSTEMS AFFECTED
• Polyarteritis nodosa can affect virtually any tissue or organ in the body and as a result its signs and symptoms can resemble numerous disease processes.
• Involvement of the kidneys, liver, heart, and GI tract are most common. May also involve joints, muscles, skin, GU tract, and CNS.
• Oral mucosal involvement is rare, but presents as an ulceration that may become secondarily infected.
Eyes
  ◇ visual compromise or loss.
Vestibulo-cochlear
  ◇ hearing loss.

DIAGNOSIS

SYMPTOMS AND SIGNS
General
  ◇ weakness, anorexia, weight loss, chills, fever, malaise, abdominal and extremity pain, myalgia, arthralgia.
CNS
  ◇ headache, paresthesias, convulsions, organic psychosis.
Vestibulo-cochlear
  ◇ difficulty hearing or deafness, tinnitus, vertigo, nausea.
Eyes
  ◇ ocular inflammation, hemorrhage, redness, edema, exophthalmos, floaters, papillitis.
Oral Mucosa
  ◇ ulceration, spontaneous bleeding.
Lips
  ◇ ulceration, crusting, spontaneous bleeding.
Gastrointestinal Tract
  ◇ bloody diarrhea, hepatomegaly.
Kidney
  ◇ oliguria, hematuria, hypertension.
Skin
  ◇ palpable subcutaneous nodules are common, purpura, erythema, ulcers, bullae, livido reticularis.
Other
  ◇ chronic persistent sinusitis.

LABORATORY
• Leukocytosis, proteinuria, hematuria are the most common laboratory findings. Elevated sedimentation rate and hypergammaglobulinemia.
• Uremia, Anemia, thrombocytosis. Presence of HBsAg (30% of cases), positive rheumatoid factor, anti-nuclear factor.

IMAGING/SPECIAL TESTS
• Angiography may reveal aneurysmal changes in affected medium-sized vessels.
• Biopsy of affected tissue reveals necrotizing inflammation of vessels. Infiltration of neutrophils through vessel wall.

DIFFERENTIAL
• Churg-Strauss syndrome
• Wegener's granulomatosis
• Cryoglobulinemias
• Henoch-Schönlein purpura
• Giant cell arteritis
• Systemic lupus erythematosus
• Other forms of vasculitic syndrome

TREATMENT

General
◊ Plasma exchange when there is no response to immunosuppressants and circulating immune complexes are present.
◊ Relief of denture if oral ulcerations are present.
Management of specific problems as a result of organ system involvement; renal impairment, fluid balance, transfusion if indicated, antihypertensive therapy.

MEDICATIONS
• Long-term corticosteroid therapy.
• Immunosuppression (chlorambucil, cyclophosphamide, and azathioprine)
0.2% chlorhexidene mouth rinses if oral ulcerations present.

CONSULTATION SUGGESTIONS
Rheumatologist

REFERRAL SUGGESTIONS
Rheumatologist, Primary Care Physician

PATIENT INSTRUCTIONS
Contact Arthritis Foundation (404) 872-7100 for patient information.

COURSE/PROGNOSIS
• If untreated, the disease is usually fatal due to failure of one or more vital organs.
• Early diagnosis and treatment can significantly improve prognosis.

 CODING

ICD-9-CM
446.0 Polyarteritis (nodosa)

CPT
40808 Biopsy, vestibule of mouth
99000 Transport specimen to outside laboratory

 MISCELLANEOUS

SEE ALSO
Giant cell arteritis

REFERENCES
Ankova YA, Jabba NS, Foster S; Ocular presentation of polyarteritis nodosa. Ophthalmol 100:1775-1781, 1993.

Cowpe JG, Hislop WR: Oral presentation of polyarteritis nodosa. J Oral Maxillofac Surg 56:597-601, 1983.

Burkett PR: Sinusitis and polyarteritis nodosa. Ear, Nose Throat J 64:47-50, 1985.

Goodless DR, Dhawam SS, Wiszniak J: Cutaneous periarteritis nodosa. Intl J Derm 29:611-614, 1990.

Ozen S, Besbas N, Saatci U, Bakkaloglu A: Diagnostic criteria for polyarteritis nodosa in childhood. J Ped 120:206-209, 1992.

Minkowitz G, Smoller B, McNutt S: Benign cutaneous polyarteritis nodosa. Arch Dermatol 127:1520-1522, 1991.

AUTHOR
Paul A. Danielson, DMD

Polycythemia Vera

BASICS

DESCRIPTION
• Polycythemia vera (PV) is a chronic, clonal blood stem cell disorder characterized by excessive proliferation of erythroid, myeloid, and megakaryocytic elements within bone marrow. There is a resultant increase in red blood cell mass and potentially a possible elevated peripheral granulocyte and platelet counts.
• Those with Jewish ancestry may have increased incidence.

ETIOLOGY

• A special clonal proliferation of a marrow population, which has a single enzyme component that forms a single clone of cells, presumably at the level of the pluripotential stem cell. A second (normal) clone of cells remains inactive in the marrow and is overshadowed by the transformed PV cells. This autonomous abnormal clone has no response in vitro to erythropoietin.
• It is thought that the erythrocytosis induced by proliferation of the abnormal (neoplastic) stem cells suppresses the production of erythropoietin.

SYSTEMS AFFECTED
Hematologic
◇ multiple abnormalities, including increased blood viscosity and hypervolemia due to increased erythrocyte mass and hematocrit, thrombocytosis, and leukocytosis in the absence of fever or infection. Thrombotic episodes and hemorrhage occur secondary to hyperviscosity, thrombocytosis, and platelet dysfunction. There is an increased incidence of severe hemorrhage following surgical procedures. Splenomegaly appears to reflect extramedullary hematopoiesis. Some patients develop acute myeloblastic leukemia.
Cardiovascular
◇ increased incidence of hypertension, angina, intermittent claudication, arterial and venous thrombosis.
Cerebrovascular
◇ prone to thrombosis.
Gastrointestinal
◇ possible hemorrhage. Peptic ulcer disease is prevalent.
Hepatic
◇ may be affected by occlusion of hepatic veins.
Musculoskeletal
◇ may be affected with the development of gout due to increased production of uric acid.

DIAGNOSIS

SYMPTOMS AND SIGNS
• Headaches, vertigo, weakness, tinnitus, blurred vision, diaphoresis, pruritus following bathing, finger and toe pain, epistaxis, and spontaneous bruising.
• Physical examination reveals:
Skin and oral mucosa
◇ dusky cyanosis of the face, hands, feet, and mucous membranes, ecchymoses may also be observed.
Eyes
◇ engorgement of the retinal veins and conjunctivae, retinal hemorrhages
Spleen
◇ splenomegaly
Liver
◇ hepatomegaly
Cardiovascular
◇ mild hypertension, pleural friction rub

LABORATORY
CBC with differential
◇ increased red cell mass, thrombocytosis, leukocytosis
Arterial blood gas
◇ normal oxygen saturation
Leukocyte alkaline phosphatase
◇ increased
Cholesterol level
◇ elevated
Uric acid level
◇ increased
Lactate dehydrogenase (LDH) level
◇ increased
Serum vitamin B_{12} level and vitamin B_{12}-binding protein level
◇ elevated.

IMAGING/SPECIAL TESTS
Bone marrow biopsy
◇ red cell hyperplasia, absent iron stores radioactive chromium labeled erythrocytes.
CT
◇ splenomegaly

DIFFERENTIAL
• Stress erythrocytosis (Gaisbock's syndrome)
• Primary erythrocytosis

• Secondary polycythemia
  • Generalized hypoxia
  • High altitude
  • Chronic obstructive pulmonary disease
  • Cardiovascular shunt
  • Pickwickian syndrome
  • High-oxygen affinity hemoglobin
  • Smoking
  • Local hypoxia
  • Renal cysts
  • Hydronephrosis
  • Renal artery stenosis
  • Autonomous erythropoietin production
• Tumor
• Renal carcinoma
• Hepatoma
• Cerebellar hemangioblastoma
• Uterine fibroid tumors
• Recessive familiar polycythemia

Polycythemia Vera

TREATMENT

General
Venesection (phlebotomy)
◇ remove 500 to 2000 mL of blood per week until the hematocrit reaches 45%, and repeat phlebotomy whenever hematocrit rises 4 to 5%. Iron supplements are contraindicated.

MEDICATIONS
• Radioactive phosphorous
◇ indicated when periodic phlebotomy is inadequate to control the hematocrit at 40 to 45%, and patients older than 70. This should be given parentally or orally every 3 to 4 weeks until remission occurs. When the blood counts return to normal, the patients are re-examined every 3 months. Remission may last 6 months to several years; relapse is treated by the total initial effective dose.
• Chemotherapy
◇ Hydroxyurea may produce remission. Intermittent maintenance therapy is usually required.
• Gout is treated with the usual therapy.

SURGERY
In patients with PV, hematologic remission before elective surgery is necessary to reduce the risk of hemorrhage.

CONSULTATION SUGGESTIONS
Hematologist

REFERRAL SUGGESTIONS
Primary Care Physician

COURSE/PROGNOSIS
• In treated patients, survival rate is approximately 13 years.
• Three stages of the disease are recognized: 1) the florid stage, with high hematocrit and hemoglobin lasting many years; 2) compensated myelofibrosis, not requiring treatment for a few years; 3) the anemic phase, with megakaryocytic hyperplasia, and severe myelofibrosis lasts up to 2 years.
• Approximately 5% of patients die of acute leukemia.

CODING

ICD-9-CM
238.4 Polycythemia vera

CPT
85102 Bone marrow needle biopsy

MISCELLANEOUS

SYNONYMS
Primary polycythemia
Vaquez disease

SEE ALSO
Leukemia
Myeloproliferative Disorders

REFERENCES
Gardner FH, Weiss GB: Polycythemia. In: Internal Medicine for Dentistry, 2nd ed. Rose LF, Kaye D (ed), St. Louis, CV Mosby, 1990, pp. 307-309.

Berk TP: Erythrocytosis and Polycythemia. In: Cecil's Textbook of Medicine 19th ed. Wyngaarden JB, Smith LG, Bennett JC (eds), Philadelphia, WB Saunders, 1992, pp. 925-929.

AUTHOR
Daniel S. Sarasin, DDS.

Polymyalgia Rheumatica (and Associated Giant Cell Arteritis)

BASICS

DESCRIPTION
• Polymyalgia rheumatica (PMR) and giant cell arteritis (GCA) are common and closely associated rheumatic diseases of middle-aged and older patients. Women are affected twice as frequently as men: Some believe that PMR and GCA represent the full spectrum of a single disease.
• PMR is characterized by aching and morning stiffness in the neck, torso, shoulder and hip girdles, and the proximal extremities; symptoms may be insidious or of acute onset.
• GCA affects medium and large-sized vessels that branch from the proximal aorta supplying the extracranial head, neck and arms; Headaches, scalp tenderness, visual symptoms, and claudication of the jaw muscles, and a painful, burning tongue are commonly seen.

ETIOLOGY

The etiology of PMR and GCA is unknown although a genetic predisposition (eg, not found in Afro-Americans) with an environmental trigger seems most feasible.

SYSTEMS AFFECTED
Musculoskeletal
◇ myalgia and, in some cases, polyarthritis (PMR); masseter claudication and tongue pain with function (GCA).
Hematologic
◇ normochromic, normocytic anemia (PMR).
Liver
◇ abnormal liver enzymes (PMR).
Cardiovascular
◇ granulomatous form of arteritis that may lead to occlusion of arteries causing scalp tenderness and headaches (GCA).
Visual
◇ blurring, diplopia, or blindness in one-third of the patients due to narrowing or occlusion of the ophthalmic or posterior ciliary arteries (GCA).

DIAGNOSIS

SYMPTOMS AND SIGNS
• Myalgia, especially in the morning or after inactivity, fatigue, sense of weakness, weight loss, and a low-grade fever (PMR).
• Vascular-system related, consisting of headache, scalp tenderness (may not be able to comb hair or wear a hat), visual loss (including blindness), fatigue or pain in masticating muscles when chewing tough foods and pain in tongue and throat while eating or repeated swallowing; the tongue may appear blanched or blue indicating an impending infarction (GCA).

LABORATORY
• Elevation of erythrocyte sedimentation rate greater than 30 mm per hour. Normochromic, normocytic anemia (PMR).
• Elevation of fibrinogen, C-reactive protein, alpha 2-globulin, alanine aminotransferase (ALT), and aspartate aminotransferase (AST) in PMR.
• Normal rheumatoid arthritis factor and antinuclear antibody (PMR and GCA).

IMAGING/SPECIAL TESTS
• Biopsy of superficial temporal artery (GCA).
• Microscopy of an affected artery shows thickening of the intima of the vessel with narrowing, thrombosis and multinucleated giant cells (GCA).

DIFFERENTIAL
• Rheumatoid arthritis
• Systemic lupus erythematosus
• Fibromyalgia
• Polymyositis
• Tendinitis
• Viral myalgia
• Occult infection
• Occult malignancy
• Drug excess (alcohol, heroin, amitriptyline, and phenothiazines).
• Hypothyroidism
• Polyarteritis nodosa
• Arteriosclerosis

Polymyalgia Rheumatica (and Associated Giant Cell Arteritis)

 TREATMENT

MEDICATIONS
• Mild PMR
◇ nonsteroidal anti-inflammatory drugs; if not effective, 10 to 20 mg of prednisone per day with decreasing doses.
• Moderate to severe PMR
◇ 10 to 20 mg of prednisone per day with decreasing doses.
• GCA
◇ 40 to 60 mg of prednisone per day with decreasing doses after improvement of symptoms and sedimentation rate returning to normal.

CONSULTATION SUGGESTIONS
Rheumatologist

REFERRAL SUGGESTIONS
Primary Care Physician, Rheumatologist

FIRST STEPS TO TAKE IN AN EMERGENCY
• If symptoms of visual changes occur, initiate steroid therapy immediately.

PATIENT INSTRUCTIONS
Possibility of permanent blindness makes proper therapy critical.

COURSE/PROGNOSIS
• PMR is considered a self-limited illness that runs its course in 1 to 5 years; severe debility may occur without treatment; when GCA not present, there is no increase in mortality.
• In GCA, blindness, cerebrovascular accident, myocardial infarction, claudication of extremities, and ischemic manifestations occasionally are seen.

 CODING

ICD-9-CM
446.5 Giant cell (temporal) arteritis
725 Polymyalgia rheumatica

CPT
20200 Biopsy, muscle; superficial
20205 deep
20206 Biopsy, muscle, percutaneous needle
37609 Ligation or biopsy, temporal artery
99000 Transport of specimen

 MISCELLANEOUS

SYNONYMS
Temporal arteritis

SEE ALSO
Giant-cell arteritis
Rheumatoid arthritis

REFERENCES
Friedlander AH, Runyon C: Polymyalgia rheumatica and temporal arteritis. Oral Surg Oral Med Oral Path 69:317-321, 1990.

Andreali TE, Bennett JC, Carpenter CCJ, Plum F, Smith LH Jr: Polymyalgia rheumatica and giant cell arteritis. In: Essentials of Medicine, 3rd ed. Philadelphia, WB Saunders, 1993, pp. 587-588.

Klinghofer JF: Polymyalgia rheumatica and temporal arteritis. In: Internal Medicine for Dentistry, 2nd ed. Rose LF, Kaye D (eds), St. Louis, CV Mosby Co., 1990, pp. 63-64.

AUTHOR
Dennis L. Johnson, DDS, MS

Porphyria

BASICS

DESCRIPTION
• Group of inherited or acquired disorders of various enzymes in the heme (of hemoglobin) biosynthetic pathway. Classified as either hepatic or erythropoietic, based on the main site of overproduction or accumulation of porphyrin precursor. Results in neuropsychiatric, abdominal, or dermatologic problems.
• Many symptoms of porphyrias are nonspecific, thus diagnosis may be delayed.
• Types
  Acute intermittent porphyria (AIP)
  Congenital erythropoietic porphyria (CEP)
  Hereditary coproporphyria (HCP)
  Porphobilinogen synthetase deficiency (PBD)
  Porphyria cutanea tarda (PCT)
  Protoporphyria (PP)
  Variegate porphyria (VP)
• PCT most common in U.S. AIP, PP, and VP next in frequency.
• PCT a disease of middle age, while AIP, VP, HCP, PBD seen in young adults. PP a disease of late childhood.

ETIOLOGY
Hereditary cause for most forms of porphyria.
Autosomal dominant
  ◊ AIP, PCT, HCP, PP, VP
Autosomal recessive
  ◊ PBD, CEP
PCT can also be acquired by:
  1) Exposure to ethanol, steroids, hormones, polyhalogenated hydrocarbons.
  2) Lead poisoning
  3) HIV
  4) Hepatitis C
Acute crisis can be precipitated in patients with AIP, VP and HCP by:
  1) Drugs (barbiturates, sulfa drugs in AIP)
  2) Estrogens
  3) Steroids
  4) Liver disease
  5) Fasting
  6) Infection
  7) Menstrual periods

SYSTEMS AFFECTED
• GI
• Neurologic
• Dermatologic
• Hematologic

DIAGNOSIS

SYMPTOMS AND SIGNS
Abdominal
  ◊ generalized severe pain, often mimicking an acute abdomen but without fever, chronic constipation. Urine turns dark red or brown on standing.
Neurologic
  ◊ may cause almost any neurologic symptom or sign. May be seizures and eventual quadriplegia.
Dermatologic
  ◊ photosensitivity, ulcerations, hyperpigmentation, scarring.
Psychiatric
  ◊ may cause almost any psychiatric symptom or sign, psychosis, hallucinations, disorientation, chronic depression.

LABORATORY
Stool and urine porphyrins, plasma for fluorescence omission, saliva for porphyrins.

DIFFERENTIAL
Porphyria symptoms mimic a huge variety of conditions

TREATMENT

General
◇ Prevention of attacks involves avoidance of known precipitants, including drugs, ethanol, sunshine, ultraviolet lights, and toxins. Intravenous or oral carbohydrates.

MEDICATIONS
For neuropsychiatric and abdominal symptoms
Hematin (ferriprotoporphyrin)
• Clonazepam for seizure prevention
• Serotonin reuptake inhibitors for depression
For dermatologic symptoms
• Oral carotenoids (beta-carotene)
• Avoid use of methohexital (Brevital) for anesthesia.

CONSULTATION SUGGESTIONS
Hematologist, General Surgeon (to rule out other causes of acute abdomen)

REFERRAL SUGGESTIONS
Primary Care Physician, Hematologist

PATIENT INSTRUCTIONS
Eat a high carbohydrate diet and avoid precipitating factors. Can contact American Porphyria Foundation for useful information (713)266-9617.

COURSE/PROGNOSIS
Asymptomatic or minimally symptomatic patients tend to do well. Those with neurologic symptoms may be permanently affected.

CODING

ICD-9-CM
277.1 Porphyria

MISCELLANEOUS

SYNONYMS
Erythropoietic porphyria
Günther's disease
Hepatoerythropoietic porphyria

REFERENCES
Dickstein E: Porphyria. In: Griffith's 5 Minute Clinical Consult. Dambro MR (ed), Baltimore, Williams & Wilkins, 1995, pp. 830-831.

Desnick RJ: The Porphyrias. In: Harrison's Principles of Internal Medicine. 13th ed. Isselbacher KJ, et al (eds), New York, McGraw-Hill, 1994, pp. 2073-2079.

Tefferi A, Colgan JP, Solberg, Jr. LA: Acute Porphyrias: Diagnosis and Management. Mayo Clin Proc 69:991-995, 1994.

AUTHOR
James R. Hupp, DMD, MD, JD, FACS

Potassium Disorders

BASICS

DESCRIPTION
Potassium is a predominantly intracellular ion, with usual serum concentrations ranging from 3.5 to 5.0 mEq/L. Abnormal serum concentrations lead to cardiac dysrhythmias, GI disorders, and muscle weakness.

ETIOLOGY

Potassium concentration is regulated primarily by the kidney, so renal disease or failure, or diuretic use are prime causative factors; other factors affecting potassium levels include insulin, glucagon, beta-adrenergic activity, hydrogen ion concentration, and potassium intake. Factitious hyperkalemia can occur if red cells hemolyze during or after venipuncture.

SYSTEMS AFFECTED
• Cardiac conduction
• Neuromuscular junction
• Gastrointestinal
• Renal

DIAGNOSIS

SYMPTOMS AND SIGNS
Hypokalemia
◇ weakness, paralysis, dysrhythmias, muscle cramps, paralytic ileus.
Hyperkalemia
◇ weakness, paralysis, paresthesias, dysrhythmias, ventricular fibrillation.
Note: patients with chronic hyperkalemia are often asymptomatic.

LABORATORY
While serum potassium is the definitive diagnostic test, it cannot be used to reliably measure total body potassium since 98% is intracellular. A chronic reduction in serum potassium of 1 mEq/L may represent a total body deficit of 600 to 800 mEq.

IMAGING/SPECIAL TESTS
ECG shows distinct changes that can help diagnose potassium disorders:
Hypokalemia
◇ decreased T wave voltage, increased U wave voltage, ST depression
Hyperkalemia
◇ peaked T waves, absent P waves, prolonged PR interval, widened QRS complex.

DIFFERENTIAL
Hypokalemia
◇ inadequate dietary intake, malnutrition, diuretic effects (eg, furosemide), aldosterone excess, vomiting, diarrhea, renal acidosis, excess insulin, beta-adrenergic effects, hypothermia, trauma.
Hyperkalemia
◇ excessive dietary intake, iatrogenic (eg, intravenous fluids), inadequate excretion (eg, renal disease), diuretic effects (eg, ACE inhibitors, potassium-sparing), beta-blockers, aldosterone deficiency, cell destruction (hemolysis, rhabdomyolysis).

TREATMENT

MEDICATIONS
• Hypokalemia
◇ increased oral intake using potassium salts or intravenous administration using fluids containing potassium supplementation (60 to 80 mEq/L) at 0.5 to 0.7 mEq/kg/hr, not to exceed 1 mEq/kg/hr. Continuous ECG monitoring must be used to help avoid cardiotoxicity from inadvertent overcorrection.
• Hyperkalemia
◇ discontinue potassium administration; increase excretion with osmotic or loop-acting diuretics. To push potassium into the cells, administer 500 mL 10% dextrose plus 10 units regular insulin over 1 hr, and sodium bicarbonate 50 to 150 mEq.
◇ Consider oral or rectal use of cationic exchange resins (eg, Kayexalate).
◇ Calcium chloride 500 mg may be given over 5-10 min.; this does not change potassium level but attenuates the potassium effect on excitatory tissues. Hemodialysis may be necessary if other treatments fail or cannot be used.

CONSULTATION SUGGESTIONS
Nephrologist, Dietitian

REFERRAL SUGGESTIONS
Primary Care Physician

FIRST STEPS TO TAKE IN AN EMERGENCY
• See medications section. Potassium 6.0 mEq/L or more is serious emergency.

PATIENT INSTRUCTIONS
• Use potassium sparing diuretics for hypertension.
• Consume diet rich in potassium if potassium wasting diuretics used.

COURSE/PROGNOSIS
Of the two, hyperkalemia (especially if acute) can be potentially life-threatening, especially if not diagnosed prior to administration of a general anesthetic.

CODING

ICD-9-CM
276.7 Hyperkalemia
276.8 Hypokalemia

MISCELLANEOUS

SYNONYMS
Hyperkalemia
Hypokalemia

SEE ALSO
Renal insufficiency
Cardiac dysrhythmias

REFERENCES
Tonnesen AS: Crystalloids and colloids. In: Anesthesia, 3rd ed. Miller RD (ed), New York, Churchill Livingstone, 1990.

Levinsky NG: Fluids and electrolytes. In: Harrison's Principles of Internal Medicine, 13th ed., Isselbacher KJ, et al (eds), New York, McGraw-Hill, Co., 1994.

Sendak MJ: Monitoring and management of perioperative fluid and electrolyte therapy. In: Principles and Practice of Anesthesiology. Rogers MC, Tinker JH, Covino BG, et al (eds), St. Louis, CV Mosby, 1993.

AUTHOR
Jeffrey B. Dembo, DDS, MS

Pregnancy

BASICS

DESCRIPTION
The condition of having a developing embryo or fetus in the body for a duration of approximately 40 weeks. It is marked by significant increases in blood volume, cardiac output, and hormone levels. Organogenesis occurs in the first trimester, which is thus the time that the fetus is most susceptible to injury.

ETIOLOGY

SYSTEMS AFFECTED
Virtually every system is affected to an extent. Pregnant patients become slightly hypotensive and anemic and develop dyspnea on exertion. Gingival response to local irritants (plaque, calculus) is exaggerated with pyogenic granuloma formation and is presumed to be due to hormonal changes. Most of the gingival changes (inflammation, bleeding, pregnancy tumors) regress at the end of pregnancy. There is no evidence that pregnancy contributes directly to the development of dental caries.

DIAGNOSIS

SYMPTOMS AND SIGNS
The most common signs of pregnancy include cessation of menses, and moderate enlargement of the thyroid and mammary glands. Flushing, tachycardia, weight gain, increased appetite, urinary frequency, and polydipsia.

LABORATORY
• Urine pregnancy test to confirm that missed period due to pregnancy.
• Serum pregnancy test more reliable but adds cost.

IMAGING/SPECIAL TESTS
• The measurement of chorionic gonadotropin (NCG) is the most common test and is reportedly 97 to 98% accurate. It becomes positive between day 35 to 40 following the first day of the last menstrual period. Fetal heart sounds can be heard as early as 12 weeks.
• Sonogram used to assess fetal size and health.
• Avoid all radiographs that are not absolutely necessary.

DIFFERENTIAL
• Normal weight gain.
• Menstrual disturbance.
• Ectopic pregnancy.

TREATMENT

General
◇ early in the pregnancy patients should be advised of the periodontal response to poor oral hygiene. Scaling, polishing, and improved oral hygiene will help to prevent adverse periodontal response. Dental treatment is safest in the 2nd trimester. However, emergency treatment (pain, infection) should be performed promptly. As hypertension can be a serious complication of pregnancy, routine monitoring of the blood pressure of the pregnancy patients is indicated. Avoidance of treatment in the 3rd trimester is primarily for patient comfort. It should also be remembered that urinary frequency increases during this trimester. Radiographs are not contraindicated, but clinical judgment will significantly decrease the number of films taken during pregnancy. A lead apron must be used. Supine chair position is to be avoided to prevent supine hypotensions which may result from the pressure of the fetus on the inferior vena cava.

MEDICATIONS
• Any medication used during pregnancy may cross the placenta to the fetus. Care must be taken in prescribing drugs that are not teratogenic. The advantages of use of drugs must outweigh the risk to the fetus (FDA risk factor).

CONSULTATION SUGGESTIONS
Obstetrician, Primary Care Physician

REFERRAL SUGGESTIONS
Obstetrician, Primary Care Physician

FIRST STEPS TO TAKE IN AN EMERGENCY
• If patient becomes hypotensive while laying back, turn onto side to relieve fetal pressure on inferior vena cava.

PATIENT INSTRUCTIONS
• Strict attention to oral hygiene will decrease chance of serious dental problems occurring during pregnancy.
• Maintain good dietary calcium intake during pregnancy and post-partum.

CODING

ICD-9-CM
522.6 Pyogenic granuloma maxillary alveolar ridge
528.9 Pyogenic granuloma oral mucosa

CPT
40808 Biopsy, vestibule of mouth
41825 Excision of lesion, dentoalveolar structures, no repair
70300 Periapical of teeth, single view

MISCELLANEOUS

SEE ALSO
Pyogenic granuloma

REFERENCES
Pregnancy and breast-feeding. In: Dental Management of the Medically Compromised Patient. 4th ed. Little JW, Falace DA (eds), St. Louis, CV Mosby, 1993, pp. 383-389.

AUTHOR
C. Daniel Overholser, DDS, MSD

Pressure Sores

BASICS

DESCRIPTION
• Soft tissue ulcerations over bony prominences or dependent areas resulting from prolonged immobilization in the hospitalized, bedridden, or paralyzed person.
• Occurs in 3 to 4% of all acute care hospital admissions, 45% in chronic care facilities.
• Mortality increased four times in hospitalized elderly.

ETIOLOGY

• Prolonged recumbency, immobilization
• Shear forces, friction
• Sustained pressure
• Inflamed tissues
• Compromised healing state
• nutritional, sepsis, diabetics, hepatic failure, etc.

SYSTEMS AFFECTED
Paraplegics (in decreasing order of frequency)
    ◇ ischial > trochanteric > sacral > heel
    90% all pressure sores below waist
    2/3 of those in hips, buttocks
    1/3 in lower extremity
• Subcutaneous and muscle tissue more susceptible to sustained or heavy pressure.
• Shear forces exacerbate condition in deep tissues
• Dermis more resistant but excessive friction and moisture will compromise skin integrity.
• Underlying bone may become infected

DIAGNOSIS

SYMPTOMS AND SIGNS
• Often no pain/discomfort due to paralyzed state or no sensation in tissues.
• First sign may be erythema of skin if pressure prolonged up to 2 hours.
• Hyperemia present in tissue for up to 24 to 36 hours if pressure persists 2 to 6 hours.
• Extension of ulcer may be greater in subcutaneous and muscle than overlying skin.

LABORATORY
CBC with differential; electrolytes

IMAGING/SPECIAL TESTS
Cultures
    ◇ swabs; tissue; (anaerobic)
Bone scan if extension to bone suspected.

DIFFERENTIAL
• Osteomyelitis with draining fistula
• Chronic ulcer may be cancer (Marjole's ulcer)
• Stasis ulcers (more common below knee)
• Septic thrombi with abscess formation

TREATMENT

- Prevention is mainstay.
- Vigilance for care givers.
- Precautions in elderly, bedridden or paralyzed, immuno-compromised or diabetics when hospitalized.
- Skin care
  - Turning every 2 hours
  - Weight dispersion measures, eg, cushions, air-fluid beds
  - Talc to reduce friction
  - Barrier dressings, eg, Duoderm, on hyperemic area

MEDICATIONS
- Antibiotics if cellulitis present.
- Debriding agents
  ◇ collagenase, trypsin, papain, sutilains used to remove necrotic tissue to keep ulcer clean.

SURGERY
Optimize preoperative
  ◇ antibiotics, nutrition status
Surgical debridement
  - Total bursal/eschar removal (stain with methylene blue)
  - Bone removal until bleeding surface obtained
Primarily closure with tension-free, well-vascularized myofascial tissue
  - Local muscle flaps
  - Myocutaneous free flaps
Postoperative care
  ◇ pressure relief 2 to 3 weeks; nutrition; hematocrit > 30; antibiotics as indicated
Amputation in extensive, infected ulcers or recalcitrant, non-healing ulcers.

CONSULTATION SUGGESTIONS
General Surgeon, Plastic Surgeon

REFERRAL SUGGESTIONS
General Surgeon, Plastic Surgeon

PATIENT INSTRUCTIONS
- Bedridden patients with paralysis need to remind caregivers to turn regularly and pad pressure points.
- Maintain high calorie, high protein diet if ulcers occur.

COURSE/PROGNOSIS
Pressure Sore Grading
Grade I
  ◇ Skin
Grade II
  ◇ Skin and subcutaneous
Grade III
  ◇ Underlying muscle
Grade IV
  ◇ Bone involved

CODING

ICD-9-CM
707.0 Pressure ulcer

MISCELLANEOUS

SYNONYMS
Decubitus ulcer
Bedsore
Trophic ulcer
Pressure sore

REFERENCES
CI Price, F Nahai: Trauma and Reconstruction. In: Plastic Surgery. A Core Curriculum. Ruberg RL, Smith DJ, (eds), St. Louis, CV Mosby Co., 1994. pp. 547-552.

Mulder GD, LaPan M: Decubitus ulcers: update on new approaches to treatment. Geriatrics 43:44-57, 1988.

Allman RM: Pressure ulcers among the elderly. N Engl J Med 320:850-853, 1989.

AUTHOR
Bruce Horswell, DDS, MD

Pseudomembranous Colitis

BASICS

DESCRIPTION
A species of enterocolitis that may develop in hospitalized, elderly, or debilitated patients, usually in conjunction with antibiotic administration.

ETIOLOGY

- Compromised patient:
  - Hospitalized
  - Elderly or debilitated
  - Immunocompromised
- Antibiotic administration:
  - Clindamycin (first identified)
  - Cephalosporins
  - Penicillins
- Antibiotics-initiate change in bowel flora:
  - Clostridium difficile (minor commensal in gut).
  - Antibiotics rid competing organisms, allowing clostridial overgrowth.
- Clostridial overgrowth (2 days after antibiotics to 3 weeks after stoppage of antibiotics).
  - Elaboration of enterotoxin:
- Shigella, Staph., C. perfringens may cause enteritis with pseudomembrane formation.
- Person-to-person transmission may also play role, which may explain occasional outbreaks in hospitals and wards.

SYSTEMS AFFECTED
- Predominantly colonic mucosa.
- Rarely, ileum may be involved or primary site of infection.

DIAGNOSIS

SYMPTOMS AND SIGNS
- Loose, dark diarrhea; occasionally bloody.
- Abdominal cramps and tenderness to palpation.
- Nausea, vomiting, (secondary to toxemia).
- Fever
- Hypotension, tachycardia, decreased urine secondary to fluid loss.
- Distended, quiet abdomen may herald toxic megacolon.

LABORATORY
- CBC/differential
- Electrolytes

IMAGING/SPECIAL TESTS
- Stool extracts to detect C. difficile toxin
- Quantitative stool culture (several days).
- Sigmoidoscopy:
  - Mucinous, fibrin plaques on colonic mucosa.
  - Composed of inflammatory cells and necrotic debris.
  - Underlying, hyperemic or erosive mucosa.
  - Late in disease, plaques coalesce to form the characteristic pseudomembranes.
- Barium enema
- Radiographs if toxic megacolon suspected.

DIFFERENTIAL
- Ulcerative colitis
- Crohn's enterocolitis
- Ischemic colitis
- Infectious diarrhea (gastroenteritis)
- Radiation enterocolitis

Pseudomembranous Colitis

TREATMENT

- Stop antibiotics
- Fluid and electrolyte replacement
- Supportive care when necessary

MEDICATIONS
- Oral vancomycin, 500 mg q.i.d. for 7 to 10 days.
- Metronidazole, 500 to 750 mg t.i.d. for 7 to 14 days.
- Oral cholestyramine to bind toxin (4 g q6h for 5 days).
- (Do not give antidiarrheals, may prolong illness).

SURGERY
Surgical intervention when necrotic (toxic megacolon) or perforated colon occurs.

CONSULTATION SUGGESTIONS
Infectious Disease Specialist, Gastroenterologist

REFERRAL SUGGESTIONS
Primary Care Physician

FIRST STEPS TO TAKE IN AN EMERGENCY
- If vital signs show hypotension and/or tachycardia, consider hypovolemia and hydrate patient.

PATIENT INSTRUCTIONS
Maintain hydration and carefully follow medication instructions.

COURSE/PROGNOSIS
Most early or mild cases resolve after a few days with stoppage of antibiotics and supportive care. Severe cases require the above and administration of vancomycin or metronidazole. Mortality 10 to 20% in compromised, hospitalized patients with severe colitis.

CODING

ICD-9-CM
008.45 Pseudomembranous colitis

CPT
90780 Intravenous infusion therapy
90784 Intravenous injection

MISCELLANEOUS

SYNONYMS
Antibiotic-associated colitis

SEE ALSO
Diarrhea
Gastroenteritis
Inflammatory bowel disease

REFERENCES
McFarland LV, et al: Nosocomial acquisition of Clostridium difficile infection. N Engl J Med 320:204-209, 1989.

Shrock TR: Large Intestine. In: Current Surgical Diagnosis and Treatment. LW Way, (ed), Norwalk, CT, Appleton and Lange. 1991, p. 674.

Silva J, Jr: Treatment of Clostridium difficile colitis and diarrhea with vancomycin. Am J Med 71:815-818, 1981.

AUTHOR
Bruce Horswell, DDS, MD

Psoriasis

BASICS

DESCRIPTION
A skin disease characterized most commonly by symmetrical rashes that spontaneously resolve and exacerbate. Associated arthropathy may occur.

ETIOLOGY

• A genetic predisposition occurs that is most likely due to multiple loci, one of which is the HLA locus.
• Precipitating factors include infections, hormonal influences, medications, trauma, and psychogenic causes.

SYSTEMS AFFECTED
Skin
  ◇ raised red scaly patches that are sharply demarcated are the most common form.
Joints
  ◇ psoriatic arthropathy ranges from asymmetrical oligoarthropathy to severe mutilating joint disease.
Cardiovascular
  ◇ high output cardiac failure may occur.

DIAGNOSIS

SYMPTOMS AND SIGNS
• Thick, scaling, well-demarcated symmetrical lesions.
• Pruritis
• Nail pitting
Joint involvement
  ◇ pain, swelling, stiffness. May involve TMJ.
• Red, raised scaly patches on scalp, extensor surfaces of knee and elbows.
• Flaking of skin
• Rare oral lesions consisting of plaques.

LABORATORY
• HLA antigens
• Rheumatoid factor (negative)
• Leukocytosis and increased sedimentation rate

IMAGING/SPECIAL TESTS
Biopsy
  ◇ epidermis exhibits microabscesses, parakeratosis, lack of a granular layer, thinning of the suprapapillary plate, clubbing and elongation of the rete ridges.

DIFFERENTIAL
• Seborrheic eczema
• Lichen planus
• Lichen simplex
• Discoid eczema
• Intraepidermal carcinoma
• Mycosis fungoides
• Pityriasis rubra pilaris
• Basal cell carcinoma

Psoriasis

 ## TREATMENT

General
◇ Solar radiation but avoid excessive amount.
   ◇ Skin moisturizers
   ◇ Oatmeal bath for pruritis
   ◇ Cool compresses

MEDICATIONS
Primary Topical
- Topical corticosteroids
- Tar compounds
- Dithranol
- Ultraviolet radiation
- Keratolytic agents: topical salicylates

Secondary Systemic
- Etretinate alone
- PUVA (psoralen plus ultraviolet light)
- Etretinate with PUVA

Tertiary Systemic
- Methotrexate
- Cyclosporine
- 5-Hydroxyurea
- Azathioprine
- Isotretinoin
- Systemic corticosteroids

CONSULTATION SUGGESTIONS
Dermatologist, Rheumatologist

REFERRAL SUGGESTIONS
Primary Care Physician

FIRST STEPS TO TAKE IN AN EMERGENCY
- If patient shows pustule formation, should be immediately sent for emergency care.

PATIENT INSTRUCTIONS
Patients can receive useful information from the National Psoriasis Foundation (503)297-1545.

COURSE/PROGNOSIS
- Spontaneous remission may occur in 40% of cases.
- Early onset, wide-spread rash, and appearance of new lesions indicates a poorer prognosis.
- Psoriatic arthropathy appears to have a better prognosis than rheumatoid arthritis.

 ## CODING

ICD-9-CM
696.0 Psoriatic arthropathy
696.1 Other psoriasis

CPT
11100 Biopsy, skin
40490 Biopsy, lip
99000 Handling and transport of specimen

 ## MISCELLANEOUS

SEE ALSO
Lichen planus
Dermatitis

REFERENCES
Elder JT, Nair RP, Guo SW, Henseler T, Christophers E, Voorhees JJ: The genetics of psoriasis. Arch Dermatol 130:216-224, 1994.

Koorbusch GR, Zeitler DL, Fotos PG, Doss JB: Psoriatic arthritis of the TMJ with ankylosis. Oral Surg, Oral Med, Oral Path 71:267-274, 1991.

Pyle GW, Vitt M, Nieusma G: Oral psoriasis: Report of a case. J Oral Maxillofac Surg 74:185-187, 1994.

AUTHOR
Deborah L. Zeitler, DDS, MS

Pulmonary Edema

BASICS

DESCRIPTION
An accumulation of pulmonary interstitial alveolar fluid due to increased venous pressure. Lungs become less compliant, the resistance of small airways increases, and there is an increase in lymphatic flow and pulmonary extravascular liquid volume.

ETIOLOGY

• Usually due to left ventricular heart failure, mitral stenosis, or aortic valve disease. Any process that increases pulmonary venous pressure can result in pulmonary edema including cardiac septal defects, cardiac tamponade, constrictive pericarditis, or hypertensive crisis.
• May also result from respiratory distress syndrome.

SYSTEMS AFFECTED
• Cardiovascular
• Pulmonary

DIAGNOSIS

SYMPTOMS AND SIGNS
• Dyspnea
• Tachypnea
• Tachycardia
• Cardiomegaly
• Weakness
• Fatigue
• Anxiety
• S3 gallop
• S4 present
• Jugular venous distention
• Moist rales
• Wheezing
• Cough with or without pink frothy sputum
• Pulsus alternans
• Peripheral edema
• Orthopnea

LABORATORY
Blood gas
◊ hypoxia, hypercarbia, respiratory acidosis, increased A-a gradient.

IMAGING/SPECIAL TESTS
Chest radiograph changes
◊ Kerley B lines and loss of distinct vascular margins.
• In later stages with increased intravascular pressure, there is a disruption of junctions between alveolar lining cells and alveolar edema occurs with liquid that contains red blood cells and macromolecules. Alveolar edema occurs with bilateral wet rales and rhonchi. Chest radiograph shows diffuse haziness of lung fields with increased density in hilar regions.
• ECG
• Pulmonary function tests show increased obstruction to airflow.
• 2-D echocardiogram
• Cardiac catheterization
• Swan-Ganz catheter to determine etiology (cardiogenic versus noncardiogenic) Mixed venous oxygen saturation determination.

DIFFERENTIAL
• Congestive heart failure
• Aspiration pneumonitis
• Myocardial infarction
• Cardiomyopathy
• Anaphylaxis

TREATMENT

General
◊ Fluid Retention
  • Acute pulmonary edema is usually caused by left ventricular failure or mitral stenosis. This is life-threatening and a medical emergency.
  • With more chronic forms of pulmonary edema, attention must be directed to removing any precipitating causes of decompensation, such as dysrhythmia or infection.
◊ Patient placed in sitting position to decrease venous return.
◊ While other measures are being employed, rotating tourniquets can be applied to the extremities.

MEDICATIONS
• Morphine
  ◊ 2 to 5 mg IV (reduces anxiety, reduces adrenergic vasoconstriction stimuli to arteriolar and venous beds, and decreases venous return).
• 100% O_2
  ◊ preferably with positive pressure to increase oxygen diffusion and reduce pulmonary capillary pressure.
• Furosemide (20 to 80 mg), ethacrynic acid (40 to 100 mg) or bumetanide (1 mg) reduce circulating blood volume, exert a venodilator action, and reduce venous return.
• Sodium nitroprusside or nitroglycerin IV for afterload reduction.
• Digoxin if component of heart failure.
• Aminophylline (240 to 480 mg) is effective in diminishing bronchoconstriction.

CONSULTATION SUGGESTIONS
Cardiologist

REFERRAL SUGGESTIONS
Primary Care Physician

FIRST STEPS TO TAKE IN AN EMERGENCY
• Activate EMS, administer oxygen, monitor vital signs, administer morphine.

PATIENT INSTRUCTIONS
• Comply with physician recommendation.
• Notify physician immediately if symptoms appear or worsen.

COURSE/PROGNOSIS
Highly dependent upon etiology and its management. Mortality 50% for noncardiogenic and up to 80% for cardiogenic pulmonary edema.

CODING

ICD-9-CM
  428.1 Acute pulmonary edema due to heart disease
  518.4 Acute pulmonary edema, noncardiogenic

MISCELLANEOUS

SEE ALSO
Heart failure
Respiratory distress syndrome
Pneumonitis aspiration

REFERENCES
Internal Medicine for Dentistry 2nd ed. Rose LF, Kaye D (eds). St. Louis, CV Mosby, Co., 1990.

Ingram RH, Braunwald E: Dyspnea and Pulmonary Edema. In: Harrison's Principles of Internal Medicine 13th ed. Isselbacher, et al (eds). New York, McGraw-Hill, Inc., 1994, pp. 174-178.

Colice GL: Detecting the presence and cause of pulmonary edema. Postgrad Med 93:161-169, 1993.

Crapo JD: New concepts in the formation of pulmonary edema. Am Rev Respir Dis 147:790, 1993.

AUTHOR
Jerry L. Jones, DDS, MD

Pulmonary Embolism

BASICS

DESCRIPTION
Pulmonary embolism occurs when a thrombus, formed in a large systemic vein (usually a lower extremity or pelvic vein), detaches from the vessel wall, travels through the right side of the heart, and becomes lodged in the pulmonary artery on its immediate branches. Acute pulmonary embolism is a major cause of morbidity and mortality today, and the diagnosis remains one of the most challenging dilemmas in clinical medicine.

ETIOLOGY

Deep Venous Thrombosis (DVT):
- Virchow's triad (three predisposing factors for DVT)
- Venous stasis
- Abnormality of the vessel wall
- Disorders of blood coagulation (hypercoagulability)

Conditions associated with a high risk of DVT:
- Prolonged surgical procedures
- Pregnancy/postpartum period
- Biventricular failure
- Lower extremity injury/fracture
- Prolonged immobilization/bed rest
- Chronic venous insufficiency/ vasculitis of the lower extremities.
- Peripheral vascular disease
- Obesity
- Estrogen use
- Neoplastic disease
- Blood dyscrasias/ hemoglobinopathy
- Burns/soft tissue trauma
- Advanced age
- Diabetes mellitus

SYSTEMS AFFECTED
- Cardiovascular-hemodynamic compromise/collapse.
- Pulmonary-mechanical obstruction and pulmonary infarction.

DIAGNOSIS

SYMPTOMS AND SIGNS
- Apprehension
- Sweating
- Fever (>38.5 degrees C)
- Dyspnea
- Tachypnea (respiratory rate > 20 breaths/min)
- Cough
- Hemoptysis
- Chest pain, pleuritic
- Pleural friction rub
- Dullness to percussion over involved lung parenchyma
- Decreased breath sounds
- Occasional wheezing
- Inspiratory rales
- Tachycardia (heart rate > 100 beats/min)
- Accentuation of the pulmonic component of the 2nd heart sound
- Jugular venous distention
- Cyanosis
- Syncope
- Phlebitis

Evidence of DVT
◊ leg pain/swelling, cord palpable in popliteal fossa, positive Homan's sign (tenderness of the calf muscles upon dorsiflexion of the foot).

LABORATORY
Arterial blood gas (ABG)
◊ Increased alveolar
◊ arterial PO_2 gradient, arterial hypoxemia ($PO_2 < 80$ mm Hg), hypocapnia (low $PCO2$), respiratory alkalosis (due to hyperventilation).
CBC
◊ Leukocytosis
Erythrocyte sedimentation rate (ESR)
◊ Elevated (nonspecific).

IMAGING/SPECIAL TESTS
Electrocardiogram (ECG)
◊ most cases normal. May show sinus tachycardia, and signs of right heart strain and pulmonary hypertension, including right axis deviation, poor R wave progression in the anterior leads, right bundle branch block, abnormal S wave in lead I, abnormal Q wave in lead III (S1Q3T3 pattern).
Chest radiograph
◊ Usually normal. May show decreased vascular markings, plate-like atelectasis, wedge-shaped pleural radiopacity (Hampton's hump), pleural effusion, unilateral elevated hemidiaphragm, oligemia (hyperluceny) of lung fields (Westermark sign), and/or bulging pulmonary artery (knuckle sign).
Transthoracic echo
◊ Doppler studies
◊ may show right ventricular hypertrophy or identify thrombi.
Transesophageal echocardiography
◊ may detect emboli.
CT scanning with contrast.
MRI

Pulmonary nuclear scanning {Ventilation/ Perfusion scan, (V/Q scan)}
◊ the perfusion scan is performed before the ventilation scan. A normal perfusion scan essentially rules out a pulmonary embolism. Ventilation scanning increases the specificity of the perfusion scan; areas that are well ventilated but not perfused are suggestive of pulmonary embolism (V/Q mismatch). The results of a V/Q scan are categorized as low, intermediate, high, and indeterminate for a pulmonary embolus. Equivocal results of a V/Q scan warrant further evaluation.
Pulmonary angiography
◊ considered the gold standard because it is the most sensitive and specific test for establishing the diagnosis of pulmonary embolism. This test gives precise anatomic information about the pulmonary vasculature.
Digital subtraction angiography
◊ can produce a view of the pulmonary vascular tree with less contrast than an angiogram, and without a pulmonary arterial catheter.
Contrast venography (venogram)
◊ gold standard for detection of DVT.
Noninvasive venous studies
◊ impedance plethysmography (IPG), radiofibrinogen thigh/leg scanning studies, Doppler ultrasound examinations ("duplex scanning")
◊ may demonstrate stasis and thrombosis in the lower extremities.

DIFFERENTIAL
- Acute myocardial infarction
- Pneumothorax
- Pneumonia
- Congestive heart failure
- Pulmonary edema
- Primary pulmonary hypertension
- Aortic dissection
- Acute pericarditis
- Cor pulmonale
- Angina pectoris
- Mediastinal emphysema
- Peptic ulcer disease
- Parenchymal lung disease
- Neoplastic disease
- Trauma

TREATMENT

General
◊ Prompt anticoagulation is the treatment of choice.
◊ Supportive care should be considered, including supplemental oxygen, volume expansion with intravenous fluids, possible vasopressor agents, and bed rest.
◊ Because the best treatment for acute pulmonary embolism is the prevention of deep venous thrombosis, prophylaxis is important and may consist of any of the following: low-dose (mini-dose) heparin, coumadin, intermittent pneumatic compression devices to the lower extremities, or a combination.
◊ Dental treatment of a patient on chronic anticoagulation warrants consultation with the physician. Coagulation studies (PT/PTT) should be performed, local hemostatic measures used, and elective procedures delayed. Consideration should be given to discontinuation of anticoagulation for a short time prior to dental treatment, or alternatively, employing the use of tranexamic acid as a local antifibrinolytic agent.

MEDICATIONS
• Anticoagulants
◊ heparin is the drug of choice. Continuous intravenous heparin is given in a dose of approximately 1000 units/ hr, and guided by serial measurements of partial thromboplastin time (PTT) in an attempt to maintain levels at approximately 1.5 to 2.0 times the control values. Heparin may also be given in intermittent intravenous or subcutaneous administration (intramuscular injections are avoided because of the risk of hematoma formation). Heparin does not dissolve a clot, which is already formed, but prevents further clot formation while the body's fibrinolytic system attempts to slowly lyse the clot over several weeks. Heparin is continued usually for the first 7 to 10 days. Oral coumadin therapy should be initiated several days prior to discontinuation of heparin, and should be guided by prothrombin time (PT) measurements. The duration of therapy with coumadin is controversial, but should continue for approximately 3 months, or indefinitely, depending upon the individual patient.

• Thrombolytic (fibrinolytic) therapy
◊ systemic therapy with streptokinase, urokinase, or recombinant human tissue plasminogen activator (tPA) is controversial in the management of acute pulmonary embolism, but may hasten resolution of emboli. Unlike heparin, these agents are capable of clot lysis. They do not replace anticoagulants in the treatment of pulmonary embolism. These agents carry the significant risk of hemorrhage; therefore, they are reserved for patients with significant hemodynamic instability.
• Inferior vena caval interruption (Greenfield filter)
◊ these devices, resembling umbrellas, are placed percutaneously, and are reserved for those patients in whom emboli continue despite anticoagulation, or who have a contraindication to the use of anticoagulation.
• Alternative is inferior vena caval ligation via laparotomy.
• Pulmonary embolectomy
◊ is reserved for patients with documented pulmonary embolus by angiogram, significant hemodynamic compromise, and contraindications to anticoagulation. This procedure carries a significant degree of morbidity and mortality.

SURGERY
In rare cases, open thoractomy for removal of massive emboli performed. In patients with recurrent or serious risk of recurrent emboli from lower extremities, inferior vena cava filters can be positioned transvenously to block massive emboli.

CONSULTATION SUGGESTIONS
Primary Care Physician, General Surgeon

REFERRAL SUGGESTIONS
Primary Care Physician

FIRST STEPS TO TAKE IN AN EMERGENCY
• Administer oxygen, endotracheal intubation if necessary for proper oxygenation, transport to emergency facility or call for medicine consult, if in hospital already.

PATIENT INSTRUCTIONS
Prevention depends on avoiding prolonged stasis of blood in lower extremities. Ambulate as soon as possible after surgery and often during the day. While in bed, exercise legs by pointing toes several times every few minutes on a regular basis.

COURSE/PROGNOSIS
In cases when prompt recognition is made and therapy instituted immediately, the prognosis is excellent. Many episodes of pulmonary embolism could be avoided with adequate prophylaxis. Recovery from the embolic event is usual, and few patients progress to pulmonary hypertension or infarction, or develop other significant complications. Recurrence rates are variable.

CODING

ICD-9-CM
415.1 Pulmonary embolism
453.8 Deep or superficial vessel thrombophlebitis

MISCELLANEOUS

SYNONYMS
PE

SEE ALSO
Thrombophlebitis

REFERENCES
Sindet-Pedersen S, Ramstrom G, Bernvil S, Blomback M: Hemostatic effect of tranexamic acid mouthwash in anticoagulant-treated patients undergoing oral surgery. N Engl J Med 320: 840-843, 1989.

Thomas SH, Shepherd SM, Allison EJ: Thrombolytic therapy in review. J Emerg Med 11:83-89, 1993.

Goldhaber SZ: Recent advances in the diagnosis and lytic therapy of pulmonary embolism. Chest 99 (Suppl 4): 173S-179S, 1991.

Ryu JH, Rosenow EC: Acute pulmonary embolism. Cardiovascular Clinics 22: 103-112, 1992.

Wolfe MW, Skibo LK, Goldhaber SZ: Pulmonary embolic disease: Diagnosis, pathophysiologic aspects, and treatment with thrombolytic therapy. Current Prob Cardiol 18: 587-633, 1993.

AUTHOR
Michael Miloro, DMD, MD

Pyogenic Granuloma

BASICS

DESCRIPTION
• A small, elevated nodule that represents a reactive proliferation of granulation tissue on the oral mucosa. The lesion is friable and often has a hemorrhagic or ulcerated appearance.
• These lesions are common, accounting for 1 to 2% of all oral biopsies.
• Female to male ratio is 7:3.

ETIOLOGY

• A reactive lesion produced in response to some chronic irritation, which provides a pathway for the invasion of nonspecific micro-organisms.
• Lesions often noted during pregnancy when the levels of circulating estrogens are high, subsequently shrinking postpartum.
• Common local irritants are plaque, calculus, and overhanging restoration margins.

SYSTEMS AFFECTED
Gingiva
◊ 75% occur in gingiva, with the majority seen in the maxillary anterior facial gingiva. Hemorrhage may be spontaneous or easily provoked, but rarely is there dental pain, mobility, or loss of teeth.
Lips
◊ 10%
Tongue
◊ 5%, in this site may have an effect on speech and mastication.
Buccal mucosa
◊ 4%.

DIAGNOSIS

SYMPTOMS AND SIGNS
Mouth
◊ occasional localized pain to the affected mucosal structures affecting mastication and speech. Frequent oral bleeding.
Oral mucosa
◊ all lesions are similar and may be represented as a pedunculated or sessile mass. The surface may be smooth, lobulated, or even warty in appearance. Lesions may have a reddish or purplish color depending on the vascularity. Hemorrhage is usually spontaneous or easily provoked. Purulent exudate is uncommon.

LABORATORY
Urine pregnancy test.

IMAGING/SPECIAL TESTS
Excisional biopsy
◊ lobular masses of tissue containing numerous capillaries, inflammatory cells, and loose connective tissue stroma.

DIFFERENTIAL
• Small, ulcerative benign or malignant mesenchymal tumors.
• Exophytic capillary hemangioma
• Peripheral giant cell granuloma
• Peripheral odontogenic fibroma
• Acute periodontitis
• Periodontosis
• Epulis fissuratum
• Epulis granulomatosum
• Parulis
• Myxofibroma
• Traumatic (irritation) fibroma

Pyogenic Granuloma

TREATMENT

General
◇ Improved oral hygiene.
◇ Scaling and root planing.
◇ Repair of defective restorations.
◇ Removal of other identifiable chronic irritations.

MEDICATIONS
• Chlorhexidine mouth rinse to minimize plaque accumulation.
• Antibiotics, if associated with a more generalized periodontal infection.

SURGERY
Biopsy of lesions that do not spontaneously regress.

CONSULTATION SUGGESTIONS
Oral-Maxillofacial Surgeon

REFERRAL SUGGESTIONS
Oral-Maxillofacial Surgeon

PATIENT INSTRUCTIONS
Excellent oral hygiene and replacement of old or defective restorations important for prevention.

COURSE/PROGNOSIS
Improvement in oral hygiene, removal of chronic irritants, and waiting until pregnancy has come full term will usually result in spontaneous regression of the lesions. Lesions that do not respond to conservative treatment should be excised and examined histologically.

CODING

ICD-9-CM
522.6 Maxillary alveolar ridge granuloma
523.8 Peripheral giant cell reparative granuloma of gingiva
528.9 Oral mucosa pyogenic granuloma
686.1 Pyogenic granuloma of skin
998.8 Granuloma secondary to suture

CPT
11440 Excision lesion, face, ear, lid, nose, lip, membrane, 0.5 cm or less.
11441 Excision lesion, face, ear, lid, nose, lip, membrane, 0.6 to 1 cm.
40490 Biopsy of lip.
40808 Biopsy vestibule of mouth
40810 Excision, lesion mucosa/submucosa without repair
41100 Biopsy tongue, anterior 2/3
41110 Excision lesion of tongue without closure
41112 Excision lesion of tongue with closure, anterior 2/3
41825 Excision lesion/tumor without repair
41826 Excision lesion/tumor with simple repair
99000 Handling and transport of specimen

MISCELLANEOUS

SYNONYMS
Pregnancy tumor
Pregnancy epulis
Granuloma pyogenicum

SEE ALSO
Hemangioma
Fibroma

REFERENCES
Daley TD, Nartley NI, Wysocki GP: Pregnancy tumor: An analysis. Oral Surg Oral Med Oral Path 72:196-199, 1991.

Burket's Oral Medicine Diagnosis and Treatment, 9th ed. Lynch MA, Brightman VJ, Greenberg MS. (eds), Philadelphia, JB Lippincott Co., 1994, pp. 260-261.

AUTHOR
Dale J. Misiek, DMD

Rabies

BASICS

DESCRIPTION
• An acute infectious disease characterized by travel of the rabies virus along the involved peripheral nerve to the central nervous system. The virus attacks neurons in the spinal cord and brainstem producing an encephalitis and death.
• In human rabies infection, there is a five-stage clinical course: incubation, prodrome, neurologic stage, coma, and death.

ETIOLOGY

• Most naturally occurring rabies infection is the result of the bite of a rabid animal. Among wild animals, carnivorous (ie, skunks, raccoons, foxes, and bats) are more suspect unless proven uninfected. Rabbits, squirrels, chipmunks, rats, mice, and other rodents are rarely infected. Rare cases are transmitted by infected saliva. The virus travels from the site of entry via peripheral nerves to the spinal cord and the brain, where it multiplies. It then continues through efferent nerves to the salivary glands and into the saliva. Human rabies virus infection is characterized by a highly variable incubation period from 13 days to 9 months, with an average of 30 days.
• Length of incubation is determined by severity of lacerations due to bite, amount of virus at wound site, and distance virus must travel to reach the brain.
• Head and neck wounds usually have shorter incubation periods.

SYSTEMS AFFECTED
<u>Salivary glands</u>
  ◊ excessive salivation
<u>Central nervous system</u>
  ◊ acute disseminated encephalomyelitis characterized by autonomic dysfunction and seizures.
<u>Gastrointestinal</u>
  ◊ hydrophobia due to excruciatingly painful spasms of accessory muscles of neck and diaphragm.

DIAGNOSIS

SYMPTOMS AND SIGNS
<u>General</u>
  ◊ early headache, nausea, sore throat, followed by a period of excitation and nervousness. This stage of encephalitic rabies is characterized by hydrophobia, aerophobia, periods of agitation, hyperexcitation, confusion, hyporeactivity, and drowsiness, followed by convulsions, coma, and death. During paralytic stage, there is usually a high and constant fever.
<u>Salivary glands</u>
  ◊ excess salivation
Sensitivity around bite wound.

LABORATORY
<u>Lumbar puncture to test spinal fluid</u>
  ◊ protein normal or elevated normal or elevated cell count.
An asymptomatic animal that bites a human should be confined and observed by a veterinarian for 10 days. If animal remains healthy, one can be assured the animal was not infectious. If animal appears rabid, or was a wild animal, it should be sacrificed and submitted to a diagnostic laboratory.

IMAGING/SPECIAL TESTS
Detection of rabies virus by the indirect fluorescent assay technique has a sensitivity and specificity of 96 and 97%, respectively.
In patients, the diagnosis is suggested by a history of compatible animal bite and confirmed by viral testing. Impression smears of the cornea, as well as viral cultures of nasal and salivary secretion, may be useful.

DIFFERENTIAL
• Acute disseminated encephalomyelitis
• Guillain-Barré syndrome

Rabies

 ## TREATMENT

General
◊ Local wound treatment may be most important preventive measure.

◊ The wound should be cleansed immediately and thoroughly, and may be closed if on the face. Otherwise, leave open to drain and granulate.

◊ If rabies develop, treatment is symptomatic with vigorous supportive measure and expert consultation from the State Health Department or the Centers for Disease Control in Atlanta, Georgia.

MEDICATIONS
• Systemic postexposure prophylaxis should be started immediately if animal is rabid or demonstrates rabid behavior.
• Administration of rabies immune globulin for passive immunization, followed concurrently by active immunization.
• Rabies Immune Globulin (RIG) should be used for passive immunization only once at the beginning of prophylaxis.
• Human Diploid Cell Rabies Vaccine (HDCV) should be used for active immunization. This vaccine provides complete protection after only five injections, and allergic reactions seldom occur.
• Up to one-half of the dose of RIG should be infiltrated around the wound.
• Active immunization with HDCV should also begin immediately. The vaccine is given in a series of five injections into the deltoid area. A sixth injection should be given 90 days after the first injection.

CONSULTATION SUGGESTIONS
Infectious Disease Specialist

REFERRAL SUGGESTIONS
Infectious Disease Specialist

FIRST STEPS TO TAKE IN AN EMERGENCY
• Seek immediate medical care if bitten and carefully clean wound.

PATIENT INSTRUCTIONS
Avoid contact with wild animals or strangely behaving domestic animals.

COURSE/PROGNOSIS
Once encephalitis has developed, rabies may be fatal. Fortunately, postexposure passive and active immunization are highly effective. Because the incubation period is relatively long, these preventive measures may be used. In addition, recent vaccines have few side effects.

 ## CODING

ICD-9-CM
071.0 Clinical rabies
V01.5 Rabies exposure
V04.5 Inoculation or prophylactic vaccination

CPT
12011 Simple repair of superficial wounds of face, lip, mucous membrane 2.5 cm or less
12013 2.6 to 5.0 cm
12051 Layered closure of wounds of face, lip, 2.5 cm or less
12052 2.6 to 5.0 cm
13131 Complex repair of forehead, cheeks, chin, mouth 1.1 to 2.5 cm
13132 2.6 to 7.5 cm
13150 Repair complex, eyelids, nose, ears, lips, 1 cm or less
13151 1.1 to 2.5 cm
13152 2.6 to 7.5 cm

 ## MISCELLANEOUS

REFERENCES
Peter JB: Use and Interpretation of Tests in Medical Microbiology, 2nd ed. Santa Monica, CA, Specialty Labs, pp. 121-122.

Tsiang H: Pathophysiology of rabies virus infection of the nervous system. Adv Virus Res 42:375-413, 1993.

Hupp JR: Infections of the soft tissues of the maxillofacial and neck regions. In: Oral Maxillofacial Infections. 3rd ed.

Topazian RG, Goldberg M (eds), Philadelphia, WB Saunders, 1994, pp. 338-359.

Gonzalez-Scarano F, Tyler K: Molecular pathogenesis of neurotropic viral infections. Ann Neurol 22:565, 1987.

AUTHOR
John Jandinski , DMD

Ranula

BASICS

DESCRIPTION
A mucous retention or mucous extravasation phenomenon located in the floor of the mouth. It is most often a unilateral fluid-filled swelling, with a bluish cast, but it can also be located in the midline.

ETIOLOGY

• Occurs when mucin accumulates in the tissues of the floor of the mouth. It is thought to be due to a blockage or a partial blockage in the sublingual glands, or less commonly in the submandibular glands. Usually no sialolith can be demonstrated.
• Ranula can be due to rupture of a salivary duct or from dilation of a salivary duct. Microscopically, the walls of the lesion are most often granulation tissue, but may have an epithelial lining.
• Of note is the plunging or cervical ranula. This rare variant herniates through the mylohyoid musculature and presents as a swelling in the upper neck. More common in children.

SYSTEMS AFFECTED
• Oral mucosa is thinned and often has a bluish cast.
• Salivary flow is occluded if a major salivary gland duct is involved.

DIAGNOSIS

SYMPTOMS AND SIGNS
• Asyptomatic swelling in the floor of the mouth.
• Unilateral fluctuant swelling in the floor of the mouth, usually located near the submandibular duct.
• Overlying mucosa normal in appearance, often with a bluish cast when superficial.
• If a major salivary gland duct is involved, no saliva can be expressed from that gland.

LABORATORY
Microscopic examination reveals thick mucoserous fluid surrounded by granulation tissue. Retention mucocele features lining derived from duct epithelium.

IMAGING/SPECIAL TESTS
Aspiration of fluid to test for amylase and total protein present in plunging ranulas but not cystic hygromas.

DIFFERENTIAL
Floor of mouth swelling
  ◇ dermoid cyst
Neoplasms
Neck swelling
  ◇ branchial cleft cyst
    thyroglossal duct cyst
    cystic hygroma

TREATMENT

MEDICATIONS
• Not indicated

SURGERY
Marsupialization is the initial treatment of choice, packing the cavity with gauze may be useful.
In refractory cases, removal of the sublingual gland may be necessary.

CONSULTATION SUGGESTIONS
Oral-Maxillofacial Surgeon

REFERRAL SUGGESTIONS
Oral-Maxillofacial Surgeon

PATIENT INSTRUCTIONS
Even if lesion spontaneously drains, will recur if not surgically managed.

COURSE/PROGNOSIS
Occasionally recurs even if excision performed.

CODING

ICD-9-CM
527.6 Mucocele-Ranula

CPT
42325 Fistulization of sublingual salivary cyst (ranula)
42326 with prosthesis
42409 Marsupialization of sublingual salivary cyst (ranula)
42440 Excision of submandibular gland
42450 Excision of sublingual gland

MISCELLANEOUS

SYNONYMS
Mucocele

SEE ALSO
Dermoid cyst

REFERENCES
Regezi JA, Sciubba J: Oral Pathology, 2nd ed. Philadelphia, WB Saunders, 1993, pp. 246-247.

Baurmash H: Marsupialization for treatment of oral ranula. J Oral Maxillofac Surg 50:1274-1279, 1992.

AUTHOR
Michael J. Dalton, DDS

Raynaud's Phenomenon

BASICS

DESCRIPTION
• Spasm of arterioles, with intermittent pallor or cyanosis of the skin usually in the digits and toes (and occasionally other acral parts such as nose and tongue).
• Raynaud's disease most often begins in young women.

ETIOLOGY

• May be idiopathic (Raynaud's disease) or secondary to rheumatic or connective tissue disorders and drugs (ergot, methylsergide, β-adrenergic blockers).
• Vasoconstriction of digital and palmar or plantar arteries.
• An intimal proliferation of the blood vessel wall and hypertrophy of muscle layers may occur later in disease.
• Thromboses may form in small arteries.
• In secondary Raynaud's, the pathologic changes of the underlying disease are apparent.
• Vasospastic response is triggered by anything that activates sympathetic outflow or releases catecholamines (emotion) in addition to exposure to cold.
• Raynaud's phenomenon may be associated with the following factors:
    Connective tissue disorders
    Scleroderma
    Rheumatoid arthritis
    Systemic lupus erythematosus
    Dermatomyositis
    Obstructive arterial disease
    Thromboangiitis obliterans
    Thoracic outlet syndrome
    Dysproteinemia
    Trauma (occupational)
    Construction workers
    Pianists
    Typists
Drugs associated
    Ergot, methysergide
    Sympathomimetic drugs
    β-Adrenergic blockers
Mental State
   ◇ Stress/tension may precipitate attacks

SYSTEMS AFFECTED
Oral mucosa
   ◇ spasms of lips and tongue may occur.
Teeth
   ◇ extraction sockets slow to heal and more susceptible to complications.
Digits and toes
   ◇ ischemic changes with possible focal gangrene of the tips.
Ear lobes, nose, cheeks and chin
   ◇ may also present with ischemic changes.

DIAGNOSIS

SYMPTOMS AND SIGNS
Mouth
   ◇ spasms of lips/tongue
Digits and toes
   ◇ paresthesia, stiffness and, less commonly, pain.
• Digits are cold/numb during vasoconstriction and painful during reactive hyperemia. Painful ulcers on digits/toes.
• Pallor, followed by cyanosis and rubor (hyperemia) precipitated by exposure to cold or emotional stress.
• Focal gangrene of tips of fingers and toes.
• Signs of underlying disease in Raynaud's phenomenon.

LABORATORY
• Raynaud's disease is differentiated from secondary Raynaud's phenomenon by bilateral involvement, a history of symptoms without progression (less than 2 years and no evidence of an underlying cause).
• CBC, erythrocyte sedimentation rate, rheumatoid factor, antinuclear antibody, cryoglobulins, serum protein electrophoresis, and muscle enzyme determinations to rule out underlying disease.

DIFFERENTIAL
• Connective tissue disorders
• Peripheral arterial disease
• Hematologic abnormalities
• Occupational hazards
• Drugs

TREATMENT

General
◇ Protection of extremities from cold (ie, wear gloves, do not touch cold door knobs, avoid putting hand in refrigerator).
◇ Discourage smoking (vasoconstriction).
◇ Biofeedback or relaxation techniques to reduce stress.

MEDICATIONS
• Reserpine 0.1 to 0.5 mg orally b.i.d. to q.i.d. (may cause depression).
• Methyldopa 1 to 2 g/day orally
• Prazosin 1 to 2 mg h.s. and in morning, if necessary.
• Nifedipine -10 to 30 mg orally t.i.d.

SURGERY
Regional sympathectomy in patients with progressive disability.

CONSULTATION SUGGESTIONS
Rheumatologist

REFERRAL SUGGESTIONS
Primary Care Physician

FIRST STEPS TO TAKE IN AN EMERGENCY
• Administer vasodilator and warm part of body experiencing the problem.

PATIENT INSTRUCTIONS
Avoid precipitating factors and stop smoking.

COURSE/PROGNOSIS
• Although no cure, treating the underlying cause of Raynaud's phenomenon is extremely important.
• Proper preventive measures usually diminish ischemia, alleviate symptoms, and prevent dystrophic changes.

CODING

ICD-9-CM
443.0 Raynaud's disease or phenomenon

MISCELLANEOUS

SEE ALSO
Claudication
Thromboangiitis obliterans
Scleroderma
Systemic lupus
Rheumatoid arthritis

REFERENCES
Rademaker M, et al: The antiplatelet effect of nifedipine in patients with systemic sclerosis. Clin Exp Rheumatol 10:57, 1992.

Katz WA: Raynaud's phenomenon. In: Internal Medicine for Dentistry 2nd ed. Rose LF, Kaye D. (eds), St. Louis, Mosby, 1990, pp. 55-56.

Giunta JL: Raynaud's disease with oral manifestations. Arch Derm 111:78-80, 1975.

Bonnette GH, Arrentz RE: Raynaud's disease and extraction wound healing. J Oral Surg, 26:185-187, 1968.

AUTHOR
John Jandinski, DMD

Reiter's Syndrome

BASICS

DESCRIPTION
A multisystem disease that includes arthritis, conjunctivitis, urethritis, skin lesions, and oral mucosal lesions similar to aphthous ulcers. It has a striking predilection for white males in their third decade, and is the most common cause of arthritis in young men.

ETIOLOGY

• Precise cause is unknown, but genetic factors and abnormal immune response to infectious agents appear important.
Genetic factors
◇ up to 90% of patients are positive for HLA-B27 histocompatibility antigen.
• The disease usually follows infection of the digestive or urogenital tract.

SYSTEMS AFFECTED
Urogenital
◇ disease usually begins with urethritis.
Eyes
◇ conjunctivitis lasts a few days or weeks.
Skeletal
◇ arthritis is acute, asymmetrical, involves multiple joints, usually of the lower extremities.
Skin
◇ lesions occur mainly on palms, soles and glans penis.
Oral mucosa
◇ aphthous-type ulcers may occur.

DIAGNOSIS

SYMPTOMS AND SIGNS
Urogenital
◇ urethritis is typically asymptomatic. May have intermittent urethral discharge.
Eyes
◇ itching, erythema, and burning of conjunctiva, or may be asymptomatic.
Arthritis
◇ joints are painful, warm and erythematous, and accompanied by fever and malaise. Acute episode lasts days to several months.
Skin lesions
◇ nonpainful, crusted, scaling papules on palms, soles, and glans penis. Keratin build-up under nails.
Oral mucosa
◇ aphthous-like ulcers are relatively painless. Ulcers appear almost anywhere on oral mucosa.

LABORATORY
• No specific tests for Reiter's syndrome . Diagnosis is based on signs and symptoms.
• Rheumatoid factor and antinuclear antibodies are negative.

DIFFERENTIAL
• Aphthous ulcers of oral mucosa
• Gonococcal urethritis
• Viral conjunctivitis
• Psoriasis of skin
• Rheumatoid or psoriatic arthritis

TREATMENT

General
◇ No cure is available. Goal of treatment is relief of symptoms. When joint problems occur, bed rest, physical therapy, and NSAIDs are needed.
◇ Oral lesions are mild and usually require no treatment.
◇ Patient education, physical therapy, and nonsteroidal anti-inflammatory medications for arthritis.

MEDICATIONS
• Ibuprofen, 400 to 800 mg, 4 times a day, up to a maximum of 3200 mg per day, is an example of a regimen for arthritis. Maximum dose may be associated with prolonged bleeding time and gastric upset.
• Eye involvement may necessitate use of steroids.
• Sulfasalazine is experimental.

CONSULTATION SUGGESTIONS
Rheumatologist, Ophthalmologist, Urologist

REFERRAL SUGGESTIONS
Primary Care Physician

PATIENT INSTRUCTIONS
Contact Arthritis Foundation for useful patient information (404) 872-7100.

COURSE/PROGNOSIS
• Arthritis is usually the most difficult problem.
• Duration is weeks to months.
• One third of patients may have recurrences.

CODING

ICD-9-CM
099.3 Reiter's syndrome (listed as a venereal disease).
528.2 Aphthous ulcers

MISCELLANEOUS

SYNONYMS
Arthritis urethritica
Urethro-oculo articular syndrome.
Idiopathic blennorrheal arthritis.
Reactive arthritis

SEE ALSO
Rheumatoid Arthritis
Psoriasis
Conjunctivitis

REFERENCES
Moutsopoulos HM, Taurog JD, Lipsky PE: Reactive arthritis. In: Harrison's Principles of Internal Medicine, 13th ed. Isselbacher KJ, et al, (eds), New York, McGraw-Hill, 1994, pp. 1664-1669.

AUTHOR
Michael W. Finkelstein, DDS, MS

Renal Disease, Dialysis, and Transplantation

BASICS

DESCRIPTION
• Renal disease results from a kidney's inability to function as a filter to eliminate metabolic waste via the urine, maintain the body's fluid, acid/base and electrolyte balance, secrete the hormones renin and angiotensin (responsible for the control of blood pressure), and manufacture erythropoietin, which modulates red blood cell maturation.
• Results in acidosis, anemia, and nitrogen retention.
• Affects 60,000 Americans each year.

ETIOLOGY

• Renal disease may be either acute or chronic. Causes of acute renal disease include trauma, ischemia, septicemia, or adverse reaction to medications or toxic chemicals. Causes of chronic renal failure include conditions that result from either malfunction of the kidney or systemic disease such as hypertension, diabetes mellitus, drug-induced nephropathies, polycystic renal disease, and chronic glomerulonephritis.
• A healthy kidney is capable of compensatory hypertrophy, which allows it to carry out normal function by increasing in its size to compensate for the loss, damage, or disease of the other kidney. Therefore, the ill effects of renal failure typically require dysfunction of both kidneys.

SYSTEMS AFFECTED
Renal
◊ renal output may be increased but ineffective or decreased, both with resulting accumulation of waste products.
Cardiovascular
◊ hypertension, congestive heart failure, pericarditis, or myocarditis.
Dermatologic
◊ facial edema, pallor or greenish hue to skin, periorbital or labial edema, pruritus, bruising, and hyperpigmentation.
Lip
◊ patients with renal transplants have increased incidence of squamous cell carcinoma of the lip, leukoplakia, and oral mucosal dysplasia.
Hematologic
◊ anemia, increased susceptibility to infection, lymphopenia, abnormal bleeding times.
Metabolic
◊ glucose intolerance, lipid abnormalities, thyroid and pituitary disorders.

DIAGNOSIS

SYMPTOMS AND SIGNS
• The dentist should take a careful history of patients at risk for or with suspected or known renal disease. The review of systems and evaluation of the patient's blood pressure and sun-exposed skin for signs of renal disease as described above will provide invaluable diagnostic information. If undiagnosed renal disease is suspected, evaluation of the patient's medication list may provide information related to drugs known to cause acute renal failure. Patients may complain of dysgeusia or oral ulceration and discomfort.
• Intraoral signs of renal disease may present as:
Halitosis
◊ breath may smell like ammonia. Gingival bleeding from impaired platelet function.
Acute necrotizing ulcerative gingivitis (ANUG).
Graft-versus-host disease
◊ lichen planus-like lesions of the buccal mucosa noted in patients who are rejecting a renal transplant.
Uremic stomatitis
◊ nonspecific aphthous-like lesions of the oral mucosa. These lesions tend to be painful and are often covered by a pseudomembrane.
Parotid inflammation and enlargement.

LABORATORY
CBC
◊ normochromic, normocytic anemia, thrombocytopenia.
Glomerular filtration rate (GFR)
◊ decreased
Blood urea nitrogen (BUN)
◊ elevated
Creatinine
◊ elevated (gives good estimate of degree of renal insufficiency).
Electrolytes
◊ elevated potassium, phosphate, and depressed calcium.
Urinalysis
◊ proteinuria, casts of red cells, white cells, hyaline.
Glucose
◊ elevated serum level

IMAGING/SPECIAL TESTS
Renal biopsy
◊ may reveal glomerulonephritis and/or interstitial nephritis.
24 urine collections to gauge creatinine clearance, protein, and electrolyte loss.
• Decreased Vitamin D levels when elevated parathyroid hormone levels present.
• Renal imaging (IVP, CT, tomograms, retrograde pyelograms, angiography) and/or ultrasound.

• Dental radiographs may show signs of renal osteodystrophy, which include loss of lamina dura, scanty or fine trabeculation, thinning of the inferior mandibular cortex and/or thinning of the cortices surrounding the inferior alveolar canal. A decrease in bone density may be revealed by evaluating serial radiographs.

DIFFERENTIAL
• ANUG
• Aphthous stomatitis
• Candidiasis
• Erythema multiforme
• Gingivitis
• Mucositis
• Periodontitis
• Stomatitis, idiopathic

TREATMENT

General
Hemodialysis
◊ metabolic waste products are removed from the patient by passing their blood through a thin semipermeable membrane. The patient's blood is then heparinized and returned to them. An arterio-venous fistula (AV fistula) is usually surgically formed in the patient's arm for this purpose.
Peritoneal dialysis
◊ this procedure is slower as the abdominal peritoneum serves as the semipermeable membrane. The waste fluid is periodically drained from the abdomen.
◊ Oral Manifestations of Renal Disease
◊ The best time to provide dental care is the day after dialysis.
◊ Blood pressure must not be taken on the arm of the renal transplant patient who has an AV fistula. The resultant increase in intravenous pressure may cause the fistula to rupture.
◊ Attention must be paid to modifying prescription of medications, which might build up in the blood stream due to impaired excretion such as antibiotics that depend upon renal excretion.
◊ Avoidance of nephrotoxic medications such as streptomycin, neomycin, and gentamicin is mandatory. Tetracyclines can cause marked elevation of BUN. Oral or intravenous penicillins containing a potassium salt should be avoided due to the risk of hyperkalemia. Salicylate and NSAID medications should also be avoided, as they can be nephrotoxic and result in bleeding and fluid retention.
◊ Determination of bleeding times prior to elective surgery is necessary.

Need for antibiotic prophylaxis, especially those with an indwelling catheter or AV fistula. Vancomycin (1 gram over 20 minutes) can be given to the patient during dialysis and will remain effective until their next dialysis appointment.

◊ Avoid dental therapy the day of hemodialysis due to prolonged bleeding tendencies from residual heparin, unless protamine reversal of heparin is done.

◊ Supplemental steroid therapy may be necessary on patients on an immunosuppressive regimen following renal transplantation.

◊ Treatment of mucous membrane ulceration is dependent on the cause. Discontinuance or adjusting the dose of an offending medication (such as cyclophosphamide in the transplant patient) if identified, will usually resolve the ulcerative stomatitis. If the lesions are not found to be of infectious origin (bacterial, viral or fungal), a burst of systemic steroids may be appropriate. Topical anesthetics such as 2% viscous lidocaine or 0.5% dyclonine hydrochloride may be applied prior to meals to allow the patient to eat more comfortably. Sucralfate suspension may be used between meals as a means of covering the ulceration(s), thereby providing relief from pain and irritation.

MEDICATIONS
• Hypertension controlled with antihypertensives, including diuretics and angiotensin converting enzyme inhibitors.
• Vitamin D and calcium to manage secondary hyperparathyroidism.
• Vitamin E or quinine for muscle cramps.
• Erythropoietin (recombinant) for anemia.
• DDAVP, cryoprecipitate, platelets, dialysis for problems with excessive or spontaneous bleeding.
• Antihistamines and skin moisturizers for pruritus.
• Insulin for glucose intolerance.

SURGERY
Renal transplantation
◊ kidney transplantation is a means of improving the quality of life for the recipient. Renal transplants are ideally procured from a close relative with a good histocompatibility profile. However, cadaver kidneys are also used. Immunosuppressive drugs such as cyclosporine-A, cyclophosphamide, or azathioprine are employed to prevent rejection.

CONSULTATION SUGGESTIONS
• The patient's Primary Care Physician or Nephrologist should be contacted to ascertain the patient's systemic health pertaining to:
• Anemia
• Bleeding abnormalities

• The need for antibiotic prophylaxis due to either an indwelling catheter, AV fistula, or renal transplantation.
• The need for steroid augmentation therapy for renal transplant patients.
• The infectious disease status for HIV and hepatitis C, if renal transplantation was performed prior to 1985 or 1987, respectively.

REFERRAL SUGGESTIONS
Primary Care Physician

FIRST STEPS TO TAKE IN AN EMERGENCY
• Toxic accumulation of substances usually eliminated by the kidneys may necessitate emergency dialysis.

PATIENT INSTRUCTIONS
Contact National Kidney Diseases clearing house for useful patient information (301) 468-6345.

COURSE/PROGNOSIS
• Routine dental care is usually uneventful in the well-controlled renal patient. The oral cavity usually reflects the control of the renal disease. Therefore, more oral problems with a worse prognosis would be expected with the poorly controlled patient.
• Graft-versus-host disease is an ominous prognostic sign and generally portends the ultimate rejection of a renal transplant.

CODING

ICD-9-CM
101.0	ANUG
112.0	Candidiasis
285.9	Anemia
288.0	Mucositis
523.1	Gingivitis
523.4	Periodontitis
527.2	Parotitis
528.0	Stomatitis
528.2	Aphthous stomatitis
695.1	Erythema multiforme
784.9	Halitosis
996.80	Graft-versus-host disease
996.81	Renal transplant

MISCELLANEOUS

SYNONYMS
Uremia
Chronic renal failure

SEE ALSO
Glomerulonephritis
Potassium disorders
Hyperparathyroidism
Anemia

REFERENCES
Naylor GD, Hall EH, Terezhalmy GT: The patient with chronic renal failure who is undergoing dialysis or renal transplantation: another consideration for antimicrobial prophylaxis. Oral Surg Oral Med Oral Path 65:116-121, 1989.

Sampson E, Meister F, Jr: Dental complications in the end-stages of renal disease. Gen Dent 32:297-299, 1984.

Sonis ST, Fazio RC, Fang L: Chronic renal failure, dialysis and transplantation. In: Principles and Practice of Oral Medicine, 2nd ed. Philadelphia, WB Saunders, 1994, pp. 293-304.

AUTHOR
Michael A. Siegel, DDS, MS

Respiratory Distress Syndrome (RDS)

BASICS

DESCRIPTION
RDS is typically an intensive-care symptom-complex, with numerous potential initiating events, but few precise explanations regarding its pathophysiology.

ETIOLOGY

Sepsis and trauma are the most common pre-existing conditions. However, it may be precipitated by a variety of other factors, including pulmonary gastric aspiration, fat embolus, shock, drug injury, burns, drowning, pneumonia, multiple transfusions, inhaled toxins, pancreatitis, head injury, eclampsia, and air embolism.

SYSTEMS AFFECTED
RDS is a respiratory disease characterized by diffuse pulmonary cell injury with accompanying increased capillary permeability, edema, inflammation, and infiltrates. Blood-borne substances are thought to initiate and/ or sustain the process, which include complement, free fatty acids, fibrin degradation products, histamine, lysozyme, platelets, serotonin, leukotrienes, and neutrophils. Persistent hypoxemia is seen in the later states, caused by intrapulmonary shunting, increased dead space, decreased functional residual capacity, and microatelectasis.

DIAGNOSIS

SYMPTOMS AND SIGNS
• Increasing respiratory difficulty with or without obvious cause.
• Within the first 6 hours in the development of tissue injury, there may be no specific clinical signs. Twelve to 24 hours later, respiratory insufficiency begins, characterized by tachypnea and rales. Other signs include: clammy skin, cyanosis, use of accessory muscles of respiration, lethargy, agitation.

LABORATORY
Early stages may show no changes on chest radiograph. After 12 to 24 hours, diffuse radiographic alveolar and interstitial infiltrates are seen. Hypoxemia and hypercarbia persist despite administration of 100% oxygen.

IMAGING/SPECIAL TESTS
Arterial blood gases combined with sequential chest radiographs are needed to help confirm the diagnosis.

DIFFERENTIAL
• The diagnosis is usually one of exclusion, with several criteria necessary to confirm the presence of RDS:
• $PaO_2 < 50$ mm Hg when using > 40% O_2 with 5 cm H_2O positive end-expiratory pressure (PEEP).
• New bilateral and changing pulmonary infiltrates.
• Pulmonary capillary wedge pressure < 18 mm H_2O.
• Appropriate risk factors present (described above).
• No other explanation for above findings.

TREATMENT

General

◇ Ventilatory support is the most important type of treatment for RDS, involving intubation, mechanical ventilation, and PEEP. This support is needed until alveolar-capillary membrane integrity is re-established. Fluid restriction may be needed, but this needs to be balanced with maintaining adequate urinary output to prevent renal failure. Pulmonary toilet is needed to clear the airway of secretions. Use of corticosteroids, while generously used in the past, are used with discretion and often in the later stages of RDS.

MEDICATIONS

- Vasodilators
- Anxiolytics
- Anticoagulants
- H-2 antagonists

CONSULTATION SUGGESTIONS

Pulmonologist

REFERRAL SUGGESTIONS

Primary Care Physician, Pulmonologist

FIRST STEPS TO TAKE IN AN EMERGENCY

• Administer oxygen, intubate if possible, transport to emergency facility or, if in hospital, to intensive care unit.

COURSE/PROGNOSIS

Mortality from RDS may range from 50 to 75%. Patients rarely die from RDS itself; the usual cause of death is sepsis or infection. While there may be underlying sepsis as the initiating event, nonseptic patients with RDS are at greater risk for developing sepsis, so it appears RDS and sepsis are almost always coexistent.

CODING

ICD-9-CM

518.5 Respiratory distress syndrome post-trauma or surgery

518.82 Respiratory distress syndrome associated with other conditions

MISCELLANEOUS

Current research is aimed at evaluating the role of a variety of substances to limit or reverse the process, including prostaglandins (PGE1), antioxidants, nonsteroidal anti-inflammatory drugs, anti-adhesion molecules, and thrombolytics.

SYNONYMS

Adult respiratory distress syndrome (ARDS).
Shock lung
Wet lung

SEE ALSO

Aspiration pneumonitis
Pneumonia, bacterial

REFERENCES

Dembo JB: Surgical critical care. Oral Maxillofac Surg Clin N Am 4:709, 1992.

Bresler MJ, Sternbach GL: The adult respiratory distress syndrome. Emerg Med Clin N Am 7:419, 1989.

Chapman MJ: Adult respiratory distress syndrome an update. Anaesth Intens Care 22:255, 1994.

AUTHOR

Jeffrey B. Dembo, DMD

Retinitis Pigmentosa

BASICS

DESCRIPTION
A group of hereditary disorders in which progressive retinal degeneration occurs that usually leads to blindness. Retinitis pigmentosa (RP) is divided into two major categories: 1) isolated RP, in which the retina and other ocular tissue show abnormalities; and 2) associated RP, in which similar ocular findings are associated with other abnormalities in a multisystem disease.

ETIOLOGY

RP is a set of diseases caused by abnormal genes at various loci within the human genome. Genetic loci have been found on the short arm of the X chromosome, as well as chromosomes 3, 6, and 8. RP is inherited as an autosomal dominant, autosomal recessive, and X-linked recessive, or can occur spontaneously. The pathogenesis of the genetic change is unknown.

SYSTEMS AFFECTED
Ocular
◇ photoreceptors are diffusely and profoundly affected initially followed by degenerative pigment epithelial changes. The rod function is affected earlier than the cone function. The abnormalities of RP are symmetrical, including decreased peripheral visual fields, decreased visual acuity and color vision, as well as refractive errors. There is an increased prevalence of fundus, macular, optic disc, and vitreous abnormalities in patients with RP. Cataracts occur frequently in all types of RP.

DIAGNOSIS

SYMPTOMS AND SIGNS
• Progressive night blindness, increased loss of peripheral vision, decreased visual acuity, light flashes, and loss of color vision. There is variability in vision from day to day.
• Myopia, astigmatism, progressive decreased visual acuity, tritanopia (blue blindness), narrowed retinal vessels, depigmentation of the retinal pigment epithelium, intraretinal bone spicule pigmentation, waxy pale optic disc, vitreous abnormalities, posterior subcapsular cataracts, and maculopathy.

LABORATORY
Serologic test for syphilis.

IMAGING/SPECIAL TESTS
Electroretinograms, fluorescein angiography, static perimetry, dark adaption testing.

DIFFERENTIAL
Neurologic disease, gyrate atrophy of the choroid and retina, choroideremia, stationary night blindness, cone dystrophies, cone-rod dystrophies, inherited macular dystrophies, primary choroidal dystrophies, pseudo-RP, infectious retinopathies (rubella, syphilis), retinal trauma.

TREATMENT

General
◊ genetic counseling is important to reduce the incidence of RP.
◊ Optical devices are used to maximize remaining vision.
◊ Psychologic and vocational counseling is recommended.
◊ Sunglasses are recommended to prevent damage of the retina from excessive sunlight.
◊ Follow-up examinations are conducted every 2 years to monitor the course of the disease.
◊ No medical or surgical treatment has proven to be effective for the cure or amelioration of the diseased retina associated with RP.

MEDICATIONS
• Acetazolamide is used for patients with cystoid macular edema.

SURGERY
Cataract surgery is performed without any effect on the basic disease process.

CONSULTATION SUGGESTIONS
Ophthalmologist

REFERRAL SUGGESTIONS
Ophthalmologist, Primary Care Physician

PATIENT INSTRUCTIONS
Useful patient information available from RP Foundation (800)638-2300.

COURSE/PROGNOSIS
Progressive loss of peripheral vision and eventual blindness will occur, although in most instances vision is retained for 20 to 40 years in most individuals. The rate of progression is related to the genetic type of RP. In autosomal dominant RP, which is considered the mild form, it has a later onset of major symptoms and longer preservation of central vision. In X-linked RP, loss of vision is more rapid.

CODING

ICD-9-CM
362.74 Pigmental retinal dystrophy

M MISCELLANEOUS

SYNONYMS
Rod-cone degeneration

REFERENCES
Merin S: Inherited Eye Disease: Diagnosis and Clinical Management, New York, Marcel Dekker, 1991, pp. 219-279.

Berson EL: Retinitis Pigmentosa and Allied Disease. In: Principles and Practice of Ophthalmology: Clinical Practice. Albert DM, Jakobiec FA (eds), Philadelphia, WB Saunders, 1994, pp. 1214-1236.

AUTHOR
Daniel S. Sarasin, DDS

Rheumatic Fever

BASICS

DESCRIPTION
A serious nonsuppurative sequela of infection with group A β-hemolytic streptococcus. It possibly represents an autoimmune reaction triggered by a preceding pharyngitis with a rheumatogenic strain of group A streptococcus.

ETIOLOGY

Group A β-hemolytic streptococcus can be classified into a variety of types based on the M protein in the cell wall. Various M proteins share certain epitopes with components of cardiac muscle, while others have epitopes associated with joint tissue. Following a pharyngeal infection with one of these group A streptococci, an autoimmune reaction may develop. Antibody formed to the M protein attacks host tissue of the heart, leading to cardiac injury (rheumatic heart disease), and of the joint, leading to polyarthritis. Most common in children aged 5 to 15.

SYSTEMS AFFECTED
• Musculoskeletal (joints)
• Cardiac tissue-mitral valve/aortic valve
• Skin
• Central nervous system

DIAGNOSIS

The diagnosis of this process is elusive because of the variety of signs and symptoms, and also because the streptococcal infection usually occurs 20 days or more prior to onset.

SYMPTOMS AND SIGNS
Diagnosis made by presence of either two major or one major and two minor signs/symptoms outlined in the "revised Jones criteria."
Major Criteria
• Carditis (65%)
• New or changed murmur
• Arthritis (75%)
  • Polyarticular and migratory
  • Tender, red, hot, swollen joints that resolve in 3 to 4 weeks.
• Chorea (10-15%)
  • Adolescent female
  • Better prognosis
  • Moodiness
  • Lack concentration, clumsiness, involuntary movement, and ataxia.
• Rash (Erythema marginatum) (<5%)
  • Red, macular, truncal
  • Transient
  • Migratory, non-pruritic
  • Never on face
  • Rare except in severe rheumatic fever
• Subcutaneous nodules (5 to 10%)
  • Extensor surface, elbow, knee, wrists, spinous process of vertebrae and occipital region.
  • Painless, freely movable
Minor Criteria
  • Fever >38C
  • Positive serology streptococcal infection
  • ECG changes
  • Fatigue, irritability, weight loss, anemia, epistaxis
  • Abdominal pain
  • Facial tics and grimacing
  • History of epistaxis

LABORATORY
• Serologic tests for streptococcal infection
    antistreptolysin O
    antistreptokinase
    antideoxyribonuclease B
• Anemia
• Increased erythrocyte sedimentation rate
• Increased C-reactive protein

IMAGING/SPECIAL TESTS
    Throat culture for β-hemolytic
    ECG prolonged PR interval
    2-D Echocardiogram
    Pulsed doppler

DIFFERENTIAL
• Viral pharyngitis/systemic viral infection
• Lupus erythematosus
• Juvenile rheumatoid arthritis
• Myocardial infarction
• Malignancy

TREATMENT

• Prevent initial episode of rheumatic fever by diagnosis and treatment of acute streptococcal pharyngitis with antibiotic therapy as outlined below.
• Prevent recurrent rheumatic fever by prophylaxis and avoid crowded living conditions.

MEDICATIONS
• <u>Primary prophylaxis</u>
  ◊ treat acute pharyngitis
• Penicillin V 250 mg p.o., q.i.d. x 10 days or
• Erythromycin 250 mg p.d., q.i.d. x 10 days or
• Clindamycin 150 mg p.o., q.i.d. x 10 days or
• Benzathine penicillin 1.2 million units IM x 1 dose
• <u>Secondary prophylaxis</u>
• Benzathine penicillin 1.2 million units IM every 3 to 4 weeks or
• Erythromycin 250 mg p.o., b.i.d.

CONSULTATION SUGGESTIONS
Primary Care Physician, Infectious Disease Specialist

REFERRAL SUGGESTIONS
Primary Care Physician

FIRST STEPS TO TAKE IN AN EMERGENCY
• If disease suspected immediately, refer to emergency facility or personal physician.

PATIENT INSTRUCTIONS
After recovery, have determination made whether endocarditis prophylaxis necessary for dental procedures.

COURSE/PROGNOSIS
• Acute rheumatic fever rarely fatal.
• Carditis only permanent sequelae.
• Cumulative valve injury may lead to congestive heart failure.
• Chronic prophylaxis needed for prevention of recurrence.
• In cases of valvular damage, prophylaxis necessary to prevent infective endocarditis.

CODING

ICD-9-CM
390 Rheumatic fever

MISCELLANEOUS

SEE ALSO
Glomerulonephritis
Endocarditis

REFERENCES
Haffaejee I: Rheumatic fever and rheumatic heart disease: the current status of its immunology, diagnostic criteria, and prophylaxis. Quar J Med 84:641-658, 1992.

Alto WA, Gibson R: Acute rheumatic fever: an update. Am Fam Physician 45:613-620, 1992.

AUTHOR
Peter E. Larsen, DDS

Rheumatoid Arthritis

BASICS

DESCRIPTION
Rheumatoid arthritis (RA) is a chronic, multisystem inflammatory disorder, characterized by a persistent polyarticular, symmetrical joint involvement of unknown etiology. The pattern of disease involves cartilaginous destruction, bony erosions, and joint deformation. The prevalence of RA is 1% of the population, with women affected three times more than men.

ETIOLOGY

Unknown
<u>Genetic predisposition</u>
  ◊ there is an association between seropositive patients [+ rheumatoid factor (RF) and various alloantigens of the major histocompatibility complex (MHC)].
<u>Infectious agent</u>
  ◊ has been suggested, but not proven. Possible agents include mycoplasma, Epstein-Barr virus, cytomegalovirus, parvovirus, and rubella virus.
<u>Products of infectious agents ("superantigens")</u>
  ◊ these are proteins capable of binding HLA-DR molecules in the host. Speculative organisms include staphylococci, streptococci, and Mycoplasma arthritides.
Alteration in normal immune response may be involved in etiology.

SYSTEMS AFFECTED
• Generalized joint involvement
• Cardiovascular
• Pulmonary
• Ocular
• Neurologic
• Hematologic
• Vascular

DIAGNOSIS

SYMPTOMS AND SIGNS
<u>Constitutional symptoms</u>
  ◊ weight loss, generalized aches, malaise, fatigue, anorexia.
<u>Symmetrical joint involvement</u>
  ◊ swelling, joint pain, tenderness to palpation, limitation of active and passive movement (worse in the morning and aggravated by movement), warmth; joint is held in flexion in an attempt to increase joint volume and decrease capsular distention.
<u>Hand and wrist</u>
  ◊ classic involvement of the proximal interphalangeal (PIP) and metacarpophalangeal (MCP) joints [DIP (distal interphalangeal) spared].
   <u>Swan neck deformity</u>
   ◊ flexion of DIP and MCP with hyperextension of PIP.
   <u>Boutonniere deformity</u>
   ◊ PIP flexion with DIP hyperextension.
   <u>Z-deformity (ulnar drift)</u>
   ◊ radial deviation at the wrist with ulnar deviation of the digits.
   <u>Hyperextension</u>
    of 1st interphalangeal joint and flexion of the 1st MCP with loss of thumb mobility.
   <u>Carpal tunnel syndrome</u>
   ◊ median nerve entrapment
<u>Elbow</u>
  ◊ flexion contractures, rheumatoid nodules on extensor surfaces of forearm, and olecranon bursitis.
<u>Shoulder</u>
  ◊ rotator cuff involvement.
<u>Hip</u>
  ◊ groin pain and limitation of hip internal rotation.
<u>Knee</u>
  ◊ popliteal cysts (Baker's cysts).
<u>Cervical spine</u>
  ◊ atlantoaxial joint subluxation, spinal cord compression.
<u>Cricoarytenoid joint</u>
  ◊ hoarseness, stridor, aspiration.
<u>Ankle and foot</u>
  ◊ angle and subtalar joint tenderness and swelling leading to pain with ambulation.

Rheumatoid Arthritis

Temporomandibular joint (TMJ)
◊ the literature is inconsistent with regard to the incidence of TMJ involvement in RA, but signs and symptoms mimic those of other involved joints. Other findings might include crepitus and limitation of mandibular opening. Juvenile rheumatoid arthritis (JRA) patients suffer from loss of mandibular growth resulting in micrognathia, apertognathia (skeletal anterior open bite), and possibly TMJ ankylosis. Radiographic changes include decreased joint space, flattened condylar heads, bony erosions, subchondral cysts, and osteopenia. Dental management of RA patients may be complicated by the neutropenia or thrombocytopenia of Felty's syndrome, as well as the hematologic and adrenocortical effects of multidrug therapy.

Extraarticular manifestations
◊ occur more commonly in patients who are seropositive (+RF):
Rheumatoid nodules (20 to 30% of RA patients)
◊ occur on periarticular structures subject to mechanical pressure. Common locations are the olecranon bursae, extensor surfaces of the forearms, proximal ulna, Archilles tendon, and occiput. They may also occur on the heart, pleura, and meninges.
Skeletal muscle weakness/atrophy.
Eye
◊ keratoconjunctivitis sicca (secondary Sjögren's syndrome) (10 to 15%), scleritis (may lead to scleromalacia perforans) and episcleritis (<1%).
Heart
◊ usually asymptomatic; acute pericarditis, may progress to chronic constrictive pericarditis or cardiac tamponade.
Pleuropulmonary
◊ pleuritis, pleural effusion (exudative
◊ low glucose and complement levels), interstitial pulmonary fibrosis, pulmonary nodules (Caplan's syndrome = pneumoconiosis and pulmonary nodules), pulmonary arteritis (pulmonary hypertension).
Neurologic
◊ vasculitis causes a peripheral neuropathy; atlantoaxial subluxation can cause nerve root impingement; entrapment neuropathies (carpal tunnel syndrome); and amyloid infiltration of nerves.
Hematologic
◊ normochromic, normocytic anemia of chronic disease; thrombocytosis or thrombocytopenia (Felty's syndrome = chronic RA, splenomegaly, neutropenia); eosinophilia; mild leukocytosis or leukopenia (selective neutropenia).

Rheumatoid vasculitis
Skin
◊ small vessel vasculitis results in splinter hemorrhages, palpable purpura, cutaneous ulceration, or distal digital gangrene.
Nerve
◊ distal sensory neuropathy or mononeuritis multiplex (sensorimotor neuropathy).
Visceral lesions
◊ coronary vasculitis can lead to myocardial infarction; other areas of involvement include lungs, bowel, liver, spleen, pancreas, and lymph nodes.
Skeletal
◊ osteoporosis.
Juvenile rheumatoid arthritis (JRA)
◊ five subgroups exist:
• Systemic onset (Still's disease)
• Polyarthritis, seropositive (same as adult RA)
• Polyarthritis, RF negative
• Oligoarthritis, early onset, ANA positive
• Oligoarthritis, late onset, HLA-B27 positive
Treatment similar to adult RA

LABORATORY
• No test is specific for the diagnosis of RA.
Rheumatoid factor (RF)
◊ autoantibodies reactive with the Fc portion of IgG or IgM. RF is not specific for RA; it is found in healthy patients as well as patients with a number of other chronic disease processes. The RF level offers prognostic significance in that patients with higher levels of IgM-RF tend to have more severe RA.
Antinuclear antibodies (ANA)
◊ 25% of RA patients.
False-positive VDRL occurs in 5 to 10% of RA patients.
• Complete blood count:
• Normochromic, normocytic anemia
• Eosinophilia
• Thrombocytosis or thrombocytopenia
• Leukocytosis or leukopenia (neutropenia)
Erythrocyte sedimentation rate (ESR)
◊ increased, but nonspecific; as well as other acute phase reactants, including serum ceruloplasmin, C-reactive protein, and ferritin. Sedimentation rate useful gauge of disease activity.
Synovial fluid analysis
◊ inflammatory fluid, reduced viscosity, increased protein, low glucose, WBC between 5000 to 50,000 (mostly neutrophils), depressed complement levels (total, C3, and C4).
Peripheral blood smear
◊ increased circulating T cells expressing HLA-DR MHC antigens.

IMAGING/SPECIAL TESTS
• Radiographic evaluation:
• Symmetrical joint involvement
• Soft tissue swelling, early
• Juxta-articular osteopenia
• Cartilage destruction
• Bone erosions at joint margins
• Narrowing of joint spaces
99mTc diphosphonate bone scanning
◊ rarely necessary. May detect early changes.
MRI
◊ rarely used.
• The American College of Rheumatology has developed a revised criteria list for the diagnosis and classification of RA (Arthr Rheum 31:315, 1988).

DIFFERENTIAL
• Ankylosing spondylitis
• Psoriatic arthritis
• Reiter's syndrome
• Enteropathic arthropathies (inflammatory bowel disease).
• Systemic lupus erythematosus (SLE)
• Progressive systemic sclerosis
• Polymyositis/dermatomyositis
• Rheumatic fever
• Polymyalgia rheumatica
• Wegener's granulomatosis
• Infectious arthritis bacterial, viral, Lyme's disease, Whipple's disease.
• Chronic tophaceous gout
• Pseudogout
• Osteoarthritis
• Reflex sympathetic dystrophy
• Sarcoidosis
• Hypertrophic pulmonary osteoarthropathy
• Fibromyalgia syndrome
• Hyperlipoproteinemia
• Hemochromatosis
• Wilson's disease
• Oral contraceptive use
• Multicentric reticulohistiocytosis
• Amyloidosis
• Multiple myeloma
• Common variable immunodeficiency (CVI)
• Malignancy

(continued)

Rheumatoid Arthritis *continued*

TREATMENT

General
◊ Patient education
◊ Pain control
◊ Reduction of inflammation
◊ Preservation of joint function
◊ Treatment of the pathogenic process
◊ Physical/occupational therapy for rehabilitation.
◊ Psychological counseling

MEDICATIONS
First-line therapy
◊ aimed at controlling the signs and symptoms, but have no direct effect on disease progression
• Aspirin
• Other nonsteroidal antiinflammatory agents
◊ fenoprofen, ibuprofen, indomethacin, ketoprofen, naproxen, meclofenamate sodium, phenylbutazone, piroxicam, sulindac, tolmetin, diclofenac, oxaprozin, flurbiprofen.
• Analgesics
◊ acetaminophen, propoxyphene, codeine.
• Corticosteroids
◊ low-dose prednisone
Second-line therapy
◊ disease modifying antirheumatic drugs (DMARDs).
• Gold salt compounds
◊ parenteral gold (myochrysine or solganal) or oral gold (auranofin). Can cause severe rash, thrombocytopenia, or granulocytopenia.
• D-penicillamine
• Antimalarial drugs {hydroxychloroquine (Plaquenil)}. May cause retinopathy.
• Sulfasalazine
• Immunosuppressive agents
◊ methotrexate (folic acid antagonist), azathioprine (purine antagonist), cyclophosphamide, and chlorambucil (alkylating agents).
Third-line therapy
◊ experimental modalities
• Total lymphoid irradiation
• Lymphoplasmapheresis
• Cyclosporine
• Monoclonal antibodies to T cells

SURGERY
• Surgical therapy may include synovectomy, tendon repairs, arthroplasty, joint fusion procedures, total joint replacement.
• If surgery necessary, may need to check CBC if bone marrow suppressing drugs in use or chronic blood loss due to NSAID use has occurred. Consider need for steroid supplements for those having received prednisone for RA.

CONSULTATION SUGGESTIONS
Rheumatologist

REFERRAL SUGGESTIONS
Primary Care Physician

PATIENT INSTRUCTIONS
Useful printed material for patients available from American Rheumatism Association (800)282-7023.

COURSE/PROGNOSIS
The course is variable, but progressive, with periods of remissions and exacerbations. Approximately 15% of patients will recover without deformity or disability. The median life expectancy of RA patients is shortened by 5 to 7 years. There are several prognostic indicators of disease progression. Caucasian females have more severe erosive disease than males. Patients with high levels of RF, C-reactive protein, and other acute phase reactants have a worse prognosis. Additionally, patients with rheumatoid nodules, radiographic evidence of bony erosions at presentation, or sustained disease activity for more than 1 year tend to have a worse outcome. The greatest progression of joint disease occurs within the first 6 years, and progresses at a slower rate thereafter, while functional disability increases. Factors correlated with increased morbidity include amount of functional disability, duration or severity of disease, corticosteroid use, advance age, and male gender.

CODING

ICD-9-CM
099.3 Arthritis with Reiter's disease
136.1 Arthritis with Bechet's syndrome
714.0 Rheumatoid arthritis
715.9 Osteoarthritis

CPT
21240 Arthroplasty, TMJ
21242 Arthroplasty, TMJ, with allograft
21243 Arthroplasty, TMJ, prosthetic joint

MISCELLANEOUS

SYNONYMS
JRA

SEE ALSO
Reiter's disease
Polymyalgia rheumatica
Ankylosing spondylitis
Rheumatic fever

REFERENCES
Arnett FC, Edworthy SM, Bloch DA, McShane DJ, et al: The American Rheumatism Association 1987 revised criteria for the classification of rheumatoid arthritis. Arthr Rheum 31:315-324, 1988.

Morgan GJ, Cow WS: Clinical features, diagnosis, and prognosis in rheumatoid arthritis. Curr Opin Rheum 5:184-190, 1993.

Porter DR, Sturrock RD: Medical management of rheumatoid arthritis. Brit Med J 307:425-428, 1993.

Trentham DE: New focus on treatment for rheumatoid arthritis. Curr Opin Rheum 5:178-183, 1993.

Wilske KR, Healey LA: The need for aggressive therapy of rheumatoid arthritis. Rheum Dis Clinics N Am 19:153-161, 1993.

Ryan DE: Temporomandibular disorders. Curr Opin Rheum 5:209-218, 1993.

AUTHOR
Michael Miloro, DMD, MD

Rhinitis, Allergic

BASICS

DESCRIPTION
• Condition characterized by a combination of nasal obstruction, watery rhinorrhea, pharyngeal itching, and sneezing. The symptoms result from immediate and delayed reactions to airborne allergens, mediated by specific antigen-responsive IgE antibody receptors generated and present on the mast cells of the nasal mucosa.
• The antigen-antibody interaction precipitates a degranulation of the mast cells leading to the release of inflammatory mediators including histamine, eosinophilotactic peptides, leukotrines, and prostaglandins.
• Seasonal allergic rhinitis frequently coincides with the pollination of offending grasses, trees, or weeds.
• Perennial allergic rhinitis commonly seen in adults and may be related to house dust, mites, mold antigens, and animal body products.

ETIOLOGY

Hereditary
  ◊ generally seen in atopic individuals, that is, in persons with a family history of a similar symptom complex and a personal history of collateral allergy (eg, asthma, urticaria).
Animal, insect, and plant proteins
  ◊ offending allergens include pollens from weeds, grasses and trees, molds, mite dust, animal dander, dried saliva, urine, cockroach droppings, and locusts.
Fumes and chemicals
  ◊ processed materials or chemicals used in an industrial setting, synthetic materials (foam mattresses, acrylics).

SYSTEMS AFFECTED
• Pulmonary
• Immune

DIAGNOSIS

SYMPTOMS AND SIGNS
• Nasal congestion that is often variable and may alternate from side to side.
• Paroxysmal sneezing
• Rhinorrhea that is spasmodic, profuse and watery
• Postnasal discharge (drip)
• Symptom-associated sleeping difficulties
• Loss or alteration of smell
• Itchy nose, eyes, ears, and palate
• Sensation of plugged ears
• Pale and boggy nasal mucosa
• Nasal polyps
• Mucosa of the turbinates usually pale or violaceous due to venous engorgement.
• Watery eyes
• "Allergic shiners" dark circles under eye
• Transverse nasal crease from rubbing nose upwards
• Mouth breathing
• Dull facies

LABORATORY
Nasal probe smear with cytologic exam
  ◊ nasal secretions of allergic patients are rich in eosinophils.
CBC with differential.
  ◊ May have slight increase in eosinophils but is often normal with uncomplicated rhinitis.
Increase in total serum IgE levels.

IMAGING/SPECIAL TESTS
• If indicated, sinus film to check for opacity, fluid levels, mucosal thickening.
• Skin tests using suspected allergens. More expensive but particularly useful in cases in which skin testing is not possible (eg, atopic dermatitis).

DIFFERENTIAL
• Nonallergic rhinitis with eosinophilia syndrome (NARES)
• Nasal polyps and tumor
• Reactive rhinitis of recumbency
• Foreign body
Chronic aspirin use or aspirin intolerance
• Prolonged use of topical nasal decongestant drops and sprays
• Angiotensin converting enzyme inhibitors
• Septal/anatomical obstruction
• Chronic rhinitis digitorum
• Chronic sinusitis

TREATMENT

General
◇ Patient education and assurance
◇ Avoidance of exposure to offending allergen (if known) and maintaining an allergen-free environment.
◇ Immunotherapy or hyposensitization consisting of repeated subcutaneous injections of gradually increasing concentrations of the specific allergen extract.

MEDICATIONS
• Antihistamines such as chlorpheniramine (4 mg orally every 6 to 8 hours) and terfenadine (Seldane) (60 mg orally b.i.d.), or astemizole (Hismanal).
• Oral decongestants such as pseudoephedrine (60 to 120 mg t.i.d.).
• Nasal sprays such as beclomethasone dipropionate or flunisolide.
• Anti-inflammatory drugs (topical) Cromolyn.

SURGERY
• Correction of septal deviation if severe.
• Removal of polyps if large and obstructive.

CONSULTATION SUGGESTIONS
Allergist, Otolaryngologist

REFERRAL SUGGESTIONS
Primary Care Physician

PATIENT INSTRUCTIONS
Avoid contact with allergens.

COURSE/PROGNOSIS
• Immune system changes over time and is often associated with a lessening of symptoms of allergic rhinitis.
• Maximal, beneficially acceptable control of symptoms is the treatment goal.

CODING

ICD-9-CM
477 Allergic rhinitis

MISCELLANEOUS

SYNONYMS
Hay fever
Pollinosis

SEE ALSO
Common Cold

REFERENCES
Wyngaarden JB, Smith LH: Cecil Textbook of Medicine. 19th ed. Philadelphia, WB Saunders Co., 1992.

Gray RF, Hawthorne M: Synopsis of Otolaryngology. 5th ed. Oxford, Butterworth-Heinemann Ltd., 1992.

Tierney LM, McPhee SJ, Papadakis MA, Schroeder SA: Current Medical Diagnosis & Treatment. East Norwalk, CT, Appleton & Lange, 1993.

Dix J: Rhinitis. In: Griffith's Five Minute Clinical Consult. Dambro M, Griffith J. (eds). Baltimore, Williams & Wilkins, 1995, pp. 926-927.

AUTHOR
Vivek Shetty, DDS, DMD

Salivary Gland Tumors

BASICS

DESCRIPTION
Tumors arising from ductal, myoepithelial, or acinar cells of the major or minor salivary glands. The percentage of benign to malignant tumors is 80% in the parotid, approximately 50% in the submandibular and minor salivary glands, and 10% in the sublingual gland.

ETIOLOGY

• Etiology is unknown for most salivary gland tumors.
• Exposure to radiation increases the incidence of parotid cancer.
• Warthin's tumor is felt to arise from salivary duct epithelium enclaved in lymph nodes. A possible relationship to smoking is reported.
• Eskimos have a high incidence of undifferentiated parotid cancer.
• There is a relationship between parotid cancer and breast cancer in women.

SYSTEMS AFFECTED
Salivary glands, major or minor
Bone, muscle, and other local tissues can be infiltrated by malignant lesions.
• Local nerves can be infiltrated.
• Cervical nodes are involved by metastatic disease.
• Lungs, liver, and bone may be involved by hematogenous metastasis, eg, adenocystic carcinoma.

DIAGNOSIS

SYMPTOMS AND SIGNS
• Usually a painless, slow-growing mass. Pain is commonly associated with malignancy.
• A firm discrete mass without fixation in the major glands sign of benign neoplasm.
• Ulceration, skin fixation, facial palsy, or hard cervical nodes are signs of malignancy.

IMAGING/SPECIAL TESTS
CT scan for all palatal lesions, for bony involvement, deep lobe parotid tumors, and to assess cervical nodes.
MRI
◇ useful to delineate soft tissue spread and nerve infiltration. Fine Needle Aspiration Biopsy (FNAB) useful in the parotid in which open biopsy is contraindicated.
Biopsy
◇ incisional biopsy for all oral tumors.
  Controversial
◇ what about excisional biopsy of small lesion when size location documented
◇ ie, small mass palate with slow growth
◇ suspicion is mixed tumor.

DIFFERENTIAL
In the major salivary glands
◇ cysts, lymphocytic infiltration, sarcoid, parotid lymph nodes, non-epithelial salivary tumors, monomorphic adenoma, pleomorphic adenoma, acinic cell carcinoma, mucoepidermoid carcinoma, adenocystic carcinoma, ductal papillomas, papillary cystadenoma lymphomatosum (Warthin's tumor).
In the oral cavity,
◇ other benign or malignant tumors eg, neurofibroma, lymphoma.

TREATMENT

SURGERY
In the parotid, superficial, total or radical parotidectomy. In the oral minor salivary glands, resection with margins dictated by the histopathology. Neck dissection where indicated.

IRRADIATION
Adjuvant radiotherapy is used for high grade cancer.

CONSULTATION SUGGESTIONS
Oral-Maxillofacial Surgeon, Otolaryngologist, General Surgeon

REFERRAL SUGGESTIONS
Oral-Maxillofacial Surgeon, Otolaryngologist

COURSE/PROGNOSIS
Benign tumors are 100% curable with adequate excision. Prognosis for malignant salivary tumors depends on the ability to surgically eradicate the disease.

CODING

ICD-9-CM
142.0 Malignant neoplasm, parotid
142.1 Malignant neoplasm, submandibular gland
142.2 Malignant neoplasm, sublingual gland
142.8 Malignant neoplasm of continuous or overlapping sites of salivary glands and ducts whose point of origin cannot be determined
142.9 Malignant neoplasm of major salivary gland not otherwise specified
Malignant neoplasm of minor salivary glands:
145.0 Buccal mucosa
145.2 Hard palate
145.3 Soft palate
145.9 Not otherwise specified
Benign tumors of major salivary glands:
210.2 Parotid, submandibular, sublingual
Benign neoplasms of minor salivary glands:
210.0 Lips
210.4 Lip, oral cavity and pharyngx

CPT
31305 Incisional biopsy salivary tumor
42100 Biopsy of palate
42104 Excision lesion of palate without closure
42106 Excision lesion of palate with simple primary closure
42107 Excision lesion of palate with local flap closure
42120 Resection of palate or extensive resection of lesion

42400 Needle biopsy of salivary gland
42410 Superficial parotidectomy without nerve dissection
42415 Superficial parotidectomy with preservation of the facial nerve
42420 Total parotidectomy with preservation of facial nerve
42425 Total en bloc removal and sacrifice of facial nerve
42426 Total parotidectomy with unilateral neck dissection
42440 Excision of submandibular gland
42450 Excision of sublingual gland
42550 Injection for sialography
70390 Sialography
99000 Transport specimen to laboratory

MISCELLANEOUS

SEE ALSO
Parotid Swelling
Salivary Gland Calculi
Cancer, general concepts
Sialadenitis

REFERENCES
Langdon JD, Henk JM: Management of salivary gland tumours. In: Malignant Tumours of the Mouth, Jaws and Salivary Glands. Langdon JD, Henk JM, (eds), London, Edward Arnold. 1995, pp. 207-221.

Spiro, RM: Salivary-neoplasm: overview of 35 year experience with 2,807 patients, Head Neck Surg 8:177-184, 1986.

Million R, Cassisi NJ, Mancuso AA: Major salivary gland tumors. In: Management of Head and Neck Cancer. 2nd ed. Philadelphia, JB Lippincott, 1994, pp. 711-736.

AUTHOR
Robert A. Ord, DDS, MD, FACS, FRCS

Sarcoidosis

BASICS

DESCRIPTION
A chronic, non-infectious granulomatous disease involving multiple sites whose manifestations are protean. Most common areas of involvement are peripheral and mediastinal lymph nodes, liver, lungs, spleen, eyes, phalangeal bones, parotid glands, and skin. Tends to affect young and middle-aged adults. Acute form often termed Löfgren's syndrome.

ETIOLOGY

• Remains unknown despite extensive efforts to implicate some of the following possibilities:
- Infection with mycobacteria, M. tuberculosis, phage-infected mycobacteria, viruses, mycoplasma, and fungi have all been proposed.
- Various allergic and environmental considerations, such as exposure to hair sprays, pine pollen, peanut dust and clay consumption.
- Granulomatous reaction to various agents like beryllium, zirconium and silica.

• Hereditary link associated with susceptibility related to human leukocyte antigens (HLA) has been studied.

• The most current theory proposes that specific environmental and host factors interact to allow for the disease to manifest.

SYSTEMS AFFECTED
Pulmonary
  ◇ the most characteristic of the disease. Radiographic findings include hilar and paratracheal lymphadenopathy and/or fibrosis.
Cutaneous
  ◇ seen in 25% of cases and manifesting similar to erythema nodosum, lupus pernio, skin plaques, maculopapular eruptions, subcutaneous nodules, alopecia and erythema multiforme.
Ocular
  ◇ seen in 15 to 25% of cases. Granulomatous uveitis or inflammation of the anterior uveal tract is most common.
Hepatic
  ◇ 60% of patients have granulomatous lesions on liver biopsy.
Osseous
  ◇ 5% of patients have punched-out lesions of the distal phalanges and show destruction of alveolar bone with tooth mobility.
Oral mucosa
  ◇ nodular lesions similar to those seen in Crohn's disease.
Parotid glands
  ◇ unilateral or bilateral swelling may occur.
Upper aerodigestive tract
  ◇ may see granulomas in the nasal mucosa, sinuses, pharynx, epiglottis, and larynx.

DIAGNOSIS

SYMPTOMS AND SIGNS
• Many cases are asymptomatic. May see lethargy, chronic fatigue, anorexia, cough, shortness of breath, eye pain, fever, night sweats, and various other complaints depending upon the organ system involved.
Mouth
  ◇ nodular mucosal lesions and/or maxillary or mandibular tooth mobility with destruction of alveolar bone.
Skin
  ◇ plagues of various types on head, torso and limbs.
Salivary glands
  ◇ parotid and other salivary gland involvement with painless enlargement.
Eye
  ◇ granulomatous uveitis.
• Many other organ systems can be involved with a wide range of accompanying signs and symptoms.

LABORATORY
• Anemia, leukopenia, lymphopenia, abnormal liver functions, hypercalciuria.
• Serum angiotensin converting enzyme (ACE) elevated, Kveim-Siltzbach skin test fairly sensitive, highly specific.
• Biopsy for noncaseating granulomata, (lip, lymph node).

IMAGING/SPECIAL TESTS
• Chest radiographs, bilateral hilar lymphadenopathy or pulmonary fibrosis.
• Classification based on presence or absence of adenopathy and/or fibrosis.
• CT scans looking for hilar nodes.
• Gallium scinti-scanning, looking for uptake in parotid glands, lymph nodes, chest.
• Oral radiographs.
• Ophthalmologic exam.

DIFFERENTIAL
• Sarcoidosis
• Tuberculosis
• Leprosy
• Foreign body reactions
• Cat-scratch disease
• Fungal infections
• Parasitic diseases
• Granulomas associated with beryllium or talc exposures
• Lymphoma

Sarcoidosis

 ## TREATMENT

General
◇ Eliminating exposure to potential causative agents.
◇ Comprehensive dental and periodontal care.
◇ Psychological counseling.
◇ Regular medical exams with close follow-up care.
◇ Use ACE levels to monitor disease activities.

MEDICATIONS
• Corticosteroids for treating symptomatic pulmonary sarcoidosis. Usual dose not to exceed 40 mg of prednisone daily.
• Intralesional injections of corticosteroids often used for cutaneous and oral granulomas.
• Chloroquine used in management of lupus pernio, pulmonary fibrosis, and hypercalcemia.
• Immunosuppressive drugs such as methotrexate, hydrochloroquine, or chlorambucil are used when no response to corticosteroids.
• Immunomodulators (ie, levamisole) for management of arthritic symptoms.

CONSULTATION SUGGESTIONS
Rheumatologist, Pulmonologist

REFERRAL SUGGESTIONS
Primary Care Physician

PATIENT INSTRUCTIONS
Disease has no malignant potential. Avoid calcium in diet.

COURSE/PROGNOSIS
Generally good, but close patient monitoring with chest radiographs and serum angiotensin-I-converting enzyme levels must be followed. When spontaneous resolution has occurred clinical relapses are rare. 80% have spontaneous resolution in 2 years.

 ## CODING

ICD-9-CM
135.0 Sarcoidosis
425.8 Cardiac sarcoid
517.8 Lung sarcoid

CPT
40490 Lip biopsy
42405 Biopsy, salivary gland, incisional

 ## MISCELLANEOUS

SYNONYMS
Noncaseating granulomatous disease
Loeffgren's syndrome
Desnier-Boeck disease
Boeck's sarcoid
Schaumann's disease

SEE ALSO
Tuberculosis
Cat-scratch disease
Salivary gland disease

REFERENCES
Regezi JA, Sciubba J: Oral Pathology, 2nd ed. Philadelphia, WB Saunders, 1993, pp. 255-257.

Pollack CV, Jorden RC: Recognition and management of sarcoidosis in the emergency department. J Emerg Med, 11:297-308, 1993.

Rubin MM, Sanfilippo RJ, Pliskin A: Maxillary alveolar bone loss in a patient with sarcoidosis. J Oral Maxillofac Surg, 49:1351-1353, 1991.

AUTHOR
Lawrence T. Herman, DMD

Schizophrenia

BASICS

DESCRIPTION
• Presence of psychotic symptoms in the active phase: either 1, 2, or 3, for at least 1 week:
  1. Two of the following: a) delusions (erroneous beliefs); b) prominent hallucinations (auditory are most common); c) disorganized thinking (incoherence or marked loosening of associations) and/or communication; d) catatonic behavior; and e) flat or grossly inappropriate affect.
  2. Bizarre delusions (ie, being controlled by outside forces)
  3. Prominent hallucinations (ie, a voice that keeps a running commentary or voices conversing with each other).
• Social relations, work, and self-care are markedly below behaviors before onset of disturbance. Among children and adolescence behaviors are below expected level of social development.
• Schizoaffective disorder and mood disorder with psychotic features are ruled out (ie, major depressive or bipolar syndrome).
• Continuous signs for at least 6 months.
• Organic factor did not initiate or maintain the disturbance.
• If there is a history of autism, the additional diagnosis of schizophrenia is appropriate only when prominent delusions or hallucinations are also present.
• Associated features: inappropriate affect (eg, smiling, laughing, or a silly facial expression in the absence of an appropriate stimulus; anhedonia (loss of interest); dysphoric mood (depression, anxiety or anger); disturbances in sleep patterns; lack of appetite; psychomotor activity (ie, rocking, pacing); physically awkward (eg, poor coordination, left/right confusion); difficulty concentrating; confusion; nicotine dependency; somatic concerns.
Types include:
  ◇ Catatonic stupor or mutism, rigidity, or bizarre posturing;
Disorganized
  ◇ incoherence or disorganized behavior and flat or inappropriate affect;
Paranoid
  ◇ preoccupation with auditory delusions with unfocused anxiety, anger and violence, as well as extreme formal or intense interpersonal interactions;
Undifferentiated
  ◇ prominent delusions, hallucinations, incoherence or disorganized behavior; or residual type in which there are an absence of symptoms but continued evidence of the disorder exist. Onset is usually in the 20's. Is equally prevalent in men and women.

ETIOLOGY
• Unknown, no evidence due to organic factor.
• Higher prevalence in first degree biologic relative than in the general population. Higher concordance rate in monozygotic than in dizygotic twins; yet development of the illness indicated the importance of nongenetic factors.

SYSTEMS AFFECTED
Nervous

DIAGNOSIS

SYMPTOMS AND SIGNS
• (See description section above)
• Hallucinations
• Delusions
• Flat affect
• Catatonia
• Dysphoric mood
• Paranoia
• Withdrawal from reality
• Loose thought processes

LABORATORY
None conclusive. Rule out organic disease with CBC, blood chemistries, thyroid studies, urinalysis, drug screen.

IMAGING/SPECIAL TESTS
• Psychological tests
• EEG
• CT or MRI.

DIFFERENTIAL
• Psychotic disorder due to a general medical condition, delirium or dementia.
• Substance-induced psychotic disorder.
• Organic mental disorder
• Mood disorder (particularly bipolar disorder with psychotic features)
• Pervasive developmental disorder
• Schizophreniform disorder
• In obsessive compulsive disorder and hypochondriasis, the person may have distinct ideation that may appear delusional, but these individuals often acknowledge that their symptoms and thinking are irrational.

TREATMENT

General
Inpatient
◊ hospitalize for initial work-up; and treatment of psychotic conditions.
Outpatient
◊ with medications and ongoing extensive psychotherapy if not dangerous to self or family and cooperative with treatment regimen. Vocational rehabilitation; day hospital. A complete history is recommended to ascertain as much information regarding dental behavior and receptivity to treatment. Patients may have extreme responses to the sight of blood. Suicide ideation is a significant issue
◊ approximately 10% of individuals with schizophrenia commit suicide (risk profile includes males under 30 years old, depressive symptoms, and recent hospital discharge). Preventive dental education is important. Use of positive verbal reinforcement and use of a mirror can be helpful for demonstration. However, some patients will be resistant
◊ do not persist if patient becomes combative; do not persist during that appointment. Increased likelihood of a gag reflex has been reported, therefore keeping the airway protected is advised.

MEDICATIONS
• Benzodiazepine and/or neuroleptics used based on presenting conditions.
• Neuroleptic medications may induce agranulocytosis, leukopenia, and thrombocytopenia (rule out with CBC) with secondary ulceration, infection, bleeding, candida or stomatitis. Dental treatment should not be undertaken if there is significant bone marrow suppression (WBC < 3000 per mm or granulocyte count < 1500 per mm).
• Neuroleptics induce extrapyramidal side effects including xerostomia and movement disorders (tardive dyskinesia, mandibular tics, spasm of perioral and jaw muscles, and dysphagia with secondary drooling). High dose or long-term use of neuroleptics may cause tachycardia, orthostatic hypotension or blood pressure fluctuations. Anticholinergics, antihistamines, and beta blockers may be used to control these side effects (diphenhydramine (Benadryl) 25 to 50 mg IM).
• Anticholinergic properties may contribute to sedation, hypotension, and body temperature elevations. Check for alcohol use which can further compromise bone marrow function and cause thrombocytopenia and leukopenia.

• Drug interactions in dentistry with neuroleptics
Epinephrine
◊ severe hypertension;
CNS depressants
◊ additive sedation;
Atropine
◊ increased anticholinergic effect. Limit local anesthetic with vasoconstrictor to 3 cartridges. Aspirate before injecting. No topical epinephrine in retraction cord. Avoid use of atropine. Decrease dosage of sedatives, hypnotics, or narcotics.
• Patients who are delusional may have paranoid (persecutory) or bizarre delusions, sense of exaggerated severity of their condition (monosymptomatic hypochondriacal psychosis) and may be extremely noncompliant. Hypochondriacal delusions centering on the mouth are common; somatic concerns may be extreme. Complaints may include worms in the mouth or hearing voices in their fillings. Acts of orofacial self-mutilation and burning gingiva have been reported. Recommend having another person in the operatory at all times.

CONSULTATION SUGGESTIONS
Consultations with other specialists may be indicated to ensure the patient that their concerns are being taken seriously. When resistance to treatment is significant, further consultation with a mental health specialist is warranted.

REFERRAL SUGGESTIONS
Mental Health Professional, Primary Care Physician

FIRST STEPS TO TAKE IN AN EMERGENCY
• Use diphenhydramine (25 to 50 mg IM) for tardive dyskinesia.
• Use benztropine (Cogentin) 0.5 mg b.i.d. for pseudoparkinsonism.

PATIENT INSTRUCTIONS
Contact National Alliance for the Mentally Ill (703)524-7600 for useful patient and family information.

COURSE/PROGNOSIS
Range from chronic (greater than 2 years) to subchronic with or without exacerbation (6 months to 2 years) to in remission (free of all signs). Typically following the active stage (not due to psychoactive substance use disorder or mood disorder), significant social withdrawal and impairment in occupational status.

CODING

ICD-9-CM
295.0 Schizophrenic disorders

MISCELLANEOUS

REFERENCES
Scully C, Cawson RA: Medical problems in dentistry. Oxford. Butterworth-Heinemann, 1993.

American Psychiatric Association. Diagnostic and statistical manual of mental disorders, DSM-IV, Washington, DC, 1994.

Jeffe S: Schizophrenia. In: Griffith's 5 Minute Clinical Consult. Dambro M. (ed) Baltimore, Williams & Wilkins, 1995. pp. 948-949.

Carpenter Jr. WT Buchanan RW: Schizophrenia. In: Comprehensive Textbook of Psychiatry, 6th ed. Kaplan HI, Sodock BJ (eds), Baltimore, Williams & Wilkins, 1995, pp. 889-902.

AUTHORS
Hillary Broder, PhD, MEd
Kani Nicolls, DDS

Seizure Disorders

BASICS

DESCRIPTION
• A seizure is a sudden, uncontrolled, paroxysmal alteration in consciousness or behavior, either sensory or motor, due to an aberrant electrical discharge from cerebral cortex. Epilepsy refers to chronic, recurrent seizure episodes.

Seizure Classification
I. Partial (focal) seizures
   A. Simple partial seizures (consciousness preserved)
      1. With motor signs (Jacksonian, adversive)
      2. With somatosensory or special sensory symptoms
      3. With autonomic symptoms or signs
      4. With psychic symptoms
   B. Complex partial seizures (consciousness impaired)
      1. Simple partial onset, followed by impaired consciousness
      2. Impaired consciousness at onset
   C. Secondary generalized partial seizures
      1. Simple partial seizures evolving to generalized tonic-clonic seizures
      2. Complex partial seizures evolving to generalized tonic-clonic seizures
      3. Simple partial seizures evolving to complex partial seizures, then to generalized tonic-clonic seizures
II. Primary generalized seizures (bilaterally symmetric)
   A. Tonic-clonic (grand mal)
   B. Tonic
   C. Clonic
   D. Absence (petit mal)
   E. Atypical absence
   F. Myoclonic
   G. Atonic or akinetic
   H. Infantile spasms
III. Unilateral seizures
IV. Unclassified epileptic seizures

ETIOLOGY

• Idiopathic
• Head trauma
• Intracranial neoplasm
• Hypoglycemia
• Drug or alcohol withdrawal
• Febrile illness
• Cerebral hypoxia
• Infection
• Uremia
• Hepatic failure
• Electrolyte abnormalities
• Toxemia of pregnancy
• Alcoholism
• Cerebrovascular disease/stroke
• Exogenous stimuli (lights, sounds, tactile)
• Ingestion of toxic substances (lead, strychnine)
• Inadequate level of anticonvulsant medication
• Genetic factors

SYSTEMS AFFECTED
Central nervous system

DIAGNOSIS

SYMPTOMS AND SIGNS
• CNS-confusion, loss of consciousness, coma
• Behavior and personality changes
• Headache
• Muscle aches
• Stupor, memory loss, amnesia
• Hallucinations
• Impaired cognitive abilities
• Generalized or focal seizure activity
• Fever
• Papilledema
• Impaired consciousness
• Generalized muscle rigidity (tonic phase)
• Uncoordinated movements of head & limbs (clonic phase)
• Incontinence of urine or feces
• Muscle contractions (diaphragm, limbs, jaws, etc.)
• Frequent eye-blinking and nystagmus or other eye deviations
• Dyspnea
• Stridor

LABORATORY
• Complete blood count (infection).
• Electrolytes, calcium, phosphorus, magnesium, glucose, blood urea nitrogen, ammonia.
• Anticonvulsant levels
• Toxicology screen (including alcohol)

IMAGING/SPECIAL TESTS
• Electroencephalogram (EEG) not diagnostic
• MRI
• CT scan

DIFFERENTIAL
• Syncopal episode
• Transient ischemic attack (TIA)
• Migraine headache
• Stroke (cerebrovascular accident)
• Intracranial hemorrhage

TREATMENT

General
◇ Protection of the airway
◇ Protection of the head
◇ Position patient on side with head extended
◇ Treat cause of seizure
◇ Compliance with anticonvulsant medication administration schedule needs to be stressed to patients.

MEDICATIONS

Primary generalized tonic-clonic (grand mal):
• phenytoin 300 to 400 mg/day (therapeutic level 10 to 20 microgram/mL).
• carbamazepine 800 to 1600 mg/day (therapeutic level 6 to 12 microgram/mL).
• phenobarbital 90 to 150 mg/day (therapeutic level 15 to 35 microgram/mL).
• primidone 750 to 1250 mg/day (therapeutic level 6 to 12 microgram/mL).

Partial, including secondary generalized:
• carbamazepine
• phenytoin
• primidone
• phenobarbital

Absence (petit mal):
• ethosuximide 750 to 1250 mg/day (therapeutic level 40 to 100 microgram/mL).
• valproate 1000 to 3000 mg/day (therapeutic level 50 to 120 microgram/mL)
• clonazepam 1.5 to 20 mg/day (therapeutic level 20 to 80 ng/ml)

Atypical absence, myoclonic, atonic:
• valproate
• clonazepam

Other medications:
• methsuximide 600 to 1200 mg/day
• trimethadione 900 to 2100 mg/day
• lamotrigine 100 to 500 mg/day
• gabapentin 900 to 2400 mg/day
• felbamate 1200 to 3600 mg/day

SURGERY

May be indicated for seizure patients who fail to respond to anticonvulsant therapy, and who meet certain criteria:
(1) seizure originates in focal identifiable cerebral region.
(2) surgical margins can encompass most of epileptogenic region.
(3) resection will not impair neurologic function.

Surgical procedures:
(1) cortical resection (anterior temporal lobe).
(2) corpus callosotomy
(3) "functional" cerebral hemispherectomy.

• Dentist should monitor gingiva for hyperplasia. Minimize hyperplasia with hygiene measures and surgically reduce when size of gingiva prevents good hygiene.

CONSULTATION SUGGESTIONS
Neurologist

REFERRAL SUGGESTIONS
Primary Care Physician, Neurologist

FIRST STEPS TO TAKE IN AN EMERGENCY
• Protect patient from injury during seizure, be ready to institute basic life support and be ready with high volume suction when seizure ceases. Call EMTs for help.

PATIENT INSTRUCTIONS
• Wear medic alert jewelry if seizure prone. Carefully comply with instructions for antiseizure medications.
• If on dilantin, maintain excellent oral hygiene to minimize hyperplasia.

COURSE/PROGNOSIS
• Depends upon seizure etiology.
• Determine etiology and treat to prevent recurrence.
• Monitor anticonvulsant levels
• Monitor side effects of therapy
  phenytoin
  ◇ gingival hyperplasia
  carbamazepine
  ◇ agranulocytosis, elevated liver function tests.
  valproate
  ◇ thrombocytopenia
• Consider discontinuation of drug therapy after 2-year seizure-free period.

CODING

ICD-9-CM
345.0 Akinetic seizure
345.9 Epilepsy
780.3 Seizure
780.3 Febrile seizure

MISCELLANEOUS

SYNONYMS
Epilepsy
Convulsions

SEE ALSO
Status epilepticus

REFERENCES
Scheuer ML, Pedley TA: The evaluation and treatment of seizures. N Engl J Med 323:1468-1474, 1990.

Abramowicz M: Drugs for epilepsy. Med Letter 37(947):37-40, 1995.

Morrell MJ: Differential diagnosis of seizures. Neurologic Clinics 11:737-754, 1993.

AUTHOR
Michael Miloro, DMD, MD

Septicemia

BASICS

DESCRIPTION
Severe form of infection characterized by invasion and multiplication of large numbers of bacteria in the blood stream.

ETIOLOGY

• Sepsis results when a source of infection somewhere in the body seeds the bloodstream.
• Complement cascade is activated by toxin release.
• Common sources of sepsis are:
  Skin wounds
    ◊ staphylococcus
  Burns
    ◊ pseudomonas, serratia, staphylococcus
  IV sites
    ◊ serratia, klebsiella, bacteroides, staphylococcus
  Lung
    ◊ pneumococcus, streptococcus
  Urinary
    ◊ E. coli, proteus
  Heart valves
    ◊ staphylococcus, streptococcus
• Risk factors for sepsis are:
  Underlying disease, ie,: malignancy, renal insufficiency, congestive heart failure, diabetes mellitus; respiratory intubation; urinary catheter; immunosuppression; major surgery; multiple trauma.

SYSTEMS AFFECTED
• Any organ may be involved.
• Multisystem organ failure common in septic shock.

DIAGNOSIS

SYMPTOMS AND SIGNS
• High spiking fever
• Chills
• Rigor
• Tachycardia
• Myalgia
• Skin petechiae, erythema, embolic lesions
• Anemia
• Altered mental status
• Shock
  Early
    ◊ warm shock with decreased PVR, diaphoresis, vasodilation.
  Late
    ◊ cold shock with decreased cardiac output, vasoconstriction.
  Shock most common with Gram-negative bacteria.
• Metastatic abscess
  bone, brain, spleen
• Sign of initiating infection
  red IV site, purulent sputum, cough, rales, pleuritic pain, diarrhea, flank pain, or headache.
• Disseminated intravascular coagulation (DIC).

LABORATORY
• Left shift in differential
• Positive blood cultures
• Proteinuria
• Hyperglycemia
• Acidosis
• Decreased PaO_2
• Elevated serum potassium
• Signs of DIC

IMAGING/SPECIAL TESTS
• Chest radiograph
• Cultures from potentially infected sites
• Counterimmune electrophoresis
• Latex agglutination tests
• Gram stain of buffy coat

DIFFERENTIAL
• Cardiogenic shock
• Viral disease
• Rickettsial disease
• Protozoal disease
• Spirochetal disease
• Collagen vascular disease

Septicemia

TREATMENT

General
◊ Determine and remove source
  UA, sputum culture, CBC, wound
    culture
◊ Medically support patient
  Bed rest
  Perfuse tissue
  Fluid resuscitation
  Swan-Ganz catheter to monitor
    cardiovascular status
  Prevent end-organ damage
  Metabolic support

MEDICATIONS
• Antibiotics based on culture
• Bactericidal
• Narrow spectrum
• Intravenous route
• Begin ASAP
• Naloxone (Narcan) may be beneficial
(controversial)

SURGERY
Remove collections of pus and devices
or necrotic tissue.

CONSULTATION SUGGESTIONS
Infectious Disease Specialist, General
Surgeon

REFERRAL SUGGESTIONS
Primary Care Physician

FIRST STEPS TO TAKE IN AN
EMERGENCY
• Start IV
• Administer fluids
• Transport to emergency facility

COURSE/PROGNOSIS
Gram-negative sepsis
  ◊ 40% mortality. Presence of
neutropenia, diabetes, advanced age,
immunodeficiency, alcoholism, or major
organ failure worsens prognosis.

CODING

ICD-9-CM
  038 Septicemia

MISCELLANEOUS

SYNONYMS
Gram-negative shock
Sepsis
Septic shock

SEE ALSO
Endocarditis
Pneumonia
Shock
Disseminated intravascular coagulation

REFERENCES
Nichols RL: Surgical Infections. In:
Manual of Surgical Therapeutics, 5th ed.
Condon, Nyhyus (eds). Boston, Little,
Brown & Co., 1982, p. 241.

Dunn DL: Infection. In: Surgery:
Scientific Principles and Practice.
Greenfield (ed). Philadelphia, JB
Lippincott, 1993, pp. 148-170.

AUTHOR
Peter E. Larsen, DDS

Serum Sickness

 BASICS

DESCRIPTION

An acute allergic reaction that results from the formation of circulating complexes of antigen and antibody. Deposition of these complexes occurs mainly in arteries, renal glomeruli, and joint synovia resulting in vasculitis, nephritis, and arthritis.

 ETIOLOGY

• Reactions from horse serum occur in at least 5% of persons receiving it for the first time. Anti-venom (serum from horses immunized with venoms) may still be used in managing venomous snake and spider bites, as well as diphtheria and botulism.
• Antilymphocyte serum from horse and other species is used to suppress the immune reactions to transplanted organs.
• Such treatments may also stimulate the host immune system to make IgG antibody against the foreign serum proteins.
• Most reactions today occur after repeated exposure to a drug (sulfonamides, hydralazine, sulfonylureas, thiazides, and penicillin).
• The pathogenesis can be resolved into three phases: formation of antigen-antibody complexes in the circulation; deposition of the immune complexes in various tissues; initiation of an acute inflammatory reaction.
• It is thought that IgE antibody is also induced by the antigen shortly after injection and, therefore, facilitates deposition of complexes.
• Immune complexes are initially detected in the circulation and then deposited in tissues where they activate complement.

SYSTEMS AFFECTED

Joints
◇ polyarthritis or periarticular edema of joints, including temporomandibular, resulting in pain.
Skin
◇ urticaria or purpuric
Intestinal
◇ abdominal pain and diarrhea
Nervous
◇ peripheral neuritis
Kidneys
◇ glomerulonephritis

 DIAGNOSIS

SYMPTOMS AND SIGNS

General
◇ fever, malaise
Appear 7 to 12 days after administration of antigen. Peaks in 1 to 3 days. Symptoms may appear earlier if individual has been previously exposed.
Joints
◇ pain due to arthralgia
Temporomandibular joint
◇ periarticular edema and erythema and arthralgia.
Skin
◇ erythematous, urticaria, multiform or morbilliform presentation; rarely scarlatiniform or purpuric.
Intestinal
◇ pain, nausea, vomiting
Kidney
◇ albuminuria, decreased renal functions.
Lymph nodes
◇ lymphadenopathy in region draining injection site.
Nervous system
◇ peripheral neuropathy (usually unilateral mononeuritis) involving the shoulder girdle or arm, weakness, and sensory deficit.
Spleen
◇ splenomegaly

LABORATORY

• Detection of circulating immune complexes (CIg-binding assay).
• Polyethylene glycol (PEG) assay for circulating immune complexes.
• Complement levels (fall in early serum complement components, C1, C4 or C2).
• Circulating antibody to suspected foreign antigen such as horse serum.
• RAST
◇ test for allergic specific immunoglobulins.
• Direct immunofluorescence of vasculitis lesions demonstrating presence of immunoglobulin and complement.
Renal function
◇ albuminuria (possible reduction of renal function).
CBC
◇ leukocytosis
History
◇ exposure to foreign agent or drug.

IMAGING/SPECIAL TESTS

• PEG and Cl-9 binding assay for immune complexes.
• Detection of specific antibody against foreign antigen.

DIFFERENTIAL

• Erythema multiforme
• Anaphylaxis
• Trismus, due to other causes.
• Systemic lupus erythematosus

TREATMENT

General
◊ Immediate cessation of further treatment with the offending serum or drug.
◊ Most allergic reactions of this type begin to clear within a few days after the allergen is withdrawn.
◊ Treatment usually limited to control of pain and itching.

MEDICATIONS
• Arthralgias usually controlled with aspirin or other NSAIDs.
• Antihistamines in the usual therapeutic doses can be given for mild symptoms.
• If patient is acutely ill, with signs of multiple system involvement or with exfoliative dermatitis, an adrenal corticoid such as prednisone (40 to 80 mg/day orally) is required.
• Desensitization therapy
◊ risk of anaphylaxis may be high.
• Skin tests, using weaker serial dilutions of antigen are required to determine the starting dose.

CONSULTATION SUGGESTIONS
Allergist

REFERRAL SUGGESTIONS
Skin testing or desensitization should be carried out by an expert allergist and given subcutaneously with proper resuscitation equipment at hand.

FIRST STEPS TO TAKE IN AN EMERGENCY
• Stop administration of any serum-containing substance. If wheezing or other signs of impending anaphylaxis occur, treat with epinephrine.

PATIENT INSTRUCTIONS
Patient should keep careful record of past reactions to inoculations.

COURSE/PROGNOSIS
• The prominent symptom, glomerulonephritis, is rarely a problem.
• Unusual, but serious, manifestations include cardiac dysrhythmias, myocarditis, and peripheral neuritis. Peripheral neuritis is the only complication that may cause irreversible damage.
• Problem usually resolves in 2 to 3 weeks, with complete recovery.

CODING

ICD-9-CM
999.5 Other serum reaction

MISCELLANEOUS

SYNONYMS
Protein sickness
Inoculation reaction

SEE ALSO
Hypersensitivity
Contact dermatitis

REFERENCES
Lawley JJ, et al: A prospective clinical and immunologic analysis of patients with serum sickness. N Engl J Med 311:1407, 1984.

Manik M: Mechanisms of tissue deposition of immune complexes. J Rheumatol, 13 (Suppl. 14):35, 1987.

Erffmeyer JE: Serum sickness. Ann Allergy, 56:105, 1986.

AUTHOR
John Jandinski, DMD

Shock (Circulatory)

BASICS

DESCRIPTION
A condition in which there is inadequate tissue perfusion to meet the metabolic requirements causing dysfunction and damage.

ETIOLOGY

Physiology of Shock
• May have many causes, all of which result in inadequate tissue perfusion. The cardiovascular system is, by definition, incapable of compensating for this hypoperfusion in spite of efforts to increase cardiac output (increased rate, and stroke volume) or to increase systemic vascular resistance.
• Causes
• Cardiogenic shock (restrictive cardiomyopathy, myocardial infarction, valvular heart disease, severe dysrhythmias), also known as primary pump failure;
• Pericardial disease (tamponade, constrictive pericarditis);
• Hypovolemic shock which is due to loss of greater than 20% of circulating blood volume as in acute hemorrhage, severe dehydration (including Addisonian crisis);
• Pulmonary pathology (tension pneumothorax, pulmonary embolism) which compromises cardiac output;
• Septic shock which causes severe vasodilatation, reduced intravascular volume, and capillary leakage of intravascular fluid into extravascular sites, thereby contributing to hypovolemia;
• Neurogenic shock (spinal cord injury, peripheral neuropathies causing orthostatic hypotension, ganglionic-blocking, or other hypotensive medications);
• Anaphylaxis due to immediate hypersensitivity reaction.
• All forms of shock have in common inadequate intravascular volume and perfusion pressures for the metabolic needs of vital organs resulting in hypotension with secondary findings of altered consciousness, possible myocardial ischemia, oliguria and possible renal failure, and manifestations of tissue ischemia of various organs including hepatic, intestinal, cerebral, and peripheral tissues such as digits.

SYSTEMS AFFECTED
• Cardiovascular
• CNS
• Renal
• GI

DIAGNOSIS

SYMPTOMS AND SIGNS
Due to underperfusion
◇ altered mentation, anxiety, oliguria, peripheral cyanosis, poor capillary refill, cool skin, pallor, absence of bowel sounds, thready pulse, hypotension, postural hypotension, dysrhythmias. Tachycardia.

LABORATORY
• Hematocrit
• Serum lactate when elevated indicates anaerobic metabolism in hypoperfused tissues.
• Arterial blood gases

IMAGING/SPECIAL TESTS
• Blood cultures
• ECG
• Chest radiograph
• Reduced mixed venous oxygen measured from pulmonary artery catheterization.
• Endoscopy if GI bleeding suspected.
• Echocardiogram to look for pericardial effusion.
• Lung scan to look for pulmonary embolism.
• Swan-Ganz catheterization to measure cardiac output and other cardiac parameters.

DIFFERENTIAL
• Hypovolemia
• Cardiogenic shock
• Venous pooling
• Sepsis
• Neurogenic shock

TREATMENT

General
◊ Treatment acutely is based on volume expansion (IV fluids), correction of coagulopathies and electrolyte abnormalities, and searching for clues to etiology (history, physical exam, cultures, imaging). Hemodynamic monitoring (ECG, urine output, central venous pressure, and pulmonary wedge pressure) and serial laboratory tests (serum chemistries, CBC, urine electrolytes) are critical to guiding fluid replacement and use of vasopressors. Ultimately, treatment of the primary cause is critical to resuscitation. Primary cardiogenic shock could acutely require cardiac surgery (coronary bypass, valve replacement, pericardiectomy, intra-aortic balloon counterpulsation) and pulmonary causes may require chest tube placement (pneumothorax) or anticoagulation (embolism).

MEDICATIONS
• Vasopressors
  ◊ (dobutamine, dopamine, norepinephrine, phenylephrine, etc.)
• Empirical treatment with steroids or antibiotics may be appropriate in certain situations, but acutely anti-endotoxins may be efficacious.

CONSULTATION SUGGESTIONS
Primary Care Physician, Cardiologist, General Surgeon, Infectious Disease Specialist, Neurologist

REFERRAL SUGGESTIONS
Primary Care Physician

FIRST STEPS TO TAKE IN AN EMERGENCY
• Trendelenberg position
• Start IV and administer fluids

COURSE/PROGNOSIS
Outcome depends upon successful identification and treatment of etiology.

CODING

ICD-9-CM
785.5   Shock, nonspecific
785.51 Cardiogenic
785.59 Septic
958.4   Hemorrhagic (trauma)
998   Hemorrhagic (surgery

MISCELLANEOUS

SYNONYMS
Circulatory collapse

SEE ALSO
Heart failure
Anaphylaxis

REFERENCES
Bollaert PE, Bauer P, et al: Effects of epinephrine on hemodynamics and oxygen metabolism in dopamine-resistant septic shock. Chest 98:949-953, 1990.

Tuchschmidt J, Fried J, et al: Elevation of cardiac output and oxygen delivery improves outcome in septic shock. Chest 102:216-220, 1992.

AUTHOR
Robert Chuong, MD, DMD

Sialadenitis

BASICS

DESCRIPTION
• A painful infection or inflammation of one or all of the six major salivary glands occurring as a result of a bacteria or virus, and presenting as a chronic or acute swelling.
• The parotid gland is most commonly affected.
• Flow rate from the salivary gland is reduced.
• Saliva becomes thicker and more viscous.
• Dehydration (secondary to surgery or drugs) encourages bacterial sialadenitis.

ETIOLOGY

Viral
• Mumps paramyxovirus the most common viral infection.
• Cytomegalovirus
• HIV-related salivary gland disease.
Bacterial
• Occurs in dehydrated, debilitated often postsurgical patients.
• Staphylococcus aureus is the most common infecting organism.
• Streptococcus viridans has also been implicated.
• Can be secondary to salivary gland stones.

SYSTEMS AFFECTED
Salivary glands
  ◇ swelling of the salivary glands and decrease in the quantity of salivary flow. Expression of pus from the salivary gland orifice, in particular Stenson's duct. Pain upon eating sour or tart foods.
Skin
  ◇ redness and warmth of the skin overlying the gland.
Oral mucosa
  ◇ inflammation of the opening of the duct.
Teeth
  ◇ limitation of opening and decreased salivary flow lead to decrease in oral hygiene and higher plaque levels.
General
  ◇ patient may be febrile.
Genitourinary
  ◇ mumps can cause orchitis and epididymitis in postpubertal males and oophoritis in women.

DIAGNOSIS

SYMPTOMS AND SIGNS
• Pain in the salivary glands when eating tart foods or opening widely.
• Pain when touching the region of the affected gland.
• Presence of a stone in the gland can lead to increased swelling and pain before or during mealtimes.
• Swelling of the parotid gland will present as a swelling at the angle of the mandible and frequently displaces the ear upwards.
• Pus can be expressed from the ductal orifice of the affected gland.
• The overlying skin is red and warm to the touch.
• Difficulty of expressing saliva from the affected gland.

LABORATORY
Leukocytosis

IMAGING/SPECIAL TESTS
• Diagnosis of mumps in children is rarely difficult.
• Mumps in adults can be diagnosed by a negative history of mumps or mumps vaccination and a minimum of a four-fold increase of the antibody titers following the acute infection.
• Bacterial sialadenitis can be diagnosed by the expression of pus from the orifice of the gland and suitable aerobic and anaerobic cultures being performed.
• The presence of an obstructing stone can be visualized with flat plane films (ie, panorex, antero-posterior, or occlusal view).

DIFFERENTIAL
• Sjögren's syndrome
• Sarcoid
• Neoplasm

TREATMENT

General
◇ Hydration
◇ Moist heat
◇ Antibiotics
◇ Incision and drainage may be required if intra-oral drainage does not occur with bacterial sialadenitis.
◇ Supportive therapy is the only treatment for mumps.
◇ Removal of stone and/or gland indicated when sialolithiasis is the cause.

MEDICATIONS
• Mumps
◇ inoculation with a live attenuated vaccine for prevention.
• Bacterial sialadenitis
◇ use of appropriate antibiotic following culture and sensitivity.
• Should antibiotic coverage be required prior to availability of culture and sensitivity, the use of antibiotics active against penicillin-resistant Staphylococcus is advised.
• Cefalexin 500 mg p.o. q6h.

SURGERY
Infections of major glands should be treated medically and allowed to resolve before gland removal is considered. If stone present, may consider stone removal if necessary to allow gland to drain.

CONSULTATION SUGGESTIONS
Oral-Maxillofacial Surgeon, Oral Medicine

REFERRAL SUGGESTIONS
Oral-Maxillofacial Surgeon

FIRST STEPS TO TAKE IN AN EMERGENCY
• If patient becomes septic from salivary infection, consider hospitalization, high-dose intravenous staphylocidal antibiotics, and hydration.

COURSE/PROGNOSIS
Most cases of mumps are self-limiting and last 1 to 2 weeks. Cytomegalovirus (CMV) infection of gland can occur with immunosuppression (ie, during immunosuppressive therapy, AIDS, or with hematologic malignancies.

CODING

ICD-9-CM
072.9 Mumps
527.2 Sialadenitis
527.5 Sialolithiasis
527.8 Sialosis

CPT
42300 Drainage of parotid abscess
42310 Drainage of submandibular abscess, intraoral
42320 Drainage of submandibular abscess, extraoral
42330 Sialolithotomy, intraoral uncomplicated
42335 Sialolithotomy intraoral submandibular, complex
42340 Sialolithotomy, parotid extraoral or complicated intraoral
42400 Biopsy of salivary gland
42550 Injection procedure for sialography
42650 Dilation of salivary duct
42660 Dilation and catheterization of salivary duct, with or without injection
42699 Unlisted procedure, salivary glands
70355 Panorex

MISCELLANEOUS

SYNONYMS
Mumps

SEE ALSO
Salivary gland neoplasms
Sialolithiasis

REFERENCES
Nevill BW, et al: Oral and Maxillofacial Pathology. Philadelphia, WB Saunders, 1995.

AUTHOR
Janet E. Leigh, BDS, DMD

Sialolithiasis

 BASICS

DESCRIPTION
- The presence of calcified concretions in salivary gland ducts or glands.
- Can affect any minor salivary gland, with those in the upper lip and buccal mucosa most frequently involved.
- Most common in middle age but can occur at any age.

 ETIOLOGY

Calcified concretions are formed by the deposition of calcium salts, primarily $Ca(PO_4)_2$ and $CaCO_3$, about a central nidus of mucin, bacteria, desquamated epithelial cells, or a foreign body.

SYSTEMS AFFECTED
- Can affect either major or minor salivary glands.
- The submandibular gland affected most often, followed by the parotid and sublingual.

 DIAGNOSIS

SYMPTOMS AND SIGNS
- Pain and swelling about the area of the affected major salivary gland in the periprandial period.
- May have diffuse swelling over major salivary gland.
- May have pain over major salivary gland. If infected, skin over gland also warm and erythematous.
- Inability to express saliva from the affected duct.
- May palpate firm mass in the duct or see yellowish mass transmucosally within the duct.
- May palpate firm movable mass in minor salivary gland.
- Purulence may appear at duct orifice if secondarily infected.

IMAGING/SPECIAL TESTS
- Mandibular occlusal films for submandibular or sublingual glands, panoramic for parotid involvement, looking for radio-opacity in duct or hilum of gland.
- Sialography using water soluble agents looking for filling defects, obstruction, or dilatation. Avoid sialography in presence of probable infection.
- Technetium-99 scan or CT scan may be helpful if reason for facial swelling unclear.

DIFFERENTIAL
- Neoplasm of gland or compressing duct
- Cyst
- Salivary duct obstruction by mucous plug
- Sialadenitis, non-obstructive
- Stricture of duct
- Foreign body, minor salivary glands

TREATMENT

MEDICATIONS
• Analgesics for discomfort.
• Staphylocidal antibiotics if infection suspected.

SURGERY
• Use lacrimal probes or dilators to increase duct size and then digitally manipulate stone out.
• Surgically remove stone from duct by direct opening into site of obstruction, leaving catheter in place as temporary stent.
• Sialectomy (gland excision) if pain, induration, lack of function persist, or if some portion of stone is located in the parenchyma of the gland.

CONSULTATION SUGGESTIONS
Radiologist, Oral-Maxillofacial Surgeon

REFERRAL SUGGESTIONS
Oral-Maxillofacial Surgeon

FIRST STEPS TO TAKE IN AN EMERGENCY
• If infection present, begin staphylocidal antibiotics and hydration.

PATIENT INSTRUCTIONS
Avoid sour or bitter foods and beverages. Avoid dehydration.

COURSE/PROGNOSIS
Sialoliths rarely recur unless anatomic abnormality of duct present.

CODING

ICD-9-CM
527.2 Sialoadenitis
527.5 Sialolithiasis

CPT
42330 Sialolithotomy; Submandibular, sublingual, or parotid uncomplicated intraoral.
42335 Submandibular, complicated intraoral
42340 Parotid extraoral or complicated intraoral
42440 Excision of submandibular gland
42450 Excision of sublingual gland
42550 Injection for sialography
70355 Panorex
70380 Radiologic exam for salivary calculus
70390 Sialography

MISCELLANEOUS

SYNONYMS
Salivary duct stone
Salivary duct calculus

SEE ALSO
Sialadenitis

REFERENCES
Lutcavage G, Schaberg S: Bilateral submandibular sialolithiasis and concurrent sialoadenitis: A case report. J Oral Maxillofac Surg 49: 1220-1222, 1991.

AUTHOR
Michael J. Dalton, DDS

Sinusitis

 BASICS

DESCRIPTION
• Acute, subacute, or chronic inflammatory condition within the paranasal sinuses, as the sinus ostium becomes obstructed by inflammatory exudates and the normal drainage of the sinus is inhibited.
• Classified as acute or chronic depending on duration of infection.

 ETIOLOGY

• Invasion of microorganisms from neglected dental infections, common colds, influenza, frontal or ethmoidal infections, traumatic injuries, and allergies are most frequent causative factors.
• Dental foci associated with sinusitis; 10 to 23% of all sinusitis
  ◇ periapical abscess and periodontitis of maxillary premolars or molars, antral perforation by the extraction of molars and dental implants, sinus lift for implants, and maxillary osteotomies.
• Causative organisms; mostly mixed infection with Streptococcus pyogenes, Staphylococcus aureus, or Haemophilus influenzae.
• Anaerobic microorganisms such as Bacteroides have been isolated in as many as 88% of culture positive specimens.

SYSTEMS AFFECTED
• Maxillary sinus (antrum)
• Ethmoidal sinus, frontal sinus.
• Sphenoid sinus

 DIAGNOSIS

SYMPTOMS AND SIGNS
• Constant pain with swelling overlying the sinus.
• Frontal or temporal headache in the chronic forms.
• Toothache or referred pain, tenderness of maxillary posterior teeth.
• Midfacial pain when head held upside-down.
• Nasal stuffiness, obstruction.
• Stuffy sensation of the affected area.
• Dizziness, nausea
• Fetid breath or odor
• Tenderness of the anterior wall of the sinus.
• Tenderness of the upper posterior teeth to percussion.
• Mucopurulent nasal discharge.
• Moderate fever and malaise which is variable with some degree.
• Increased "opacity" upon the antral trans-illumination.
• Nasal voice (hypernasality)

LABORATORY
CBC
  ◇ varying degree of leukocytosis.

IMAGING/SPECIAL TESTS
• Aspiration of sinus exudates (antral puncture) for culture and sensitivity test.
• Radiographic exam (Water's or panoramic view); antral cloudiness and thickened antral lining demonstrates the degree of fluid accumulation or hyperplastic polyps.
• Computerized tomogram to identify the involved area.
• Dental radiographs, panoramic view to find dental foci.
• Rhinoscopy to find antral polyps.
• Trans-illumination of the sinus.

DIFFERENTIAL
• Mucoceles of the antrum, retention cyst.
• Pseudocyst with degeneration of inflammatory polyps.
• Postoperative maxillary cyst (surgical ciliated cysts).
• Ethmoid infections
• Phycomycosis

TREATMENT

General
◇ Pain relief with analgesics, re-establishment of effective drainage and elimination of pathologic mucosa.
◇ Appropriate antibiotic therapy for an adequate period of time (usually 10 to 14 days).
◇ Sinus drainage by the application of nasal decongestant to the obstructed antral opening.
◇ Antihistamines and steroids may be used.

MEDICATIONS
• Nasal spray containing 2% ephedrine 0.5% phenylephrine, or long-acting agent 0.05% oxymetazoline.
• Penicillinase-resistant penicillin, amoxicillin, or dicloxacillin. Oral cephalosporins such as cephalexin, cefadroxil are considered most effective antibiotics.
• Erythromycin or trimethoprim-sulfamethoxazole for penicillin allergic patients.

SURGERY
• Antral puncture and sinus lavage (not indicated for acute sinusitis) through the inferior meatus or through the canine fossa.
• Nasal antrostomy, Caldwell-Luc operation for chronic sinusitis.
• Endoscopic approaches, short-wave diathermy for acute and subacute sinusitis.
• Removal of the cause of the infection such as offending tooth, nasal polyp.
• Eradication of local inflammation and oro-antral closure with palatal and/or buccal mucoperiosteal flaps.
• Total removal of the respiratory epithelial lining should be avoided to maintain a healthy sinus after resolution of the sinusitis.

CONSULTATION SUGGESTIONS
Oral-Maxillofacial Surgeon, Otolaryngologist

REFERRAL SUGGESTIONS
Oral-Maxillofacial Surgeon, Otolaryngologist, Primary Care Physician

PATIENT INSTRUCTIONS
Humidify air when exposed to dry air. Avoid overuse of topical decongestants.

COURSE/PROGNOSIS
• Chronic suppurative sinusitis follows repeated attacks of acute or subacute sinusitis.
• Basic pathophysiologic response involves necrosis, proliferation, and squamous metaplasia of the ciliated lining epithelium in the sinus.
• Occasionally, the long-persisting sinusitis invades the periosteum and underlying bone.

• Oro-antral fistula can occur along retained roots or at the extraction site.
• Fungal infections such as aspergillosis and phycomycosis can follow in immunosuppressed and diabetic patients.

CODING

ICD-9-CM
461.0 Acute maxillary sinusitis
461.9 Acute sinusitis
473.0 Chronic maxillary sinusitis
473.9 Chronic sinusitis

CPT
31020 Maxillary antrotomy, intranasal
31030 Caldwell-Luc antrotomy
31050 Sphenoid sinusotomy
31070 Frontal sinusotomy, simple (trephine)
70210 Radiologic exam, sinuses, less than 3 views
70355 Panorex
99000 Transport of specimen to laboratory

MISCELLANEOUS

SYNONYMS
Chronic suppurative sinusitis

SEE ALSO
Headache, migraine
Rhinitis, allergic

REFERENCES
Schow SR: Infections of the maxillary sinus. Oral Maxillofac Surg Clin N Am 3:343-353, 1991.

Lebovics R, Baker AS: Infectious diseases of the upper respiratory tract. In: Harrison's Principles of Internal Medicine. Isselbacher KJ, et al (ed), New York, McGraw-Hill, 1994, pp. 515,520.

Leonard G, Lafremiere DC: Infections of the ear, nose and throat. In: Oral and Maxillofacial Infections, 3rd ed. Topazian RG, Goldberg M (eds), Philadelphia, WB Saunders, 1994, pp. 360-366.

AUTHOR
Myung-Rae Kim, DDS, PhD

Sjögren's Syndrome

 BASICS

DESCRIPTION
• A chronic inflammatory autoimmune disorder that results in a lymphocyte mediated destruction of exocrine glands.
• There are two subclassifications:
Primary SS
◊ presence of keratoconjunctivitis sicca and xerostomia in the absence of a well-defined autoimmune or rheumatic disease.
Secondary SS
◊ associated with a variety of autoimmune diseases. Classic triad of xerostomia, keratoconjunctivitis sicca, and rheumatoid disease included.
• Disorder occurs mainly in females over the age of 40. (female/male ratio is 10:1)

 ETIOLOGY

• An autoimmune disease in which 70% of the patients test positive for specific antibodies that recognize human tissue antigens: anti-SS-A and anti-SS-B. Patients have an elevated total serum IgG and circulating rheumatoid factors.
• Genetic markers are commonly found in these patients.
• It is hypothesized that viral infection by the Epstein-Barr virus and/or other viruses may be the initiating event in those individuals genetically predisposed.

SYSTEMS AFFECTED
Eyes
◊ affected secondarily due to impaired lacrimal function.
Oral mucosa
◊ rendered more susceptible to trauma from chewing food and other benign insults.
Taste
◊ impaired secondary to reduced salivary flow.
Respiratory tract
◊ inflammation of the nasal mucosa. Respiratory infections may be common.
Skin
◊ may become dry and develop chronic urticaria.
Subcutaneous nodules may develop as a result of associated vasculitis.
General
◊ other organ systems may become involved and additional diseases present: vaginal dryness, atrophic gastritis, pseudolymphoma, non-Hodgkin's lymphomas.

 DIAGNOSIS

SYMPTOMS AND SIGNS
Mouth
◊ dry, painful, difficulty eating, speaking and swallowing, difficulty with removable prostheses, loss of taste, halitosis.
Eyes
◊ dry, burning, foreign body sensation, itching, ocular soreness, decreased visual acuity, photophobia, difficulty in tolerating low humidity.
Nose
◊ nasal crusting can lead to mucosal ulceration and nasal septum perforation. Olfactory sense decreased.
Oral mucosa
◊ dry, erythema, fissuring, ulceration, white streaks or plaques, leathery feel, easily traumatized, poor wound healing. Difficulty in swallowing due to lack of saliva.
Salivary glands
◊ often bilateral swelling of major glands that is smooth, firm, and tender. Difficulty or inability to manually express saliva from ducts. Calculi present in ducts.
Tongue
◊ may be red, fissured, and absent of papillae.
Teeth
◊ cervical caries, staining, periodontal disease, and bleeding.
Lips
◊ chapped, angular cheilitis.
Eyes
◊ redness, thick strands of mucous secretions, corneal ulcers.
Skin
◊ dry, subcutaneous nodules.

LABORATORY
Antinuclear antibodies, rheumatoid factors, anti-SS-A, anti-SS-B, elevated erythrocyte sedimentation rate, polyclonal hyperglobulinemia.

IMAGING/SPECIAL TESTS
Labial salivary gland biopsy
◊ infiltrate of lymphocytes, histiocytes, and often plasma cells. Criteria includes at least two foci of periductal lymphocytes per 4 mm^2.

DIFFERENTIAL
• Age-related decrease in lacrimal or salivary gland function.
• Dehydration
• Graft versus host disease
• Medication induced
• Anxiety, emotional problems
• Therapeutic radiation

Sjögren's Syndrome

TREATMENT

General
◇ Sialagoguesto stimulate salivary flow in those patients who have some functioning salivary tissue. Usually of limited value.
◇ Artificial salivary replacement. Artificial tears when indicated.
◇ Frequent recall for dental hygiene and bitewing radiographs.
◇ Topical fluoride in a custom tray 5 minutes/day.
◇ Soft diet
◇ Education and counseling, particularly in home-based oral hygiene.
◇ Monitor for development of lymphoma or carcinomas.

MEDICATIONS
• Avoid drugs with anticholinergic effect
• Artificial saliva
• Oral candidiasis: Clotrimazole (Mycelex) 10 mg, troche dissolved in mouth five times per day for 14 days.
• Topical anesthetics for oral discomfort.

SURGERY
Labial salivary gland biopsy

IRRADIATION
Not indicated.

CONSULTATION SUGGESTIONS
Oral Medicine, Ophthalmology

REFERRAL SUGGESTIONS
Rheumatologist, Primary Care Physician

PATIENT INSTRUCTIONS
• Strict oral hygiene with topical fluoride applications
• Soft diet

COURSE/PROGNOSIS
• There is no cure for Sjögren's syndrome. Treatment is palliative. Development of pseudolymphomas and malignant non-Hodgkin's lymphoma is often a major complication and occurs in 6 to 7% of cases.

CODING

ICD-9-CM
527.7 Mikulicz's
527.7 Xerostomia
710.2 Sjögren's

CPT
42405 Biopsy, salivary gland
42699 Salivary gland, unlisted procedure

MISCELLANEOUS

SYNONYMS
Dry mouth, dry eyes
Sicca Syndrome

SEE ALSO
Xerostomia
Conjunctivitis

REFERENCES
Abaza N, Torreti M, Miloro M, Balsara G: The role of labial salivary gland biopsy in the diagnosis of Sjögren's syndrome. J Oral Maxillofac Surg 51:574-580, 1993.

Atkinson J, Fox P: Sjögren's syndrome. JADA 124:74-82, 1993.

Vitali C, et al: Preliminary criteria for the classification of Sjögren's syndrome. Arthr Rheum 5:340-347, 1993.

AUTHOR
Paul A. Danielson, DMD

Sleep Apnea, Obstructive

 BASICS

 ETIOLOGY

 DIAGNOSIS

DESCRIPTION
The persistent and progressively increasing diaphragmatic efforts with no exchange of air at the nose and mouth (to be differentiated from central sleep apnea which is secondary to decreased respiratory muscle activity).

• Anatomic anomalies such as narrowing of the upper airway involving one or more sites, including the soft palate, the base of the tongue, and the lateral pharyngeal wall, or adjacent skeletal discrepancies such as mandibular or maxillary deficiencies.
• Associated with predominance in males, obesity, hypersomnolence, and excessive snoring.
• Associated with many conditions: upper airway allergies, enlargement of lymphoid tissues in the upper airway resulting from repetitive infections, hemopathy, Down's syndrome, hormone-related enlargement of the soft tissues of the upper airway as in myxedema, pituitary adenoma, cortico-adrenal tumors. Steroid treatment.
• Associated with mandibular abnormalities such as in acromegaly, Pierre Robin sequence, Crouzon's disease, Treacher Collin's syndrome, and idiopathic micrognathia.

SYSTEMS AFFECTED
Cognitive and psychological functions:
  • excessive daytime sleepiness due to repetitive apneic events and frequent arousals.
  • deterioration of memory and judgment.
  • irritability
  • morning headaches
  • personality changes, including sudden episodes of inappropriate behavior, jealousy, suspicion, anxiety, or depression.
  • in children, enuresis, failure to thrive, weight loss, problems in growth, misbehavior, poor school performance, and nightmares.
Cardiopulmonary systems:
  • systemic and pulmonary arterial pressures increase, later, hypertensive while awake.
  • oxygen desaturation
  • significant cardiac dysrhythmias: sinus bradycardia, sinus arrest, atrioventricular block, premature ventricular contractions, and tachycardia.
  • anoxic seizure, cardiac arrest, and sudden death.

SYMPTOMS AND SIGNS
• Hypersomnolence and excessive snoring.
• Obesity and history of eating habits and diet.
• Increasing frequency and prolongation of apneic episodes due to central nervous system depressant drugs, including alcohol and hypnotics and tranquilizers or aggravation by respiratory allergies, smoking, and dusty working environment.
• Physical examination of upper airway tract: significant septal deformity or turbinate enlargement, macroglossia, mandibular or maxillary deficiencies, long soft palate, enlarged tonsils, a large, floppy base of tongue, redundant mucosa with fatty infiltration, ruling out obstructive tumors and masses.

IMAGING/SPECIAL TESTS
• Polysomnography, including electroencephalogram (EEG), electro-oculogram (EOG), electromyogram (EMG), and electrocardiogram (ECG, lead V2).
• Plethysmography of respiration or diaphragmatic function.
• Thermistor monitoring of nasal and oral air flow.
• Transcutaneous monitoring of oxygen saturation.
• Recordings of cessation of respiration (RDI above 20%), oxygen desaturation (below 85%).
• Radiographic evaluation by cephalometrics and three-dimensional computed tomography (3D-CT).
• Fiberoptic endoscopy of nasopharynx, oropharynx, hypopharynx, and larynx.

DIFFERENTIAL
Central and mixed sleep apnea.

TREATMENT

General
◇ Nonsurgical:
- weight loss
- normalization of genioglossus function with weight loss.
- avoidance of alcohol and other central nervous system depressant drugs.
- avoidance of androgenic drugs
- tricyclic antidepressants
- nasal continuous positive airway pressure (CPAP).
- appliances such as nasal trumpets, tongue retaining devices, and head position holding apparatuses.

MEDICATIONS
- Confer with family physician about possible modification of drug regimens, and perhaps include tricyclic antidepressants.

SURGERY
- Tonsillectomy and adenoidectomy
- Nasal surgery (septoplasty, partial turbinectomy)
- Tongue reduction
- Tracheostomy
- Uvulopalatopharyngoplasty (UPPP)
- Mandibular osteotomy including hyoid myotomy and suspension, and maxillary, mandibular, and hyoid advancement.

CONSULTATION SUGGESTIONS
Oral-Maxillofacial Surgeon, Neurologist, Orthodontist

REFERRAL SUGGESTIONS
Oral-Maxillofacial Surgeon

PATIENT INSTRUCTIONS
Variety of treatments available, depends upon source of problem.

COURSE/PROGNOSIS
OSAS remains a therapeutic challenge, despite a substantial increase in the understanding of the pathophysiology and in the subsequent new modalities of treatment.

CODING

ICD-9-CM
780.51 Sleep apnea with insomnia
780.53 Sleep apnea with hypersomnia

CPT
21144 LeFort I osteotomy
21195 Sagittal advancement of mandible
21196 Sagittal advancement of mandible with rigid fixation
30462 Rhinoplasty
30520 Septoplasty
30930 Turbinate fracture to improve airway
31600 Tracheostomy
42145 Palalopharyngoplasty
70350 Cephalogram
70355 Panorex
70360 Soft tissue x-ray, neck
95805 Sleep testing

MISCELLANEOUS

SYNONYMS
Pickwickian syndrome
Nocturnal upper airway

REFERENCES
Siebert J: Obstructive sleep apnea. In: Plastic Surgery, Vol. 4, Cleft lip and palate and craniofacial anomalies. McCarthy JG, (ed), Philadelphia, WB Saunders, 1990, pp. 3147-3160.

Kimoff RJ, et al: Clinical features and treatment of obstructive sleep apnea. Can Med Assoc J 144:689-695, 1991.

Douglas NJ, Polo O: Pathogenesis of obstructive sleep apnoea/hypopnoea syndrome. Lancet 344:656-660, 1994.

Rintala A, et al: Cephalometric analysis of the obstructive sleep apnea syndrome. Proc Fin Dent Soc 87:177-182, 1991.

Riley RW, et al: Obstructive sleep apnea and the hyoid: a revised surgical procedure. Otolaryngol Head Neck Surg, 111:717-721, 1994.

Petri N, et al: Predictive value of Müller maneuver, cephalometry and clinical features for the outcome of uvulopalatopharyngoplasty. Acta Otolarynga (Stockh) 114:565-571, 1994.

AUTHOR
Irene H. S. So, DMD

Sodium Disorders

BASICS

DESCRIPTION
Body sodium is contained intracellularly and in bone, but is predominantly found as an extracellular electrolyte with a normal serum concentration of 135 to 145 mEq/L. An apparent sodium disorder is not necessarily due to an absolute deficit or excess of body sodium.

ETIOLOGY

The kidney normally regulates total body sodium through glomerular filtration and tubular reabsorption, modulated by the sympathetic nervous system, the renin-angiotensin-aldosterone systems, and antidiuretic hormone. These systems should balance the ordinary dietary fluid and sodium intake, and disruption of any of the above can cause disorder of sodium concentration.

    Causes of hyponatremia: water excess or inadequate free water excretion, sodium deficiency by inadequate intake or excessive loss (vomiting, diarrhea).

    Causes of hypernatremia: water deficiency or excessive loss of free water, excess consumption or administration of sodium, or inadequate excretion.

SYSTEMS AFFECTED
Because sodium is an essential ion for excitable tissues, changes in sodium concentration tend to cause symptoms related to nerve and muscle.

DIAGNOSIS

SYMPTOMS AND SIGNS
Hyponatremia
  ◊ hyperactivity, seizures, peripheral edema, muscle cramps, mental status changes, hypotension, tachycardia, elevated central venous pressure, lethargy, disorientation, decreased reflexes, Babinski present.
Hypernatremia
  ◊ thirst, irritability, restlessness, motor weakness, mental status changes, including CNS depression ranging from lethargy to coma, hyperreflexia, peripheral edema, ascites.

LABORATORY
Hyponatremia
  ◊ serum sodium is less than 135 mEq/L. A rapid drop of > 10 to 15 mEq/L or an absolute value of < 125 mEq/L is considered severe and requires immediate treatment.
Hypernatremia
  ◊ serum sodium is greater than 145 mEq/L.
• It is also necessary to measure serum osmolality and urine sodium concentration. These tests can help determine: (1) if the abnormality real or artifactual; (2) if the toxicity normal or abnormal; and (3) if the extracellular fluid volume normal or abnormal.
• This helps pinpoint the apparent disorder. If the abnormality is artifactual (eg, hypovolemia causing an apparent hypernatremia), this will also be reflected in other laboratory abnormalities (elevated hematocrit, potassium, protein levels).

DIFFERENTIAL
Hyponatremia:
vomiting and/or diarrhea, burns, "third spacing," diuretic effects, renal disease or failure, adrenal insufficiency, hypoproteinemia, emotional stress, polydipsia, hypothyroidism (myxedema), syndrome of inappropriate secretion of antidiuretic hormone (SIADH).
Hypernatremia:
neurogenic or nephrogenic diabetes insipidus, trauma, neoplasms of the pituitary, CNS infections, renal disease (polycystic, pyelonephritis), hyperaldosteronism.

Sodium Disorders

TREATMENT

General
1. Review water and sodium balance and hemodynamics.
2. Correct underlying problem.
3. Hyponatremia:
correct hypovolemia as needed with 0.9% NaCl, water restriction; use of diuretics to prevent circulatory overload and help increase water loss. In severe cases, 3% or 5%, NaCl is given based on calculated deficit.
Hypernatremia:
replacement of extracellular fluid with D5W or 0.45% NaCl replacing no more than half the deficit in the first few hours; restrict sodium and avoid hypertonic fluids; increase sodium excretion.
4. In either case, abnormal sodium concentrations should not be corrected too rapidly, no more than 6 to 8 mEq/day; serum electrolytes and osmolality should be checked frequently.

MEDICATIONS
• Chronic hyponatremia may respond to demeclocycline.
• While correcting hypernatremia, add calcium gluconate to IV solutions.
• Neurogenic diabetes insipidus managed with desmopressin acetate.

CONSULTATION SUGGESTIONS
Nephrologist, Critical Care Physician

REFERRAL SUGGESTIONS
Nephrologist, Primary Care Physician

FIRST STEPS TO TAKE IN AN EMERGENCY
• Hyponatremia
◇ administer IV 0.9% NaCl
• Hypernatremia
◇ administer IV DSW

COURSE/PROGNOSIS
Of the two, hypernatremia is of greater clinical significance owing to potential for CNS symptoms. In either case, only gross correction of sodium abnormalities can be achieved within the first few hours; finer adjustment may take several days.

CODING

ICD-9-CM
276.0 Hypernatremia
276.1 Hyponatremia

MISCELLANEOUS

Sodium requirement (in mEq) = total body water × (140 − actual serum sodium).
Total body water = (wt in kg × 0.6).

SEE ALSO
SIADH
Diabetes insipidus

REFERENCES
Tonnesen AS: Crystalloids and colloids. In: Miller RD (ed). Anesthesia, 3rd ed. Miller RD (ed), New York, Churchill Livingstone, 1990.

Levinsky NG: Fluids and electrolytes. In: Harrison's Principles of Internal Medicine 13th ed. Isselbacher KJ, et al (eds), New York, McGraw-Hill, Co., 1994.

Sendak MJ: Monitoring and management of perioperative fluid and electrolyte therapy. In: Principles and Practice of Anesthesiology. Rogers MC, Tinker JH, Covino BG, et al (eds), St. Louis, CV Mosby, 1993.

AUTHOR
Jeffrey B. Dembo, DDS, MS

Squamous Cell Carcinoma of Floor of Mouth

BASICS

DESCRIPTION
Malignant epithelial neoplasm involving oral mucosa of the floor of the mouth.

ETIOLOGY

• Tobacco abuse is associated with squamous cell carcinoma at all oral cavity sites.
• Alcohol abuse is also associated with squamous cell carcinoma of the oral cavity.
• Alcohol, when combined with tobacco use, acts synergically to greatly increase the risk of oral cancer.
• Leukoplakia of the floor of the mouth is a poor prognostic sign and malignant change in these lesions is much higher than for other leukoplakias. All floor of mouth leukoplakias, especially "speckled leukoplakia," should be regarded as premalignant.

SYSTEMS AFFECTED
• Oral mucosa of the floor of mouth, anteriorly and midline most common.
• Involvement of Wharton's duct orifices.
• Anterior invasion of the mandible can cause bone destruction and involve anterior teeth.
• Posterior invasion may involve the tongue, affecting speech and swallowing with subsequent weight loss.

DIAGNOSIS

SYMPTOMS AND SIGNS
• Usually a painless ulcer in floor of mouth frequently attributed to loose dentures. Ulceration has indurated, rolled edges, granular base, often with associated leukoplakia.
• In more advanced disease, problems with speech and swallowing.
• Invasion of mandible with losing of teeth.
• Tongue tethering if musculature involved.
• Swelling of the neck either due to blockage of the submandibular ducts or cervical node metastasis.
• Hard palpable cervical nodes or swollen, tender submandibular glands.

IMAGING/SPECIAL TESTS
• Biopsy mandatory for diagnosis of all nonhealing ulcers of 3 or more weeks. Fine needle aspiration biopsy (FNAB) for suspected cervical nodes.
• Plain radiographs of the mandible Panorex or lower occlusal helpful if mandibular bone involvement suspected.
• Bone scans (technetium) show earliest bone invasion, but false positive common.
• CT scan good for mandible and cervical nodes.
MRI good for muscle and soft tissue invasion.

DIFFERENTIAL
• Chronic traumatic ulcers (such as denture ulceration).
• Tumor of sublingual gland
• Fungal ulcer

TREATMENT

General
◊ Treatment will depend on the stage.

MEDICATIONS
• The role of chemotherapy as a curative modality is not defined for this disease.

SURGERY
• Early disease Stage I or II may be treated with either surgery or radiation with comparable 5-year survivals.
• Treatment of the N0 (non-enlarged or hard nodes) neck is controversial for T2 lesions involving either a supra-omohyoid staging neck dissection or a "watch and wait" policy. 50 Gy of external beam radiation may also be used where microscopic disease is suspected.
• Stages III and IV disease is best treated with radical surgery followed by radiotherapy.

IRRADIATION
See surgery discussion.

CONSULTATION SUGGESTIONS
Medical Oncologist, Radiation Oncologist, Oral Maxillofacial Surgeon, Head and Neck Surgical Oncologist

REFERRAL SUGGESTIONS
Medical Oncologist, Head and Neck Surgical Oncologist, Oral-Maxillofacial Surgeon

PATIENT INSTRUCTIONS
Stop smoking and ethanol consumption.

COURSE/PROGNOSIS
Prognosis will be dependent on the stage of disease. While small T1 lesions may have a 5-year survival of greater than 95%, advanced stage IV lesions will have a less than 10% survival. The presence of a positive node is the most important factor, decreasing percentage of survival by 50%.

CODING

ICD-9-CM
144.0 Malignancy, anterior floor of mouth
144.1 Malignancy, lateral floor of mouth
144.8 Malignancy, other sites, floor of mouth
144.9 Malignancy, unspecified site, floor of mouth

CPT
41108 Biopsy floor of mouth
41116 Excision lesion floor of mouth
41150 Composite resection floor of mouth and mandible without neck dissection
41153 Composite resection floor of mouth with suprahyoid neck dissection
41155 Composite resection floor of mouth, mandibular resection and radical neck
99000 Transport specimen to outside laboratory

MISCELLANEOUS

SYNONYMS
Mouth Cancer

SEE ALSO
Squamous cell carcinoma of tongue
Cancer, in general

REFERENCES
Shaw HJ, Hardingham M: Cancer of the floor of the mouth: surgical management. J Laryngology 91:467, 1977.

Kolson H, Spiro RH, Rosewit B, Lawson W: Epidermoid carcinoma of the floor of the mouth. Arch Otolaryngol 93:280, 1971.

Florin EH, Kolbosz RV, Goldberg LH: Verrucous carcinoma and the oral cavity. Intl J Derm 33: 618-622, 1994.

Million RR, Cassisi NJ, Mancuso AA: Oral cavity. In: Management of Head and Neck Cancer. 2nd ed. Philadelphia, JB Lippincott, 1994, pp 321-400.

AUTHOR
Robert A. Ord, MD, DDS, FACS, FRCS

Squamous Cell Carcinoma of Tongue

 BASICS

DESCRIPTION
A malignant tumor of epithelial origin involving the tongue, most commonly the lateral border of the anterior two-thirds.

 ETIOLOGY

• Smoking
• Alcohol Abuse
• Syphilis
• Associated with premalignant lesions, leukoplakia, and erythroplakia.

SYSTEMS AFFECTED
• Tongue mucosa and musculature.
• Local spread to the floor of mouth, anterior pillar, mandible.
• Cervical nodes involved by metastases.
• Lungs, liver, and bone involved (late) by hematogenous spread.

 DIAGNOSIS

SYMPTOMS AND SIGNS
• Painless or painful ulcer or mass of the tongue. Indurated ulcer with everted rolled edges.
• Pain radiating to the ear.
• Alteration in speech or swallowing. Impaired mobility of the tongue due to muscle infiltration.
• Lump in the neck. Firm, hard cervical lymphadenopathy.

LABORATORY
FTA to exclude syphilis.

IMAGING/SPECIAL TESTS
• CT scan for neck nodes.
• MRI scan for tongue infiltration and neck nodes.
• Incisional biopsy.
• FNAB of cervical nodes, if necessary.

DIFFERENTIAL
• Traumatic ulcer
• Malignant salivary gland
• Tumor of tongue (benign)
• Syphilis

TREATMENT

MEDICATIONS
• Chemotherapy has not been shown to increase survival, but has been used as an adjuvant therapy and for palliation.
• Unresectable disease will require palliative treatment, including pain control.

SURGERY
Surgery or radiation therapy are both valuable in this disease. T1 and T2 lesions can be treated with either surgery or radiation, using external beam or brachytherapy. Five-year survival rates are similar. Stages III and IV disease are best treated with surgery and radiation therapy in combination.

IRRADIATION
50 to 70 Gy of irradiation used for regional therapy.

CONSULTATION SUGGESTIONS
Radiation Oncologist, Speech Pathologist, Oral-Maxillofacial Surgeon, Head and Neck Surgeon

REFERRAL SUGGESTIONS
Oral-Maxillofacial Surgeon, Head and Neck Surgeon

PATIENT INSTRUCTIONS
Cease smoking and ethanol consumption.

COURSE/PROGNOSIS
Survival rates vary depending on the TNM Stage
◇ 5 year survival for Stage I disease is 72% and for Stage IV, 18%.
Local regional recurrence is the largest cause of failure.
Tumors in the tongue base present late and have a much worse prognosis than tumors that are more anterior. Between 8 to 20% of patients with tongue cancer will develop a second primary cancer in the upper aero-digestive tract.

CODING

ICD-9-CM
141. Malignant neoplasm of tongue
141.0 Base of tongue
141.1 Dorsal surface of tongue
141.2 Tip and lateral border of tongue
141.3 Ventral surface of tongue
141.4 Anterior two-thirds of tongue, part unspecified
141.5 Junctional zone
141.6 Lingual tonsil
141.8 Other sites of tongue
141.9 Tongue, unspecified site

CPT
41000 Biopsy of tongue; anterior two thirds
41105 Biopsy of tongue; posterior one third
41120 Glossectomy; less than one-half tongue
41130 Hemiglossectomy
41135 Partial glossectomy with unilateral radical neck dissection
41140 Total glossectomy without radical neck dissection
41145 Total glossectomy with unilateral radical neck dissection

MISCELLANEOUS

SYNONYMS
Tongue cancer

SEE ALSO
Squamous cell carcinoma of floor of mouth
Glossitis
Cancer, in general

REFERENCES
Rice DH, Spiro RH: Current Concepts in Head and Neck Cancer. American Cancer Society, 1989.

Thawley SE, Panje WR: Comprehensive Management of Head and Neck Tumors. Part IV. Tumors of the Oral Cavity. Philadelphia, WB Saunders, 1987, pp. 460-613.

Frazell EL, Lucas JC: Cancer of the tongue: Report of the management of 1,554 patients. Cancer 15:1085, 1962.

Cade S, Lee ES: Cancer of the tongue. A study based on 653 patients. Brit J Surg 44:433-446, 1957.

Million RR, Cassisi NJ, Mancuso AA: Oral Cavity. In: Management of Head and Neck Cancer. 2nd ed. Philadelphia, JB Lippincott, 1994, pp 321-400.

AUTHOR
Robert A. Ord, MD, DDS, FACS, FRCS

Status Epilepticus

BASICS

DESCRIPTION
Status epilepticus is defined as two or more tonic-clonic convulsive seizures occurring in rapid succession without a period of recovery between attacks, or continuous absence, complex partial, or partial seizure activity for 30 minutes or longer. This phenomenon may occur with any form of partial or generalized seizure, and can be a life-threatening emergency unless prompt treatment is instituted.

ETIOLOGY

• Unknown in large number of cases.
• Idiopathic
  ◊ 50% of cases have no previous history of seizure disorder.
• Other causes:
• Sleep deprivation
• Cyclic recurrence (sleep-wake cycle or menstrual cycle).
• Reaction to specific stimulus (reflex epilepsy).
• Alcohol abuse
• Abrupt anticonvulsant or alcohol withdrawal.
• Dehydration/electrolyte imbalance
• Metabolic disturbances
• Hypoglycemia/hyperglycemia
• Hypocalcemia
• Hyponatremia
• Drug intoxication [isoniazid (INH), tricyclic antidepressants, neuroleptics, strychnine].
• Excessive physical exertion
• Renal failure
• Hepatic failure
• Hypoxic encephalopathy
• CNS infection meningitis/encephalitis (most common childhood cause of status epilepticus).
• Radiation therapy
• Pregnancy/delivery
• Intracranial hemorrhage
• Tumor
Cerebrovascular disease

SYSTEMS AFFECTED
CNS
  ◊ irreversible brain damage
Pulmonary
  ◊ aspiration pneumonia
Cardiac
  ◊ dysrhythmias

DIAGNOSIS

SYMPTOMS AND SIGNS
CNS
  ◊ confusion, impaired consciousness, loss of consciousness, frequent eye-blinking and nystagmus or other eye deviations, generalized or focal seizure activity, coma.
• Behavior and personality changes
• Memory loss, amnesia
• Hallucinations
• Impaired cognitive abilities
• Fever
• Muscle aches
• Dyspnea
• Stridor

LABORATORY
• Complete blood count.
• Electrolytes, calcium, phosphorus, magnesium, glucose, creatinine, blood urea nitrogen to help define etiology.
• Arterial blood gas determination to check if acidosis or hypoxia is cause.

IMAGING/SPECIAL TESTS
EEG monitoring
  ◊ may show periodic lateralized epileptiform discharges (PLEDS).

DIFFERENTIAL
• Stroke (cerebrovascular accident)
• Intracranial hemorrhage
• Other seizure activity

TREATMENT

General
  ◊ Immediate treatment can be life-saving
  ◊ ABCs of basic life support
  ◊ Protection of the airway
  ◊ Provide supplemental oxygen
  ◊ Check blood pressure and pulse
  ◊ Position patient on side, with head extended and cushioned
  ◊ Protection of the head
  ◊ Intravenous access
  ◊ Send blood for laboratory evaluation

MEDICATIONS
• Bolus of D5W (50% glucose in water).
• Second IV access with 0.9% normal saline [diazepam (Valium) and phenytoin (Dilantin) are poorly soluble in D5W].
• Place ECG monitors
• Diazepam 10 mg intravenously, then at a rate of 2.5 mg/minute until the seizure stops or to a maximum of 20 to 25 mg. Other benzodiazepines commonly used in status epilepticus include midazolam, clonazepam, or lorazepam.
• Phenytoin 1000 to 1500 mg (18 to 20 mg/kg) slow IV push (<50 mg/min).
• Phenobarbital 10 to 20 mg/kg (up to 1 gm), divided in 2 to 4 doses at 30 to 60 minute intervals. The use of phenobarbital immediately after diazepam might result in severe respiratory depression. Other barbiturates used in the treatment of status epilepticus include pentobarbital and thiopentone.
• If convulsions persist beyond 30 to 60 minutes, administer general anesthesia with halothane and neuromuscular blockade, or lidocaine 100 mg IV. Use EEG monitoring, if available.
Protocol for Management of Convulsive Status Epilepticus
• (after Walsh GO, Delgado-Escueta AV: Neurologic Clinics 11:850, 1993).
• Time from initial observation and treatment (min.)
Procedure:
  0: Assess cardiorespiratory function. If unsure of diagnosis, observe 1 tonic-clonic seizure and verify the persistence of unconsciousness after the seizure. Insert oral airway and administer O_2 if necessary. Obtain IV access. Draw blood for anticonvulsant levels, glucose, electrolytes, and urea. Draw ABG. Monitor respiration, BP, HR, ECG, and EEG if available.
  5: Start IV infusion of 0.9% normal saline with thiamine 100 mg. Infuse 50 ml of 50% dextrose to rule out hypoglycemic seizures (child-glucose dose is 2 ml/kg of 25% dextrose).

10 to 20: Administer either lorazepam 0.1 mg/kg at 2 mg/min, or diazepam 0.2 mg/kg at 2 mg/min IV. If diazepam is given, it can be repeated if seizures do not stop after 5 minutes.

21 to 60: If status persists, administer phenytoin 15 to 20 mg/kg no faster than 50 mg/min in adults, and 1 mg/kg/min in children IV. Monitor ECG and BP during the infusion. Phenytoin is incompatible with glucose-containing solutions; the IV line should be purged with normal saline before the phenytoin infusion.

60+: If status does not stop after 20 mg/kg of phenytoin, give additional doses of 5 mg/kg to a maximum dose of 30 mg/kg. If status persists, endotracheal intubation is mandatory. Give phenobarbital 20 mg/kg IV at 100 mg/min. When phenobarbital is given after benzodiazepine, the risk of apnea is great, and assisted ventilation is usually required. If status persists, give anesthetic doses of drugs such as phenobarbital or pentobarbital. Ventilatory assistance and vasopressors are almost always necessary.

Options for Drug-Resistant Convulsive Status:

• If seizures continue, general anesthesia can be instituted with either:

1. IV pentobarbital, loading dose of 15 mg/kg over 1 hour is followed by maintenance infusion of 1 to 2 mg/kg/hr until seizures stop or EEG burst suppression.

2. IV phenobarbital, additional 5 to 10 mg until seizures stop or EEG burst suppression.

3. Thiopentone may be given at 2 mg/min in normal saline by a microdrip set for 30 to 60 minutes. Reduce dosage to 0.5 mg/min when controlled. Dose can be increased to anesthetic levels, if necessary, to achieve control. EEG monitoring to ascertain at "burst-suppression" pattern and seizure control is required. Alternatively, other anesthetic barbiturates could be used.

• Once control is achieved, EEG monitoring is recommended continuously or as frequently as is technically possible in the obtunded patient, to ensure that EEG status has not recurred.

SURGERY
Only indicated in rare cases when epileptic focus can be precisely localized.

CONSULTATION SUGGESTIONS
Neurologist

REFERRAL SUGGESTIONS
Neurologist, Primary Care Physician

FIRST STEPS TO TAKE IN AN EMERGENCY
• See treatment section above.

PATIENT INSTRUCTIONS
If taking antiseizure medications, take them properly and have blood levels checked periodically.

COURSE/PROGNOSIS
• After seizure cessation, it is necessary to determine the etiology to prevent recurrence.
• If the status episode persists beyond 30 to 60 minutes, the chance of serious neurologic sequelae or death increases significantly.
• Tonic-clonic status epilepticus is the most serious condition, with a mortality rate of 10%, and morbidity rates of permanent neurologic disability of 10 to 30%.

CODING

ICD-9-CM
345.3 Status epilepticus
780.3 Febrile seizures, Repetitive seizures

CPT
90782 Therapeutic injection, SQ or IM
90784 Therapeutic injection, IV

MISCELLANEOUS

Classification of Status Epilepticus
• Primary Generalized Convulsive Status
• Tonic-clonic status (Grand Mal Status) (most common and most serious form).
• Myoclonic status
• Clonic-tonic-clonic status
• Secondary Generalized Convulsive Status
• Tonic-clonic status with partial onset
• Tonic status
• Subtle generalized convulsive status
• Simple Partial status
• Partial motor status
• Unilateral status
• Epilepsia partialis continua
• Partial sensory status
• Partial status with vegetative autonomic or affective symptoms.
• Nonconvulsive status
• Absence status-typical or atypical
• Complex partial status

SEE ALSO
Seizure disorders
Stroke

REFERENCES
Walsh GO, Delgado-Escueta AV: Status epilepticus. Neurologic Clinics 11:835-856, 1993.

DeLorenzo RJ: Status epilepticus: Concepts in diagnosis and treatment. Sem Neurol 10:396-405, 1990.

Bone RC: Treatment of convulsive status epilepticus. Recommendations of the Epilepsy foundation of America's Working Group on Status Epilepticus. JAMA 270:854-859, 1993.

Brown JF, Hussain IH: Status epilepticus. I: Pathogenesis. Develop Med Child Neurol 33: 3-17, 1991.

Brown JF, Hussain IH: Status epilepticus. II: Treatment. Develop Med Child Neurol 33:97-109, 1991.

AUTHOR
Michael Miloro, DMD, MD

Stevens-Johnson Syndrome

BASICS

DESCRIPTION
A severe form of erythema multiforme that displays regional mucosal surface involvement and is often "explosive" in its presentation. Erythema multiforme is an acute dermatologic and mucosal disorder that displays variation in lesional and as clinical presentation. It is often a disease of exclusion due to an often nondescript histopathologic picture. Most commonly seen in adolescents and young adults.

ETIOLOGY

• Thought to most likely be an antigen-antibody response that reacts preferentially at submucosal and subepidermal blood vessels. IgM and C3, which are a part of many early antibody responses, have been detected by immunofluorescent studies in early lesions.
• Cytotoxic CD8 lymphocytes have also been seen to be associated with the individual cell necrolysis of keratinocytes. This would point to a cellular rather than humoral immune response.
• Erythema multiforme/Stevens-Johnson syndrome is most likely a result of a complex, overzealous immune response, possibly involving both cellular and humoral immune systems.
• There are literally scores of possible antecedent infections and predisposing medicaments/substances that have been reported to cause erythema multiforme.
• Drugs and vaccinations are thought to be the most common cause of major cases.

SYSTEMS AFFECTED
Oral mucosa
 ◊ all mucosal surfaces may be affected. Lips, buccal mucosae, palate, and tongue are the most commonly involved. Mucosal lesions are most often ulcerative.
Skin
 ◊ classic lesion is called a target lesion. These lesions have alternating areas of erythematous skin alternating with normal colored (centrally healed) skin. Bullous skin lesions more likely in this severe form. Perianal involvement possible.
Joints can be painful
Systemic
 ◊ low grade fever
Conjunctiva- inflammation, ulceration, and possible uveitis. Blindness a possible consequence.
Uro-genital mucosa-urethritis, vaginal ulceration.

DIAGNOSIS

SYMPTOMS AND SIGNS
• Low-grade febrile complaints.
• Acute, possibly "explosive," onset usually rules out autoimmune vesiculo-bullous diseases such as pemphigus and pemphigoid.
• Joint pain.
• Acutely painful ulcerations. Severe concomitant skin and multiple mucosal ulcers.
Mucosal
 ◊ ulcerations that can range from a few aphthae-form lesions to large 2 to 3 cm lesions.
Lips
 ◊ can be extensively involved with crusting and necrosis not being uncommon.
Skin
 ◊ target lesion is classic though macular, papular, vesicular, and bullous lesions can be seen all in the same patient or as the presenting lesion. Most common areas of involvement are the extremities (with more severe involvement in the more distal areas) and face.
• Positive orthostatic hypotension if patient has become dehydrated.

LABORATORY
CBC, culture, or cytologic exam for Herpes simplex; serologic tests if pemphigus highly suspected; toxicologic tests if drug history dictates; liver panel if hepatitis symptoms were/are present; and glucose level if steroid therapy anticipated and diabetes suspected.

IMAGING/SPECIAL TESTS
Biopsy to rule out other possibilities in differential diagnosis. Biopsy may need to be divided into pieces with one-half in 10% formalin and the other half fresh frozen or placed in Michel's solution. Immunofluorescent study if autoimmune disease is high in the differential.

DIFFERENTIAL
• Acute drug reaction
• Reiter's syndrome
• Behcet's syndrome

TREATMENT

General
◇ Must rule out or take into account the possibility of other disease processes, especially infectious causes.

◇ Dehydration is a major complication that will most likely necessitate hospital admission. Check for skin turgor and do postural blood pressure measurements. IV fluids to treat or prevent dehydration.

◇ Lesions can become secondarily infected.

MEDICATIONS
• Glucocorticosteroids are necessary. IV or oral dosing is needed, as topical preparations will not address the systemic nature of the process. Tapering or maintenance dosing of oral glucocorticosteroids may be necessary depending on disease course.

• Steroids almost absolutely contraindicated in the presence of active infection. Consult physician/infectious disease specialist in face of this possibility.

• Because steroids lower immune response, the immunocompetency of the patient must be taken into account.

• Steroids will elevate glucose levels in diabetics.

SURGERY
Biopsy if needed.

CONSULTATION SUGGESTIONS
Oral Medicine, Oral-Maxillofacial Surgeon

REFERRAL SUGGESTIONS
Primary Care Physician, Oral Medicine, Oral-Maxillofacial Surgeon

FIRST STEPS TO TAKE IN AN EMERGENCY
• Consider IV hydration if any sign of dehydration.

PATIENT INSTRUCTIONS
Maintain hydration orally if possible.

COURSE/PROGNOSIS
Self-limiting disease, but it may last 4 to 6 weeks. It is usually of acute onset with the patient being very uncomfortable due to oral/palmar/planter involvement and the fact that these areas are routinely traumatized in everyday activities. Disease is most commonly seen in young adults and adolescents.

CODING

ICD-9-CM
276.0 Dehydration, hypotonic
695.1 Erythema multiforme
995.2 Adverse drug reaction (see table of drugs for specific drug)

CPT
11100 Biopsy, skin
40808 Biopsy, mouth intraoral

MISCELLANEOUS

SYNONYMS
Major erythema multiform
Erythema multiforme exudativum

SEE ALSO
Erythema Multiforme
Oral Ulcers

REFERENCES
Regezi JA, Sciubba J: Oral Pathology, 2nd ed. Philadelphia, WB Saunders, 1993, pp. 61-65.

Patterson R, Dydewicz MS, Gonzales A, et al: Erythema multiforme and Stevens-Johnson syndrome. Descriptive and therapeutic controversy. Chest 98:331-336, 1990.

Moschella SL, Hurley HJ: Dermatology. 3rd ed. Philadelphia, WB Saunders, 1991, pp. 580-585.

AUTHOR
John W. Hellstein, DDS

Subdural Hematoma

BASICS

DESCRIPTION
A subdural hematoma (SDH) results from tearing of the bridging veins passing from the brain to the dural sinuses, or laceration of the brain that tears the overlying pia arachnoid. Signs and symptoms may appear immediately within minutes of injury, or as late as 6 to 8 weeks later. There are three distinct patterns of SDH, each with different symptoms, clinical findings, treatments, and prognoses: acute SDH, subacute SDH, and chronic SDH.

ETIOLOGY

- Head trauma
- Acceleration/deceleration injury
- Whiplash
- Concurrent medical conditions:
    - Atherosclerosis
    - Cardiovascular disease
    - Cerebrovascular disease
    - Hypertension
    - Bleeding disorders
    - Coagulopathy
    - Diabetes mellitus
    - Hyperlipidemia

SYSTEMS AFFECTED
CNS
  ◇ aphasia, weakness, sensory and motor disturbances, headaches, visual changes, paralysis.

DIAGNOSIS

SYMPTOMS AND SIGNS
Acute SDH
- Symptoms develop within minutes to 48 hours from the time of injury.
- Confusion, drowsiness, stupor, unresponsiveness
- Progressive deterioration in neurologic signs
- Unilateral headache
- Comatose
- Unilateral pupillary dilation (5 to 10% contralateral)
- Ipsilateral hemiparesis

Subacute SDH
- Symptoms occur between 48 hours and 2 weeks after injury.
- Usually less severe level of neurologic deficit than acute SDH.
- History of head trauma with loss of consciousness.
- Episodes of gradual improvement, then deterioration, with fluctuating levels of consciousness.

Chronic SDH
- Unclear history of preceding trauma
- Headaches
- Slowed though processes
- Confusion, drowsiness, inattentiveness
- Personality changes
- Progressive alteration in level o consciousness and mentation over 4 to 6 weeks out of proportion to the focal neurologic deficit.
- Mild hemiparesis
- Seizures
- Dementia, rapid onset
- Aphasia

LABORATORY
CBC with platelets, PT/PTT

IMAGING/SPECIAL TESTS
CT scan with contrast
- Can localize the specific site of hemorrhage.
- May be difficult to identify subacute SDH because they become isodense within 2 weeks of injury.
- Can identify midline and ventricular shift, or mass effect.
- Bilateral chronic SDHs may show no midline shift

MRI.
- May fail to show acute hemorrhage.
- May show subacute SDH better than CT.

Cerebral angiography
- May localize a persistent hemorrhage.
- May show compression of adjacent structures.

EEG monitoring
  • May reveal epileptiform activity
Lumbar puncture (LP) with measurement of opening pressures and examination of spinal fluid.
Intracranial pressure (ICP) monitoring

DIFFERENTIAL
- Cerebrovascular accident (stroke)
- Brain tumor
- Drug or alcohol intoxication
- Senile dementia

TREATMENT

General
◊ Acute SDH
  • Emergent craniotomy to evacuate clot.

◊ Subacute SDH
  • Depends on patient condition
  • Unresponsive patient with solid clot-emergent craniotomy with clot evacuation.
  • Stable patient with clot liquefaction
  • Small craniectomy or burr holes to evacuate the clot externally.

◊ Chronic SDH
  • Drainage through perforator openings
  • Some advocate removal of fibrous pseudomembranes through a craniotomy to prevent fluid reaccumulation.

MEDICATIONS
• Glucocorticoids may be helpful in select situations.
• Antiseizure medications, if necessary.

SURGERY
• See general treatment above.
• Surgery is the treatment of choice, and some medications could have disastrous consequences if used inappropriately. For example, the use of thrombolytic, anticoagulant, or antiplatelet agents for presumed cerebral ischemia or stroke.

CONSULTATION SUGGESTIONS
Neurologist, Neurosurgeon

REFERRAL SUGGESTIONS
Neurosurgeon

FIRST STEPS TO TAKE IN AN EMERGENCY
• Monitor vital signs, institute BLS if needed, administer O_2, immediately transport to emergency facility.

PATIENT INSTRUCTIONS
After recovery from subdural, elective dentistry should be deferred for about six months.

COURSE/PROGNOSIS
• Acute SDH carries a 100% mortality if not treated with prompt surgical intervention.
• Chronic SDH, if small, resorb on their own, leaving only the organizing pseudomembranes, which calcify after many years.
• If appropriately diagnosed and surgically treated, subdural hematomas rarely lead to long-term sequelae.

CODING

ICD-9-CM
432.1 Nontraumatic subdural hematoma
852.2 Subdural hematoma
852.3 Subdural hematoma with open intracranial wound

MISCELLANEOUS

SYNONYMS
Subdural hemorrhage

SEE ALSO
Stroke
Seizure disorder

REFERENCES
Hamilton MG, Frizzell JB, Tranmer BI: Chronic subdural hematoma: The role of craniotomy reevaluated. Neurosurg 33: 67-72, 1993.

Kaminski HJ, Hlavin ML, Likavec MJ, Schmidley JW: Transient neurologic deficit caused by chronic subdural hematoma. Am J Med 92: 698-700, 1992.

Ellis GL: Subdural hematoma in the elderly. Emerg Med Clinics N Am 8: 281-294, 1990.

AUTHOR
Michael Miloro, DMD, MD

Syphilis

BASICS

DESCRIPTION
Syphilis is an infectious disease with numerous systemic manifestations, which appear in three general stages over months to years. The causative bacterial agent is a spirochete which most often is transmitted through sexual contact (venereal).

ETIOLOGY

• Dating back to the 15th century, syphilis had a world-wide distribution as an endemic venereal disease with records of several historical epidemics. The infection is almost exclusively caused by the spirochete Treponema pallidum.
• The bacterium is an approximately 10 x 0.5 micron, slender, tightly coiled motile cell that can be maintained in laboratory rabbits. Speciation largely depends on association with clinical illness.
• Transmission is through sexual contact, transplacental passage, accidental parenteral injury, transfusion, or other contact involving wet mucosa (kissing).
• Patients are most infectious in the early disease stages (especially in which a mucous patch or chancre is present). As the disease progresses into later stages, transmissibility decreases dramatically. An extremely low inoculum (as few as 4 spirochetes in laboratory animals) can produce infection. Following mucosal or skin penetration, the bacterium disseminates through the lymphatics and bloodstream.

SYSTEMS AFFECTED
• All organ systems can be affected after a 3 to 90 day incubation period.
• Clinically, syphilis is divided into five major states: (1) incubating, (2) primary, (3) secondary, (4) latent, and (5) tertiary, and 3 stages. The primary stage refers to the development of the initial lesion (chancre) which characteristically heals spontaneously in 2 to 8 weeks. The secondary (disseminated) stage usually becomes evident in 3 to 14 weeks, and demonstrates high antigen load with resulting immune complex disease and associated kidney, CNS, and dermal abnormalities. Periods of acute exacerbations followed by long-term remission occur throughout this stage. Tertiary (late) syphilis develops in over 1/3 of untreated patients, and most commonly involves more severe immune-complex disease, obliterative endarteritis (gumma) at any site, and neurosyphilis (ie, dementia, tabes dorsalis, seizures).

DIAGNOSIS

SYMPTOMS AND SIGNS
<u>Early Congenital</u>
◊ rash, mucous patches, jaundice, lymphadenopathy, anemia, osteochondritis, vague neurologic abnormalities.
<u>Late Congenital</u>
◊ frontal bossing, short maxilla, mandibular protrusion, saddle nose, 8th nerve dysfunction, Hutchinson's incisors, Clutton's joints, mulberry molars, interstitial keratitis, saber shins.
<u>Secondary Syphilis</u>
◊ rash and pruritus, oral aphthae, oral mucous patches, condyloma lata, fever, malaise, anorexia, weight loss, arthralgia, pharyngitis and laryngitis (neurologic signs occur in approximately 1/3 of patients).
<u>Tertiary and Neurosyphilis</u>
◊ hemiplegia, aphasia, tremors, slurring, ataxia, Argyll Robertson pupils, impotence, incontinence, Romberg sign (deranged postural sense), and cardiovascular disease (endarteritis obliterans).

LABORATORY
Unlike other spirochetes (ie, Leptospira, Borrelia), Treponema pallidum has not been successfully cultured on artificial media. However, organisms successfully isolated from clinical lesions or blood can be grown in rabbits and demonstrated microscopically or serologically.

IMAGING/SPECIAL TESTS
• Specific anti-treponemal antibody tests such as the indirect immunofluorescent antibody test (FTA-abs) is the standard for detecting syphilis. In addition, Treponema pallidum hemagglutination assays (TPHA) are also valuable for measuring specific treponemal antibody.
• The classical nonspecific assay for syphilis is the VDRL slide test, which involves the heating of serum on a glass slide to determine its ability to flocculate a suspension of cardiolipin-cholesterol-lethicin antigen. This screening tool has been replaced by a rapid plasma reagin (RPR) card test or the automated reagin test (ART).
• Dark field microscopy is the fastest, most direct laboratory method for the detection of treponemes obtained from nodal aspirations or skin lesions. Spirochetes demonstrated from oral specimens are not diagnostic because other spirochetal genera and species are found as normal flora in the oral cavity.

DIFFERENTIAL
• It has been stated that "he who knows syphilis, knows medicine," because this infectious disease may include a wide range of signs and symptoms exhibited as acute, chronic, or recurrent episodes over months to years.
• Autoimmune or immune-complex disorders.
• Viremias (ie, HIV, EBV, Arboviruses)
• Other spirochetal disease (ie, Lymes, Leptosporosis).
• Degenerative neurologic processes {ie, multiple sclerosis (MS), Alzheimer's, chronic alcoholism}.

TREATMENT

MEDICATIONS
• Benzathine penicillin 2.4 million units given IM as a single dose for early stage disease, or same given weekly for three doses in late disease. Alternatively, 600,000 units of procaine penicillin can be administered IM daily for 8 to 15 days.
• Penicillin-allergic patients can be given either tetracycline 500 mg or erythromycin stearate or ethyl succinate 500 mg p.o., q.i.d. for 15 to 30 days.
• More than 50% of patients initially treated with antibiotic therapy will exhibit a Jarisch-Herxheimer reaction within 8 hours following the beginning of therapy. This generally consists of fever, adenopathy, arthralgia, exacerbation of any skin lesions, and hypotension. This reaction rarely lasts longer than 24 hours and is thought to result from massive Treponemal destruction and release of bacterial antigens. Administer NSAIDs if reaction occurs.

SURGERY
Biopsy of mucous patch if diagnosis unclear.

CONSULTATION SUGGESTIONS
Infectious Disease Specialist

REFERRAL SUGGESTIONS
Primary Care Physician, Infectious Disease Specialist

PATIENT INSTRUCTIONS
Chancre and mucous patch highly infectious. Those with infection should notify previous sexual partners and public health authorities.

COURSE/PROGNOSIS
• Untreated syphilis demonstrates a highly variable course characterized by acute exacerbations followed by periods of remission over weeks, months, or years. Ultimately, the disease progresses to cardiovascular disease (ie, hypertension) and/or neurosyphilis (ie, dementia, paralysis).
• Syphilis is an extremely treatable disease if therapy is started prior to irreversible neurologic or cardiovascular damage.
• Unfortunately, while the organism can be eradicated in children born with congenital syphilis, physical anomalies persist depending on the level of fetal development when the infection occurs.

CODING

ICD-9-CM
090.5 Late congenital syphilis, symptomatic (Hutchinson's teeth, Saddle nose)
091.2 Primary syphilis, lip
091.3 Secondary syphilis of mucous membrane
094.0 Neurosyphilis
095.8 Other specified forms of late symptomatic syphilis
097.9 Syphilis unspecified

MISCELLANEOUS

SYNONYMS
Lues
The Great Imposter
Clap

SEE ALSO
Dementia
Human Immunodeficiency Virus
Alzheimer's
Multiple Sclerosis

REFERENCES
Mandell GL, Douglas RG, Bennett JE: Principles and Practices of Infectious Disease, 4th ed. New York, Churchill Livingston, 1995.

Holms KK, Mardh PA, Sparling PF, Stamm WE: Sexually Transmitted Diseases, 2nd ed. New York, McGraw-Hill, 1990, pp. 213-263.

Lukehart SA, Holmes KK. Syphilis. In: Harrison's Principles of Internal Medicine, 13th ed. Isselbacher KJ et al (eds) NY, McGraw-Hill, 1994, pp. 726-737.

AUTHOR
Peter G. Fotos, DDS, MS, PhD

Systemic Lupus Erythematosus

BASICS

DESCRIPTION
A chronic, multisystem autoimmune disease in which antibodies are formed to a variety of cells and tissues. Antibodies directed against cell nuclei (antinuclear antibodies) are found in the blood of almost all patients. Over 80% of cases involve women of childbearing age.

ETIOLOGY

• The causes of the immune abnormalities are unknown, but both genetic and environmental factors appear important.
• Some clinical features are due to vasculitis resulting from deposition of immune complexes in smaller vessels.
• Other clinical features are due to antibodies directed against cell-surface molecules in blood.

Drug-induced lupus
◊ certain medications, such as procainamide, hydralazine, and isoniazid can cause a disease similar to systemic lupus, except that the disease is milder and resolves when the drug is removed.

SYSTEMS AFFECTED
Skin
◊ rash, photosensitivity, Raynaud's phenomenon, ulcers.
Oral mucosa
◊ ulcers
Musculoskeletal
◊ arthritis
Neurologic
◊ psychosis and seizures
Kidney
◊ glomerular disease, kidney failure.
Serosa
◊ inflammation of serosa
Hematologic
◊ reduction in circulating blood cells.

DIAGNOSIS

SYMPTOMS AND SIGNS
Early affective symptoms
◊ chronic fatigue, anxiety, depression. Arthritis and dermatitis are most common clinical features.
Arthritis
◊ involves multiple joints, migratory, nonerosive.
Skin
◊ photosensitivity, erythematous malar ("butterfly") rash. Discoid lesions: red to purple plaques covered by scale; follicular plugging; atrophic scarring; hyperkeratosis; hyper- or hypopigmentation; telangiectasia; alopecia.
• Raynaud's phenomenon- cold or stress causes acute transient vascular changes of fingertips. Blanching, numbness, or pain followed by cyanosis and finally hyperemia.
Oral mucosa
◊ painful ulcers, and erosions with white rough epithelial thickening or white striae similar to lichen planus at periphery. Candidiasis is common.
Kidney
◊ persistent proteinuria and/or cellular casts.
Central nervous systems
◊ seizures, atypical migraine headaches, psychosis.
Serositis
◊ pleuritis, pericarditis, peritonitis.
Hematologic
◊ hemolytic anemia, leukopenia, thrombocytopenia.

LABORATORY
• Biopsy of skin and/or oral mucosal lesions for histopathology and immunopathology. Shows collagenous swelling, fibrinoid change, cellular necrosis, periarterial sclerosis, granulomatous reaction.
• Antinuclear antibodies and anti-DNA antibody almost always present in blood. Increased serum complement, abnormal CBC present in blood. Increased serum complement, abnormal CBC and differential (anemia, leukopenia, lymphopenia, thrombocytopenia), positive rheumatoid factor, elevated sedimentation rate, false-positive serologic test for syphilis, elevated serum creatinine, and protein and casts in urine.

IMAGING/SPECIAL TESTS
• Cerebral angiography
• Chest radiograph
• Echocardiogram

DIFFERENTIAL
• Oral lichen planus
• Oral carcinoma in situ, early squamous cell carcinoma.
• Discoid lupus erythematosus

TREATMENT

General
◇ refer patient to physician for management of skin lesions and systemic disease.
◇ Infection is a serious problem; consider prophylactic antibiotic coverage for seriously ill patients or patients on chronic, high-dose corticosteroids.
◇ Educate patient that oral lesions cannot be cured but can usually be controlled with medications.
◇ Minimize UV exposure, use sunscreens.

MEDICATIONS
• Skin lesions: topical steroids, intralesional injection of steroids, antimalarial drugs.
• Oral mucosal lesions topical and/or systemic steroids.
• Systemic: prednisone 40 to 60 mg 1 hour after arising for 5 days followed by 10 to 20 mg every other day. Systemic corticosteroids are contraindicated for patients with peptic ulcers, active infections, and other conditions. Confer with the patient's physician before initiating treatment.
• Topical corticosteroids may be used as initial treatment, as an adjunct to systemic corticosteroids, or to maintain remissions. Triamcinolone acetonide 0.1% aqueous suspension, rinse with 5 ml and expectorate, four times a day, nothing by mouth for 1 hour. (Directions to pharmacist: Dilute injectable triamcinolone 40 into 200 ml of water for irrigation, add 5 ml of 95% ethanol).

CONSULTATION SUGGESTIONS
Rheumatologist

REFERRAL SUGGESTIONS
Primary Care Physician

PATIENT INSTRUCTIONS
Patient can contact Lupus Foundation for useful literature (800)558-0121.

COURSE/PROGNOSIS
• Clinical course is variable and unpredictable. 10-year survival rate is almost 90%.
• Kidney disease and systolic hypertension indicate a poorer prognosis. Most common causes of death are infection and kidney failure.

CODING

ICD-9-CM
710.0 Systemic lupus erythematosus

CPT
11100 Biopsy of skin
99000 Transport of specimen to a laboratory

MISCELLANEOUS

SYNONYMS
Disseminated lupus erythematosus
SLE
Raynaud's Candidiasis

SEE ALSO
Lichen planus
Discoid lupus erythematosus
Raynauds candidiasis

REFERENCES
Habif TP: Clinical Dermatology. A Color Guide to Diagnosis and Therapy, 2nd ed. St. Louis, The CV Mosby Co., 1990, pp. 425-435.

Mills JA: Systemic lupus erythematosus. N Engl J Med 330:1871-1879, 1994.

AUTHOR
Michael W. Finkelstein, DDS, MS

Taste Disorders

BASICS

DESCRIPTION

Taste disorders can be classified as ageusia (total inability to taste one or more taste qualities, including salt, sweet, sour, and bitter); hypogeusia (decreased ability to taste one or more taste qualities); dysgeusia or parageusia (abnormal taste perception, generally unpleasant); hypergeusia (increased sensitivity to one or more taste qualities); and gustatory agnosia [inability to verbally identify taste(s)].

ETIOLOGY

• Taste disorders can be due to a variety of underlying local, behavioral, and systemic problems.
• Decreased transport/access or taste stimuli to the taste receptors can cause complaints of taste dysfunction, but are relatively uncommon because there is much overlap in the taste system (ie, taste buds have such widespread distribution in the oral cavity that it is difficult to block all receptors). Suggested causes of decreased access are poor oral hygiene and altered salivary flow.
• Damage to taste receptors, taste nerves, or central nervous system structures can be due to viral infections, tumors, or lesions of the taste nerves or central nervous system, head trauma, cancer, radiation therapy, drugs (particularly those that affect cell turnover), epilepsy, psychiatric disorders, metabolic disorders (such as hypothyroidism), diabetes, liver and kidney diseases, and rare conditions such as familial dysautonomia.

SYSTEMS AFFECTED

Oral mucosa
  ◊ etiologies related to decreased salivary flow, radiation therapy, antineoplastic drugs, and poor oral hygiene may be related to alterations in oral mucosa.
• Appetite and subsequent nutritional status may be affected by taste disorders.
• Social and psychological status, including coping skills, sexual function, etc, have been linked to taste disorders.

DIAGNOSIS

SYMPTOMS AND SIGNS
• Changes in ability perceive the flavor of food.
• Perception of a foul or abnormal taste.
• Altered appetite
• Burning sensation in mouth or dry mouth.
Oral mucosa
  ◊ poor oral hygiene, inflamed mucosa, evidence of infection.
Gingiva
  ◊ evidence of suppurative exudate.
• Foul odor
• Absence/abnormality of taste buds and/ or taste papillae.
• Weight change due to altered appetite.

LABORATORY
No definitive laboratory tests except those used to determine underlying systemic metabolic disorders.

IMAGING/SPECIAL TESTS
• Taste testing should involve evaluation of perception of quality and intensity of taste stimuli as well as localization of taste sensitivity. Testing should use taste stimuli dissolved in water or electric testing.
• Imaging of teeth and supporting structures may be indicated in cases of dysgeusia/parageusia.
• Imaging of the head is rarely indicated in taste disorders unless a peripheral nerve or central nervous system lesion is suspected.
• Biopsy of the taste buds may be helpful.

DIFFERENTIAL
• Olfactory disorders are the primary cause of altered food perception and must be clearly differentiated from taste problems.
• Burning mouth syndrome sometimes confused with a salty/bitter dysgeusia.
• Psychiatric disorders, including depression, sometimes associated with taste disorders.
• Sjögren's syndrome/dry mouth due to drug therapy sometimes associated with taste disorders.

TREATMENT

General
◇ There are no known treatments of primary taste disorders. Treatment of the underlying medical or systemic etiology should result in resolution of the complaint.

◇ Treatment of oral conditions such as infected teeth/abscesses should resolve dysgeusia.

MEDICATIONS
• Topical anesthetics such as a combination of 0.1% Benadryl and 0.1% dyclonine HCl dissolved in isotonic saline for a 1 minute rinse have been used to alleviate the symptoms of dysgeusia and burning mouth syndrome.

CONSULTATION SUGGESTIONS
Oral Medicine, Neurologist, Otolaryngologist

REFERRAL SUGGESTIONS
Oral Medicine

PATIENT INSTRUCTIONS
Necessary to rule out olfactory disorders before attributing taste disorders directly to primary taste problem.

COURSE/PROGNOSIS
• Little is known about the course and prognosis of primary taste disorders.
• For those taste disorders caused by systemic or other etiologies, removal of etiologic agent should allow taste function to return to normal.

CODING

ICD-9-CM
112.0 Candidiasis of mouth
300.4 Anxiety
311.0 Depression
527.0 Xerostomia
710.2 Sjögren's
781.1 Ageusia, dysgeusia
782.0 Disturbance, sensory
990.0 Radiotherapy, adverse effect
995.2 Medicinals, adverse effect

CPT
70220 Radiologic examination of sinuses, complete, minimum of three
87060 Culture of throat or nose
87070 Culture of any source
95904 Sensory nerve evaluation

MISCELLANEOUS

SYNONYMS
Ageusia
Hypogeusia
Dysgeusia
Parageusia
Hypergeusia

SEE ALSO
Xerostomia
Burning mouth syndrome
Sjögren's syndrome
Halitosis

REFERENCES
Deems DA, Doty RL, Settle RG, Moore-Billon V, et al: Small and taste disorders, a study of 750 patients from the University of Pennsylvania Smell and Taste Center. Arch Otolaryngol Head Neck Surg 117:519-528, 1991.

Doty, RL : Handbook of Olfaction and Gustation. New York, Marcel Dekker, Inc., 1995.

Getchell TV, Doty RL, Bartoshuk LM, Snow, Jr. JB : Smell and Taste in Health and Disease. New York, Raven Press, Ltd., 1991.

Goodspeed RB, Gent JF, Catalanotto FA: Chemosensory dysfunction: Clinical evaluation results from a taste and smell clinic. Postgrad Med 81:251-258, 1987.

Mott AE, Grushka M, Sessle BJ: Diagnosis and management of taste disorders and burning mouth syndrome. Dent Clinics N Am 37:33-71, 1993.

Mott AE, Leopold DA: Disorders in taste and smell. Med Clinics N Am 75:1321-1353, 1991.

Scott AE: Clinical characteristics of taste and smell disorders. Ear, Nose, Throat J 68:297-315, 1989.

Ship JA: Gustatory and olfactory considerations: examination and treatment in general practice. JADA 124:55-62, 1993.

AUTHOR
Frank A. Catalanotto, DMD

Teething

BASICS

DESCRIPTION
Teething alludes to eruption of teeth in the infant and its associated symptoms. It is a natural process that usually occurs without complications. Although the timing of eruption of teeth can usually be predicted, its occurrence often surprises new parents, particularly when accompanied by signs of systemic distress in the child.

ETIOLOGY

Normal eruption of primary teeth begins between ages 6 to 9 months with the eruption of the mandibular primary incisors. This is followed by the mandibular lateral incisors, succeeded next by the maxillary central and lateral incisors. Lower and upper first primary molars arise around age 12 to 15 months, followed by the lower and upper canines between age 16 to 18 months. Finally, the lower and upper second primary molars erupt sometime between months 20 to 24. All of the primary teeth generally have erupted by 24 to 36 months of age.

SYSTEMS AFFECTED
• Dentition
• GI tract
• Central nervous system possible irritability of child during eruption process.
• Skin

DIAGNOSIS

SYMPTOMS AND SIGNS
Increased salivation is a frequent characteristic of teething. Temperature, diarrhea, dehydration, skin eruptions, and gastrointestinal disturbances may be observed in some cases.

IMAGING/SPECIAL TESTS
If eruption pattern seems abnormal imaging of alveolus indicated.

DIFFERENTIAL
If symptoms persist for more than 24 hours, the infant should be examined by a physician to rule out upper respiratory infection and other common diseases and conditions of infancy.

TREATMENT

General
◇ Increased fluid consumption and palliative care to reduce the symptoms.

MEDICATIONS
• A non-aspirin analgesic can be given to the child for symptomatic discomfort. Also, over-the-counter topical anesthetics are available containing benzocaine (Baby Anbesol gel) apply small amount on gingiva in area of discomfort prn. Comes in 0.25 oz. tubes.

SURGERY
The need for incision of soft tissues overlying erupting teeth is extremely rare.

CONSULTATION SUGGESTIONS
Pediatric Dentist, Pediatrician (if symptoms persist)

REFERRAL SUGGESTIONS
Family Dentist, Pediatric Dentist

FIRST STEPS TO TAKE IN AN EMERGENCY
• If teething accompanied by high fever or seizures, consider alternative explanations for infant irritability.

PATIENT INSTRUCTIONS
Palliative care apply cold and pressure to the affected areas using teething rings. Reassure parents.

COURSE/PROGNOSIS
Discomfort is transient, abating once teeth appear in mouth.

CODING

ICD-9-CM
520.7 Teething

CPT
41899 Unlisted procedure, dentoalveolar structures

MISCELLANEOUS

SYNONYMS
Teething syndrome

SEE ALSO
Disturbances of tooth eruption

REFERENCES
McDonald RE: Eruption of the teeth: factors that influence the process. In: Dentistry for the Child and Adolescent. 5th ed. St. Louis, CV Mosby, 1987, pp. 189-196.

King NM, Lee A: Prematurely erupted teeth in the newborn infant. J Ped 114:807, 1989.

AUTHOR
Maria Rosa Watson, DDS, MS, MPH

Temporomandibular Joint Disorders - Extracapsular

BASICS

DESCRIPTION
• Extracapsular disorders of the temporomandibular joint (TMJ), include pathology of the hard and soft tissue structures contiguous to that joint which may contribute to or mimic intracapsular disorders.
• Extracapsular tissues include the muscles of mastication, the extracapsular portion of the mandibular ramus (coronoid process and distal ramus), the extracapsular portion of the zygomatic arch and zygoma, the ear canal and middle ear, the paranasal sinuses, the naso- and oropharynx, and the overlying skin and subcutaneous tissues with their enclosed nerves and blood vessels. The temporal lobe of the brain resides immediately superior to the TMJ fossa.

ETIOLOGY

Pathology of the Extracapsular Tissues:
Muscles of Mastication
◇ atrophy, hypertrophy, fibrosis, contusions, tears, rupture, fatty infiltration, contracture; may contribute to hypomobility, muscle weakness or fatigue, facial pain.
Bony Structures
◇ hypertrophy or elongation of the coronoid process may restrict movement and cause pain; elongated styloid process may cause facial pain (Eagle's syndrome); osteomas or other causes of bony expansion of the zygomatic arch may restrict mobility.
Ear Structures
◇ infections of the external or middle ear, mastoiditis, tumors or tumor-like growth (eg, cholesteatoma) may cause pain around the TMJ, tinnitus, hypomobility.
Nasal and Paranasal Structures
◇ lesions of nasopharynx may cause otalgia, trismus, facial pain.
Central Nervous System Lesions
◇ headache and facial pain may be the initial presentation of multiple sclerosis, cerebral neoplasms (eg, trigeminal schwannoma), trigeminal neuralgia or other forms of neuralgia;
Peripheral Nervous System Disorders
◇ consider reflex sympathetic dystrophy (RSD).

SYSTEMS AFFECTED
• Musculoskeletal
• Central Nervous System

DIAGNOSIS

Maintain a proper index of suspicion for non-TMJ causes of trismus, facial pain, headache, weight loss or other constitutional symptom. Thorough history and physical examination.

SYMPTOMS AND SIGNS
Facial or ear pain, headache, restricted mouth opening, facial swelling, facial numbness, tinnitus, or occlusal change.

IMAGING/SPECIAL TESTS
Screening panoramic image, possibly TMJ radiographs (transcranial, tomography). MRI of cranium should be considered if history and exam are not sufficiently consistent with primary intracapsular disorder. TMJ MRI can show pathologic changes of muscle, bone, and contiguous paranasal sinus and mastoid structures. Electromyography may be useful in diagnosis. MRI of brain may be diagnostic for multiple sclerosis by demonstrating demyelinization.

DIFFERENTIAL
• Myofascial pain dysfunction
• Eagle's syndrome
• Neoplasm
• Rheumatoid arthritis
• Temporal arteritis
• Otitis externa or media

TREATMENT

General
◇ Directed to specific etiology: Non-TMJ disorders require proper referral for further evaluation and treatment. Pain due to or triggered by anxiety-provoking activities improve with anxiety-reduction measures.
◇ Occlusal splint may assist those with parafunctional habits such as bruxism.
◇ Physical therapy using heat, ultrasound, massage, and TENS may be beneficial.

MEDICATIONS
• Analgesics, anti-inflammatory agents, muscle relaxants, antidepressants.
• Amitriplyline (Elavil) 50 mg h.s. often effective.
• Nonsteroidal anti-inflammatory drugs more effective if etiology inflammatory in nature and therapeutic blood levels attained and maintained.
• Reflex sympathetic dystrophy may respond to stellate ganglion blockade.

SURGERY
Coronoidectomy may resolve hypomobility by relieving mechanical obstruction of ramus movement; resection of bony interferences around the TMJ fossa; treatment of infection; muscle release procedures may be helpful (temporalis myotomy, lateral pterygoid myotomy).

CONSULTATION SUGGESTIONS
Oral-Maxillofacial Surgeon, Oral Medicine, Orthodontist, Dentists with special training in facial pain, Psychologist

REFERRAL SUGGESTIONS
Oral-Maxillofacial Surgeon, Oral Medicine, Orthodontist, Dentists with special training in facial pain, Physical Therapist

PATIENT INSTRUCTIONS
• Avoid eating hard or chewy foods or other vigorous uses of muscles of mastication. Use NSAIDs, apply heat, and avoid clenching.
• Follow medication instructions.

COURSE/PROGNOSIS
• Pain due to temporary, anxiety-provoking situation likely to quickly resolve.
• Pain accompanying chronic anxiety-provoking activities less likely to improve even with aggressive therapy.

CODING

ICD-9-CM
350.2 Atypical facial pain
524.60 TMJ pain syndrome
784 Facial pain

CPT
20605 Arthrocentesis
21085 Impression and custom preparation, oral surgical splint
21116 Injection for TMJ arthrography
21497 Interdental wiring, for other than fracture
21499 Unlisted musculoskeletal procedure, head
64450 Diagnostic injection
70328 Radiologic exam, TMJ, open and closed mouth, unilateral
70330 bilateral
70332 TMJ arthrography
70336 MRI, TMJ
70355 Panorex
90799 Unlisted therapeutic injection
90900 Biofeedback training
95867 Needle EMG, cranial nerve supplied muscle unilateral
95868 bilateral
97010 Physical medicine, hot or cold packs
97014 Electrical stimulation
97110 Physical medicine therapeutic exercises
97124 Massage
97128 Ultrasound

MISCELLANEOUS

SYNONYMS
MPD
TMJ

SEE ALSO
TMJ
◇ Intracapsular
Trigeminal neuralgia
Eagle's syndrome
Otitis

REFERENCES
Schellhas KP: MR imaging of muscles of mastication. Am J Neurorad 10:829-837, 1989.

Isberg A, Isaacsson G, Nah K-S: Mandibular coronoid process locking: A prospective study of frequency and association with internal derangement of the temporomandibular joint. Oral Surg Oral Med Oral Path 63:275-279, 1987.

Markoff M, Farole A: Reflex sympathetic dystrophy syndrome. Case report with a review of the literature. Oral Surg Oral Med Oral Path 61:23-28, 1986.

AUTHOR
Robert Chuong, MD, DMD

Temporomandibular Joint Disorders - Intracapsular

BASICS

DESCRIPTION
• Intracapsular temporomandibular joint (TMJ) disorders are pathologic changes of the mandibular condyle or fossa, articulating disc, the synovial membrane, the articular capsule, and/or the intracapsular portion of the lateral pterygoid muscle. Thus, hard and soft tissue components may be affected, and often, both are simultaneously involved.
• Intracapsular Disorders:
• Internal derangement (ID) refers to displacement of the articulating disc from the normal alignment relative to condyle and fossa; typical direction of displacement is anteromedial due to pull of lateral pterygoid muscle, although lateral displacement has been reported. Consequences of ID may include localized or regional pain, TMJ noise, mechanical restriction of translation, synovitis, joint effusion, acute or chronic changes of condylar position or morphology, and their effects on the dental occlusion, changes of the mandibular condyle (regressive remodeling, osteoarthrosis, and possibly osteonecrosis). Bone changes vary from early stages of marrow edema to focal or generalized necrosis; articular surface irregularity ranges from chondromalacia to osteoarthrosis to collapse secondary to subchondral osteonecrosis; localized form of osteonecrosis is osteochondritis dissecans (OCD).

• ID is characterized by stages based on degree of disc displacement and whether the disc is reducing or nonreducing (reflecting degree of displacement and deformity of the disc.) Chronic, advanced stages of ID are often characterized by short, deformed, immobile discs, and secondary degenerative bone changes. If the dentoalveolar structures are able to compensate by extrusion or intrusion, the gross occlusion will be maintained in spite of condylar morphologic changes. Failure to compensate may be manifested by anterior open bite, mandibular retrusion, and/or lateral asymmetry. Lateral pterygoid muscle fibrosis and foreshortening are accompaniments of chronic ID. Alterations of synovial fluid composition may influence its lubrication characteristics which may impede disc mobility and therefore joint mobility, possibly contributing to acute closed lock. Synovitis or inflammation of the synovium is commonly encountered in painful ID and may be accompanied by transudation of fluid into the joint space causing an effusion. Capsular fibrosis may develop in response to chronic synovitis and TMJ hypomobility due to pain and/or mechanical restriction. Chronic synovitis may potentiate intracapsular joint space adhesions; depending on density of such adhesions, ankylosis may develop (fibrous or osseous), further restricting mobility.
• Intracapsular disorders may include traumatic injuries, including condylar fractures, hemarthrosis, disc dislocation secondary to "whiplash" or to direct blows to the mandible. May also include mandibular hypermobility due to laxity of capsular ligaments, often resulting in recurrent open locking of the jaw unrelated to disc disturbances.

ETIOLOGY

• Controversial
• Macro and microtrauma
• Bruxism
• Anxiety-produced parafunctional habits
• Estrogen-associated ligamental laxity

SYSTEMS AFFECTED
Musculoskeletal

DIAGNOSIS

Largely through history

SYMPTOMS AND SIGNS
• Limited jaw mobility, acute occlusal alterations, swelling, local capsular tenderness, joint noises such as crepitus or click (noted by palpation or auscultation), masticatory and cervical muscle tenderness are supportive of the diagnosis.
• Most TMJ disorders present with local or regional pain (headaches, otalgia, cervical pain), sometimes with decreased jaw mobility, occlusal changes, or joint noise. Tinnitus and ear pressure are common. Progressive facial skeletal change (apertognathia, mandibular retrognathia, lateral asymmetry) may be a reflection of chronic TMJ disorders, sometimes not marked by protracted periods of pain or disability. Facial numbness is an occasional complaint which, if persistent, should prompt investigation of possible unrelated causes. Marked weight loss, malaise, and other constitutional symptoms may occur, but extreme presentations should again provoke further investigation of possible non-TMJ causes.

LABORATORY
If other joints symptomatic, consider rheumatoid work-up.

IMAGING/SPECIAL TESTS
• Screening radiographs (panoramic, transcranial, etc.) are appropriate to evaluate for degenerative bone changes. Magnetic resonance imaging (MRI) using T1 and T2 images allows visualization of disc position, effusions, muscle fibrosis, marrow edema, and possible osteonecrosis.
• Arthrograms (radiopaque dye into joint spaces) permit excellent visualization of disc position.
• Diagnostic injections (eg, auriculotemporal block) may assist in defining origin of pain.

DIFFERENTIAL
• Myofascial dysfunction syndrome
• Neoplasm
• Infectious arthritis
• Rheumatoid changes

TREATMENT

General
◇ Basic treatment includes joint rest (soft diet) and ice application. Physical therapy may help with cervical or masticatory muscle contraction pain. Occlusal splint devices (centric relation) may unload the TMJs by diminishing masticatory muscle spasm. Narcotic analgesics may be appropriate in some cases.

MEDICATIONS
• Anti-inflammatory drugs, possibly muscle relaxants.
• Intra-articular injection of local anesthetic may be helpful acutely; steroid injection is rarely indicated.
• Nonsteroidal anti-inflammatory medications work best for articular disease when given continuously over a few weeks, then taper and stop. Monitor for signs of gastrointestinal side effects (pain, bleeding).

SURGERY
• Surgical treatment appropriate for severe pain and/or severe restriction of jaw movement if other therapies fail.
• Arthroscopic surgery allows lavage of upper space, debridement of adhesions and chondromalacia, and possible improvement in disc position.
• Arthroplasty involves a direct open approach to the TMJ and is appropriate for severe ankylosis, advanced stages of ID, advanced stages of bone degeneration, and for removal of previously placed implants. Various grafts or flaps have been used as disc replacements (temporalis fascia or muscle, auricular cartilage, dermis), but none proven superior. Core decompression of the condyle has been discussed as possibly effective for early stages of osteonecrosis. Advanced condylar degeneration may require costochondral graft reconstruction or total prosthetic joint replacement. Condylar core decompression with marrow graft may be considered. Aggressive mobilization postoperatively is mandatory following surgery. Splint treatment is typically helpful before, as well after surgery.

CONSULTATION SUGGESTIONS
Oral-Maxillofacial Surgeon, Orthodontist, Other dentists with special training

REFERRAL SUGGESTIONS
Oral-Maxillofacial Surgeon, Orthodontist, Other dentists with special training

FIRST STEPS TO TAKE IN AN EMERGENCY
• Acute dislocation of jaw can be managed with sedation with diazepam, and manual reduction using downward and backward pressure on posterior mandibular teeth.

PATIENT INSTRUCTIONS
• Limit use of jaw for chewing
• Begin NSAIDs

COURSE/PROGNOSIS
Acute pain or locking that fails to resolve in 1 to 2 weeks likely to run protracted course. Degenerative changes often occur that may leave patient with limited jaw function.

CODING

ICD-9-CM
524.60 TMJ pain/dysfunction

CPT
20605 Arthrocentesis
21010 Arthrotomy TMJ
21050 Condylectomy TMJ
21060 Menisectomy TMJ
21085 Impression and custom preparation, oral surgical splint
21110 Application of interdental fixation
21116 Injection for TMJ arthrography
21240 Arthroplasty TMJ (autograft)
21242 Arthroplasty TMJ (alloplast)
21243 Arthroplasty prosthetic TMJ replacement
29800 Arthroscopy
64450 Diagnostic injection
70328 Radiologic exam, TMJ, open and closed mouth, unilateral
70330 bilateral
70332 TMJ arthrography
70336 MRI, TMJ
70355 Panorex
90799 Unlisted therapeutic injection
97010 Physical medicine, hot or cold packs
97014 Electrical stimulation
97110 Physical medicine therapeutic exercises

MISCELLANEOUS

SYNONYMS
Internal derangement

SEE ALSO
TMJ
◇ Extracapsular
Rheumatoid arthritis

REFERENCES
Israel HA: Current concepts in the surgical management of the temporomandibular joint. J Oral Maxillofac Surg 52:289-294, 1994.

Nickerson JW, Moystad A: Observations on individuals with radiographic bilateral condylar remodeling. A clinical study. J Craniomand Pract 1:21-37, 1983.

Chuong R, Piper MA: Avascular necrosis of the mandibular condyle
◇ pathogenesis concepts of management. Oral Surg Oral Med Oral Path 75:428-32, 1993.

AUTHOR
Robert Chuong, MD, DMD

Tetanus

BASICS

DESCRIPTION
An acute life-threatening infection caused by the bacterium Clostridium tetani.

ETIOLOGY

• Laceration/puncture wound contaminated by C. tetani spores.
• Associated with pregnancy or abortion if uterine contents contaminated with C. Tetani-containing instruments.
• Parental drug abuse another means of acquiring disease.

SYSTEMS AFFECTED
Spinal Cord
  ◇ toxin suppresses spinal reflex, which are inhibitory pathways, leading to generalized muscle spasms.
Mouth
  ◇ trismus results from closing muscle dominance over opening muscles.

DIAGNOSIS

SYMPTOMS AND SIGNS
General
  ◇ restlessness, fever
Cardiovascular
  ◇ tachycardia, hypertension, dysrhythmias.
Muscle
  ◇ muscle spasm, rigidity with stiffness of back, neck, thighs, abdomen, chest.
Face
  ◇ trismus, stiffness of facial muscles (risus sardonicus), dysphagia from pharyngeal spasm, laryngeal spasm.
Respiratory
  ◇ respiratory arrest from diaphragmatic, intercostal, glottal, or laryngeal spasm.
Neurologic -
  • Exaggerated deep tendon reflexes
  • Generalized muscle rigidity/spasm with flexion in upper extremities
  • Extensor posturing in torso and lower extremities.
  • Sudden noise, bright light may precipitate tonic seizures
Cephalic tetanus
  ◇ special form with effects of toxin limited to brain stem following introduction of spores into head and neck. Trismus is early sign.

LABORATORY
CBC
  ◇ leukocytosis
Cultures
  ◇ C. tetani only isolated 30% of time.

IMAGING/SPECIAL TESTS
ECG
  ◇ supraventricular tachycardia, bradycardia, multifocal premature ventricular contractions (PVCs).
EEG
  ◇ sleeping pattern

DIFFERENTIAL
• Tetanus
• Acute strychnine toxicity
• Encephalitis with trismus
• Trismus associated with masticator space infection
• Hepatic encephalopathy with muscular stiffness, rigidity
• Hysteria
• Dystonic response to phenothiazines

TREATMENT

General
◇ Avoid sudden stimuli that may precipitate muscle spasms.
◇ Enteral nutrition as oral feeding may trigger pharyngeal or laryngeal spasm, consider tube feeding or parenteral nutrition.
◇ May require nasoendotracheal intubation or tracheotomy to manage/protect airway.
◇ wound debridement only after immunoglobulin and control of spasms.

MEDICATIONS
Antitoxin
◇ neutralize circulating toxin.
• Antitoxin (Human tetanus immunoglobulin)
    • Local infiltrations at wound and intramuscular. Neutralized circulating toxin.
• Sedatives/muscle relaxants
    ◇ diazepam.
• Non-depolarizing muscle relaxants
• Beta adrenergic blocker
    ◇ propranolol
• Penicillin 10 to 15 million units/day
    ◇ Eliminate bacteria that could produce additional toxin.
• Tetanus toxoid
    ◇ Immunize against future infections.

CONSULTATION SUGGESTIONS
Critical Care Physician, Neurologist

REFERRAL SUGGESTIONS
Primary Care Physician, Neurologist

FIRST STEPS TO TAKE IN AN EMERGENCY
• Patient must be admitted to intensive care unit immediately if tetanus suspected.

PATIENT INSTRUCTIONS
Stay current with tetanus immunizations. Receive boosters if contaminated and/or deep puncture wound occurs.

COURSE/PROGNOSIS
Following inoculation, symptoms begin by 12 weeks in 80% of cases. Mortality is related to length of incubation with high mortality for short incubation periods. In 60% of cases, generalized spasms occur in 72 hours or less. After peak, illness symptoms will persist for a week, then decrease over several weeks. Survival depends on adequate airway management and management of sympathetic hyperactivity. Mortality is 35 to 40% when the incubation period is greater than 10 days.

CODING

ICD-9-CM
037.0 Tetanus

CPT
11000 Excision of infected skin (up to 10% of body surface)
90703 Tetanus toxoid immunization

MISCELLANEOUS

SYNONYMS
Lock jaw

REFERENCES
Simon HB, Swartz MN: Anaerobic Infections. In: Scientific American Medicine, Section 7, Subsection V. Rubenstein E, Federman DD (eds), New York, Scientific American, Inc., 1989, pp. 8-12.

Hupp JR: Infections of Soft Tissues of the Maxillofacial and Neck Regions. In: Oral and Maxillofacial Infections, 3rd ed. Topazian RG, Goldberg MH (eds), Philadelphia, WB Saunders Co., 1994, pp. 338-359.

AUTHOR
Samuel J. McKenna, DDS, MD

Thromboangiitis Obliterans, Buerger's Disease

BASICS

DESCRIPTION
• A segmental thrombotic occlusion of small and medium-sized arterial vessels, most commonly affecting the distal arms and legs. The ischemia results in pain, tissue loss, and potential limb loss.
• The overall incidence in North American is 11.6 per 100,000. Large numbers of cases are reported in the Middle East, Asia, and Far East. The median age at onset is 34 years with a male to female ratio of 7.5:1. Upon presentation, 30 to 40% have presence of superficial thrombophlebitis or Raynaud's phenomenon.

ETIOLOGY

Currently, the cause of this process is unknown. Strongly linked to smoking as a permissive factor. It also has a distinct geographic distribution around the world. The pathology of this disease was felt to be a vasculitis, but now there exists controversy regarding this issue. The histopathology of the acute lesion is a hypercellular intraluminal thrombus with inflammation of the vessel wall and giant cell foci. No inflammation or destruction of the elastic lamina occurs as is seen in a true vasculitis.

SYSTEMS AFFECTED
• The upper and lower distal extremity arterial vasculature.
• Rarely the abdominal mesentery.

DIAGNOSIS

SYMPTOMS AND SIGNS
• Usually presentation is of a 25 to 35 year old male with relatively sudden lower extremity rest pain with ensuing tissue loss. When claudication occurs, it affects the instep of the foot involved. Extremity coolness or sensitivity to cold, paresthesias.
• Pulses beyond the brachial and popliteal are diminished or entirely absent. Usually two to four limbs are affected at presentation, with signs of ischemic pain, cold, pallor, neurosensory changes, possible mottling. Raynaud's phenomenon, pedal edema, on elevation of extremity.

LABORATORY
• Hypercoagulable evaluation: Protein C, Protein S, anti-Thrombin III, antiphospholipid levels, lupus anticoagulant, platelet aggregometry, and reactivity
• Biopsy

IMAGING/SPECIAL TESTS
• Segmental arterial Doppler pressures and waveforms nonspecific
• Hand radiographs (rule out calcinosis).
• Arteriography multiple areas of segmental occlusion (skip areas may be present).
• Digital cold sensitivity

DIFFERENTIAL
• Diabetes peripheral neuropathy
• Renal disease
• Hypercoagulable state eg, secondary to occult malignancy
• Raynaud's disease
• Atherosclerotic disease
• Peripheral vasculitis
• Scleroderma
• Gout
• Polyarteritis nodosa

TREATMENT

General
◇ The single most important factor is to have the patient stop smoking. The entire basis of treatment for this disease is based upon the observation that cessation has been found to have the most important prognostic factor in successful treatment of this disease. Even users of snuff and chewing tobacco are at risk. Therefore, all tobacco use must be immediately curtailed.

◇ Treatment is aimed to be supportive and conservative in nature. For the ischemic pain, narcotics and reverse Trendelenberg are necessary. Usually lower extremity outcome is worse than the upper extremities.

MEDICATIONS
• If gangrene is present, hospital admission and systemic anticoagulation with heparin is instituted. Infections of affected toes or fingers are treated with standard antibiotic protocols.

• Medical therapy consists of calcium channel blockers, anti-platelet therapy, and pentoxyfilline. None of these has been conclusively shown to have beneficial effect, but are used due to the minimal side-effect profile. Corticosteroids are of questionable use and do not appear to alter the prognosis.

SURGERY
• Bypass surgery is not successful due to obliteration of distal arterial vasculature.

• Approximately 20% of patients with affected lower extremity have toe or transmetatarsal amputation. An overlapping population of 20% need either above the knee or below the knee amputation.

CONSULTATION SUGGESTIONS
Primary Care Physician

REFERRAL SUGGESTIONS
Primary Care Physician

PATIENT INSTRUCTIONS
Curtail or stop smoking critical

COURSE/PROGNOSIS
The life expectancy of patients with Buerger's disease approaches that of age-matched control population.

CODING

ICD-9-CM
443.1 Thromboangiitis obliterans

MISCELLANEOUS

SEE ALSO
Diabetes mellitus
Polyarteritis nodosa

REFERENCES
Creager MA, Dzau VJ: Vascular Diseases of the Extremities. In: Harrison's Principles of Internal Medicine, 13th ed. Isselbacher KJ, et al (eds). New York, McGraw-Hill Inc., 1994, p. 1137.

Mills JL, Porter JM: Buerger's Disease: A Review and Update, Sem Vascular Surg 6:14-23, 1983.

Young JF: Treatment of Upper Extremity Vasospastic Disorders. In: Current Therapy in Vascular Surgery. Philadelphia, BC Decker Inc., 1991, pp. 193-198.

Nonatherosclerotic Vascular Disease. BC in: Vascular Surgery: A Comprehensive Review, Moore WS (ed). Philadelphia., WB Saunders Co., 1993, pp. 119-121.

AUTHOR
Roger S. Badwal, DMD, MD

Thyroglossal Duct Cyst

 BASICS

DESCRIPTION
A slowly expanding cyst of the midline upper anterior neck midline that forms from remnants of the embryologic descent of the thyroid gland into the lower neck. It can become secondarily infected.

 ETIOLOGY

Forms from remnants of the thyroglossal duct, the embryologic tract that the thyroid gland follows as it descends from the posterior tongue to the anterior neck.

SYSTEMS AFFECTED
<u>Integumentary</u>
◊ secondary infection can produce chronic draining sinus through overlying skin.
<u>Immune</u>
◊ secondary infection can result in serious infection with development of neck abscess, requiring hospitalization.
<u>Endocrine</u>
◊ thyroglossal duct cyst can harbor functioning thyroid tissue.

 DIAGNOSIS

SYMPTOMS AND SIGNS
<u>Neck</u>
◊ painless mass in region of hyoid bone.
- pain is present if secondary infection has occurred.
- rapid enlargement can be noted following upper respiratory infection.
- cystic lesion of upper anterior neck, most often seen in children, but may be found at any age.
- moves on tongue protrusion and with swallowing.
- location is characteristically at or near midline, in area of hyoid bone, although cyst(s) can potentially occur at any point between tongue base and thyroid gland.

LABORATORY
- Elevated WBC if cyst infected.
- Thyroid function tests are not affected.

IMAGING/SPECIAL TESTS
<u>CT Scan</u>
◊ will clearly demonstrate lesion, although not absolutely required for treatment .
<u>Thyroid scan</u>
◊ will demonstrate location of functioning thyroid tissue. In approximately 7% of cases, the thyroid gland will fail to fully descend into the neck and the thyroglossal duct cyst will be the only functioning thyroid tissue in the body.
- Histologic examination reveals either stratified squamous or columnar epithelium lined cyst. Thyroid tissue may be seen within connective tissue wall. Inflammatory cells may be present if infected.

DIFFERENTIAL
- Dermoid cyst
- "Plunging" ranula
- Lymphadenopathy involving submental lymph nodes
- Epidermoid cyst of neck skin
- Teratoma

Thyroglossal Duct Cyst

TREATMENT

MEDICATIONS
• Antibiotic treatment of secondary infection based on cultures and sensitivity of aspirate.

SURGERY
• Drainage is reserved for acute infection with abscess formation.
• Comprehensive surgical removal requires removal of the central 1/3 of the hyoid bone, (Sistrunk procedure).

CONSULTATION SUGGESTIONS
Oral-Maxillofacial Surgeon

REFERRAL SUGGESTIONS
Oral-Maxillofacial Surgery, Otolaryngology

COURSE/PROGNOSIS
• Recurrence rate of approximately 3% following Sistrunk operation.
• Removal of central 1/3 of hyoid bone produces minimal discomfort and no adverse functional sequelae.

CODING

ICD-9-CM
759.2 Cyst, thyroglossal (duct) (infected) (persistent)

CPT
60000 Incision and drainage of thyroglossal cyst, infected
60280 Excision of thyroglossal duct cyst or sinus
60281 Recurrent

MISCELLANEOUS

SYNONYMS
Thyroglossal cyst
Thyroglossal tract cyst

SEE ALSO
Dermoid cyst
Neck masses

REFERENCES
Pincus RL: Congenital neck masses and cysts. In: Head & Neck Surgery
◇ Otolaryngology. Bailey BJ (ed). Philadelphia, JB Lippincott Co., Philadelphia, 1993, p 755.

AUTHOR
Eric J. Dierks, DMD, MD

Tonsillitis

BASICS

DESCRIPTION
• Condition is characterized by inflammation of the palatine tonsils.
• More common in children and adolescents.

ETIOLOGY

• β-hemolytic streptococci
• Adenoviruses

SYSTEMS AFFECTED
Gastrointestinal

DIAGNOSIS

SYMPTOMS AND SIGNS
• Sore throat
• Pain on swallowing and radiating to the ear (bacterial infections)
• Headache
• Malaise
• Nausea
• Swelling and hyperemia of the tonsils
• Purulent exudate or yellow stippling
• Cervical adenopathy
• Rigors, marked toxemia, thirst, and oliguria (severe cases)
• Slight difficulty opening mouth
• Thickened speech

LABORATORY
• Elevated ESR
• Shift to left (WBCs)
• Culture

IMAGING/SPECIAL TESTS
Referral for cardiovascular examination and renal function tests may be indicated if Streptococcal infection discovered.

DIFFERENTIAL
• Viral versus Bacterial
• Diphtheria
• Infectious mononucleosis
• Agranulocytosis
• Leukemia
• Herpangina
• Scarlet fever
• Vincent's angina

TREATMENT

General
◇ Rest
◇ Fluids
◇ Salt water gargles
◇ Analgesics

MEDICATIONS
• Penicillin is the drug of choice and is administered as Penicillin V, 500 mg q.i.d. (25 to 50 mg/kg/day) for 7 to 10 days.
• For patients allergic to penicillin, give erythromycin ethyl succinate 300 to 400 mg t.i.d. (30 mg/kg/day) or cephalexin 500 mg q.i.d. (30 mg/kg/day).

SURGERY
Repeated attacks of acute tonsillitis may necessitate tonsillectomy.

CONSULTATION SUGGESTIONS
Otolaryngologist

REFERRAL SUGGESTIONS
Primary Care Physician

FIRST STEPS TO TAKE IN AN EMERGENCY
• If airway compromised or patient septic, arrange immediate transport to emergency facility.

COURSE/PROGNOSIS
• Resolves uneventfully in most cases.
• Complications include peritonsillar abscess, laryngeal edema, septicemia, otitis media, mastoiditis, sinusitis.
• Streptococcal tonsillitis can lead to rheumatic fever and glomerulonephritis if not adequately treated.

 ## CODING

ICD-9-CM
034.0 Streptococcal tonsillitis
463 Viral tonsillitis

 ## MISCELLANEOUS

SEE ALSO
Pharyngitis
Herpangina

REFERENCES
Wyngaarden JB, Smith LH (eds): Cecil Textbook of Medicine. 19th ed. Philadelphia, WB Saunders Co., 1992.

Gray RF, Hawthorne M: Synopsis of Otolaryngology. 5th ed. Oxford. Butterworth-Heinemann Ltd., 1992.

Tierney LM, McPhee SJ, Papadakis MA, Schroeder SA (eds): Current Medical Diagnosis & Treatment. East Norwalk, CT, Appleton & Lange, 1993.

AUTHOR
Vivek Shetty, DDS, DMD

Tori/Exostosis

BASICS

DESCRIPTION
• Benign, bony, circumscribed protuberances located on the lingual aspect of the mandible opposite the premolars (mandibular tori), midline of the palate (palatal tori), and buccal or labial aspect of the mandibular or maxillary alveolus (exostoses).
• The overlying soft tissues are usually thin and may appear pale.
• Trauma to the soft tissues may result in a painful, slowly healing ulceration.
• Seldom of clinical significance unless ulcerated; may cause speech difficulties (mandibular tori), interfere with prosthetic reconstruction (mandibular, maxillary tori, and exostoses), or difficulties with oral hygiene (exostosis).
• Tori commonly occur before the age of 30 years of age.
• Mandibular tori usually bilateral.

ETIOLOGY
• Mandibular tori show an inherited pattern, are equally distributed among the sexes, and are found in 5 to 10% of the adult population; they are commonly found in Aleuts and Alaskan Eskimos (up to 80%).
• Palatal tori show an inherited pattern with a prevalence of 20 to 25% in the United States, and a female to male ratio of 2 to 1.
• Exostoses are less common than tori with an unknown etiology; some investigators have proposed that the bony growths represent a reaction to abnormal occlusal forces.

SYSTEMS AFFECTED
• Oral mucosa is more susceptible to trauma, resulting in painful ulceration.
• In the dentulous state, may interfere with oral hygiene and periodontal health.
• In the edentulous or partially edentulous state, may interfere with prosthetic reconstruction and, therefore, mastication.
• Extremely large maxillary or mandibular tori may interfere with speech.

DIAGNOSIS

SYMPTOMS AND SIGNS
• Most patients are asymptomatic and may be unaware of their presence.
• If large, may interfere with speech or mastication.
• Hard, nodular protuberances of bone in the respective areas of the mandible, palate, or facial alveolus of mandible or maxilla.

IMAGING/SPECIAL TESTS
Radiographs of large mandibular tori or mandibular/maxillary exostoses may demonstrate radiopaque masses. Imaging usually unnecessary unless diagnosis in doubt.

DIFFERENTIAL
• Palatal abscess of odontogenic origin (palatal tori).
• Salivary gland tumor (palatal tori).
• Lymphoma (palatal tori).
• Neoplasm of the maxilla or maxillary sinus (palatal tori or maxillary exostoses).
• Neoplasm of mandible (mandibular torus or exostoses).

TREATMENT

SURGERY
• Surgical treatment usually not necessary.
• Excision or reduction indicated if:
  1) Difficulty with speech or mastication
  2) Interference with construction of a prosthesis
  3) Chronic irritation/ulceration of overlying soft tissues
  4) Inability to maintain adequate oral hygiene or
  5) Fear of cancer (cancerophobia)

CONSULTATION SUGGESTIONS
Oral-Maxillofacial Surgeon, Prosthodontist

REFERRAL SUGGESTIONS
Oral-Maxillofacial Surgeon, Prosthodontist
• Patient Instructions
• Reassure process completely benign.

COURSE/PROGNOSIS
Benign condition with infrequent complications or need for surgery.

CODING

ICD-9-CM
528.9 Exostosis of Jaw

CPT
21031 Excision of torus mandibularis
21032 Excision of maxillary torus palatinus

MISCELLANEOUS

SYNONYMS
Torus palatinus
Torus mandibularis

SEE ALSO
Benign jaw tumors

REFERENCES
Regezi JA, Sciubba J: Oral Pathology Clinical Pathologic Correlations, 2nd ed. Philadelphia, WB Saunders, 1993, pp. 416-418.

Eckles RL, Miller RI: Tori. A common but neglected entity. Gen Dent 36:417-420, 1988.

Rezal RF, Jackson JT, Salamat K: Torus palatinus, an exostosis of unknown etiology: Review of the literature. Compend Cont Ed 6:149-152, 1985.

Peterson LJ, Ellis E, Hupp JR, Tucker MR: Contemporary Oral and Maxillofacial Surgery, 2nd ed. St. Louis, CV Mosby Co., 1993, pp. 310-316.

AUTHOR
Dennis L. Johnson, DDS, MS

Torticollis

BASICS

DESCRIPTION
The sign or symptom of torticollis (literally "twisted neck") denotes a fixed or posturing of the head and neck in a tilt, rotation, or flexion. It may be due to congenital and acquired deformities of both organic and psychogenic origin.

ETIOLOGY
Congenital muscular torticollis
   ◊ possibly a venous occlusion in utero involving a firm, cartilaginous-like "tumor" of the sternocleidomastoid muscle
Congenital vertebral maldevelopment
Acquired torticollis
   Traumatic
   ◊ rotary subluxation, fracture/ dislocation, muscular injury, basilar skull fracture.
   Infection
   ◊ cervical osteomyelitis, discitis, tuberculosis, retropharyngeal abscess, vestibular infection (most commonly otitis media), cervical adenitis.
   Calcified cervical disc
   Ligamentous laxity and synovitis due to adjacent inflammation
   ◊ pseudosubluxation.
   Juvenile rheumatoid arthritis
   Tumor of cervical spine
   ◊ metastasis, osteoid osteoma/ osteoblastoma, eosinophilic granuloma, rare primary bone/ muscle tumors.
   Other tumors
   ◊ midbrain tumor, posterior fossa/ other cranial tumors, cervical cord tumor, lymphoma, acoustic neuroma, orbital tumor.
   Atlanto-occipital subluxations
   ◊ associated with Down's syndrome, mucopolysaccharidosis, and other conditions causing ligamentous laxity.
   Vestibular
   ◊ mastoiditis, paroxysmal torticollis of infancy, peripheral vestibular disease.
   Miscellaneous
   ◊ migraine headache, myasthenia gravis, associated gastrointestinal reflux, syringomyelia, habitual/ hysterical, oculogyric crisis (phenothiazine overdose).

SYSTEMS AFFECTED
Congenital muscular torticollis
   ◊ short, inelastic sternocleidomastoid muscle, cervical vertebrae normal.
Congenital vertebral maldevelopment:
Acquired torticollis
   Orthopedic abnormalities
   Ocular abnormalities
   ◊ abnormal head tilt to compensate for strabismus.
   Otolaryngologic abnormalities
   ◊ dysfunction of the vestibular system.
   Neurologic abnormalities
   ◊ long tract and cerebellar signs, or cranial nerve palsies in conjunction with torticollis.

DIAGNOSIS

SYMPTOMS AND SIGNS
Congenital
   ◊ residual torticollis and possible facial asymmetry.
Acquired
   ◊ head tilt, mild to moderate pain in cervical spine.

LABORATORY
Rule out inflammatory conditions with white blood count, ESR, and rheumatoid factor.

IMAGING/SPECIAL TESTS
Bone scanning, computed tomography (CT), magnetic resonance imaging (MRI), myelography, plain roentgenography.

DIFFERENTIAL
 • Congenital, birth injury versus severe maldevelopment of the cervical vertebrae; ocular, secondary, and spasmodic (adult), and benign paroxysmal (child 1 to 5 years old) torticollis.
 • Acquired structural and acquired nonstructural torticollis.
 • CNS infections
 • Soft or hard tissue neoplasms
 • Myositis of cervical musculature
 • Cervical disk lesions (eg, spondylosis)

TREATMENT

General
◇ A meticulous and thorough search for the etiology important because problems associated with torticollis that can be serious or life-threatening. If due to birth injury, a short-term use of soft cervical collar may help. Spasmodic torticollis benefits from physical therapy, heat, massage, NSAIDs. Psychiatric care may be indicated.

MEDICATIONS
• Some now trying use of botulinum toxin injections for muscle induced torticollis.

CONSULTATION SUGGESTIONS
Orthopedic Surgeon, Neurologist, Ophthalmologist, Otolaryngologist, Pediatrician, Plastic Surgeon

REFERRAL SUGGESTIONS
Primary Care Physician

PATIENT INSTRUCTIONS
Patient can apply own physical therapy measures, in addition to those provided by therapist.

COURSE/PROGNOSIS
Prognosis excellent when etiology is not structural.

CODING

ICD-9-CM
300.11 Hysterical torticollis
306.0 Psychogenic torticollis
333.83 Spasmodic torticollis
714.0 Rheumatoid torticollis
723.5 Intermittent torticollis
754.1 Congenital torticollis
767.8 Torticollis due to birth injury

CPT
97010 Physical medicine (hot or cold packs)
97110 Physical medicine treatment to one area 30 minutes
97112 Neuromuscular reeducation
97118 Electrical stimulation
97124 Massage
97128 Ultrasound
97260 Cervical manipulation
97799 Unlisted physical medicine procedure

MISCELLANEOUS

SYNONYMS
Wryneck
Spasmodic torticollis

SEE ALSO
Cervical adenopathy

REFERENCES
Cronin TD, Barrera A: Deformities of the Cervical Region In: Plastic Surgery, Vol. 3. McCarthy JG (ed), Philadelphia, WB Saunders, 1990, pp. 2085-2093.

Kahn ML, et al: Acquired torticollis in children. Orthopaedic Rev 20:667-674, 1991.

Tachdjian M: Pediatric Orthopedics. 2nd ed. Philadelphia, WB Saunders, 1990.

Akazawa H, et al: Congenital muscular torticollis: long-term follow-up of 38 partial resections of the sternocleidomastoid muscle. Arch Orthop Trauma Surg 112:205-209, 1993.

AUTHOR
Irene H.S. So, DMD

Toxoplasmosis

BASICS

DESCRIPTION
• Disease caused by infection with the protozoan Toxoplasma gondii. Primary infection of fetus damages vital organs.
• Mononucleosis-like infection occurs with acute toxoplasmosis, in immunocompetent patients.
• May result in necrotizing encephalitis, myocarditis, pneumonitis, and death when organism reactivated in immunocompromised patients.

ETIOLOGY

• Infection with the protozoan Toxoplasma gondii , endemic in most of the U.S. Acquired by eating uncooked infected meat containing cysts filled with organisms.
• Toxoplasma gondii exists in three forms
  1) Oocyst-form in mucosa of domestic cat intestines.
     Oocysts are excreted in the feces and remain infectious up to one year.
  2) Tachyzoite-invasive form of the disease that penetrates and replicates in all nucleated mammalian cells.
  3) Cysts-formed in organs (skeletal muscle, heart, and central nervous system) of infected animals including humans.

SYSTEMS AFFECTED
Eye, heart, lung, liver, brain, muscle.

DIAGNOSIS

The diagnosis varies as signs and symptoms are significantly different depending on the immunocompetence of the individual.

SYMPTOMS AND SIGNS
• Vary from none in immunocompetent people to severe, usually in immunocompromised patients.
• May include abdominal pain, confusion, malaise, stiffness, myalgia, arthralgia, headache, sore throat, and blurred vision.
• May persist for months.
• Immunocompetent patient:
   Mononucleosis-like presentation with cervical lymphadenopathy and fever.
   Hepatosplenomegaly
   Maculopapular rash
   Chorioretinitis with blurred vision, scotoma, pain, photophobia, epiphora, strabismus and decreased vision.
• Immunocompromised patient:
   Rapidly fatal with CNS involvement as the first presenting sign (50% of patients)
   Headache, focal neurological deficit, seizures, mental status changes.

LABORATORY
• Isolate Toxoplasma gondii from body fluid, blood, or tissues.
• Trophozoites in histologic specimens.
• Serology: IFA, IHA, ELISA

IMAGING/SPECIAL TESTS
• Sabin-Feldman dye test
• Skin test using Toxoplasma antigen
• CT scan may show CNS involvement
• Lymph node biopsy reveals reactive follicular hyperplasia with irregular clusters of epithelioid histiocytes.

DIFFERENTIAL
• Lymphoma
• Infectious mononucleosis
• Cytomegalovirus
• Sarcoidosis
• TB
• Leukemia
• Fungal disease
• Herpes encephalitis
• Cat scratch disease

TREATMENT

• The need and duration of treatment determined by the severity.
• Immunocompetent patients with lymphoadenopathic toxoplasmosis require no treatment.
• Patients with chorioretinitis require specific treatment.
• All patients with immunocompromise require aggressive treatment.

MEDICATIONS
• Combination treatment with pyrimethamine (Daraprim) and sulfadiazine (Microsulfon).
• Bone marrow depression with pyrimethamine, so weekly CBC, folinic acid supplementation indicated.
• Treat for 4 to 6 weeks beyond resolution of signs and symptoms. Clindamycin and corticosteroids may be useful for ocular involvement.

SURGERY
Lymph node biopsy

CONSULTATION SUGGESTIONS
Ophthalmologist (if eye involved)

REFERRAL SUGGESTIONS
Infectious Disease Specialist, Primary Care Physician

PATIENT INSTRUCTIONS
Prevention by adequate preparation of meats and avoid contact with cat feces, particularly by pregnant individuals.

COURSE/PROGNOSIS
Immunocompetent patient
◇ excellent chance for complete recovery.
Immunocompromised patient
◇ poor prognosis.

CODING

ICD-9-CM
130.9 Toxoplasmosis

MISCELLANEOUS

SEE ALSO
Human immunodeficiency virus (HIV)

REFERENCES
Marr JJ: Toxoplasmosis. In: Textbook of Internal Medicine. Kelly WN (ed). Philadelphia, JB Lippincott, 1989, pp. 1690-1694.

Decker CF, Tuazon CU: Toxoplasmosis: An update on clinical and therapeutic Prog Clin Parasitol 3:21-41, 1993.

AUTHOR
Peter E. Larsen, DDS

Tracheitis

BASICS

DESCRIPTION
• Acute viral tracheitis is a poorly defined but common clinical condition that is often associated with bronchitis (tracheobronchitis) or laryngitis (laryngotracheobronchitis).
• Bacterial tracheitis, also called pseudomembranous croup, is an uncommon disease of childhood, with rapid onset and severe progressive course.

ETIOLOGY

• Viral tracheitis
  Parainfluenza viruses
  Influenza A and B viruses
  Respiratory syncytial virus
  Adenovirus
• Bacterial tracheitis
  Staphylococcus aureus
  Haemophilus influenzae
  Streptococcus species (usually β-hemolytic group A)

SYSTEMS AFFECTED
Respiratory

DIAGNOSIS

SYMPTOMS AND SIGNS
• Cough
• Retrosternal pain
• Difficulty breathing (dyspnea), especially in children
• Symptoms of upper respiratory tract infection
• Fever
• Hoarse voice
• Harsh breath sounds audible over the trachea
• Toxic appearance
• Inspiratory stridor
• Copious tracheal secretions that are initially mucus and then purulent with expectoration.
• Edema of the larynx

LABORATORY
• Culture of secretions or aspirates during endoscopy.
• Leukocytosis with shift to left (WBCs)

IMAGING/SPECIAL TESTS
• Diagnostic imaging with survey radiographs of the cervical and thoracic soft tissues, eventually CT and MRI.
  Subglottic narrowing
  Hypopharyngeal distention
  Shaggy laryngeal wall
  Laryngoscopy
• Tracheobronchoscopy
  Adherent membrane on larynx
  Subglottic inflammation

DIFFERENTIAL
• Croup or laryngotracheobronchitis
• Diphtheria
• Bronchopneumonia
• Epiglottitis
• Bronchial foreign bodies
• Specific tracheobronchial infections (tuberculosis, sarcoidosis, syphilis)

TREATMENT

General
Viral tracheitis
Usually short-lived and takes a
benign course.
Treatment is mainly symptomatic,
aimed at controlling cough, chest
discomfort and fever.
Increase fluids.
Bacterial tracheitis
Rest and reassurance
Humidification of inspired air
Tracheal suctioning
Oxygen
Nasotracheal tube or tracheotomy
may be necessary
Monitoring of blood gases
Intravenous hydration

MEDICATIONS
• Relieve cough with hydrocodone,
codeine, or dextromethorphan.
• In viral tracheitis, systemic antibiotics
given only in patients with underlying
chronic obstructive pulmonary disease
or those with persistent cough
productive of purulent sputum, which
suggests possible secondary bacterial
infection.
• In bacterial tracheitis, the broad-
spectrum antibiotics are given
parenterally.
• Emperic antibody therapy usually
consists of amoxicillin (500 mg t.i.d.);
ampicillin, erythromycin, or tetracycline
(each in a dose of 250 to 500 mg
q.i.d.), or trimethoprim-sulfamethoxazole
(160/800 mg b.i.d.) given for 7 to 10
days.

CONSULTATION SUGGESTIONS
Primary Care Physician, Otolaryngologist

REFERRAL SUGGESTIONS
Primary Care Physician

FIRST STEPS TO TAKE IN AN EMERGENCY
• If symptoms of impending airway
compromise, accompany patient to
emergency facility.

PATIENT INSTRUCTIONS
Seek definitive care immediately.

COURSE/PROGNOSIS
Acute viral tracheitis
◊ complete recovery within 7 to 10
days.
Bacterial tracheitis
◊ complete recover, but may be
associated with complications, including
subglottic stenosis, sudden respiratory
arrest, pneumonia, and airway
granulomas.

CODING

ICD-9-CM
464.1 Acute tracheitis

MISCELLANEOUS

SYNONYMS
Bacterial tracheitis
Pseudomembranous croup

SEE ALSO
Tracheobronchitis
Epiglottitis

REFERENCES
Gray RF, Hawthorne M: Synopsis of
Otolaryngology. 5th ed. Oxford,
Butterworth-Heinemann Ltd., 1992.
Tierney LM, McPhee SJ, Papdakis MA,
Schroeder SA (eds): Current Medical
Diagnosis & Treatment. Norwalk, CT,
Appleton & Lange, 1993.
Dambro MR. Tracheitis. In: Griffith's Five
Minute Clinical Consult. Dambro M,
Griffith J (eds). Baltimore, Williams &
Wilkins, 1995, pp. 1066-1067.

AUTHOR
Vivek Shetty, DDS, DMD

Transfusion Reaction

BASICS

DESCRIPTION
An acute or delayed reaction occurring in response to intravenous administration of blood or blood products. While infectious sequelae (hepatitis, AIDS, cytomegalovirus) may also result from transfusions, these are not included in this description.

ETIOLOGY

An acute hemolytic reaction, the most severe, is usually due to blood group incompatibility; donor cells are directly attacked by antibodies and complement, leading to intravascular hemolysis. Fatality can occur through renal failure and/or disseminated intravascular coagulation (DIC). It is most common caused by error at the time of blood administration. Less severe reactions include delayed hemolytic reaction (recipients sensitized from previous transfusions possessing lower antibody levels) and nonhemolytic reactions (anaphylactoid, caused by foreign proteins in the transfused blood).

SYSTEMS AFFECTED
Cardiovascular, renal, and reticuloendothelial.

DIAGNOSIS

SYMPTOMS AND SIGNS
Fever, chills, flank and/or chest pain, headache, coughing, nausea and vomiting, dyspnea, flushing, hypotension, hemoglobinuria, bleeding diathesis.

LABORATORY
Hemoglobin/hematocrit, platelet count, partial thromboplastin time, serum fibrinogen level.

IMAGING/SPECIAL TESTS
Urine hemoglobin concentration, urine pH (must be kept alkaline to prevent precipitation of acidic hematin).

DIFFERENTIAL
When onset of symptoms is temporally related to the blood product administration, a transfusion reaction should be assumed until proven otherwise.

TREATMENT

General

1. At the first suspicion of a transfusion reaction, stop the transfusion. The severity of the reaction can be diminished by minimizing the volume of blood transfused.

2. Confirm the diagnosis of hemolysis through the presence of hemoglobin in urine and blood specimens.

3. Maintain oxygenation and perfusion, taking care to prevent hypotension.

4. Return unused blood products to blood bank along with new specimen of recipient blood for new cross-match.

5. Maintain urine output (75 to 100 mL/hr) with fluid boluses, diuretics (furosemide, mannitol), or dopamine.

6. Alkalinize the urine with 40 to 70 mEq/kg sodium bicarbonate.

7. Monitor coagulation profiles through serial PT, PTT, platelet count, and fibrinogen level.

MEDICATIONS
See general treatment above.

CONSULTATION SUGGESTIONS
Hematologist

REFERRAL SUGGESTIONS
Primary Care Physician

FIRST STEPS TO TAKE IN AN EMERGENCY
• See general treatment section

PATIENT INSTRUCTIONS
Patients having received blood products during early 1980s should consider being tested for infectious diseases such as HIV and hepatitis.

COURSE/PROGNOSIS
While the incidence of hemolytic transfusion reaction is about 1:5000, mortality can occur in 20% to 60% of patients when severe hemolysis occurs.

CODING

ICD-9-CM
999.8 Transfusion reaction

MISCELLANEOUS

The FDA requires all fatal transfusion reactions to be reported within 7 days.

SEE ALSO
Serum sickness

REFERENCES
Murray DJ: Blood component therapy: indications and risks. In: Principles and practice of anesthesiology. Rogers MC, Tinker JH, Covino BG, el al (eds), St. Louis, CV Mosby, 1993.

Miller RD: Transfusion therapy. In: Anesthesia, 3rd ed. Miller RD (ed), New York, Churchill Livingstone, 1990.

AUTHOR
Jeffrey B. Dembo, DDS, MS

Transient Ischemic Attack (TIA)

BASICS

DESCRIPTION
Acute cerebral ischemia resulting in the abrupt onset of a focal neurologic deficit with complete resolution in less than 24 hours.

ETIOLOGY

• Atherosclerotic narrowing of the carotid or vertebral arteries with release of platelet emboli into the cerebral circulation.
• Emboli from heart valve vegetation.
• Emboli associated with atrial fibrillation or acute myocardial infarction.
• Compression of carotid or vertebral artery by vertebral osteophyte.
• Transient decrease in blood pressure.
• Cardiac dysrhythmia that temporarily limits cardiac output.

Occult cardiac lesion
◇ patent foramen ovale, septal defect that permit emboli from venous side of circulation to reach the brain.

SYSTEMS AFFECTED
Cerebral hemispheres
◇ sudden, contralateral cerebral ischemia from carotid artery distribution occlusion.

Brainstem, cerebellum, occipital lobes
◇ sudden neurologic deficit from ischemia of areas in the distribution of the vertebral arteries.

Retina
◇ sudden unilateral retinal ischemia from carotid artery distribution occlusion (amaurosis fugax).

DIAGNOSIS

SYMPTOMS AND SIGNS
Cerebral hemisphere ischemia
◇ contralateral neurologic symptoms of muscle weakness, sensory loss, aphasia, visual disturbance.

Brainstem, cerebellum, occipital cortex ischemia
◇ dimming of vision or total transient blindness, vertigo, nausea, vomiting, dysarthria, dysphagia, perioral numbness, weakness and/or sensory disturbance of all extremities, abrupt memory loss, and confusion.

Eye
◇ retinal ischemia with transient unilateral blindness often described as shade being pulled over one eye. Possible cholesterol and/or platelet emboli in retinal vessels.

Neck
◇ possible carotid and/or vertebral artery bruit(s).

LABORATORY
• CBC
• Prothrombin time for those patients taking an anticoagulant.
• Antiphospholipid antibodies.

IMAGING/SPECIAL TESTS
ECG
◇ to investigate for possible cardiac dysrhythmia.

Head CT
◇ will show areas of focal ischemia in 20% with TIA.

Neck and transcranial doppler ultrasound
◇ non-invasive technique to diagnose stenotic vessels and effect on blood flow.

Cerebral arteriography
◇ used selectively to visualize stenotic vessels, especially in those patients considered for endarterectomy.

Magnetic resonance angiography
◇ new MRI technique for imaging blood vessels.

Echocardiography
◇ if heart suspected as source of emboli.

Holter monitoring for transient dysrhythmias.

DIFFERENTIAL
• Atherosclerotic cerebrovascular disease.
• Emboli associated with cardiac valvular lesions, occult cardiac lesion, dysrhythmia, myocardial infarction.
• Osteophyte compression of blood vessel.
• Transient drop in blood pressure
• Evolving stroke (50% with stroke have premonitory TIA).
• Migraine
• Hypoglycemia
• Focal seizure

TREATMENT

General
Modify risk factors
◇ control hypertension, cessation of smoking, modify risk factors for ischemic heart disease.

MEDICATIONS
• Antiplatelet agents
◇ enteric coated aspirin, ticlopidine (250 mp p.o. b.i.d.).
• Coumadin
◇ in patients at risk for emboli of cardiac origin.

SURGERY
Carotid endarterectomy
◇ decreases risk of major and/or fatal stroke in patients with 70 to 99% narrowing of symptomatic internal carotid artery. Also recommended for large ulcerative carotid plaques and recurrent TIAs in spite of medical therapy.

CONSULTATION SUGGESTIONS
Neurologist, Cardiologist, Vascular Surgeon

REFERRAL SUGGESTIONS
Neurologist, Primary Care Physician

PATIENT INSTRUCTIONS
Patients can contact National Stroke Association for helpful information: 300 E. Hampden Ave., Suite 240, Englewood, CO 80110. 303-771-1700.

COURSE/PROGNOSIS
Patients with TIAs are at high risk for recurrent cerebral ischemic attacks. Reduction of blood pressure, cessation of smoking, use of antiplatelet drugs, and selective application of carotid endarterectomy can reduce the risk of stroke.

 CODING

ICD-9-CM
434.0 Occlusion of cerebral arteries
435.0 Transient cerebral ischemia
438.0 Late effects of cerebrovascular disease

 MISCELLANEOUS

SYNONYMS
Mini-stroke

SEE ALSO
Stroke

REFERENCES
Cutler WP: Cerebrovascular Disease. In: Scientific American Medicine, Section II, Subsection X. Rubenstein E, Federman D (eds), Scientific American, Inc., New York, 1994. pp. 1-5.

Nadeau SE: Stroke. Med Clin N Am, 73: 1351 1367, 1989.

Little JW, Falace DA: Neurologic disorders. In: Dental Management of the Medically Compromised Patient, 4th ed. St. Louis, CV MOsby, 1993, pp. 325-340.

AUTHOR
Samuel J. McKenna, DDS, MD

Traumatic Brain Injury

BASICS

DESCRIPTION
Damage to intracranial structures that results from skull penetration, direct nonpenetrating blow, or from brain acceleration and deceleration.

ETIOLOGY

Primary injury includes lacerations or contusions of the brain substance and direct disturbance of brain tissue by shearing of axons. Secondary injuries to the brain are caused by effects of an expanding hematoma or from the biochemical insults caused by increased intercranial pressure (ICP) and tissue hypoxia. Often secondary to traumatic episodes, ranging from assault to high-speed motor vehicle accidents (MVA). Few head injuries occur in isolation and in most cases require simultaneous attention to other seriously traumatized parts of the body.

SYSTEMS AFFECTED
Brain
   ◊ focal injuries — localized to limited areas of the brain and are the result of mechanical injury produced at the time of immediate or secondary impacts. Types of focal injuries include intercranial hematoma (subdural, epidural, intraparenchymal), contusions (bruising of the brain), laceration (frank disruption of brain tissues), and variable degrees of brain swelling. Intercranial hematoma can be defined as acute (less than 24 hours after injury), early subacute (within 3 days), subacute (3 days to 10 days), or chronic (more than 2 weeks after injury, with manifestations seen immediately after injury or appearing hours to days after injury).
Neck
   ◊ severe head injuries are often associated with cervical spine injuries.

DIAGNOSIS

SYMPTOMS AND SIGNS
• Drowsiness, confusion, loss of consciousness, headaches, amnesia.
• Hemiplegia, hemiparesis, irregular respirations, dilated and/or unequal pupils, unreactive pupils, decorticate or decerebrate rigidity of extremities, coma, bloody cerebral spinal fluid.

LABORATORY
Screening for ethanol and other toxins.

IMAGING/SPECIAL TESTS
• Glasgow coma scoring
• Head radiographs, head CT scans, head MRI, angiography, C-spine evaluation.

DIFFERENTIAL
• Stroke
• Septic shock
• Diabetic shock
• Alcohol/drug intoxication

TREATMENT

General
◊ airway, breathing, and circulation maintenance. Careful assessment of state of consciousness and neurologic status using the Glasgow coma scale.

Observation
◊ all head injuries should be observed for a variable length of time.
◊ Maintain systolic blood pressure above 100 but keep mean blood pressure less than 110.
◊ Patients unable to care for their dental hygiene needs should have them provided by nurse or aide. Use chlorhexidine rinses and mechanical cleansing with toothbrush. Consider topical fluoride application if coma prolonged. If signs of bruxism or tongue trauma, prepare occlusal appliance.

MEDICATIONS
• Increased ICP controlled through hyperventilation to induce hypocarbia (PCO_2 = 28 to 33) and controlled dehydration by osmotic diuresis (mannitol), possible megadose steroids (controversial if beneficial), pancuronium for paralysis, barbiturate coma.
• Dilantin for seizure prevention, particularly if depressed skull fracture present.
• Patients with past history of head injury and steroid use may need steroid supplementation prior to invasive dental surgery.

SURGERY
Surgical intervention includes burr hole decompression and craniotomies for intracranial hematomas. Direct measuring of intracranial pressure.

Scalp
◊ should be inspected for associated lacerations.

CONSULTATION SUGGESTIONS
Neurosurgeon, Neurologist

REFERRAL SUGGESTIONS
Neurosurgeon, Neurologist

FIRST STEPS TO TAKE IN AN EMERGENCY
• Neurosurgery consultation

PATIENT INSTRUCTIONS
Refer to National Head Injury Foundation (800)444-6443 for information.

COURSE/PROGNOSIS
Depending on severity, range from transient loss of consciousness without permanent injury to chronic vegetative state which may last for years. Recovery from vegetative state rare after 3 years. Rehabilitation assists in regaining some or all affected neurologic functions.

CODING

ICD-9-CM
800-804 Skull fracture
850 Concussion
851 Contusion
852 Cerebral Hematoma
854 Other cerebral injury

M MISCELLANEOUS

SYNONYMS
Head injury

Glasgow Coma Scale
Sum of score for 3 areas of assessment.
1. Eye-opening (E)
   a) spontaneous - 4
   b) to speech - 3
   c) to pain - 2
   d) none - 1
2. Verbal (V)
   a) oriented - 5
   b) confused - 4
   c) inappropriate - 3
   d) incomprehensible - 2
   e) none - 1
3. Motor (M)
   a) obeys - 6
   b) localizes - 5
   c) withdraws - 4
   d) abnormal flexion - 3
   e) extensor posture - 2
   f) no movement - 1

GCS ≤ 8
   severe head injury in coma
GCS = 9-12
   moderate head injury
GCS = 13-15
   mild head injury

REFERENCES
Cooper PR (ed): Head Injury, 2nd ed. Baltimore, Williams & Wilkins, 1987.

Pitts LH: Neurological evaluation of the head injury patient. Clin Neurosurg 29:203-224, 1982.

Ropper AH: Trauma of the Head and Spine. In: Harrison's Principles of Internal Medicine, 13th ed. Isselbacher KJ, et al (eds). New York, McGraw-Hill, Inc., 1994, pp. 2320-2327.

Traumatic Fibroma

BASICS

DESCRIPTION
• The most common exophytic lesion of the oral soft tissues ranging from a few millimeters to 1 to 2 cm.
• Painless, firm, well-demarcated, sessile, or pedunculated soft tissue mass involving buccal mucosa, tongue, or lower lip.
• Usually covered with pink mucosa, but may be white due to hyperkeratosis.
• Surface may be ulcerated.

ETIOLOGY

Not a true tumor but reactive hyperplasia secondary to repeated trauma.

SYSTEMS AFFECTED
Oral mucosa only in most cases. Speech or mastication may be compromised if lesion extremely large.

DIAGNOSIS

SYMPTOMS AND SIGNS
Palpation reveals a painless, freely movable, moderately firm, pink to whitish mass involving oral mucosa; may be ulcerated.

IMAGING/SPECIAL TESTS
Biopsy
  ◇ usually excisional.
Dense fibrous tissue with fibroblasts, minimal inflammatory cells, and thinned, sometimes hyperkeratotic epithelium.

DIFFERENTIAL
• Mucocele
• Minor salivary gland tumor
• Neurilemmoma
• Granular cell tumor
• Lipoma

TREATMENT

SURGERY
Surgical excision with microscopic examination.

CONSULTATION SUGGESTIONS
Oral-Maxillofacial Surgeon

REFERRAL SUGGESTIONS
Oral-maxillofacial Surgeon

PATIENT INSTRUCTIONS
Lesion completely benign. Excision indicated to avoid repeated trauma.

COURSE/PROGNOSIS
• Although of benign nature, may recur if trauma continues.
• No known malignant potential.

CODING

ICD-9-CM
528.9 Other and unspecified diseases of oral soft tissues; irritative hyperplasia.

CPT
40810 Excision of lesion of mucosa and submucosa, vestibule of mouth; without repair
40812 With simple repair
41110 Excision of lesion of tongue without closure
41112 Excision of lesion of tongue with closure; anterior two-thirds
99000 Transport specimen to outside laboratory

MISCELLANEOUS

SYNONYMS
Irritation fibroma
Focal fibrous hyperplasia
Hyperplastic scar

SEE ALSO
Pyogenic granuloma

REFERENCES
Regezi JA, Sciubba J: Oral Pathology Clinical Pathologic Correlations, 2nd ed. Philadelphia, WB Saunders, 1993, pp. 202-204.

Bouquot JE, Gundlach KK: Oral exophytic lesions in 23, 616 white Americans over 35 years of age. Oral Surg Oral Med Oral Path, 62:284-91, 1986.

Dilley DC, Siegel MA, Budnick S: Diagnosing and treating common oral pathologies. Pediar Clin N Am 38:1227-1264, 1991.

AUTHOR
Dennis L. Johnson, DDS, MS

Trigeminal Neuralgia

BASICS

DESCRIPTION
• A disorder of the somatosensory component of the 5th cranial nerve. Characterized by momentary episodes of paroxysmal, lancinating facial pain that may be precipitated by light touch, movement, cold drafts, speaking, or mastication.
• Symptoms are unilateral and dermatomal in distribution, with the second and third divisions being the most commonly affected.
• The areas adjacent to the oral commissure and next to the alar base are common trigger points.
• To lessen the likelihood of triggering an attack, patients may avoid known triggers by shielding the trigger zone from drafts or attempting to hold the face still during speech or mastication.
• Condition is seen more frequently in females than in males.
• Age of onset is usually between 30 to 50 years.

ETIOLOGY

Compression of the semilunar ganglion by the basilar artery.
• Compression of the semilunar ganglion secondary to space occupying lesion such as posterior fossa or brain stem neoplasm.
• Focal demyelinization is a common finding in cases associated with multiple sclerosis.

SYSTEMS AFFECTED
Nervous
◊ severe, lancinating paroxysmal pain in affected dermatome.
Skin
◊ patient may avoid cleaning trigger zone resulting in localized accumulation of food, dirt, or debris. This may lead to lichenification, inflammation, and ulceration.
Teeth
◊ to avoid contact with trigger zone, patient may neglect to maintain proper oral hygiene. Resultant plaque accumulation may promote caries and periodontal disease.

DIAGNOSIS

SYMPTOMS AND SIGNS
• Severe, lancinating pain in V1, V2, or V3 dermatome.
• Pain elicited by light touch, cold drafts, speech, or mastication.
Neurosensory system
◊ no associated neurosensory deficit in affected dermatome.
Eyes
◊ lacrimation during attack
Skin
◊ flushing during attack

IMAGING/SPECIAL TESTS
CT scan, MRI and/or arteriography if compression suspected.

DIFFERENTIAL
• Neoplasm
• Multiple sclerosis
• Postherpetic neuralgia
• Atypical facial pain
• Traumatic peripheral neuropathy

TREATMENT

General
◇ Avoidance of stimulation of trigger areas.
◇ Pharmacologic management is initial/ preferred means of treatment.
◇ If unresponsive to, or unable to tolerate medications:
  Posterior fossa exploration/ microvascular decompression (Jannetta procedure).
  Glycerol injection into trigeminal cistern.
  Radiofrequency rhizotomy.

MEDICATIONS
Drugs of choice
• Baclofen (10 to 100 mg/day) and/or carbamazepine (Tegretol) (200 to 1600 mg/day).
• Baclofen is used for initial therapy, side effects include drowsiness, weakness, fatigue, and nausea.
• Carbamazepine is introduced if symptoms fail to respond to baclofen, side effects include drowsiness ataxia, aplastic anemia, agranulocytosis, and thrombocytopenia. Serum carbamazepine levels and complete blood count with differential must be obtained at regular intervals during chronic carbamazepine therapy.

SURGERY
Jannetta procedure to decompress pressure on semilunar ganglion from basilar artery.

CONSULTATION SUGGESTIONS
Neurologist, Oral-Maxillofacial Surgeon

REFERRAL SUGGESTIONS
Neurologist, Oral-Maxillofacial Surgeon

PATIENT INSTRUCTIONS
Patients can contact the Trigeminal Neuralgia Association, P. O. Box 340, Barnegat Light, NJ 08806, (609)361-1014 for useful information.

COURSE/PROGNOSIS
Spontaneous remissions for several months or longer may occur. As the disorder progresses, the painful episodes become more frequent, remissions become shorter and less common, and a dull ache may persist between episodes of lancinating pain.

CODING

ICD-9-CM
350.1 Trigeminal neuralgia
784.0 Pain, facial

CPT
64400 Anesthetic agent injection, trigeminal nerve, diagnostic
64600 Destruction by neurolytic agent, trigeminal nerve
64716 Decompression/ transposition, cranial nerve

MISCELLANEOUS

SYNONYMS
Tic Douloureux
Trifacial neuralgia

SEE ALSO
Glossopharyngeal neuralgia

REFERENCES
Campbell R: Diagnosis and management of chronic facial pain. In: Principles of Oral and Maxillofacial Surgery. Peterson LJ, et al (eds), Philadelphia, JB Lippincott, 1992, pp 1821-1855.

Dalessio DJ: Diagnosis and treatment of cranial neuralgias. Med Clin N Am 75:605-615, 1991.

Merrill RL, Graff-Radford SB: Trigeminal neuralgia: how to rule out the wrong treatment. JADA 123:63-68, 1992.

Robit, RL: Trigeminal neuralgia. Comp Therapy 18:17-21, 1992.

AUTHOR
Warren P. Vallerand, DDS

Tuberculosis

 BASICS

DESCRIPTION
Disease caused by bacterium Mycobacterium tuberculosis that is characterized by granuloma formation and other signs of a cell-mediated hypersensitivity reaction. Usually affects the lungs, but virtually all other organs and tissues may be involved. Extremely slow growth of organism causes long delay in onset of symptoms and signs, and makes eradication more complex.

 ETIOLOGY

• Although most mycobacteria are not pathogenic for humans, the Mycobacteria tuberculosis, leprae and avium can cause human disease.
• Mycobacterium distinguished by surface lipids and presence of many immunoreactive substances on the surface and within the cell. When the body is exposed to the M. tuberculosis organism's surface or contents, a marked cellular hypersensitivity reaction is produced.
• Organisms entering the body through inspired air or by contamination of a wound are ingested by macrophages that travel to regional lymph nodes. From there they spread via the bloodstream.
• In the U.S. 90 to 95% of healthy individuals undergo complete healing of primary TB lesions with no sequelae, without antibiotic therapy.
• TB is transmitted primarily via the respiratory route. Therefore, adequate ventilation of places where people tend to congregate is important preventive measure.
• Incidence relatively high in Hispanic, Haitian, and Southeast Asian immigrants, and in HIV positive individuals.

SYSTEMS AFFECTED
• Lung, pleural space, pericardium, peritoneum.
• Larynx
• Cervical lymph nodes (scrofula)
• Bone and joints, skin
• Kidney, ureter, bladder, ovaries, prostate, testes
• Meninges, eye, adrenals
Miliary
  ◊ generalized spread

 DIAGNOSIS

SYMPTOMS AND SIGNS
General
  ◊ night sweats, low grade fever, weight loss
Pulmonary
  ◊ asymptomatic or cough, hemoptysis, rales, pleural effusion.
Pericardium
  ◊ pericardial pain, friction rub
Larynx
  ◊ cough, hoarseness
Adenitis
  ◊ rubbery, non-tender lymph nodes in neck (scrofula); later in disease may become hard and matted and chronically draining fistulae may develop.

LABORATORY
Staining and culture
  ◊ acid-fast bacilli from sputum, fistula drainage, lymph node biopsy, body fluids or bronchoscopy. Primary isolation usually requires 4 to 8 weeks on culture media. Niacin production characterizes M. tuberculosis in culture.

IMAGING/SPECIAL TESTS
Chest radiograph
  ◊ apical areas contain cavitation due to TB. Fibrotic lesions may develop calcifications.
Serologic tests available able to detect antibodies to TB in serum of affected individuals.
Tuberculin test
  ◊ intracutaneous of tuberculin purified protein derivative (PPD). Five tuberculin units of material injected. Induration at injection site of greater than 10 mm at 48 to 72 hours considered positive.

DIFFERENTIAL
• Lymphoma
• Fungal infection
• Pneumonia, viral or other bacteria

TREATMENT

General
◇ To effect cure and prevent development of drug resistant mutants, multi-drug therapy is mainstay of care.

MEDICATIONS
• Isoniazid 300 mg PO q.d. for 9 to 12 months in combination with rifampin 600 mg PO q.d.
• Some add third drug initially, either pyrazinamide 1.5 to 2g q.d. or ethambutol 15 mg/kg q.d.
• Other less commonly used drugs are streptomycin, p-aminosalicylic acid, and thiacetazone.
• Prevention possible with isoniazid use or administration of Bacillus Calmette Guerin (BCG).

CONSULTATION SUGGESTIONS
Infectious Disease Specialist

REFERRAL SUGGESTIONS
Primary Care Physician

PATIENT INSTRUCTIONS
Usual reason for failure to cure TB is poor patient compliance with medications. Patients need to understand importance of medication therapy. Spread to others ceases within 2 weeks of starting TB chemotherapy.

COURSE/PROGNOSIS
Without drug therapy, organ involvement may lead to chronic wasting course with eventual death. Properly treated TB has excellent prognosis, but TB can become reactivated if compliance is poor.

CODING

ICD-9-CM
011.9 Tuberculosis, general
012.89 TB of sinuses
015.7 TB of jaw
017.2 Scrofula (cervical node TB)
017.9 Oral cavity TB
018.9 Miliary TB

CPT
38300 Lymph node biopsy
99000 Specimen to laboratory

MISCELLANEOUS

SYNONYMS
Scrofula
TB

SEE ALSO
Lung abscess
Pneumonia
HIV

REFERENCES
Daniel TM: Tuberculosis. In: Harrison's Principles of Internal Medicine 13th ed. Isselbacher KJ, et al (ed), NY, McGraw-Hill, 1994, pp. 710-718.

Haas DW, Des Prez RM: Mycobacterium tuberculosis. In: Principles and Practice of Infectious Diseases, 4th ed. Mandell GL, et al (eds), New York, Churchill Livingstone, 1995, pp. 2213-2243.

AUTHOR
James R. Hupp, DMD, MD, JD, FACS

Ulcerative Colitis

BASICS

DESCRIPTION
A chronic relapsing inflammatory condition of the large bowel. Signs and symptoms of this disease are frequently confused with Crohn's disease, another inflammatory gastrointestinal disease. These two diseases have overlapping clinical, radiologic, histologic, endoscopic, and epidemiologic findings. However, current evidence points to both diseases being separate entities. Ulcerative colitis (UC) affects the mucosa of the large bowel, usually beginning in the rectum (proctitis). The clinical presentation is usually one of rapid onset of rectal bleeding and diarrhea. This can be accompanied by fever and crampy abdominal pain. The range of symptoms can be classified from mild to severe. Because this is a relapsing condition, the severity, intervals between attacks, and frequency are highly variable from patient to patient. Approximately 90% of patients with distal large bowel disease (ie, proctosigmoiditis) do not go on to have generalized large bowel ulcerative colitis. It can affect persons at any age, but primarily young adults aged 20 to 24 years. Ethnicity plays significant role, as this disease occurs with greater frequency in the Jewish population.

ETIOLOGY
Genetic markers recently found to be associated with inflammatory bowel disease and UC in particular are: the presence of anti-neutrophil cytoplasmic antibodies (ANCA) in 70% (this antibody is different from that in Wegener's granulomatosis) and HLA-DR2 presence of the disease for greater than 10 years and with entire large bowel (pancolitis) involvement. A significant modifying factor is that smoking apparently reduces the risk of developing UC.

SYSTEMS AFFECTED
General
  ◊ growth retardation; malabsorption and malnutrition with vitamin/mineral deficiencies.
Skin/Mucosa
  ◊ associated pyoderma gangrenosum, erythema nodosum, apthous ulcers, pyostomatitis vegetans.
Hepatic
  ◊ fatty changes, can be associated with sclerosing cholangitis, chronic active hepatitis.
Hematology
  ◊ blood loss, iron deficiency anemia.
Skeletal
  ◊ sacroiliitis, spondylitis.
Ophthalmic
  ◊ conjunctivitis, iritis, episcleritis, and corticosteroid-induced cataracts after long-term treatment.
Psychosocial
  ◊ patients become extremely self-conscious of the unpredictable bowel movements. This can lead to difficulty with social engagements and ability to lead a normal, spontaneous lifestyle.

DIAGNOSIS

SYMPTOMS AND SIGNS
Clinical
  ◊ frequent bowel movements, rectal bleeding, weight loss, fever, tachycardia, abdominal tenderness, increased bowel sounds.

LABORATORY
• CBC with differential
• Electrolytes for loss of fluids and blood from frequent bowel movements.
• Liver function tests
• Blood cultures if bacteremia occurs.
• Stool culture ova and parasites.
• Anti-nuclear cytoplasmic antibody (ANCA) test.

IMAGING/SPECIAL TESTS
Radiologic
  ◊ initially a fine mucosal irregularity with superficial ulcers; loss of haustral markings; colonic foreshortening.
Histologic
  ◊ mucosal inflammation with infiltrate of neutrophils, lymphocytes, plasma cells, and macrophages. Invasion of the epithelium by the neutrophils leads to crypt abscesses and ulceration.
Colonoscopy with biopsy
Double contrast barium enema
Endoscopic
  ◊ skip lesions, friable mucosa, pseudopolyps.

DIFFERENTIAL
• Crohn's disease
• Infections with following organisms:
  Bacteria
    ◊ Campylobacter, Shigella, Salmonella, Clostridium difficile, Yersinia pestis, Gonorrhea.
  Viral
    ◊ H. simplex.
  Protozoal
    ◊ Amebiasis, Chlamydia.

TREATMENT

General
◇ Aimed at supportive, anti-inflammatory and immunosuppressive and is not specific for colon symptoms. Patient education. Normal diet and nutrition as much as possible.

MEDICATIONS
• Patient usually treated with sulfasalazine, which can reduce frequency of attacks and 5-ASA, helps to maintain remission.
• Oral and topical corticosteroid can aid in control of relapses, but are not preventive.
• Immunosuppressive to manage chronic active disease:
• 6-mercaptopurine
• Azathioprine
• Cyclosporine for severe, intractable cases
Investigational drug therapy:
• Lidocaine
• Smoking/nicotine derivative
• Immunotherapy with IL-1 antagonist. CD4 monoclonal antibody.
• Methotrexate early data, pending long-term studies.
• Nutritional approach perhaps fish oil in form of N-3 fatty acids, presumably divert arachidonic acid metabolites away from inflammation. LTB4 no long-term studies available.

SURGERY
100% cure with large bowel resection, good quality of life. Most systemic side effects in other systems are irreversible except for arthritis and sclerosing cholangitis.

CONSULTATION SUGGESTIONS
Gastroenterologist

REFERRAL SUGGESTIONS
Primary Care Physician

FIRST STEPS TO TAKE IN AN EMERGENCY
• If signs of volume depletion, administer fluids orally or IV.

PATIENT INSTRUCTIONS
Patient should contact National Foundation for Ileitis and Colitis for useful information (800)343-3637.

COURSE/PROGNOSIS
Have generally same life expectancy as normal population except for those presenting with fulminant colitis. Usually require life-long colon cancer surveillance.

CODING

ICD-9-CM
556.0 Ulcerative colitis

MISCELLANEOUS

SYNONYMS
Idiopathic proctocolitis

SEE ALSO
Inflammatory Bowel Disease

REFERENCES
Shanhan F: Pathogenesis of ulcerative colitis. Lancet, 342:407-411, 1993.

Hanauer SB: Medical therapy of ulcerative colitis. Lancet, 342:412-417, 1993.

Jewell DP: Ulcerative Colitis. In: Gastrointestinal Disease, 5th ed., Sleisenger, Fordtran (eds), Philadelphia, WB Saunders, 1993, pp. 1305-1327.

AUTHOR
Roger S. Badwal, DMD, MD

Urinary Tract Infection

BASICS

DESCRIPTION
• Infection of upper tract (acute pyelonephritis, renal, or perinephric abscess) or lower tract (urethritis, cystitis, and prostatitis) of urinary system. May occur together or as isolated infection.
• Defined as infection by pathogenic organisms detected in urine, urethra, bladder, kidney, or prostate. Some use growth of more than 100,000 organisms/mL of a properly collected midstream "clean catch" of urine to define infection. When urine collected from catheter or suprapubic aspiration, colony counts of 100 to 10,000/mL felt to indicate infection.
• May be difficult to determine if infection present if unable to get urine sample not contaminated by external organisms.
• Lower tract infections very common in women. Unusual in men under age 50. Asymptomatic bacteriuria common in elderly men and women, seen in up to 50% of patients.

ETIOLOGY
• Most common agents are bacteria. 80% due to E. coli. Other causative bacteria include Proteus, Klebsiella, Enterobacter, Serratia, and Pseudomonas.
• Sexually transmitted organisms such as chlamydia, N. gonorrhoeae, and herpes simplex seen in sexually active women.
• Factors contributing to infection of urinary tract include catheterization (particularly if left in place for any period of time), alteration of genital microflora by antibiotics, pregnancy, urinary tract obstruction (stones, strictures, tumors, prostatic hypertrophy), neurogenic bladder dysfunction, and vesiculoureteral reflux.

SYSTEMS AFFECTED
Urinary

DIAGNOSIS

SYMPTOMS AND SIGNS
May be asymptomatic so quantitation of bacteria in urine may be necessary to make diagnosis.
Cystitis
  ◇ presents with dysuria, urinary frequency, urgency, suprapubic pain. Cloudy, malodorous urine. May have fever, chills, nausea.
Pyelonephritis
  ◇ presents with fever, chills, nausea, vomiting, diarrhea, tachycardia, myalgias, pain on pressure over costovertebral angle area.
Urethritis
  ◇ dysuria, frequency, pyuria

LABORATORY
• Pyuria, hematuria, bacteriuria. If kidney involved, may be white cell casts.
• CBC shows leukocytosis.
• Urine Gram stain and culture, "clean catch." Can test urine for leukocyte esterase for screening. Dipstick has 75 to 90% sensitivity and 95% specificity.

IMAGING/SPECIAL TESTS
• Intravenous pyelogram (IVP) for obstructions and signs of renal enlargement.
• Catheterization or suprapubic tap for urine collection.

DIFFERENTIAL
Women
  ◇ Vaginitis
    Nephrolithiasis
    Psychogenic dysfunction
Men
  ◇ Urethritis
    Epididymitis
    Anatomic pathology

TREATMENT

General
◇ Lower urinary tract infections not due to obstruction typically resolve quickly with high turnover of urine in bladder and brief course of effective antibiotics. Single-dose therapy is gaining popularity for uncomplicated lower urinary tract infections.

◇ Upper urinary tract infections usually require resolution of obstruction and 2-week course of effective antibiotics.

MEDICATIONS
• Cystitis due to E. coli effectively treated in most cases with single dose of trimethoprim-sulfamethoxazole (400 mg/2g), amoxicillin (3g), or any of the fluoroquinolones. If patient unlikely to come for follow-up care or infection recurs, a more prolonged course of antibiotics is indicated.

• Urethritis due to chlamydia can be treated with doxycycline (100 mg b.i.d.).

• Pyelonephritis is typically treated with 14 days of trimethoprim sulfamethoxazole, a fluoroquinolone, an aminoglycoside or a cephalosporin. Severe cases may require intravenous antibiotics.

SURGERY
If renal abscess present, surgical drainage necessary in most cases.

CONSULTATION SUGGESTIONS
Nephrologist, Primary Care Physician

REFERRAL SUGGESTIONS
Primary Care Physician

FIRST STEPS TO TAKE IN AN EMERGENCY
• If signs of sepsis, hospitalization, IV fluids and antibiotics necessary

COURSE/PROGNOSIS
Most urinary tract infections in otherwise healthy patients resolve when properly treated, leaving no sequellae. Patients with anatomic or functional problems may be prone to recurrent attacks. Elderly or debilitate patients may become septic due to urinary tract infection.

CODING

ICD-9-CM
590.1 Acute pyelonephritis
595 Cystitis
595.1 Acute cystitis
595.2 Chronic cystitis
599.0 Pyuria
601.9 Prostatitis

CPT
51000 Aspiration of bladder by needle
53670 Catherization of bladder

MISCELLANEOUS

SYNONYMS
UTI
Cystitis

SEE ALSO
Renal failure

REFERENCES
Stamm WE: Urinary tract infections and pyelonephritis. In: Harrison's Principles in Internal Medicine, 4th ed. Isselbacher KJ, et al (eds), New York, McGraw-Hill, 1994, pp. 1116-1131.

Chernow B, et al: Measurement of urinary leukocyte esterase activity. Ann Emerg Med 13:150-154, 1984.

Jenkins RD, Fenn JP, Matsen JM: Review of urine microscopy of bacteriuria. JAMA 255:3397-3403, 1986.

Hooton TM, Stamm WE: Management of acute uncomplicated urinary tract infections. Med Clin N Am 75:339, 1991.

AUTHOR
James R. Hupp, DMD, MD, JD, FACS

Ventricular Fibrillation

BASICS

DESCRIPTION
Ventricular fibrillation (VF) is a chaotic cardiac dysrhythmia originating within the ventricles and needs to be treated emergently. It occurs when multiple pacing sites within the ventricles discharge asynchronously and are not superseded by a supraventricular pacemaker. This results in an uncoordinated cardiac pumping/motion that rapidly leads to cerebral hypoperfusion and loss of consciousness. VF can also be induced after administration of antidysrhythmics, which prolong the QT interval.

ETIOLOGY

• Acute myocardial infarction; cardiac arrest.
• Hypoxia; metabolic disturbances (eg, hyperkalemia).
• Wolff-Parkinson-White syndrome with atrial fibrillation and a rapid ventricular response rate.
• May begin as a ventricular tachycardic rhythm and becomes VF when the successive R wave falls on the preceding T wave (R on T phenomenon).

SYSTEMS AFFECTED
Cardiac
◇ leads to ischemia/MI and high risk of death secondary to ineffective pumping of blood.
Cerebral
◇ can cause hypoperfusion for same reason as cardiac ischemia with rapid loss of consciousness.

DIAGNOSIS

SYMPTOMS AND SIGNS
Loss of consciousness, hypotension.

IMAGING/SPECIAL TESTS
Electrocardiogram
◇ rapid chaotic pattern, QRS complexes wide and irregular.

DIFFERENTIAL
• Asystole
• ECG artifact
• Missing ECG lead

TREATMENT

General
◇ The emergent treatment of the rhythm requires an initial attempt with defibrillation. If this fails, then intravenous epinephrine 1 mg coupled with defibrillation at 360 J is necessary. This can be repeated. If this fails, other drugs such as lidocaine, and possibly bretylium, may be used.

MEDICATIONS
• Lidocaine of 1.5 mg/kg bolus intravenously, which may be repeated in 5 minutes with an additional equal bolus.
• Bretylium 5 mg/kg bolus intravenously, if lidocaine fails. If the initial bolus of bretylium fails, then it may be given in 10 mg/kg doses up to a maximum of 35 mg/kg.

CONSULTATION SUGGESTIONS
Cardiologist

REFERRAL SUGGESTIONS
Primary Care Physician

FIRST STEPS TO TAKE IN AN EMERGENCY
• Basic Cardiac Life Support

PATIENT INSTRUCTIONS
Patients with a history of cardiac arrest should consider wearing medic alert jewelry if arrest prone to recur.

COURSE/PROGNOSIS
Ventricular fibrillation is responsible for 75% of all sudden cardiac deaths. But the overall prognosis depends upon the underlying etiology. If VF occurs within 48 hours of an acute infarction, this has relatively good prognosis. Only 30% of patients resuscitated from cardiac arrest sustain transmural infarcts. These persons have recurrence rate of VF of only 2%/year. Those resuscitated without a transmural myocardial infarction have about 22% recurrence rate within 1 year and 40% in 2 years. Predictors of death include decreased ejection fraction, wall motion abnormalities; a history of congestive heart failure; a prior history of myocardial infarction, and presence of other ventricular dysrhythmias.

CODING

ICD-9-CM
427.41 Ventricular fibrillation

MISCELLANEOUS

SYNONYMS
Tachydysrhythmias
V-Fib
Cardiac arrest

SEE ALSO
Ventricular tachycardia

REFERENCES
Josephson ME, Buxton AE, Marchlinski FE: The Tachyarrhythmias. In: Harrison's Principles of Internal Medicine, 13th ed. Isselbacher KJ (ed), New York, McGraw-Hill, 1994, pp. 1029-1032.

Tierney LM, McPhee SJ, Papadakis, MA : Current Medical Diagnosis and Treatment. New York, Appleton and Lange, 1994, pp. 336-338.

Textbook of Advanced Cardiac Life Support. 2nd ed. American Heart Assoc. 1990.

AUTHOR
Roger S. S. Badwal, DMD, MD

Ventricular Tachycardia

BASICS

DESCRIPTION
Ventricular tachycardia (VT) is a cardiac dysrhythmia defined as three or more consecutive premature ventricular beats. It can occur in a sustained or nonsustained manner. Sustained VT occurs when the rhythm persists for longer than 30 seconds or cardiovascular collapse ensues. The rate is usually 100 to 240 beats/minute. There are several subtypes of VT (ie, Torsade de Pointes, accelerated idioventricular rhythm, long QT syndrome, bi-directional VT, repetitive monomorphic VT, bundle branch reentrant VT).

ETIOLOGY

Ischemic heart disease is the leading cause of disturbances of cardiac rhythm. VT usually occurs in long-standing ischemic heart disease, which produces fixed ventricular myocardial lesions. This leads to a relatively fixed area of injury, which may become the source of unstable, recurrent attacks of ventricular tachycardia.
Acute myocardial infarction
◊ dysrhythmias are quite common after an acute insult to the heart, VT may therefore occur.
Cardiomyopathies
◊ diseased myocardium leads to difficulties in conduction, therefore conduction defects. This leads to other dysrhythmogenic foci becoming the pacemakers for the heart.
Other conditions associated with VT rhythms are:
  Metabolic disturbances (eg, hypokalemia, hypomagnesemia).
  Drugs/toxins, (eg, quinidine, tricyclic antidepressants, phenothiazines).
  Hypoxia
  Mitral valve prolapse
  Myocarditis

SYSTEMS AFFECTED
Cardiac
◊ propagates ischemia. MI secondary to insufficient ventricular filling time and oxygen demand outstrips delivery.
Cerebral
◊ can cause hypoperfusion for same reason as cardiac ischemia with loss of consciousness.

DIAGNOSIS

SYMPTOMS AND SIGNS
• Dependent on rate, duration, and presence of existing cardiac disease or peripheral vascular disease palpitations, tachycardia, hypotension, presyncopal to loss of consciousness.
• Tachycardia
• Hypotension
• Weakness
• Loss of consciousness

IMAGING/SPECIAL TESTS
ECG
◊ Wide QRS complex; greater than 100 b/m (refer to cardiologist).
• Echocardiogram
• Cardiac angiographic catheterization
• Nuclear cardiac scan, (eg, stress thallium, Persantine thallium).
Electrophysiologic cardiac studies

DIFFERENTIAL
• Supraventricular tachycardia
• Ventricular fibrillation

TREATMENT

General
Sustained
◊ emergent ACLS protocol with: lidocaine; procainamide; bretylium; cardioversion.
Nonsustained
◊ refer to cardiologist

MEDICATIONS
• Class I antidysrhythmics
◊ lidocaine, quinidine drugs, procainamide.
• Amiodarone
• Other:
• Only considered when medical therapy fails, which occurs in 10%.
• Automatic implantable cardiac defibrillator (AICD).
• Surgical/radio frequency ablation VT foci of irritability after specialized electrophysiologic mapping uncommon, only specialized centers perform this kind of surgery.

CONSULTATION SUGGESTIONS
Cardiologist

REFERRAL SUGGESTIONS
Primary Care Physician, Cardiologist

FIRST STEPS TO TAKE IN AN EMERGENCY
• Basic cardiac life support, alert EMTs.

COURSE/PROGNOSIS
Depends on underlying disease. If VT develops within 6 weeks of an acute myocardial infarction, this has poor prognosis with a 75% mortality at 1 year. Nonsustained VT after a myocardial infarction has threefold greater risk of death than those which do not. However, patients without heart disease and monomorphic VT patterns have a good prognosis and low risk of death.

CODING

ICD-9-CM
427.1 Ventricular tachycardia
427.9 Cardiac dysrhythmia

SEE ALSO
Ventricular Fibrillation

MISCELLANEOUS

SYNONYMS
V-tach

REFERENCES
Josephson ME, Buxton AE, Marchlinski FE: The Tachyarrhythmias. In: Harrison's Principles of Internal Medicine, 13th ed. Isselbacher KJ, (ed), New York, McGraw-Hill, 1994, pp. 1029-1032.

Tierney LM, McPhee SJ, Papadakis, MA: Current: Medical Diagnosis and Treatment. New York, Appleton and Lange, 1994, pp. 336-338.

Textbook of Advanced Cardiac Life Support. 2nd ed. American Heart Assoc. 1990.

AUTHOR
Roger S. S. Badwal, DMD, MD

Vitamin Deficiencies

BASICS

DESCRIPTION
Vitamins are substances needed in minute quantities by the body. They act as cofactors in many metabolic reactions and are divided into fat-soluble such as Vitamin A, D, E and K, and water-soluble such as Vitamin B group and C and folate. Deficiencies in these substances lead to a wide variety of diseases.

ETIOLOGY

• Deficiencies in single vitamins are rarely seen. Deficiencies in multiple vitamins, along with protein-calorie undernutrition, are the rule when deficiencies exist at all, because any cause of protein-calorie undernutrition can result in vitamin deficiency. Deficiency is usually associated with malabsorption, alcoholism, medications, pregnancy, hemodialysis, total parenteral nutrition, food fads, inborn errors of metabolism or unbalanced diet.
• Vitamin deficiency syndromes develop gradually. Early diagnosis is difficult, as symptoms are nonspecific. Characteristic findings are seen only late in the course of the deficiency state.

SYSTEMS AFFECTED
Vitamin A
◇ loss of night vision, xerophthalmia (conjunctival drying), cutaneous hyperkeratosis, and drying of mucous membranes.
Vitamin B_1 (thiamine)
◇ deficiency causes beriberi, or in alcoholics, Wernicke-Korsakoff syndrome. Seen mostly in alcoholics and characterized by multiple neuritis. High output heart failure, generalized edema, and sudden death often follow.
Vitamin B_2 (riboflavin)
◇ mouth soreness, cheilitis, angular stomatitis, glossitis, seborrheic dermatitis, weakness, corneal vascularization, and anemia.
Vitamin B_3 (niacin)
◇ deficiency causes pellagra. Early manifestations are nonspecific, including weakness, anorexia, irritability, glossitis, stomatitis, and weight loss. Later, the classic triad of pellagra: distinctive dermatitis, diarrhea, and dementia.
Vitamin B_6 (pyridoxine)
◇ manifested as stomatitis, glossitis, cheilitis, weakness, and irritability. Severe deficiency can lead to peripheral neuropathy, anemia, and seizures.
Vitamin B_{12} and Folate
◇ deficiency causes pernicious or megaloblastic anemia. Glossitis, diarrhea, and macrocytic anemia.
Vitamin C (ascorbic acid)
◇ deficiency causes scurvy. An antioxidant and necessary for collagen synthesis. Early signs are malaise and weakness. Later, symptoms and signs include perifollicular (around hair follicles) hemorrhages, perifollicular hyperkerototic papules, petichiae, purpura, splinter hemorrhages, bleeding gingiva, joint hemorrhages, and periodontal bone loss. Anemia and impaired wound healing also occur.

Vitamin D
◇ results in secondary hyperparathyroidism. Rickets results in hypomineralized bone matrix. If seen in developing children, there may be abnormalities of dentin and enamel, delayed eruption of teeth, and misalignment of teeth. Softening and distortion of the skeleton occur at any age.
Vitamin E (alpha-tocopherol)
◇ unclear function, but thought to act as an antioxidant protecting cell membranes and other cellular structures from attack by free radicals. Areflexia, disturbances of gait, decreased proprioception, and ophthalmoplegia.
Vitamin K
◇ intimately involved in both the intrinsic and extrinsic coagulation cascade; abnormal bleeding will result from low levels. Gingival bleeding will be seen if prothrombin levels fall below 35% after brushing and spontaneous gingival bleeding will occur if levels fall below 20%.

DIAGNOSIS

Diagnosis of vitamin deficiencies is undertaken by careful history and physical exam. Laboratory test can confirm low levels of many of the vitamins. Empirical therapy with the suspected substance with improvement is sometimes all that is necessary.

SYMPTOMS AND SIGNS
See systems affected.

LABORATORY
Assays for levels of the specific substance are done if the diagnosis cannot be made from the clinical findings.

DIFFERENTIAL
Vitamin A
◇ Retinitis pigmentosa
Vitamin B_1
◇ Polyneuropathy due to other causes.
Vitamin D
◇ Syphilis, chondrodystrophy
Vitamin K
◇ Hepatic disease, anticoagulant use, NSAID use, thrombocytopenia.
Vitamin B_3
◇ Other causes of stomatitis

TREATMENT

Pharmacologic doses of the vitamin that is deficient. Proper care for Vitamin D deficiency includes exposure to sunlight. Medical treatment of the symptoms or of the cause is necessary in some cases. Alcoholics must abstain from ethanol use. Patient education in proper nutrition important.

MEDICATIONS
• Vitamin A
Fish liver oil
• Vitamin B_1
◇ Thiamine orally 5 to 30 mg t.i.d.
• Vitamin B_2
◇ Riboflavin orally 10 to 30 mg/d tapered to 2 to 4 mg/d
• Vitamin B_3
◇ Niacinamide 300 to 500 mg/d orally or IV
• Vitamin B_6
◇ Pyridoxine orally 2.5/10 mg q.d.
• Vitamin B_{12}
◇ Parenteral or sub Q cobalamin
• Vitamin C
◇ 100 to 200 mg orally q.d.
• Vitamin D
◇ Orally give Vitamin D or cod liver oil
• Vitamin E
◇ Orally 1 unit/kg/day
• Vitamin K
◇ 10 mg sub Q or IM

CONSULTATION SUGGESTIONS
Dietitian

REFERRAL SUGGESTIONS
Primary Care Physician, Psychiatrist/ Psychologist (alcoholics).

FIRST STEPS TO TAKE IN AN EMERGENCY
• If bleeding, may be due to Vitamin K deficiency, administer 10 mg sub Q or IM immediately.

PATIENT INSTRUCTIONS
Balanced diet, exposure to sunlight, limit ethanol use.

COURSE/PROGNOSIS
Prognosis is dependent on the ability to correct the cause of the vitamin deficiency and the extent to which it has progressed prior to diagnosis.

CODING

ICD-9-CM
264.9 Vitamin A
265.1 Vitamin B_1
266.0 Vitamin B_2
266.1 Vitamin B_6
266.2 Vitamin B_{12}
266.9 Vitamin B complex
267 Vitamin C
268.9 Vitamin D
269 Vitamin K
269.1 Vitamin E
269.2 Multiple deficiency

MISCELLANEOUS

SEE ALSO
Anemia
Hyperarathyroidism
Alcoholism

REFERENCES
Sherwin, McPhee, and Papadakis: Current Medical Diagnosis & Treatment. Norwalk, CT. Appleton & Lange. 1994. pp. 1039-1044.

Machlin LJ (ed): Handbook of Vitamins, 2nd Ed. New York, Marcel Dekker, 1990.

AUTHOR
Michael J. Dalton, DDS

Vitiligo

BASICS

DESCRIPTION
• An acquired, progressive pigmentary disorder, consisting of localized areas of hypopigmentation of the skin and hair due to loss of active melanocytes.
• Male and females equally affected.
• Type A (75% of cases) widespread.
• Type B (25% of cases) confined to dermatome. More frequent in childhood onset.

ETIOLOGY

• The hypopigmentation is probably the result of an autoimmune-mediated destruction of melanocytes, the cells that produce pigment. The greater the decrease in number of melanocytes, the greater the pigment loss.
• Approximately 1% of the population is affected. Autosomal dominant with variable expression and penetrance.
• Associated with hyperthyroidism, hypothyroidism, pernicious anemia, diabetes mellitus, Addisonism, and stomach cancer.

SYSTEMS AFFECTED
Skin, hair, and exocrine glands.

DIAGNOSIS

SYMPTOMS AND SIGNS
• Loss of pigmentation in discrete areas of the skin and hair that are highly susceptible to sunburning.
• Pruritis in the anogenital folds if this area is affected.
• Severe emotional problems often occur when face involved.
• Premature graying. Can involve oral and perioral tissues. Depigmentation often occurs in areas of repeated trauma.

LABORATORY
Thyroid function tests, CBC, serum glucose, and serum cortisol to rule out systemic diseases. If on psorlan with ultra-violet activation (PUVA) therapy, monitor CBC, liver, and renal function.

IMAGING/SPECIAL TESTS
• Skin biopsy reveals complete absence of melanocytes.
• Kott examination of skin scraping to rule out tinea versicolor.

DIFFERENTIAL
The differential must exclude systemic disease such as Addison's disease, hyperthyroidism or hypopituitarism, and distinguish true lack of pigment from pseudoachromia such as in tinea versicolor, pityriasis simplex, and seborrheic dermatitis. Leukoderma and partial albinism are difficult to differentiate from vitiligo. Other possible entities in small hypopigmented areas include melanoma, lupus erythematosis, leprosy, chemical exposure, and neurofibromatosis.

TREATMENT

• Sunscreen must be applied to the areas of hypopigmentation to prevent actinic damage to the skin.
• Cosmetics to cover the areas.

MEDICATIONS
• 10 to 15% of patients with true vitiligo may respond to topical or systemic psoralen treatment with methoxsalen (Oxsoralen) and ultraviolet light exposure (PUVA).
• High-potency topical steroids cream applied daily (or q.o.d.) may be useful for locally affected areas, with occasional periods of nontreatment to avoid complications.

CONSULTATION SUGGESTIONS
Dermatologist

REFERRAL SUGGESTIONS
Dermatologist, Primary Care Physician

PATIENT INSTRUCTIONS
Avoid sun exposure without sunscreen on affected areas.

COURSE/PROGNOSIS
Up to 70% respond to drug (PUVA) therapy with repigmentation.

CODING

ICD-9-CM
709.0 Dyschromia vitiligo

MISCELLANEOUS

SYNONYMS
Hypomelanosis
Depigmentation

SEE ALSO
Addison's disease

REFERENCES
Sober AJ, Fitzpatrick TB: Disturbances of Pigmentation. In: Dermatology, 2nd Ed. Moschella SL, Hurly HJ (eds), Philadelphia, WB Saunders, 1985, pp. 1261-1305.

Löntz W, et al: Pigment cell transplantation for treatment of vertigo. J Am Acad Dermatol 30: 591-597, 1994.

AUTHOR
Michael J. Dalton, DDS

Wegener's Granulomatosis

BASICS

DESCRIPTION
A disease characterized by a wide variety of clinical presentations related to systemic granulomatous vasculitis. Classic triad consists of involvement of upper airway, lung, and kidney.

ETIOLOGY

The etiology of Wegener's granulomatosis is not understood. Autoimmune phenomena suspected.

SYSTEMS AFFECTED
• Eyes
• Oral mucosa
• Skin
• Upper airway
• Pulmonary
• Renal
• Joints

DIAGNOSIS

SYMPTOMS AND SIGNS
Oral mucosa
◊ ulcers, gingival hyperplasia, and petechiae.
Skin
◊ purpura, papules, hemorrhagic bullae, ulcerations, subcutaneous nodules, pustules, vesicles, macules, petechiae, and fingernail splinter hemorrhages.
Upper respiratory track
◊ rhinorrhea, nasal crusting, epistaxis, pansinusitis, otitis media, mastoiditis, saddle nose.
Lungs
◊ hemoptysis, pulmonary infiltrates.
Kidneys
◊ hematuria, proteinuria, red cell casts, renal failure.
Joints
◊ polyarthralgias.
Eyes
◊ conjunctivitis, episcleritis, scleritis, retinal vasculitis, uveitis, proptosis.

LABORATORY
• Anemia, leukocytosis, and thrombocytosis.
• Elevated creatinine and BUN.
• Increased ESR
• Elevated C-reactive protein, immune complexes, rheumatoid factor.
• Urine analysis hematuria, casts, proteinuria.
• Sputum culture

IMAGING/SPECIAL TESTS
Radiographs and computed tomography, chest radiograph, magnetic resonance imaging, endoscopy.

DIFFERENTIAL
• Collagen vascular diseases
• Infections
• Sarcoidosis
• Lymphomatoid granulomatosis
• Pseudotumor
• Malignancy
• Necrotizing sialometaplasia
• Midline lethal granuloma

Wegener's Granulomatosis

TREATMENT

General
◇ Early appropriate treatment is extremely important and should be both local and systemic.
◇ Humidification of air and lubrication of airway.
◇ Other Treatment
◇ Plasmapheresis

MEDICATIONS
- Glucocorticoids
- Cyclophosphamide
- Azathioprine, if cyclophosphamide is contraindicated.
- Folate antagonists
- Trimethoprim-sulfamethoxazole

IRRADIATION
Local radiotherapy sometimes useful.

CONSULTATION SUGGESTIONS
Rheumatologist

REFERRAL SUGGESTIONS
Primary Care Physician

PATIENT INSTRUCTIONS
In the future, alert doctors to use of prednisone in case supplementation indicated.

COURSE/PROGNOSIS
Without adequate treatment this is a progressive mutilating disorder. Renal disease is the best predictive factor for outcome, followed by pulmonary involvement. A high rate of remission and cure is possible using steroids with cytotoxic drugs.

CODING

ICD-9-CM
446.4 Wegener's granulomatosis

CPT
30420 Rhinoplasty including major septal repair
40808 Biopsy, vestibule of mouth

MISCELLANEOUS

SEE ALSO
Polyarteritis nodosa

REFERENCES
Burlacoff SG, Wong FSH: Wegener's granulomatosis, the great masquerade: A clinical presentation and literature review. J Otolarygol 22:94-105, 1993.

Romas E, Murphy BF, d'Apice AJF, Kennedy JT, Naill JF: Wegener's granulomatosis: clinical features and prognosis in 37 patients. Aust NZ J Med 23:168-175, 1993.

AUTHOR
Deborah L. Zeitler, DDS, MS

Xerostomia

BASICS

DESCRIPTION
A sign and symptom of a dry mouth that can be due to a variety of problems relating to lack of saliva production or the subjective feeling of oral dryness.

ETIOLOGY

• Most common is medication-induced alteration in saliva production. Drugs frequently associated with xerostomia include anticholinergics (atropine), antihistamines, antidepressants (tri- and tetra-cyclics, MAO inhibitors), phenothiazines, hypotensives (diuretics, ganglionic blockers such as clonidine), anticonvulsants, antiparkinsonians, decongestants, and antineoplastic drugs.
• Radiation used for cancer therapy delivered through major salivary glands. Problem worsened by concurrent medication-induced dryness by antineoplastic drugs, phenothiazine antinausea agents, and antidepressants.
• Salivary gland diseases such as Sjögren's syndrome or Mikulicz's disease.
• Dehydration common in elderly, diseases with frequent urination such as diabetes mellitus, or diseases associated with repeated vomiting or diarrhea, including bulimia.
• Age related changes in saliva production.
• Emotionally based with anxiety-producing physiologic xerostomia, while depression may cause subjective xerostomia in the presence of objectively normal saliva flow.
• Others include AIDS, anemia, salivary duct obstruction, and chronic renal failure.

SYSTEMS AFFECTED
Oral mucosa
  ◇ rendered more susceptible to trauma from chewing food and other otherwise benign insults. Epithelial atrophy with production of inflammation, fissuring, and ulceration. Mucosa predisposed to infection and wound healing impaired.
Teeth
  ◇ become prone to caries, especially along cervical margins. Periodontal disease promoted.
Taste
  ◇ impaired due to failure of saliva to carry flavors to taste buds.
Mental state
  ◇ impacted by discomfort and inconvenience of dry mouth.

DIAGNOSIS

SYMPTOMS AND SIGNS
Mouth
  ◇ dry, burning, numbness, grittiness, tongue soreness, difficulty retaining dentures, unable to taste well, halitosis.
Oral mucosa
  ◇ dry, erythema, fissuring, ulceration, white streaks or plaques, leathery feel, easily traumatized, poor wound healing. Difficulty or inability to manually express saliva from ducts.
Teeth
  ◇ cervical caries, staining, periodontal pocketing and bleeding.
Eyes
  ◇ erythema (if xerostomia due to generalized drying process or Sjögren's).

LABORATORY
• CBC, serum immunoglobulins, rheumatoid factor, antinuclear antibodies.
• Stain and culture for candidiasis.

IMAGING/SPECIAL TESTS
Sialogram if obstruction suspected. Lip biopsy and Schirmer's test of tear production if Sjögren's suspected.

DIFFERENTIAL
• Medication induced
• Sjögren's/Mikulicz's
• Age related decrease in saliva production
• Anxiety/emotional problems
• Therapeutic radiation
• Dehydration

TREATMENT

General
◇ Saliva stimulants sugarless, citrus-flavored hard candy or gum.
◇ Saliva substitutes glycerin or gel based, frequently contain carboxymethylcellulose or mucin.
◇ Fluoride treatments and hygiene instruction with monitoring.
◇ Education about maintaining adequate hydration.
◇ Psychological counseling.
◇ Soft diet

Other
◇ acupuncture, electrical stimulation.

MEDICATIONS
- Confer with family physician about possible modification of drug regimens containing medications suspected of causing xerostomia.
- Manage mucosal candidiasis
  ◇ Clotrimazole (Mycelex) 10 mg troche dissolved in mouth five times a day for 14 days.
- Manage oral discomfort
  ◇ topical anesthetics.
- Pilocarpine to promote salivary secretion
  ◇ 5 mg capsule three times a day, side effects include sweating, flushing, urinary urgency, increased lacrimal and nasal secretions.

SURGERY
- Lip biopsy for minor salivary gland examination.
- If xerostomia due to radiation therapy, consider modification of treatment plans that involve exposure of bone or extractions.

CONSULTATION SUGGESTIONS
Oral Medicine, Oral-Maxillofacial Surgeon, Primary Care Physician

REFERRAL SUGGESTIONS
Oral Medicine, Oral-Maxillofacial Surgeon

PATIENT INSTRUCTIONS
Dentist can prescribe saliva substitute if xerostomia cannot be eliminated by altering medications.

COURSE/PROGNOSIS
Most signs and symptoms reversible if drug or emotional induced. Otherwise, unlikely to cure problem. Treatments listed above offer palliation.

CODING

ICD-9-CM
112.0 Candidiasis of mouth
276.1 Dehydration, hypotonic
300.4 Anxiety
311.0 Depression
521.0 Dental caries
527.1 Mikulicz's
527.7 Xerostomia
710.2 Sjögren's
783.6 Bulimia
990.0 Radiotherapy, adverse effect
995.2 Medicinals, adverse effect

CPT
21085 Oral surgical splint (fluoride)
42405 Biopsy, salivary gland
42699 Salivary gland, unlisted procedure
70390 Sialography

MISCELLANEOUS

SYNONYMS
Dry mouth

SEE ALSO
Schizophrenia
Bulimia
Candidiasis
Depression
Salivary gland calculi
Sjögren's/Mikulicz's
Burning mouth syndrome

REFERENCES
Sciubba JJ, Mandel ID: Sjögren's syndrome. NY State Dent J 58:39-42, 1990.

Sreebny LM: Salivary flow in health and disease. Compend Cont Educ Dent Supp 13, S461-S469, 1989.

Duxbury AJ: Systemic pharmacotherapy. In: Oral Manifestations of Systemic Disease, 2nd ed. Jones JH, Mason DK (eds), London, Balliere Tindall, 1990, pp. 438-439.

Sonis ST, Fazio RC, Fong L: Diseases of the salivary glands. In: Principles & Practice of Oral Medicine, 2nd ed. Philadelphia, WB Saunders, 1995, pp. 457-472.

AUTHOR
James R. Hupp, DMD, MD, JD, FACS

Index

Index

Index

Index

Index

Index

Index

Index

Index

Index

Index

Index

Index

Index

Index

Index

Index

H

Index

Index

Index

Index

Index

Index

Index

Index

Index

Index

Index

Index

Index

Index

Index

Index

Index

Index

Index

Index

Index

Index

Index

Index

Index

Index